You don't have to be afraid of CANCER anymore

New Therapies Promise Hope and Survival

Beyond the Failures of Conventional and Alternative Medicine to Explore a New Era of Cancer Care

by Bill Sardi

O restore me to health and let me live!

-Holy Bible, Book of Isaiah 38:16

ISBN 0-9774272-1-8

Book design by Linda Tazberikova, ATdesign.org
Printed in the United States of America
First printing 2007

ISBN 0-9774272-1-8

9 780977 427215

This book is written for information purposes only. It cannot diagnose nor prescribe. The nutritional regimens and doses published in this book are general in nature and not specifically prescribed for any individual. The author is not a doctor and does not accept consultations or examine patients. Regardless of the shortcomings of cancer doctoring today, this book is not a substitute for professional care. While readers are urged to seek other sources of information before adopting any health regimen, this book recognizes there are few health authorities available who can provide you with an up-to-date unbiased opinion. The cancer patient faces difficult choices with few sources of reliable information.

Consult with other sources before making health-related decisions.

Bill Sardi is a spokesperson for various dietary supplement companies and has an economic interest in dietary supplements.

Contents

Foreword

For everyone, cancer is the most dreaded and tear-evoking word in the dictionary. For too many, cancer is an irreversible verdict rather than just a diagnosis. But it's more than that. It's standing by and watching loved ones succumb to an awful disease right before your eyes.

There are personal experiences that every author brings to a book. These are mine.

It seems as if the first half of life is going to weddings and the last half is going to the funerals of friends and family, many who have died of cancer. Dealing with death or cancer is never easy, but this challenge is overlaid by yet another trial, the ordeal posed by cancer treatment itself.

Most of us accept all the horrors of cancer treatment in the hope that it will provide a cure or at least prolong life. We try to comfort the afflicted. But how? We really don't know what to prepare them for. Should we hope for a cure...or just a less painful death? Should we open a page in the Bible to share with a friend who has cancer as if to signal the end is near?

I recall Patti Ferguson, still a young woman, active in sales of cataract lens implants to ophthalmologists. Vibrant and energetic, her positive personality certainly dispelled the idea that a sour outlook on life has something to do with cancer. Patti was frightened when the pain in her hip was something more than just early arthritis. It was cancer that had spread to her bones. I knew little about cancer then. None of Patti's friends or family knew that there is no effective treatment for metastatic cancer.

Patti would fly by airplane from Northern California to receive gamma knife radiation treatment (radiation therapy in which high-energy radiation is aimed at a tumor from many angles) at a southern California medical center. The treatment had no chance of curing her cancer, but it was all she had to hope for.

Later, back in Northern California, Patti endured chemotherapy, and called me on the phone, not knowing who to trust any more. She was looking for a way to conquer cancer without poisoning herself, and her caregivers were telling her to suffer through more chemotherapy. It made no sense to me. Chemo would destroy her immune system in an attempt to cure her, when the immune system is what keeps cancer at bay. But who am I to second guess doctors? Patti succumbed to cancer in a relatively short period of time. Treatment seemed to quicken her passing.

I later read about Hippocrates, the Greek physician (460-377 BC) who said (paraphrased): *"It is best not to apply any treatment in cases of cancer for, if treated, the patients die quickly; but if not treated, they hold out for a long time."* [Guy B Faguet, The War on Cancer, Springer 2005, pp. 26.-27] I wondered about what Hippocrates had said in light of Patti's ordeal.

Then, there was Conny Campos, a God-loving woman, an aunt on my wife's side of the family, who struggled with chronic irritable bowel problems. Shortly after a colonoscopy found that her digestive tract was free of polyps and cancer, she was diagnosed with anemia and given iron pills. When the pills didn't resolve the anemia, she was given infusions of iron. What her doctors failed to recognize was that anemia in adulthood is often a sign of cancer. A year later a colonoscopy revealed her colon was laced with multiple tumors. Why did the doctors prescribe iron, when they should have given more thought to what was causing her iron deficiency? The anemia was caused by cancer, not by a lack of iron in her diet. What's more, iron is a primary growth factor for cancer! So not only did her doctors fail her by failing to detect the cause of her anemia, but by giving her high doses of iron they actually may have induced the tumors, thus accelerating her death.

I recall Conny singing a hymn on the front porch of my home in her last days. It's a treasured memory tainted with the realization that medical *"care"* may have hastened her passing. There are a lot of tears on the pages of my manuscript.

A book in the making

Why did I begin this crusade to understand cancer? I knew cancer care was ineffective. I knew treatments were toxic and painful. I knew that most patients never heard about any of this. And when they sought alternatives, they too were a disappointment.

As I wrote this book I became more and more outraged at the profiteering, the money made on Wall Street for the next blockbuster drug, the awards doled out to cancer researchers, the prestige derived from failure to find a cure.

I also suspected that doctors were driven more by insurance billing codes than by their concern for patients.

Watch what you say to cancer patients

Yet when I would say to others that cancer care consists of nothing more than *"slash, burn or poison,"* my comments would be met with stares of disdain. People would admonish me, *"Don't say that when someone is battling cancer." "Doctors, yes, I'm sure there are bad doctors out there, but not my family doctor, not the wonderful Mayo Clinic-trained oncologist who is taking care of me now."*

Then it struck me.

I realized patients want treatment, and hope. They don't want to hear the harsh realities of cancer, even if the treatment is ineffective. *"Don't leave us with nothing to hope for"* is what is on many cancer patients' lips.

Dr. Guy B. Faguet, in his book, The War on Cancer (Springer 2005) has said that cancer eradication is only achievable in 11 of over 200 human malignancies and meaningful prolongation of survival is possible for only another few. Despite the futility of cancer treatment, patients will fight for their right to receive it. There is no arguing with a dying cancer patient.

Doctors ready to oblige

Cancer doctors are more than willing to oblige the patient's demand for treatment, and any mention of the failings of treatment are withheld so as not to demoralize the patient any further. This is a merry-go-round I hope my loved ones never have to get on.

Cancer patients generally have no idea the treatment offered to them is of little or no value. In fact, most cancer patients succumb to the side effects of treatment before they do from their disease.

Cancer patients headed the wrong way

What makes looking for better cancer care alternatives so difficult is that the very cancer patients I was planning to write a book for are part of the problem. They not only hasten the onset of cancer with poor health habits (smoking, etc.) but they want, no, they demand, more ineffective, toxic cancer care.

Patients and their families ask, *"What are we to do, nothing?"*

Cancer patients want treatment even it means dying of it. They want the very best that modern medicine has to offer. Stand in their way and they will call attorneys and demand that health plans provide them with the most expensive treatments. Miracles happen, don't they?

Few cancer patients see how they are being used as pawns to push for public funding for a drug or treatment that only add a few days of extra life, often spent in pain and misery.

I also have been left with the impression that cancer researchers place their livelihood above that of finding a cure for cancer. Cancer research has become a jobs program – find a real cure and it would put an end to all the research grants. After talking to cancer researchers, I started to get the idea that their objective was to stretch out their research so they could make a life-long career out of finding a cure for cancer. Somehow that cure has always been just beyond their reach. Researchers always seem to conclude there is not enough evidence to prove anything about cancer. More studies are required. It is said cancer is hundreds of diseases and nobody knows its cause. If nobody knows what causes cancer, then how can it effectively be treated?

The ethics of cancer care

I'm continually puzzled over the ethics of the medical profession. In the backwards world of cancer care, an alternative medicine practitioner will be labeled a health quack for offering an unproven remedy for cancer, but a Mayo Clinic-trained doctor who performs disproven care will not be sanctioned by the state medical board.

Patients are bewildered, overwhelmed, and often too ill to make decisions for themselves. They must rely upon their doctors to make decisions for them. The most commonly prescribed treatment for those with the four most frequent cancers –colon, breast, lung and prostate — is chemotherapy. Strangely, while there is no evidence that chemotherapy is effective for solid tumors, doctors write orders for chemotherapy and patients are handed consent forms, with no questions being asked as to whether or not it will work.

What patients should be asking their physicians are: *"Doctor, do you know of others who have survived for five years or more after chemotherapy?"* and *"What are the odds that this treatment will improve survival?"* Maybe patients don't ask their doctors these questions because they are afraid to hear the real answers.

There is no way for people to differentiate an effective treatment from a false hope. There are over 3,000 references to scientific studies cited in this book. They will mean little to most cancer patients. They will take the book to their doctor and ask if any of this is true. It's an endless circle. The doctor's hands are empty, he has no proven cures, only believes alternatives interfere with treatment, yet we rely upon him/her as the final arbiter in treatment decisions.

A survey was conducted some time ago. Different types of tumors in various stages were posed to cancer doctors and they were asked which type of treatment would be best for the patient. Radiologists preferred radiation therapy. Surgeons preferred surgery. Oncologists preferred chemotherapy. Can anyone be objective?

Dr. Guy Faguet cites the fact that radiologists are 53% more likely to prescribe radiotherapy when they own a treatment facility and spend less time with patients, and charge more, for their services. Chemotherapy accounts for two-thirds of the income of oncologists in private practice. On their day of diagnosis, about 30-50% of cancer patients have tumors that have spread to other locations and only about 2% of these patients treated with chemotherapy will be cured.

Does any of the advice in this book work? Through the years, desperate cancer patients, friends and acquaintances, would call for advice because they knew of my interest in and research of cancer. They thought I might know of where to look for answers to their questions. I would offer what I knew. There were surprising prolonged remissions. Here are some of them.

- *The 77-year-old woman with colon cancer who followed a regimen of dietary supplements I had suggested nine years ago and is still alive today. At age 86, she is free of cancer as confirmed by an MRI*
- *The woman who was diagnosed with uterine cancer at age 72 and survived nine years before succumbing to its ravages.*
- *The 54-year-old advanced breast cancer patient who just wanted to endure chemotherapy without her hair failing out, and got more than she desired – life without cancer for the past seven years.*

- *A business associate who had a tumor in one kidney that was surgically removed seven years ago with no recurrence elsewhere in his body.*

- *A man with terminal cancer, so weak he could not get out of bed, whose son called to ask if there was anything that could be done for his father. The doctor consented to having a hospital nurse dispense an herbal supplement. Within two days the patient got out of bed, dressed and walked home, to live for many months thereafter.*

- *The wife of a Congressional aide with Stage IV breast cancer, who went into sudden total remission after taking a single dietary supplement.*

- *A man with a softball-sized liver tumor, who had begun taking a single dietary supplement weeks earlier, was about to receive direct injection of a toxic drug into his liver when the doctor walked into the treatment room, viewed the x-ray film in the light box, shut off the light and declared the tumor had dead cells throughout and there was no need for further treatment. His cancer was cured.*

- The 85-year-old retired genetics professor with leukemia who had only weeks to live, was receiving blood transfusions, had lost side vision, who could not walk up stairs he was so weak, who began to take a single herbal supplement and soon was able to skip blood transfusions, regained his sight, resumed driving and is alive over 36 months later.

- An Asian American woman, ex-smoker, with lung cancer, who had endured the pain and suffering of modern cancer treatment for 3 years, to the point where she could not withstand another day of it. She tried various alternative cancer treatments, spending over $20,000 on them, when by surprise she heard of simple nutritional remedies that may be effective. Within weeks she was feeling healthy and a subsequent x-ray showed her lung tumor had vanished.

- A man in South Africa with lymphoma, who read of the dietary supplement that could quell cancer. Within weeks his cancer had disappeared.

These patients didn't wait for tomorrow's cancer drugs.

Maybe the nutrients these patients took had nothing to do with these remissions. Maybe they just had tumors that were slow growing. But so many were diagnosed with Stage IV cancer and then suddenly regained a grip on life.

There is something amiss here. Why weren't doctors making these suggestions? Why were these patients suddenly beating their cancer and living normal lives? There has to be something wrong with cancer care. Without a medical degree, I was offering suggestions that were bringing about prolonged survival. My only intention at the time was to help them overcome the side effects of treatment. These patients got more than that.
Are conventional and alternative cancer treatments the only alternatives?

As I wrote this book it was taking me somewhere I didn't plan to go– to steering patients away from doctoring, or at least away from life-threatening cancer care. To do that, something else has to be substituted, something beyond the bogus or inappropriate cures offered by alternative medicine. Nutritional medicine can be that cure. Though often relegated to preventing weight loss (wasting) during the progression of cancer, it has now been found that certain foods, spices and herbs can switch cancer genes off.

Readers of this book may not initially be ready to go where this book leads. But it may at least alter their thinking and cause cancer patients to adopt a plan that has more chance of success than conventional cancer treatment does today.

This book signals a new day in cancer care, one where patients will play a more prominent role, if given proper guidance.

I've shared parts of my book with cancer patients and their families. Their responses are wide ranging and predictable.

Largely based upon prior knowledge and beliefs, some cancer readers will ardently believe what this book says, but frustratingly won't know how to sell its ideas to cancer patients or other family members.

Some patients have pre-conceived ideas about what this book represents – alternative medicine – which they are wary of.

Some cancer patients want everything thrown into the kitchen sink, the best of conventional and alternative medicine. They see no conflict between toxic cancer therapies and the natural non-toxic remedies presented in this book. The advice in this book will be of limited value to these patients.

Very few will venture on their own, away from both conventional and alternative medicine, to find a cure.

For all who do take the time to read this book, it will have been a worthy venture for this author.

Bill Sardi

CHAPTER 1

Introduction

p 14 - 30

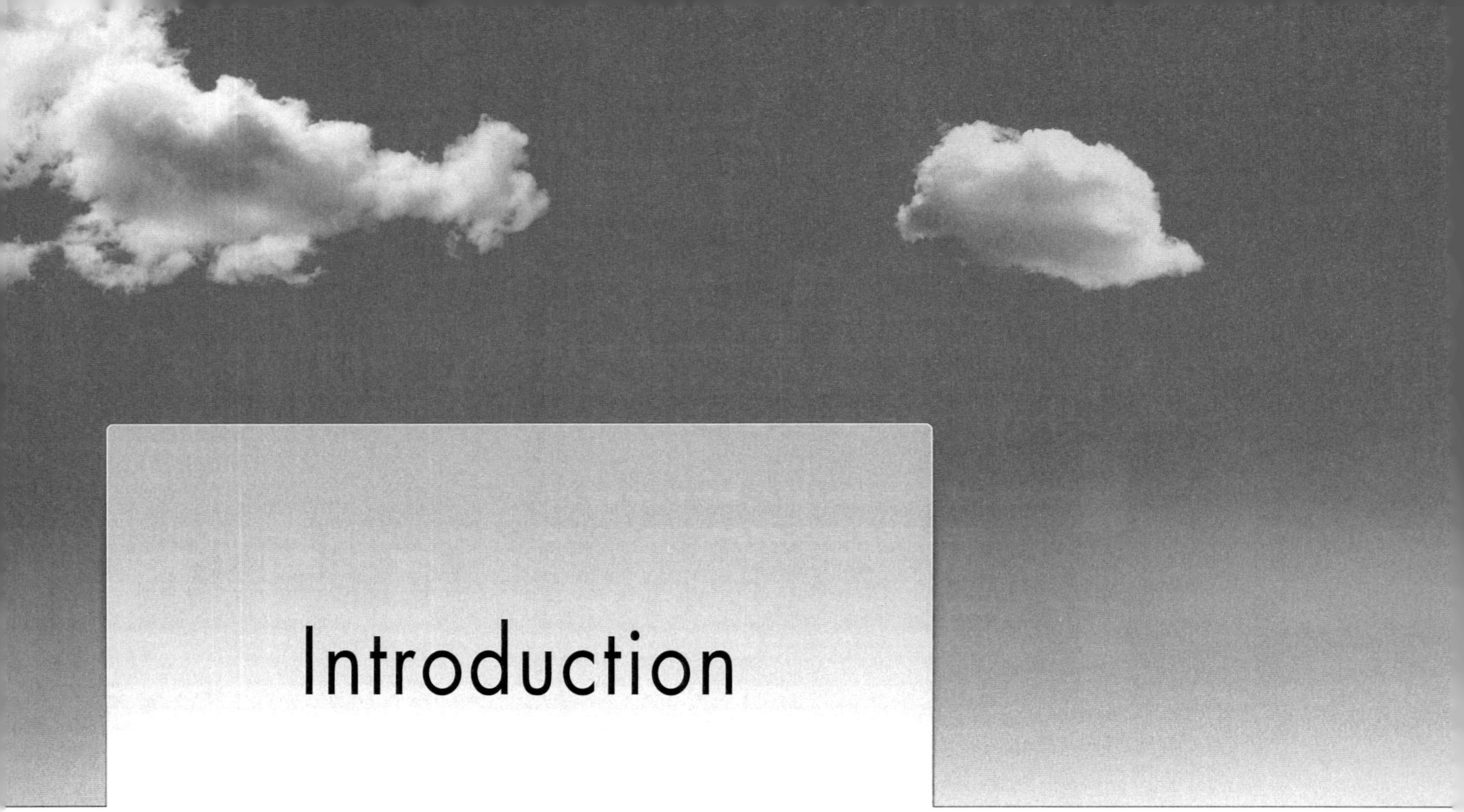

Introduction

What a time to write a book about cancer. On the one hand, the Baby Boomers are entering their most cancer-prone years with a tremendous rise in the number of cancer cases being predicted. It is estimated that as many as one in three Americans will develop cancer in their lifetime. Cancer is just now passing heart disease as the number one cause of death in the United States.

On the other hand, remarkable and unexpected developments now make it possible to place the greatest cancer-blocking molecules directly into the hands of patients so that cancer prevention can be effectively practiced for the very first time. What's more, the most potent anti-cancer treatments can be employed at home, without a doctor's prescription. These include simple remedies such as vitamin D (sunshine), rice bran, flaxseed oil, Brussels' sprouts, folic acid pill, red wine molecules and garlic cloves, which outperform the best chemotherapy drugs. You may be surprised to learn that there are no proven anti-cancer agents that can safely be prescribed to prevent cancer, that is, until now.

Concurrently, the cancer industry is in a state of chaos and uncertainty. It has begun to doubt itself. *"Doctors now wonder whether many women diagnosed with breast cancer could skip chemotherapy altogether. 'It's a slightly uncomfortable time,'* says one cancer specialist. *'If the medical profession is not even close to being of one mind, how is the patient to know?'* asks a reviewer of cancer treatment. [New York Times, May 12, 2006]

"Despite promising discoveries and multibillion-dollar investments, cancer research is quietly undergoing a crisis," says another report in the New York Times.
[NY Times, Dec. 21, 2005]

Introducing is 25-year (1990-2015) midpoint report under the title *"On the threshold of a dream,"* the American Cancer Society says cancer mortality rates have declined by about 1% per year since 1990 and if this rate of decline continues over the next decade, death rates from cancer drop by approximately 23% in the year 2015. The American Cancer Society has set a goal to reduce cancer mortality rates by 50% between 1985 - 2000. Some parts of its report made it sound like millions of lives would be saved. But the report went on to say that goals were unlikely to be reached. [Cancer, June 12, 2006 online] Much of the decline in mortality rates is imagined, extrapolated from manipulated statistics and the contrived idea that years of life are gained by early detection of cancer, when in fact most cancer patients succumb to their disease on the same calendar day whether their diagnosis is early or late.

Robert Bazell, NBC News chief science and health correspondent, says the National Cancer Institute has been too eager to claim success in the war on cancer and that medical reality doesn't match news releases issued from the agency. [Robert Bazell, When medical reality doesn't match the spin. NBC News June 20, 2006]

All this is happening at a time when the public is distracted by news reports concerning gene-targeted drugs, like Iressa, Herceptin and Erbitux, that only prolong survival by a few months, are laden with side effects, and literally cost a fortune ($1000-10,000 a month). The hype surrounding these drugs is unprecedented. The ability of these drugs to perform on Wall Street is being touted above their ability to cure cancer. *"None of these drugs prompt the kinds of dramatic tumor shrinkage or disappearance that doctors look for,"* says an Associated Press report. According to the U.S. Pharmaceutical Research and Manufacturers Association, 400 more of these types of cancer drugs are in clinical trials.

We live in an era when:

- the government-sponsored program that advocates eating 5 servings of fruits and vegetables a day has been found to be ineffective in preventing cancer
- use of sunscreen lotion has been found to be the major promoter of life-threatening skin cancer.
health authorities say breast self-examination should be abandoned.
- the occult (hidden) blood stool test for colon cancer has been declared useless.
- something as free as sunshine may prevent more cancer than any new cancer technology by virtue of its ability to produce vitamin D in the skin.
- tobacco companies want to introduce a *"safe cigarette"* that won't cause lung cancer.
- men with invasive prostate cancer were instructed by health authorities to return an herbal remedy that was saving their lives because it was *"mislabeled."*
- the PSA test for prostate cancer has been called misleading and unreliable.
- early detection of cancer is widely promoted, but waiting two years after diagnosis to treat prostate cancer doesn't make any difference in survival time.
- early cancer detection is touted, but mammography and colonoscopy still miss many early-stage tumors.
- it takes 2000 women to undergo mammography to detect one early case of breast cancer, while 10 healthy women will be inaccurately diagnosed as having breast cancer and will undergo needless treatment.
- hormone replacement therapy is abandoned when it is found to increase the risk for breast cancer.
- it is discovered, after five years of use, that Tamoxifen actually increases the risk for breast cancer.
- dogs have been trained to detect the *"scent"* of breast cancer with accuracy that rivals mammography.

- biopsies have been found to *"seed"* tumor cells and facilitate the spread of cancer.
- intravenous vitamin C, mistakenly dismissed decades ago, is found to selectively kill cancer cells without harm to healthy cells, thus vindicating research conducted by Dr. Linus Pauling.
- doctors report a disturbing trend by more and more terminal cancer patients to demand treatment that has no hope of working.
- it is suddenly realized the cancer industry has no treatment for metastasis, the chief factor that makes cancer a mortal disease.
- cancer patients are left without after-treatment plans or measures to prevent recurrence of their cancer once treatment is completed.

Dysfunctional cancer care

If you are facing cancer, you will need to learn how to navigate around a dysfunctional, self-serving, misdirected cancer care industry. It's clear that technologies of the past must be abandoned, but to be replaced by what? Health experts are unsure. You are going to have to find your own answers to cancer. This book helps you do that.

You may be shocked when you discover the most prestigious cancer centers deliver cancer care that has been disproven time and again. You may also be dismayed to learn that alternative medicine may have few answers for cancer as well. By discarding what doesn't work, or is marginal, however, you can narrow the number of options to choose from if faced with cancer or the prospect of developing cancer. This book will help you approach cancer armed with more objective information.

Don't tell me cancer treatment is ineffective

A battle with cancer causes enough anxiety. Patients don't want to hear about a failed cancer treatment system. Most cancer patients don't want to hear about all the politics and pros and cons surrounding cancer treatment today. They don't want to hear that cancer treatment is limited to *"slash, burn or poison."* After all, it is all they have to cling to.

Entering the cancer caresystem: caveat emptor

Once patients enter the cancer detection system, they may be starting on a trail that will lead to their early demise. The true story of Barry's ordeal is unfortunately typical of what happens to those afflicted with cancer.

Barry is a 60-year-old executive whose insurance company wanted him to undergo a physical exam. His wife had been nagging him to go to the doctor for some time. A PSA (prostate specific antigen) test is required. His PSA is elevated. His PSA could be elevated for a variety of reasons aside from cancer. This sends Barry to the doctor for a follow-up exam and a gloved-rectal exam to estimate the size of his prostate gland. Enlarged it is, so a biopsy is suggested.

At the urologist's office, the biopsy is performed via rectal access to the prostate gland and needles are inserted and withdrawn to obtain tissue samples. The pathologist's report says there is *"hyperplasia and neoplasia,"* pre-cancerous cells along with a few truly cancerous cells in his prostate. Barry is frightened, hears the word cancer, and wants the tumor. The urologist complies with Barry's request.

But Barry never had invasive prostate cancer and never was at mortal risk. Most men have abnormal cells in their prostate glands by age 30. Unless the cancer escapes from the prostate, these men are not at risk of dying from prostate cancer. But, because Barry had this surgery, he lost control of urinary flow and is now impotent. Did surgery eliminate the risk of prostate cancer? No. In fact, quite the contrary, the biopsy may have seeded his rectum with tumor cells when the biopsy needle was withdrawn, facilitating the spread of cancer, the most dreaded of all outcomes.

Most cancer patients will never recognize the dangers posed by cancer screening and treatment. The list includes: heart failure due to chemotherapy, radiation damage due to mammography and CT scans that can lead to cancer years later, the seeding of cancers into surrounding tissues due to biopsy, and following cancer surgery the triggering of growth factors that heal surgical wounds, but which also spur the growth of residual tumor cells.

Most cancer patients can't fathom the idea of rejecting cancer treatment or defying their doctor's orders, no matter how ineffective or toxic modern cancer treatment may be, for fear of having nowhere else to go. Cancer patients are in the dark and don't even know what questions to ask of their doctors. They want the cancer out of their body, and the delivery of timely treatment their health insurance plan promised them. Sadly, few, if any, cancer patients fully realize how ineffective those cancer treatments are. Treatment often decreases the chances of survival.

Those in the cancer care industry have become arrogant, believing that they hold the scientific high ground over alternative cancer therapy. Yet virtually all three common methods of cancer treatment– surgery, chemo and radiation therapy– do not add much in terms of survival time and have not been shown in any combination to significantly prolong the life of cancer patients. It's no wonder patients seek alternatives.

For instance, conventional cancer treatment offers the implantation of radioactive seeds to treat prostate cancer. While this is less invasive than surgical removal of the prostate, it is unproven. 5-FU is the most commonly used drug for colon cancer. It is employed for most cases of colon cancer, but only 20% of colon tumors are sensitive to this drug. There is no evidence patients live longer because they elected to receive these treatments. Treatment in itself may be of no value.

Somehow the cancer industry has managed to work itself into the undesirable position of utilizing disproven treatments while casting a condescending eye upon unproven alternative treatments. Unproven simply means there has not been sufficient investigation to come to a conclusion either way. The National Institutes of Health has not funded an adequate number of clinical trials of promising alternative therapies such as those involving vitamin D, folic acid, or intravenous vitamin C. A drawback to conducting such studies is that they take many years to complete since cancer is often a slowly developing disease.

Maybe readers need to hear about the failings of modern cancer therapy from a more *"authoritative"* source. Clifton Leaf of Forbes Magazine, normally a publication that publishes favorable information about pharmaceutical breakthroughs, wrote a chilling report on cancer therapy in 2004. Consider some of these quotations from his report:

Survival gains for the more common forms of cancer are measured in additional months of life, not years. Very little of the modest gain in survival is the result of exciting new compounds discovered by the National Cancer Institute labs or the big cancer research centers—where nearly all the public's money goes. When you break down the Big Four cancers (lung, colon and rectal, breast, and prostate) by stage—that is, how far the malignant cells have spread—long-term survival for advanced cancer has barely budged since the 1970s.

Oncologists can often shrink a tumor with chemo and radiotherapy. That sometimes makes the cancer easier to remove surgically. If not, it still may buy a little time. However, if the doctors don't get every rotten cell, the sad truth is that the regression is not likely to improve the person's chances of survival.

When most malignant solid tumors are diagnosed, they are typically quite large already—the size of a grape, perhaps, with more than a billion cells in the tumor mass. By the time it's discovered, there is a strong chance that some of those cells have already broken off from the initial tumor and are on their way to another part of the body. This is called metastasis.

So pharma companies, quite naturally, don't concentrate on solving the problem of metastasis (the thing that kills people); they focus on devising drugs that shrink tumors (the things that don't).

While it is true, 64% of cancer patients today have a 5-year survival, that doesn't mean survival can be attributed to treatment. For example, a recent review of chemotherapy employed for 22 different types of cancer found that chemotherapy is attributed to only 2.3% of the cancer patients who survived five years or more.

The point of this depressing information is not to cause dismay and shock, but to help you, as a future or current cancer patient, or caregiver, to understand you are dealing with a dysfunctional, misdirected cancer care system.

How can cancer be treated when its cause is unknown?

Cancer researchers keep saying they don't know what causes cancer.

- *Although breast cancer is the leading cause of cancer deaths for women between the ages of 35 and 54, the causes of breast cancer are unknown.*
  - Lawrence Berkeley National Laboratory's Ethical Legal and Social Issues

- *The cause of cancer of the uterus is not known.*
  - University of Michigan Health System

- *At this point, the specific cause of prostate cancer is unknown.*
  - Henry Ford Hospital

Well then, how can cancer be successfully treated if its origin is unknown? Is chemotherapy appropriate if cancer emanates from a folic acid deficiency? Is surgery appropriate if the cancer, left alone, never spreads from its place or origin and never threatens life as is often the case with prostate cancer?

Cancer can occur spontaneously, without a person being exposed to radiation or environmental carcinogens, without smoking tobacco, and without eating fatty or sugary foods. Just the age-related decline in the immune system can increase the risk for cancer. The accumulation of iron in the body also increases risk for cancer. A lack of folic acid can cause the same amount of genetic damage as exposure to atomic radiation. A deficiency of vitamin D alters the immune system, creating an environment for cancer. These causes are not addressed by the modern cancer care system.

If the riddle of cancer is to be solved, it will be a patient-driven revolution. Oncologists and cancer researchers have had 60 years and billions of dollars, and have come up with only harsh treatments that do not significantly prolong life. It's time for a change. But patients are often too fearful, too confused, too loyal to their doctors, and oftentimes too ill, to take charge of their cancer. This state of affairs needs to stop.

If you can't stand up to your doctor, and you are too fearful of the cancer to forgo treatment, at least you can adopt some of the suggestions in this book to help to minimize side effects frequently caused by cancer treatment. Dietary supplements are useful in this regard. Thousands of patients are discouraged from using dietary supplements because modern medicine's has blinders on when it comes to nutritional medicine, or what I and others prefer to call molecular medicine, or nutraceutical therapy.

Who says?

"Who said that?" is the prevailing question. Many cancer patients are likely to seek consultation with their doctor to inquire about the validity of the information in this book. Cancer patients may question the credentials of this book's author, believing if what this book says is true, then *"why didn't my Mayo Clinic-trained doctor tell me about this?"* Yes, this author wants to know the answer to that question too!

> This book attempts to provide a shortcut in your investigation concerning cancer. Your homework has been done for you.

It's interesting that a survey was once conducted where cancer doctors were asked the preferred treatment for certain types of cancer in various stages of development.

Radiologists said radiation therapy was the preferred method of treatment. Surgeons said it was removal of the tissue. Oncologists claimed chemotherapy was best. Providers of cancer care tend to steer patients toward the services they provide. The lesson here is, don't ask a doctor. You're likely to get a predictable answer.

Perhaps the simplicity of so many valid approaches to cancer prevention and treatment this book presents will befuddle readers. You may be thinking, *"Well, if it's true, why haven't I heard about it before?"* or *"It can't be that simple!"*

Would the suggestions in this book be sufficient by themselves for you to put them into practice? Probably not, because most people still want to corroborate any new information they hear from another trusted source, usually their doctor.

Readers who want to learn new ways to prevent or treat cancer need to ask themselves, *"just exactly what information do I need before I adopt a particular health regimen? What would convince me to give up on conventional medicine and adopt another course of action?"* If you are too frightened to forgo chemotherapy or radiation therapy, then what type of evidence would convince you to integrate nutritional remedies with conventional cancer care? Would your doctor need to agree before you chose to integrate any alternative therapies?

When confronted with something you have never heard before about cancer, how do you go about confirming what you heard?

A. Check on this with my doctor
B. Ask another trusted source
C. Go to the internet or public library
D. Other

Frankly, few people read books. They just like to know a book is there, and refer to the few pages that provide instruction. Many cancer patients frankly haven't the time to earn a college degree in cancer therapy. If you don't have the time to read it through, you can refer to the pages that apply to the particular type of cancer you are concerned about or look in the index to satisfy your curiosity about a cancer drug or alternative therapy.

You don't necessarily need to develop a high cancer IQ, you just need to start on a program like what is suggested in this book. For those readers who need immediate instruction on what to do, go to chapter 15 and read about universal approaches to cancer therapy.

No, all the answers aren't in. We only have access to the best available evidence. Furthermore, to reiterate, this book cannot prescribe nor supplant the advice of your physician. Cancer doctors today have the best tools to diagnose and chart the progress of your tumor.

Alternative medicine disappoints

What will be a surprise to many, upon review is that alternative medicine doesn't appear to have any better treatments for cancer than does conventional medicine. True, alternative cancer therapies are less invasive, and produce fewer side effects. But their effectiveness is in question. Alternative medicine clings to marginal or outright disproven remedies from the past, like laetrile, shark cartilage, coral calcium, or the idea that alkalinity cures cancer. (See Chapter 4 for more on this.)

While a revolution is underway in natural cancer remedies, backed by solid science, alternative medicine clings to archaic cancer treatments of the past, seemingly oblivious to the fact we now live in an era of genetic medicine where foods and dietary supplements can switch cancer genes off better than any prescription medicine.

For the first time in history, cancer patients have more powerful molecules at their direct disposal than any therapies pharmaceutical companies could even think of developing. The utter failure of modern cancer therapy to prolong survival times, and the introduction of potent non-prescription anti-cancer molecules that have broader and more potent anti-cancer activity than approved cancer drugs, signals a day in the near future when most cancer patients may be self treating their tumors at home. Here is an example.

Mike is at the forefront of this new era in cancer prevention and treatment. A stockbroker by trade, he had undergone successful radiation treatment for lymphomas, which were visible on his neck. But now the lymphomas were back and his doctor feared they were spreading. Mike knew he had to learn more than he ever wanted to know about cancer. He began supplementing his diet with extra vitamin D, some herbs (curcumin, green tea and resveratrol) along with some vitamin C. About a year later, with a large growing 3.2 centimeter lymphoma on his neck, he had to do something. He increased the amount of resveratrol. Suddenly, within days the primary lymphoma on his neck had visibly shrunk to half its size. Something remarkable was happening. While the only real measure of success against cancer is survival, and it's too early to tell his long-term outcome, Mike can see with his own eyes that natural cancer therapy has his lymphoma in retreat. This is something chemotherapy couldn't accomplish.

One of the things that cancer patients, their families and caregivers must do, is dismiss from consideration any disproven or marginal cancer therapies. Instead, create a short list of treatments that are likely to be effective.

Cancer instruction book needed

I have written this book because, sadly, there is not an adequate written guide for patients facing cancer today. There are volumes written about cancer, but so little help on how to sort out all the information. There is such so much information about cancer available today, yet so little instruction and commentary on how to go about fighting cancer.

This book is intended for four types of readers:

1. Those who are desperate to learn how to treat cancer effectively.
2. Those who want to prevent cancer from occurring in the first place.
3. Those who want to prevent cancer from recurring.
4. Those who have been freshly diagnosed with metastatic cancer that has spread to other organs and tissues and for which conventional treatments offer little or no hope.

There are many difficult choices to make once cancer is diagnosed. Should you embrace every conventional and alternative cancer therapy? Should you shun conventional cancer care and solely utilize so-called natural cancer treatment? Cancer patients often have difficulty sorting out what strategy is best for them and often decide they want to employ every anti-cancer therapy they can find, or what is called the *"kitchen sink"* approach. Sometimes alternatives aren't sought until it is too late.

You haven't the time

There is more to cancer than you would want to know. Most likely, you haven't the time to learn everything you need to know about cancer.

If you are over age 50, you need to start on an anti-cancer regimen today.

If you have cancer, and you haven't the time to read the book through to the end, skip ahead to chapter 15 and review the suggestions there.

If you have metastatic cancer, which is the life-threatening form of cancer, then you immediately need to employ measures to block the further spread of cancer since modern cancer care has no therapy that addresses metastasis.

Making the most important decisions of your life

Once cancer is diagnosed, the cancer patient and his/her family find they are not prepared to face what's next. They have to rely upon their doctor. The patient and family members are engulfed in trips for blood tests, x-rays, biopsies, doctor's office visits, and purchasing medications, without even questioning if any of this activity will result in a cure.

Many cancer patients wait until they hear the doctor's words, *"there is nothing else we can do,"* before they begin to search for alternatives. Then, grasping at straws, they often fall prey to any charlatan who offers a cancer cure.

Others cover all the bases, quickly integrating everything they hear about Essiac tea, shark cartilage, and other unproven treatments in a *"kitchen sink"* approach to surviving cancer. This trial-and-error attempt is often misdirected and fails to help the sufferer.

I interweave actual experiences into this book, to give examples of what really happens after cancer is diagnosed.

Case #1:

Mary calls to say her 80-year-old father has prostate cancer. He was healthy up until a week ago, fixing the roof on his house, she says, but the doctor detected the problem on a routine visit. I visit with her, attempting to educate her on what is happening. Based on what she tells me, her father is of advanced age and probably has the invasive form of prostate cancer that is spreading throughout his body, for which there is no effective treatment. The radiation treatment they are doing is to relieve pain and shrink the tumor at its site of origin, while nothing is being done to stop the flames of cancer from reaching the other organs in the body.

I bring her a bag of dietary supplements for her father to take, and inquire if she thinks he would be interested in using them. She says, *"yes."* But she wants me to meet with her sister, so days pass before a meeting can take place. Again, I explain the treatment their father is undergoing is not intended for cure, it is palliative, to control pain.

It's all too new for these sisters to gauge whether I know what I am talking about. The dietary supplements sit in a bag, still unused. Finally, Mary's father begins to take the supplements, but a suspicious cousin hears he is taking some pills supplied by a neighbor and suggests that a distant family member who is a physician sees her father. The distant relative examines the supplements and cautiously suggests Mary's father be wary of them. They may interfere with treatment, he warns. But what he doesn't say is that treatment has no chance of working for this advanced stage of cancer.

Mary and her sister don't know this. They believe the doctors are trying to cure their father. But it's too late. Eight weeks have passed. Mary's father has lost urinary control, has lost weight, is on morphine and is laying on his last bed.

Case #2:
At age 85, Harry has been diagnosed with leukemia, cancer of the blood. It was an advanced case. His red blood cell count was so low he lost some of his peripheral vision and couldn't walk up the stairs without fainting. Blood transfusions were frequent, just to prolong his life a few more days at a time. Then a neighbor friend suggested he begin taking a red wine molecule called resveratrol, as a dietary supplement.

Harry, a retired plant geneticist, did some research on his own. The evidence seemed convincing enough, so he began taking the red wine pills. Soon Harry was regaining his strength. His hemoglobin count rose, to the astonishment of his doctors. He didn't need any more transfusions. As his story is written here, he has survived a year beyond what doctors predicted. Harry's case is an example of the new patient-driven cancer

Lord, Please Help!

Current mood: Hurting
Category: Life

How do we feel? OVERWHELMED! We need a miracle! Raul is in terrible pain, and it is getting worse by the day (maybe even by the hour). Yes, he puts on his amazing smile and tells people he is fine, but truth be told – it is really bad. From experience in seeing this progression last May – we seem to be just days away from Raul being totally *"bed-ridden"* because of the pain.

Since arriving back home, we have had MANY people give us their opinion on what we should do. Some say we made the wrong choice and should go back to Texas. Others have shared their advice on what the *"miracle cure"* is for Raul. Honestly, since we first learned of Raul's cancer, we have been bombarded with natural cancer treatment advice. We have file drawers full of ideas. In fact, other than dealing with the pain, this is probably the most frustrating thing we face each day. We have all these people who love us VERY much and mean nothing but good by giving us their advice... but Lord, which one do we choose?

How do we know who to agree with, which theory to try? If we did everything that has been recommended to us, Raul would be taking over 1,000 pills a day, drinking around 4 gallons of stuff, doing an assortment of other very strange things, and would have visited all 50 states plus 4 other countries! Now, tell me that this not overwhelming... and I'm sure I left something out.

Currently, we (he) is on a six-day carrot juice detoxification cleanse. Basically, we drink fresh carrot juice or water all day long, then have a light organic meal based on the Oasis (similar to the Hallelujah) diet. Raul is also taking a wide variety of supplements. Since there is no way everyone would agree with what he is taking anyway – we won't bore you with those details.

Dear God, we know that You are in control of every single cell in Raul's body. We know that You are the Great Physician and Healer and that You are able to bring immediate healing. But for some reason, You have a different plan for us at this time. God, we ask that You give us patience (even without understanding), wisdom for the choices we must make every day, peace that You are still in control, and most of all, we BEG you for some relief from the pain! We know You are able, but we also know that You allow us to suffer some times. Please give us the grace to accept whatever You know is best for us right now. AMEN.

revolution. Harry's case is so unusual because rarely does any single anti-cancer agent ever quell advanced stage cancer.

Cancer patients ARE finding ways to experience prolonged remission from cancer, without chemo or radiation therapy. You will read about many of these cases in this book.

But if proven cancer remedies exist, how can patients and their families sort them out from the snake oil? Most patients, hearing of an unfamiliar cancer remedy, will run back to their doctor to inquire about it, only to find he or she dismisses these alternatives outright, without investigation, while prescribing medicine and treatments that fare no better than no care at all.

"Nutriphobia"

When it comes to cancer and nutrition, it's amazing the public misperceptions about vitamins, minerals and herbs. Truly, chemotherapy is toxic, yet cancer patients will inquire about the safety of a vitamin pill, but take toxic chemotherapy drugs without hesitation.

Mike, the stockbroker mentioned at the beginning of this chapter, has been using vitamins for years. His grandfather took vitamins and eventually died of kidney failure. He takes vitamins and has lymphoma. His family members mistakenly associate the vitamin pills with these diseases. They think Mike's melanoma was caused by taking vitamins. So many people hear TV reports or read articles in newspapers that high-dose vitamin C causes cancer, and even though these reports are later found to be in error, they leave an indelible impression upon the people who first heard them. So few Americans realize how many negative reports about nutritional therapy are planted in the news media.

According to the *Forbes Magazine* report, the best approaches to improving cancer survival are to prevent DNA mutations that initiate cancer and to halt the spread of cancer (metastasis) that is responsible for over 90% of cancer deaths. Drs. Linus Pauling and Matthias Rath have long contended that maintenance of the connective tissue and collagen prevents the spread of cancer.

Nutrients like folic acid and IP6 rice bran extract are required to repair broken DNA strands, but go unused for this purpose. Antioxidants extracted from pomegranates, onions, cranberries, grape skins, olives and cherries protect DNA from breakage by radiation or free radical bullets. The growth of cancer is inhibited by removing iron and copper from tumors through the use of rice bran extract (IP6). IP6 is also required to repair double-strand DNA breaks (where the DNA breaks at both ends). Resveratrol, known as a red wine molecule, activates a DNA repair gene (Sirtuin 1) and blocks cancer at all three stages of development (initiation, growth and spread), which is more than any anti-cancer drug can do. Resveratrol has the powerful ability to switch cancer-promoting genes off. The spread of cancer is halted by agents that thin the blood, such as fish oil, garlic, vitamin E and magnesium, and by vitamin C, which prevents cancer cells from sticking to artery walls. Cruciferous vegetables like Brussels sprouts and broccoli along with flaxseed lignans and soy phytoestrogens help to dampen the hormonal-controlled growth of cancer.

If your oncologist isn't recommending these anti-cancer agents, he is mired in the past.

If the public elects to put its guard up against cancer early on, before tumors become detectable the size of a grape), then a significant drop in mortality rates can be expected.

Cancer patients in the mirror

Cancer patients also must learn more about themselves. The greatest advances in cancer prevention lie in the hands of the patients – via smoking cessation, plant food diets and informed use of dietary supplements - not in the hands of doctors.

About half of newly diagnosed cancer patients have metastatic cancer that has spread to other organs and tissues and oncologists (cancer doctors) concede there is no proven treatment for advanced-stage cancer. By then a quick fix is impossible. Treatment is rendered because patients and their families demand it, but with little hope for cure.

The prevailing approach to cancer is to let it happen and then treat it. Beyond attempts to get smokers to stop reaching for cigarettes (20 million of 48 million Americans who use tobacco will try to quit this year, most unsuccessfully), and failed efforts to get Americans to eat more fruits and vegetables (only 9% consume 5 servings of fruits and vegetables a day), there are few proven methods employed to deter cancer before it begins.

Is cancer being overtreated?

Cancer patients and their families often demand treatment, regardless of whether it is effective. Family members often insist that the doctor do something. Cancer patients and their families have even sued medical centers for not utilizing unproven treatments, such as bone marrow transplants, to treat otherwise hopeless cases of cancer. Other patients have lobbied publicly for expensive drugs that offer no more than an extra month or two of life. Cancer doctors know this. They know that patients and their caregivers feel they have paid for health insurance and they demand treatment. For fear of telling patients *"there is nothing more that can be done,"* the patient undergoes treatment that may extend life by a few short weeks, and then are told the same thing.

Sometimes no treatment is as good as treatment. For example, small brain tumors are often left alone because surgical intervention may cause brain damage. Prostate tumors are often so slow growing that males who opt for *"watchful waiting"* live as long as patients who undergo surgical removal of their prostate.

Explaining the disturbing trend for terminal cancer patients to receive chemotherapy and other aggressive but futile treatments in the last days of their lives, Dr. Roy Herbst of the MD Anderson Cancer Center in Houston aptly says: *"Patients don't like to give up."* A survey shows nearly 12% of cancer patients who succumbed to their disease received chemotherapy in the last two weeks of life. *"Overly aggressive treatment gives false hope and puts people through grueling and costly ordeals when there is no chance of a cure,"* say cancer specialists. [Dr. Craig Earle of the Dana-Farber Cancer Institute and Harvard Medical School, American Society of Clinical Oncology, Atlanta, June 2006; Associated Press, June 2, 2006]

Surprising Facts About Cancer Care Today

Before you read the rest of this book, take the following into consideration:

1 Most patients are diagnosed with cancer when their tumors are relatively large, the size of a grape or larger, or about a billion cancer cells in size.

2 Cancer patients and their families need to immediately learn what stage of development their cancer is in. If cancer has moved from its point of origin, and is spreading to other tissues and organs (metastasis), this is an ominous condition that requires strong and immediate attention. Regardless of the stage of the tumor, the first thing to do when the diagnosis of cancer is made is to implement any measures that stop metastasis. Modern medicine has no therapies that address metastasis. Other measures must be considered, such as boosting the immune system (beta glucan, vitamin D, selenium, zinc, vitamin C, vitamin E) or keeping roaming cancer cells from adhering to other cells or getting trapped in blood clots (resveratrol, enzymes, vitamin C, allicin/garlic and omega-3 oil).

3 Cancer drugs are not approved by the Food & Drug Administration as a cure for cancer. Anti-cancer drugs do not have to demonstrate they result in cancer patients living longer or experiencing long-term remissions. Anti-cancer drugs are approved when they can demonstrate they can shrink a solid tumor by 50% or more for at least one month. However, shrinkage of tumors is not related to survival. You may be surprised to learn that cancer drugs are primarily used to manage tumor size and minimize pain rather than provide a cure. Most chemotherapy drugs work for a short time, then drug resistance sets in, and the drug becomes ineffective. For example, Tamoxifen, a breast cancer drug, actually increases the risk for cancer with long-term use. There are natural ways to reduce resistance to cancer drugs that are not being utilized.

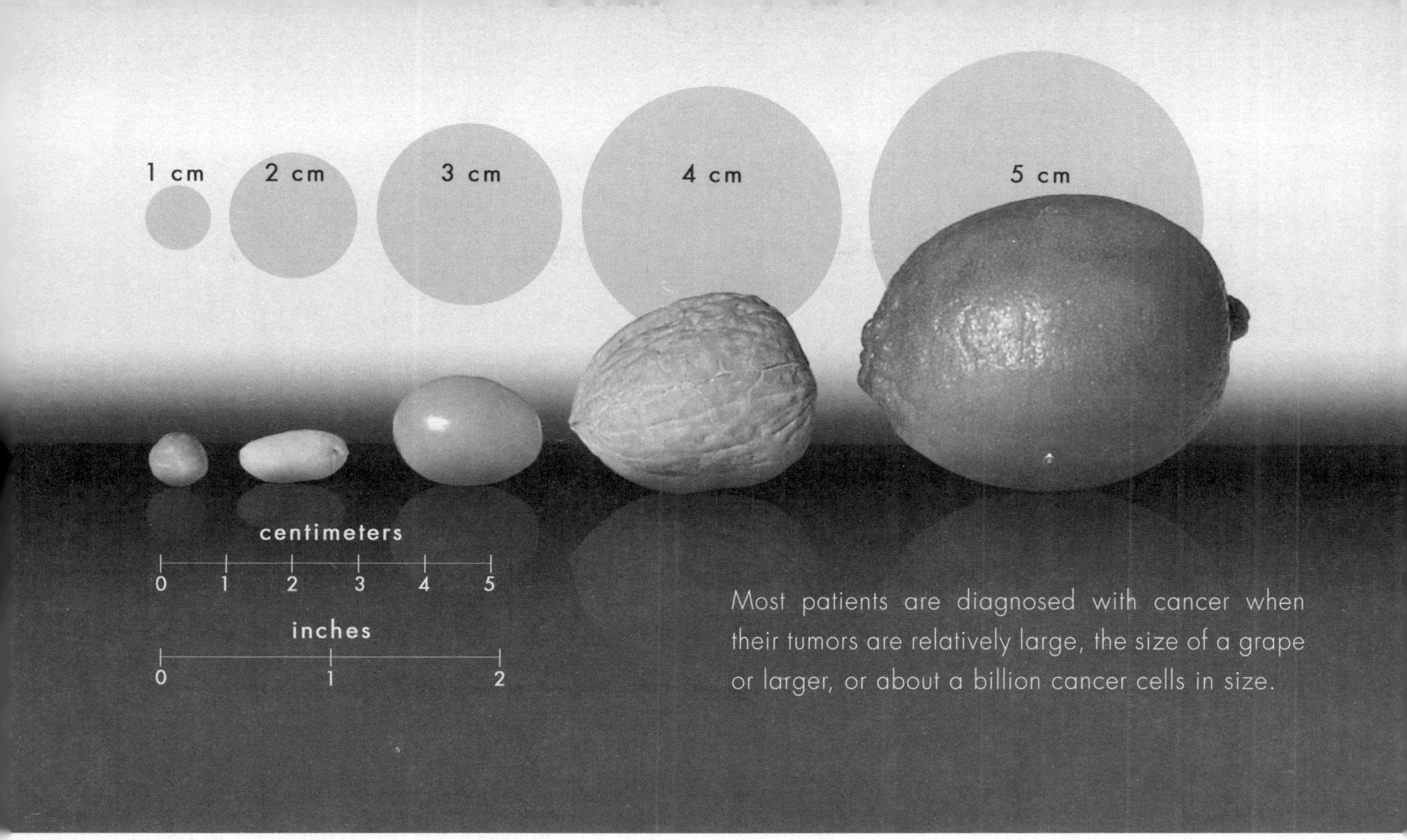

4 In regard to surgical tumor removal, there is no such thing as *"got it all."* Regardless of what cancer doctors say, if a one-millimeter ball of tumor cells (that's just 4/100ths of an inch around) remains after treatment, that means 10 million cancer cells have been left behind. A one-centimeter tumor ball (about 4/10ths of an inch around) would contain one billion tumor cells!

5 The germ theory of disease is being ignored when it comes to cancer prevention. It is now known that bacteria (example: *H. pylori* and stomach cancer) and viruses (example: Human papilloma virus and cervical cancer) induce malignancies. Stealth bacteria like *Mycobacterium tuberculosis* and *paratuberculosis* may mimic or actually trigger cancer. But little is done to put up a defense against infection. Garlic/allicin, onion/quercetin, oregano/Carvacrol, and folic acid may be helpful in this regard.

6 Cancer cells come and go. Readers will be astounded to learn that most adults harbor cancer cells from time to time. They die off in a normal fashion if the connective tissue surrounding cancer cells is maintained. For the cancer cells that do escape, less than 0.1% actually survive the immune system. Maintaining the environment that surrounds tumor cells is as important as the cancer cell itself. Modern cancer care does not address this need, but nutritional medicine does. (Chondroitin sulfate, vitamin C, proline, lysine)

7 Most cancer therapy does not discriminate between tumor cells and healthy cells. This is why cancer therapy is so toxic. However, natural nutritional therapies such as intravenous vitamin C, allicin from garlic, resveratrol and IP6 rice bran extract kill off cancer cells without harming healthy cells.

8 Cancer patients must utilize antioxidants to spare themselves the terrible side effects of chemotherapy and radiation.

9 Regardless of what you may have read elsewhere, cancer is a disease of aging, not primarily caused by environmental toxins such as pesticides or industrial chemicals, which may be cancer causing agents (carcinogens), but do not significantly contribute to cancer mortality rates. This is often difficult for cancer patients to comprehend. Carcinogens are tested in lab dishes, or administered to animals in unnaturally high doses. The human body has defenses against carcinogens. Very young children who do

not have a developed immune system, or very old adults whose immune system is not up to par, are more prone to develop cancer from exposure to cancer-causing agents than full-grown young adults.

Consider smokers, who expose their body to cadmium, a heavy metal, and to other cancer causing chemicals, yet usually do not develop cancer until the age of 50.

10 While environmentalists express outrage at the existence of cancer-causing chemicals and radiation in the daily environment, Dr. Bruce Ames of the University of California points out that nutrient deficiencies produce the same breaks in human chromosomes as does exposure to radiation. [Toxicology Letters 28: 102-03, 1998] It is estimated that between 20 and 40% of all cancer cases are caused by dietary factors, at least 35% by tobacco use, and 5% by abuse of alcoholic beverages. Exposure to cancer-causing chemicals and radiation comprises a much smaller portion of all cancer cases than most people think. [Carcinogenesis 18: 97-105, 1997] Just remember, environmental groups need to justify their cause to raise funds and maintain their jobs. While not an excuse to endure exposure to avoidable carcinogens, most programs to rid the environment of toxic agents are not likely to reduce the incidence or mortality of cancer.

11 There is too much emphasis that cancer in one location is different from cancer in another location in the body. There are universal factors involved in all cancers. An exception is cancer involving sex hormones (breast and prostate cancer). A new study shows that many cancers in different locations respond to various treatments in the same way and cancer specialists for breast, prostate, lung or colon cancer may not be necessary. More universal treatments for cancer are in store. [Washington University School of Medicine, May 2006] A universal nutritional regimen to put a halt to all cancer is provided in Chapter 15.

12 Tumors can be shrunk, removed, vaporized, and reduced in size and number, but this may not improve survival. Survival is the gold standard by which to evaluate all cancer therapy. Your doctor may show you x-ray films that confirm treatment has shrunk a tumor, but this does not equate with survival, often because treatment increases mortality rates by itself. Don't be fooled by cancer marker numbers, x-ray films or PSA tests. The only valid way to know a cancer therapy works is to measure how long the patients live.

Number of deaths from cancer per 100,000 people of specified age

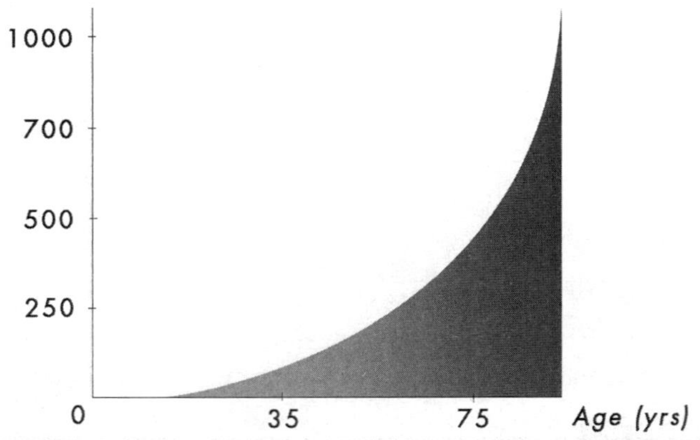

13 The cancer care industry considers that cancer screening, such as mammograms, PSA and stool tests, prevents cancer, working under the assumption early treatment will prolong survival or even lead to a cure. However, screening programs often miss detection of small tumors and sometimes indicate the patient has cancer when there is no cancer at all (called a false positive test). Cancer screening has only led to earlier detection and the false appearance of improved survival. Patients still die on about the same calendar day whether their cancer is detected early or not. In effect, screening is simply a scouting mission to find more disease to treat and bill insurance companies for, not prevent cancer from occurring in the first place. Cancer screening assumes treatment is effective. It is not.

14 Contrary to what you may read elsewhere, while a good diet is desired, the best diet (5 servings of fruits and vegetables) has utterly failed to prevent cancer. The National Cancer Institute's 5-A-Day Program has been abandoned in favor of 9 to13 servings of fruits and vegetables, which is still an unproven approach to reduce cancer mortality. While the American Institute for Cancer Research estimates 30 to 40% of all cancers are associated with a poor diet, less than 9% of Americans consume even five servings of fruits and vegetables a day and only 1 to 3% of all government funding for cancer research is devoted to cancer and nutrition.

What should be concluded is that a bad diet, filled with saturated fats, hydrogenated fats, highly absorbable iron in red meat, that is devoid of antioxidants, folic acid and other nutrients, will increase the risk of cancer. Good diets don't necessarily prevent cancer, but a bad diet certainly facilitates the early onset of malignancies. If you are trying to beat cancer, or prevent its recurrence, a bad diet must be replaced by one that is filled with dark-green leafy vegetables, berries, grapes, bran, flax, cruciferous vegetables, garlic, onions, etc.

Most of the recommended dietary measures to prevent or treat cancer help to control iron, which is the primary growth factor for cancer cells. The Gerson diet, plant food diets, fasting, whole grain diets and various dietary supplements (such as green tea, pine bark, etc.) all help to control iron. Aspirin, often suggested to reduce the risk for cancer, causes a small amount of blood loss which results in the depletion of iron. Iron chelation and control must be emphasized for adequate cancer prevention. An important lesson in this book is to learn about iron and cancer.

15 What are you going to do after cancer treatment is completed? It is estimated that there are more than 10 million Americans living with cancer. [Journal National Cancer Institute 96: 1412, 2004] An embarrassing if not distressing report reveals that many cancer patients are not provided adequate follow-up care after treatment. The problem, says a report from the National Cancer Policy Board, of the Institute of Medicine, is that cancer survivors mostly *"go it on their own."* After treatment, patients are sent back to their primary care physicians, often without a plan for follow-up care. The big problem is that doctors aren't reimbursed for follow-up care, so it gets neglected. [CA Cancer Journal Clinicians 56: 65-67, 2006] This is puzzling since a list of good health habits, dietary measures and dietary supplement regimens would suffice. A pre-printed sheet of paper with after-care instructions would go a long way. Once all the billing codes have been utilized for insurance claims, physicians virtually abandon patients in regard to secondary prevention. It must be emphasized, if your cancer is in remission, modern cancer care generally provides little advice as to how to keep it from returning. You must find ways to prevent cancer on your own. Your doctors only have surgery, chemo and radiation therapy to offer.

> Sixty years of intensive effort to remove tumors has not changed the biological outcome of the disease.
> *– G. Zajicek, Medical Hypotheses 47: 111-15, 1996*

Cancer Preparation Checklist

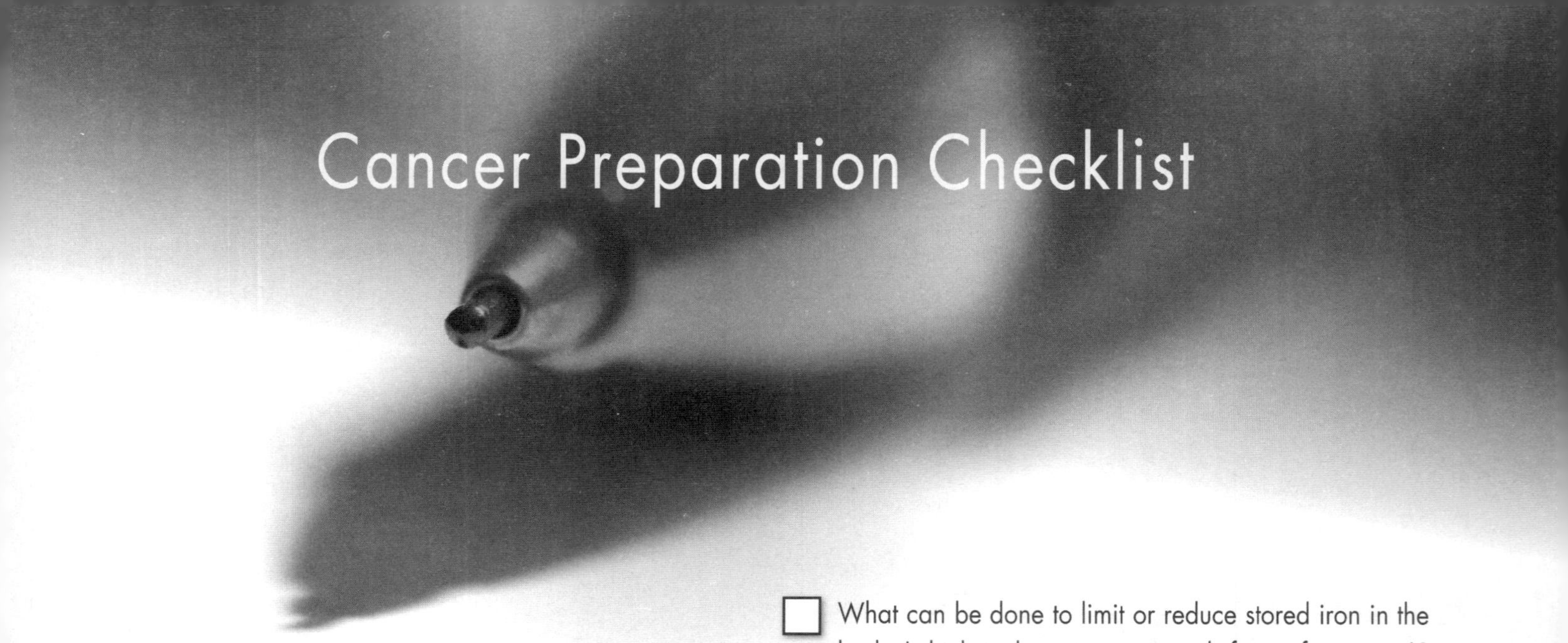

- [ ] Over age 50 – begin cancer prevention program today
- [ ] Review health habits – what can be realistically done to minimize or overcome cancer risk? (Examples: high antioxidant diets and antioxidant supplements can reduce cancer risk among smokers and alcohol drinkers; folic acid supplements can prevent colon, breast and cervical cancer.)
- [ ] Review diet. The best diet may not prevent or treat cancer, but a bad diet will certainly encourage the onset or growth of tumors. (Limit refined sugars, saturated fats, increase consumption of plant foods, limit iron intake, increase water consumption)
- [ ] Where will you turn for information once diagnosed with cancer?
- [ ] Once diagnosed with cancer, how will you make decisions regarding treatment?

    A. Rely solely upon the doctor
    B. Make independent decisions
    C. Involve family members

- [ ] If diagnosed with cancer, what will you do to prevent metastasis? (Knowing that modern medicine has no treatment that prevents the spread of cancer, which is the primary threat for mortality)
- [ ] What can be done to limit or reduce stored iron in the body (which is the primary growth factor for tumors)? (see section on IP6 rice bran in this book)
- [ ] What can be done to normalize hormone levels so they don't encourage the growth of tumors once they occur? (See Chapter on flaxseed meal, cruciferous vegetables, fermented soy – miso, tofu)
- [ ] How will you maintain a healthy immune system as you age? (refer to Chapters on selenium, zinc, magnesium, vitamin D, vitamin C, vitamin E)
- [ ] How do you maintain healthy connective tissue (collagen) that serves as a barrier against the spread of any developing tumors? (See chapter on Vitamin C, chondroitin, hyaluronic acid, proline, lysine)
- [ ] How will you prevent cancer from recurring once it goes into remission? (See sections on folic acid, vitamin D, omega-3 oil, vitamin C, vitamin E, selenium, resveratrol)
- [ ] What can be done to detect cancer in its earliest stage? Be aware: weight loss is one of the earliest signs of malignancy, yet it is mostly ignored in a population of sedentary Americans who are pleased to find that they are skinny again. Weight loss (wasting, known as cachexia) can occur when tumors are just 0.01% of body weight. [British Journal Cancer 63: 337-42, 1991]

How to use this book

1 Determine your level of interest

a. Prevent cancer from occurring or recurring
b. Treat existing cancer (non-metastatic – hasn't spread yet)
c. Treat advanced (metastatic) cancer
d. Prevent or minimize side effects of treatment

2 Acquire pertinent information on action plans

a. Location or type of cancer – refer to specific sections in this book
b. Universal regimens to prevent or treat cancer – refer to Chapter 15

3 Sort out action plan by

a. Dietary suggestions
b. Dietary supplement regimens
c. Health habits to alter
d. Compatibility with existing treatment

4 Use as a reference for new therapies that you hear about

a. Herbal or nutritional therapies
b. Alternative cancer treatments

This book is written for information purposes only. It cannot diagnose nor prescribe. The nutritional regimens and doses published in this book are general in nature and not specifically prescribed for any individual. The author is not a doctor and does not accept consultations or examine patients. Readers are urged to seek other sources of information before altering health regimens. Regardless of the shortcomings of cancer care today, this book is not a substitute for professional care. The cancer patient faces difficult choices with few sources of reliable information.

CHAPTER 2

Causes

p 32- 75

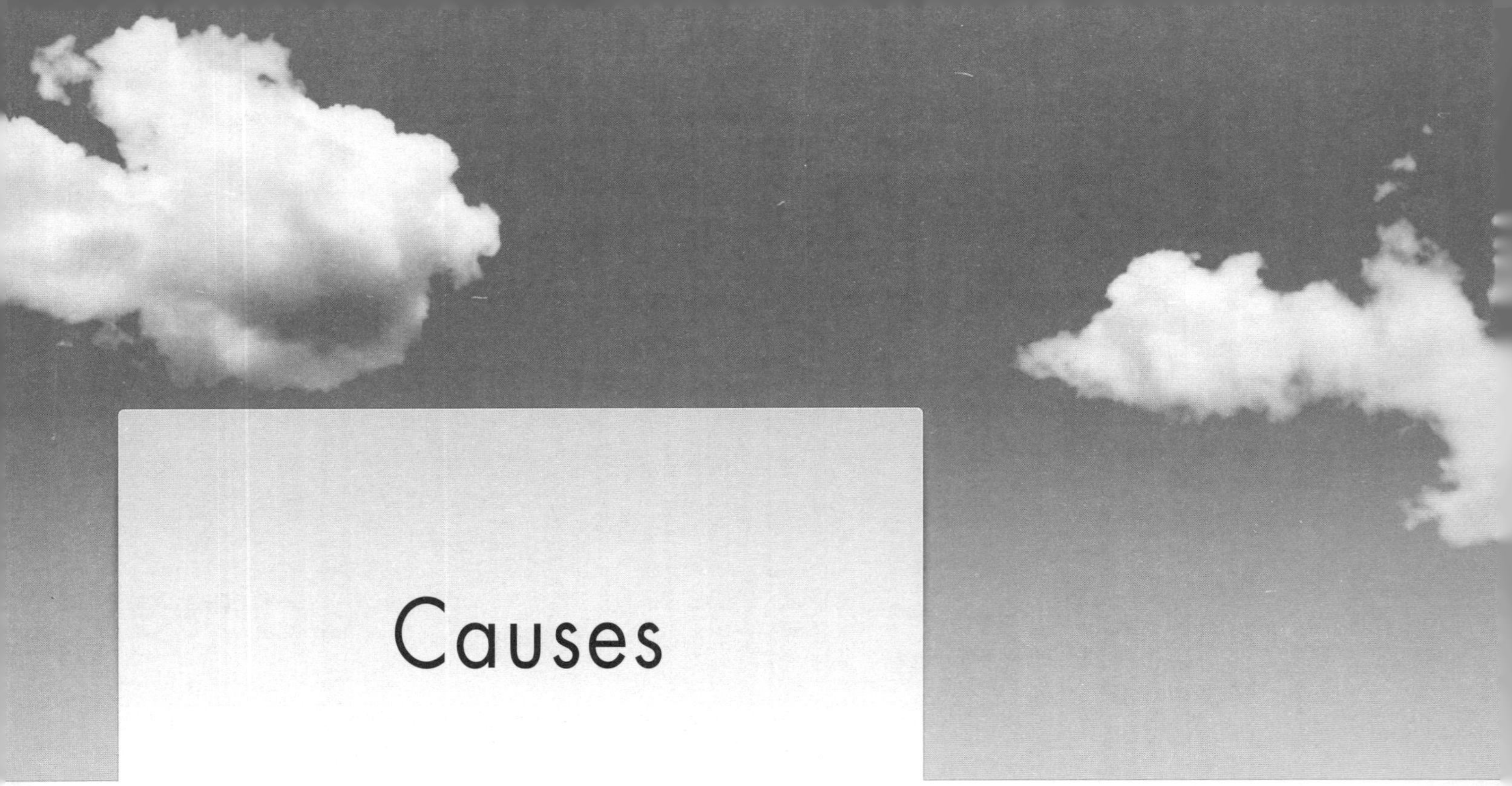

Causes

What causes cancer?

Maximal potential reduction of cancer mortality in the world by categories of factors

Factor	Percentage
Tobacco	25
Diet in adult life	15
Infection	15
Occupational factors	5
Reproductive factors	4
Environmental pollution	3
Alcohol	3
Sedentary life	2
Food additives and contaminants	1

Source: European Journal Epidemiology 20: 565-74, 2005

Exactly what causes cancer? Is it pesticides, industrial chemicals, electromagnetic fields, acidity, germs, oxygen free radicals, hormones, or all of these?

An argument can be made for all of the above causes. But the pervasive factor involved in the vast majority of cancer is **aging.**

No matter how efficient we may become at delivering health care, we must also seek to reduce demand by keeping people from developing diseases in the first place.
– Devar Lee Davis, Calum Muir, Environmental Health Perspectives, November, 1995

Sixty percent of all cancer occurs in persons over age 65 years. [Cancer 80: 1273-83, 1997] While the overall rate of cancer hovers at around 204 per 100,000 adults under age 65, it is 2,225 per 100,000 adults over age 65. [Cancer 80: 1273-83, 1997] That's 11 times greater risk!

A 70-year old is roughly 100 times more likely to be diagnosed with a malignancy as a 19 year old.
Source: Scientific American, June 9, 2003

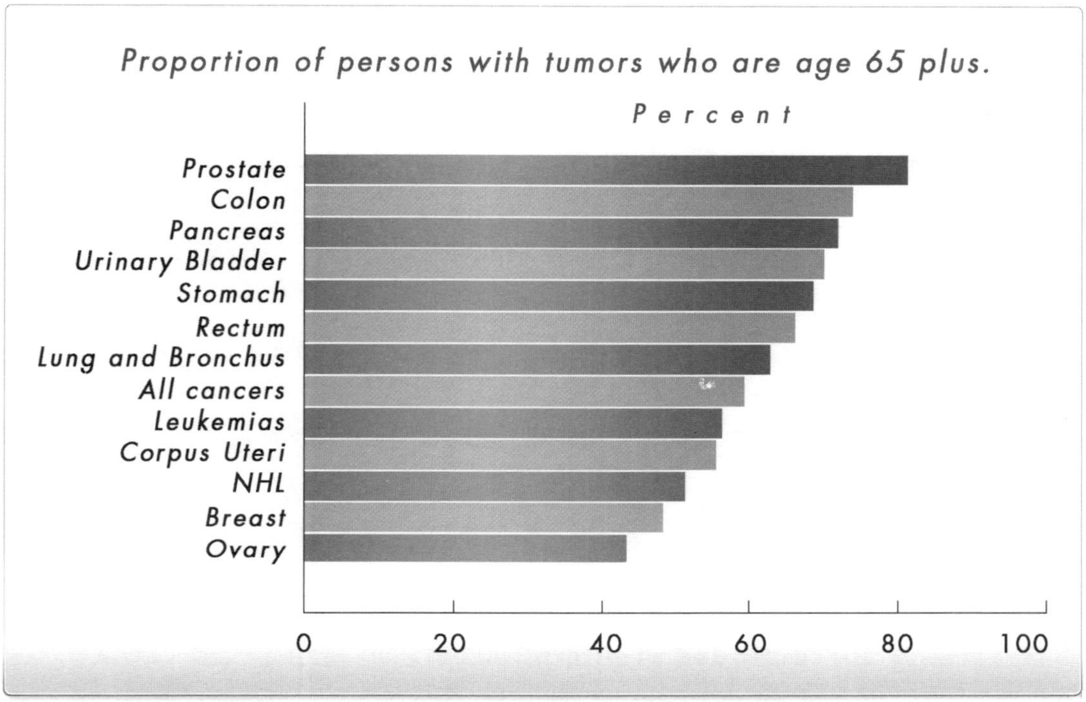

Source: Cancer 80: 1273, 1997

Many things change as the body ages.

- The immune system declines with advancing age.
- The body's primary barrier against the spread of disease – the goo that is called connective tissue that holds tumors in place so they can't spread - -also breaks down more readily with advancing age.
- Hormone levels decline as we mature.
- As oxygen is provided to living cells, a small percentage turns into oxygen free radicals or *"rusting agents"* that can damage tissues and genes and are believed to initiate DNA damage that causes cancer.
- Iron accumulates and then gets loose from binding proteins to damage DNA and cause tissue destruction.

Which of these factors is the key to preventing cancer?

Are DNA mutations the origin of cancer?

There are about 5 trillion cells in the human body. There are about 30,000 genes in each cell of your body. When uncoiled, the DNA in each cell is about six feet long. So there is a grand total of about 3 billion miles of DNA in an average-size body.

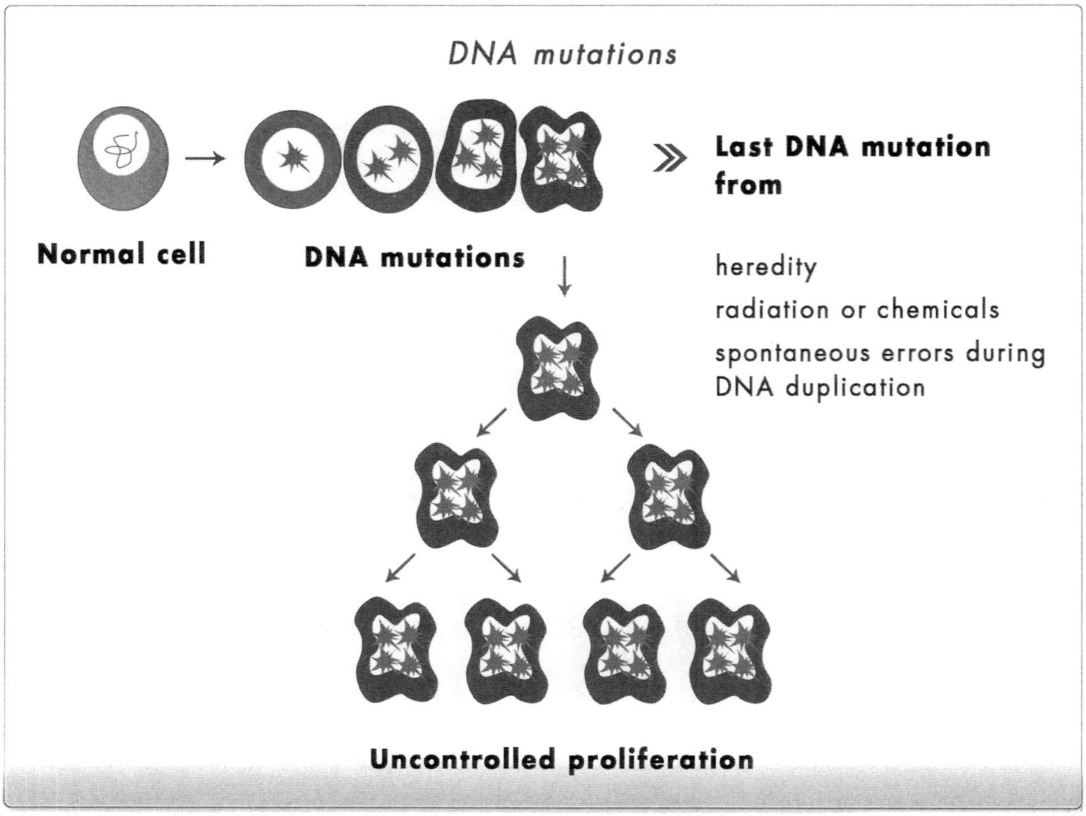

If you look at most solid tumors in adults, it looks like someone set off a bomb in the nucleus of these tumor cells, says William C. Hahn of the Dana-Farber Cancer Institute. *"No one questions that cancer is ultimately a disease of the DNA,"* says a report in Scientific American (June 9, 2003).

Early during the genesis of cancer there are enormous numbers of random mutations, 10,000 to 100,000 per cell, says Lawrence A. Loeb, University of Washington researcher. [Scientific American, June 9, 2003]

If DNA mutations spawn all cancers, then what causes abnormal DNA repair and eventually mutations?

Research conducted by Dr. Bruce Ames, of the University of California at Berkeley, suggests that whatever causes premature aging is also related to the onset of cancer.

Cancer occurs in the latter years of life. Nutritional deficiencies – shortages of vitamin B12, B6, folic acid, vitamin C, vitamin E, zinc and niacin – can equal the DNA damage caused by exposure to a dose of radiation. The provision of these nutrients to old animals, not only reduces their risk of developing cancer, but also slows their rate of aging. In some animal experiments conducted by Ames, old animals regained youthful function once provided with adequate nutrition. [Toxicology Letters 102-03: 5-18, 1998] What Ames is saying is that nutrition, aging and cancer are related.

Ames also says diet is estimated to contribute to about one-third of preventable cancers – about the same fraction as smoking. [Nature Reviews Cancer 2:694-704, 2002]

A report prepared by the Dutch Institute for Public Health and the Environment states that insufficient nutrients by poor selection of foods is as bad for human health as is smoking. [Reuters May 29, 2006]

Ames says cancer research has become distracted with avoidance of cancer-causing chemicals, which may not be relevant to preventing cancer. He says carcinogens are identified in experiments where animals are exposed to hundreds of times more of the suspect cancer-causing chemical than is found in natural human environments. Meanwhile, nutrient deficiencies are a greater cause of DNA damage that can result in cancer. Ames says huge amounts of money are being spent to examine hypothetical risks from environmental carcinogens when dietary deficiencies may pose a greater threat because they can mimic radiation damage to cells – the kind of DNA damage that leads to cancer. [Mutation Research 447: 3-13, 2000]

Ames also says it has been estimated that the United States spends 100 times more to prevent one hypothetical, highly uncertain death from a synthetic chemical than it spends to save a life by nutritional intervention. [Drug Metabolism Review 30: 201-23, 1998]

Millions of dollars of research studies conducted over recent decades cannot correlate exposure to pesticides, microwaves, smog, or electromagnetic fields to the risk for cancer. *"Unfortunately, by pushing for more study of environmental risks, the public perception of this environmental program becomes a straw man for the real issues in cancer, such as smoking, dietary habits, etc,"* says Brian E. Henderson and Susan Preston-Martin, professors of preventive medicine at the University of Southern California School of Medicine. [LA Times, June 8, 1998]

DNA damage

The human body is resilient. Only one out of three or four heavy smokers will develop lung cancer compared to one out of ten non-smokers. Cancer only develops in a fraction of patients exposed to a given cancer-causing agent. While genetic testing may indicate whether a particular individual has a mutated cancer gene, this kind of information assumes this is a static situation. In fact, it is a dynamic (ever changing) situation. For example, there is a family on record of four brothers who died of lung cancer over a 20-year period. The two brothers who did not smoke developed cancer at the age of 70 and 72 years of age, while the other two brothers who were heavy smokers became affected in their forties. There may be genetic susceptibility, but there are dynamic factors, too, that can control or delay the onset of tumors. Exposure to radiation, chemicals, tobacco, alcohol, or a lack of nutrients may increase gene mutations. Antioxidant molecules and vitamins are known to protect genes from mutations.

For example, a sample of blood serum withdrawn from a person after drinking red wine will exhibit less DNA damage than before wine consumption. [Annals New York Academy Sciences 854: 23-36, 1998] This protective effect is only attributed to the non-alcohol fraction of wine, not to alcohol. [Mutation Research August 2, 2005]

As previously stated, Dr. Bruce Ames of the University of California at Berkeley has made it clear that deficiencies of certain nutrients can be as damaging to cellular genetic material or DNA, as is exposure to strong doses of radiation. [Mutation Research 447: 3-13, 2000]

When DNA strands break, they require folic acid for repair. For instance, a shortage of folic acid will result in DNA damage to strands of the p53 tumor suppressor gene in animal colon tissue. This provides a plausible mechanism as to how folic acid deficiency results in colon cancer. [Gastroenterology 119: 151-61, 2000]

Sometimes too much of a nutrient will induce DNA damage. In a perfect state of health, there is no unbound (loose) iron in the blood circulation. But in states of inflammation or infection, iron gets loose (unbound from proteins) and can generate damage to DNA that can lead to colon cancer. [Mutation Research 519: 151-61, 2002]

Ames reports that breaks in chromosomes (groups of genes) occur when vitamin concentrations are low. The quarter of the population that consumes the fewest fruits and vegetables has about double the cancer rate for most types of cancer when compared to the quarter with the highest intake. [Annals New York Academy of Science 889: 87-106, 1999] Some researchers now propose that humans consume ample amounts of nutrients from foods and supplements that are known to prevent DNA damage. [Annals New York Academy Science 854: 23-36, 1998]

Of acute interest is the DNA genetic material found within small cell bodies called mitochondria. The mitochondria house their own set of DNA apart from the DNA found in the nucleus of living cells. Some tumors contain high numbers of mutations in mitochondrial DNA whereas none are present in healthy tissues. [Lancet 360: 1323-25, 2002]

Cancer without DNA damage

The following theory of the origin of cancer runs contrary to almost everything you may have ever read. It is such an astounding explanation, and demonstrated so convincingly that it cannot be overlooked. More remarkable, scientific experiments document that cancer can originate in living cells without DNA damage.

In 1986, Dr. O.J. Stone proposed that hyaluronic acid (HA) and the entire matrix of connective tissue is an important barrier against the growth and spread of tumors. Stone wrote that anything that helps to retain the viscosity (consistency) of HA increases the body's resistance to tumors, whereas enzymes like hyaluronidase, stimulated by infection or radiation exposure, encourage tumors. [Medical Hypotheses 20: 117-24, 1986]

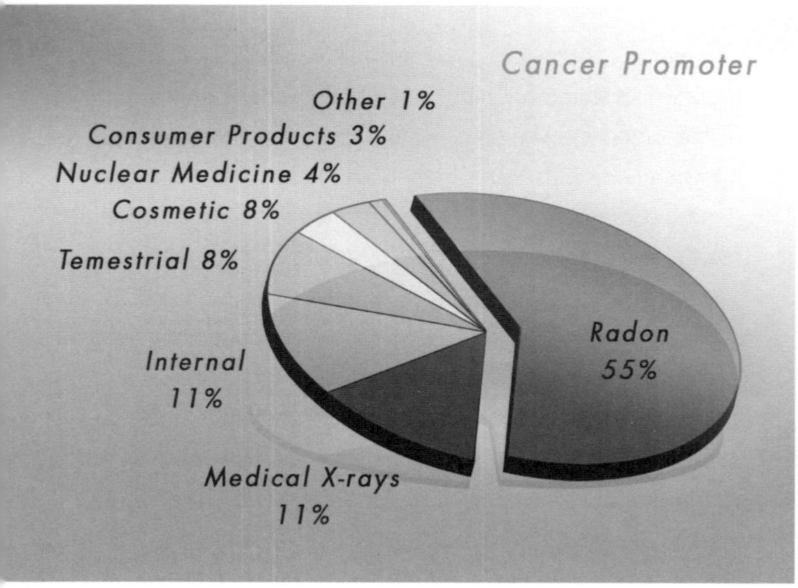

HA is a molecule comprised of glucuronic acid and glucosamine that gels water. It is a water-holding molecule that is produced by fibroblast cells. Water is the great detoxifier and diluter of the body. When young, humans produce large amounts of hyaluronic acid. Cancer occurs in the latter years of life, when HA levels in the body are low.

The research of Dr. Mary Helen Barcellos-Hoff at the Life Sciences Division, Lawrence Berkeley Laboratory, in Berkeley, California, helps to reveal the anti-cancer properties of HA and connective tissue in general. Ionizing radiation (often given off by x-rays) is a known cancer promoter, particularly in breast tissue. Radiation damages the matrix of material that surrounds cells, the HA and collagens. Even just one chest x-ray performed before the age of 20 increases the likelihood of breast cancer later on in life by 54%! [Journal Clinical Oncology, June 26, 2006 online]

In an animal experiment, supporting tissue that surrounds mammary-gland epithelial cells was exposed to low-dose ionizing radiation. Then non-irradiated breast gland cells were implanted within this matrix. A massive increase in tumors was observed in the non-irradiated mammary cells! More tumors occurred and grew larger compared to non-irradiated animals. [Cancer Research 60: 1254-60, 2000]

Only 19% of non-irradiated connective tissue produced tumors versus 81% of irradiated connective tissue. What's more the size of the tumors in the non-irradiated tissue was smaller than in the irradiated tissue. The tumors grew so fast in the healthy mammary cells implanted in irradiated connective tissue that by six weeks all of the mammary glands had tumors! But only 39% of the healthy mammary gland cells implanted in non-irradiated connective tissue expressed tumors and most were small. The study had to be halted because all of the irradiated mammary gland cells were tumorous by the sixth week. Had the study continued, the difference between the two groups would have been greater because of the tumor regression observed in the non-irradiated animals.

Previously, the connective tissue was believed to be an uninvolved bystander to cancer. It is now obvious that disrupted connective tissue permits the initial tumor cells to proliferate.

As Barcellos-Hoff says, *"Indeed, it has been suggested that cancer may be a physiological response to an abnormal environment."* Studies reveal there are many more mutated cells produced that can initiate cancer than actual number of tumors that develop. The initiation of cancer appears to be a far more frequent event than is the cases of cancer that develop. Low-dose radiation upsets the environment surrounding cells and promotes tumors, an effect that lasts for 14 days following radiation exposure. By re-establishing the matrix of supporting tissue, tumors and pre-tumorous cell processes can be reversed, even in the presence of grossly abnormal genetically damaged cells. [Cancer Research 60: 1254-60, 2000]

Barcellos-Hoff notes that conventional thought is that the ionizing radiation promotes cancer by its ability to damage DNA. But her experiments clearly show that cells undamaged by radiation, but existing in an environment of connective tissue that has been irradiated, will aggressively grow tumors of large size and numbers. Barcellos-Hoff suggests it is possible to develop blocking agents to interrupt tumor progression. [Journal Mammary Gland Biology Neoplasia 3: 165-75, 1998]

Even more evidence of HA's anti-cancer barrier effect comes from Japan. Researchers at Osaka Medical Center for Cancer and Cardiovascular Disease report that removal of an extended zone of connective tissue in addition to lymph glands surrounding pancreatic tumors increased the five-year survival rate from 8 to 25%. [Gan To Kagaku Ryoho 29: 364-69, 2002] This is an astounding improvement in survival for a type of cancer that traditionally has a very high mortality rate. To learn more about hyaluronic acid and cancer, see chapter 13 in this book on Specialized nutrients (non-vitamin).

Cancer: Is it inherited?

Can a person be genetically predisposed to develop cancer? While there are inherited genes for cancer, hereditary forms of cancer represent no more than 10% of all cases. Except for certain types of cancer that follow along family lines, such as polyps in the digestive tract, the contribution of heredity to the onset of cancer is thought to be relatively minor. [New England Journal Medicine 343: 78-85, 2000] Even those born with a genetic inclination for cancer, usually don't see tumors appear until much later in life. That is, the gene-controlled mutations that lead to cancer do not become evident for decades. Cancer genes simply increase the likelihood of developing this disease. [Seminars Cancer Biology 7: 49-53, 1996] For instance, the genes linked to ovarian cancer (BRCA1), colon cancer (hMSH2 and hMLH1), and melanoma (MLM) confer a higher lifetime risk for cancer, but represent less than 5% of these types of cancer. [British Medical Bulletin 50: 527-35, 1994]

Certainly studies of twins, who have the same genes, should help sort out whether genes or environmental factors (diet, exposure to carcinogens) play the strongest role in the onset of cancer. Among twins, inherited factors were found to be responsible for 4 to 41% of breast cancer cases and 29 to 50% of prostate cancer cases. [New England Journal Medicine 343: 78-85, 2000] While a person may inherit certain genes that may increase the risk of developing cancer later in life, this should not be looked upon as fatalistic. Women who opt to have their breasts surgically removed because they carry a gene that predisposes them to cancer is one example of a drastic over-reaction to the role of genetics.

Furthermore, while twins inherit duplicate sets of genes, they also grow up eating the same diet, drinking the same water, receiving the same amount of sun exposure. So how can inheritable or genetic factors be separated from environment factors?

So, should every human being be screened for genetic flaws that might increase their risk of developing cancer?

While there are many potential cancer-causing agents that humans come in contact with, the undeniable fact is that the two most toxic molecules that can generate genetic mutations that lead to cancer are found abundantly inside the human body – iron and oxygen. About 1-5% of the oxygen that is utilized to produce cell energy in the mitochondria of living cells lose an electron and become a destructive *"free radical"* called superoxide. About 2 kg (4.4 pounds) of superoxide is produced annually in the human body. Superoxide is converted into hydrogen peroxide (H2O2), and then with the aid of antioxidants such as catalase and glutathione, into water (H2O). However, if loose iron or copper is available, then the hydrogen peroxide is converted into the dreaded hydroxyl radical that can damage DNA and cause cancer. [Journal Molecular Medicine 74: 297-312, 1996]

Gene therapy disappoints

If mutated genes can predispose a person to cancer, then maybe insertion of a normal gene could fix the problem. That's what scientists thought. Hundreds of studies ensued after the Food & Drug Administration gave its go-ahead for the first gene therapy studies in 1989. A scientific panel criticized much of the hype surrounding these studies, some of which were of a commercial nature. Gene therapy studies have since been abandoned because of deaths associated with the gene experiments. But researchers are reluctant to call gene therapy a failure, instead characterizing it as having *"progressed slower than anticipated."* [Annals Internal Medicine 132: 549-60, 2000]

Genetic testing

A woman whose mother and older sister have developed breast cancer might want to know of her genetic predisposition for breast cancer. Knowing that the BRCA1 gene, when mutated, does increase the risk for breast cancer among women, testing can help identify at-risk individuals. However, only 5 to 10% of all cases of breast or ovarian cancer are believed to stem from defective BRCA1 and BRCA2 genes. So the test is only applicable to a small number of women. Women who do have a defective version of these genes have about an 80 to 90% chance of developing breast cancer and a 40 to 65% chance of developing ovarian cancer. Testing is likely to cost more than $2,000.

Of the 150,000 people who are diagnosed with colon/rectal cancer each year, only 5 to 10% may carry a faulty HNPCC gene.

There are obviously other factors that control cancer beyond genes. One of every 25 Caucasian American carries the gene mutation for cystic fibrosis, but far fewer actually develop this disease. [Laboratory Medicine 28: 316-22, 1997]

The problem with genetic testing is that it poses dilemmas. Should an otherwise healthy woman with a mutated BRCA1 gene undergo removal of her breasts to prevent future tumors? Should a fertile woman forgo having children for fear she would transfer a trait to her offspring? Is there an unrealistic fatalistic conclusion to be drawn from genetic testing? While there is concern that genetic testing may increase anxiety in at-risk individuals, studies do not reveal any significant psychological problems after positive identification of a mutated cancer-causing gene. [J Genet Counseling 14:349-63, 2005] However, the genetic testing is a tension-filled experience. Essentially, the at-risk patient potentially exchanges uncertainty for anxiety.

Another motive for genetic testing appears to be a way to drum up business. According to one study, more than half of the women who have the genetic marker for breast or ovarian cancer opt to have their breasts or ovaries removed. Of 411 cancer-free women who were at high-risk for breast or ovarian cancer, 48% chose to undergo genetic testing and when the tests revealed they had a genetic mutation, 51% chose double breast removal and 64% chose surgical removal of their ovaries, despite very low odds of actually getting cancer. [Lancet 355:2015-20, 2000] Only 1 in 400 women have a mutation of one of the two genes (BRCA1, BRCA2) that promote breast cancer. Yes, but the previous paragraph said that women with this gene have an 80-90% chance of getting breast cancer. It's odd that women often chose surgery over preventive measures.

Will a positive genetic test prompt individuals to change their health habits? In one study involving smokers, 65% anticipated being motivated to quit smoking upon receiving a positive genetic test result; 39% anticipated being demotivated by a negative result. [Health Education Behavior 32:640-53, 2005]

Silencing oncogenes

Genes that promote cancer are called oncogenes. Since the human genome has been mapped, the identification of oncogenes may open the way to block the activity of these genes and thereby stop cancer growth. Similarly, there are tumor suppressor genes, like p53, that researchers may be able to activate and treat cancer.

Wouldn't it be wonderful to breed a generation of humans who are resistant to cancer? Researchers have attempted to do this in the laboratory. For instance, researchers at Sloan

Kettering Memorial Cancer Center in New York bred mice with *"id"* or inactive genes. When tumor cells were injected under the skin of these animals, the mice did not develop cancer. Bravo! But now, can they do that for us humans? Well, it's a bit complicated. The *"id"* genes are vital for growth and development from fetal through childhood periods. Anything that interferes with new blood vessel formation, as does the drug thalidomide, results in birth defects. The cancer-resistant rodents in the Sloan Kettering trial had their *"id"* genes disabled during adulthood, when they were largely inactive. [Nature 401:670-7, 1999]

In another genetic experiment, researchers used telomerase, an enzyme that repairs the ends of genes, called telomeres, to produce cells that are immortal, or perpetually young. The idea was to see if youthful cells would resist cancer. After inserting the gene to produce telomerase into human breast cells, researchers found that this caused a negative reaction: harmful, cancer-producing genes, called *"c-myc"* then became active [Nature 405:755-6, 2000] This experiment casts doubts on the idea of targeting a single enzyme or gene to resist cancer. Researchers are now focusing on ways of inhibiting telomerase so that normally immortal cancer cells will grow old and die off. Researchers are also investigating small molecules, like polyphenols found in grapes, olives, tea leaves and berries, that can control telomerase. [Mutagenesis 17:539-50, 2002]

Gene targeted drugs

Researchers are also beginning to re-examine the concept behind anti-cancer drugs that target specific genes, because more than one gene is involved in cancer. Targeted cancer drugs such as Gleevec (Novartis) and Iressa (AstraZeneca), which are portrayed as *"magic bullets"* because they are designed to hit single, biological targets, have been disappointing. Gleevec ended up influencing other genes. Bryan Roth, a biochemist at Case Western Reserve University in Cleveland, says *"magic shotguns"* rather than *"magic bullets"* are what's needed. Simon Frantz, writing the lead article in an issue of Nature Magazine, says: *"Forget drugs carefully designed to hit one particular molecule – a better way of treating complex diseases such as cancer may be to aim for several targets at once."* [Nature 437: 942-43, 2005]

"Natural compounds (rather than man-made drugs) offer a less specific but perhaps more effective strategy for cancer therapy by inducing combinations of effects that may counteract the metabolic alterations related to cancer promotion" says Paolo Signorelli and Riccardo Ghidoni, researchers at the San Paolo University Hospital, School of Medicine, University of Milan.

These researchers note that cancer is not easily treated with single anti-tumor drugs. Natural compounds from plants address whole mechanisms and sets of pathways that interfere with tumors rather than just inhibiting a single enzyme which is the way synthetic drugs work.

Resveratrol: unleashes a genetic tsunami

Doctors Signorelli and Ghidoni single out resveratrol, a red wine molecule, for its unique ability to favorably control hundreds of genes at one time. [Journal Nutritional Biochemistry 16: 449-66, 2005]

Another biologist, referring to resveratrol's ability to switch hundreds of genes, says resveratrol exerts *"a whiff that induces a biologically specific tsunami."* [Cancer Biology Therapy 3: 889-90, 2004] Resveratrol's ability to influence many genes was demonstrated in a gene array experiment involving kidney cancer cells. [Cancer Biology Therapy 3: 882-88, 2004]

When referring to the many new anti-cancer technologies under development, most oncologists (cancer doctors) are reticent to use the word *"cure"* because the drugs they employ kill cancer cells but do not address the cause of malignancy. Resveratrol is as close as biologists have come to a cure for cancer.

Resveratrol overcomes gene-controlled tumor cell formation

Since the work of Nobel Prize winner Otto Warburg in the 1930s, it has been known that tumor cells are hypoxic, that is, they no longer utilize oxygen to produce energy. Rather, they generate energy by fermentation. In their relentless search for oxygen, tumor cells proceed to migrate and send signals for new blood vessels to grow towards the tumor (a process called angiogenesis). In so doing, the tumor obtains nutrients and grows at an accelerated pace.

Tumor cells produce a gene-controlled protein called hypoxia inducible factor-1 (HIF-1) that facilitates this whole process. The loss of HIF-1 activity dramatically decreases tumor growth, new blood vessel formation and energy metabolism.

A major reason for treatment failure is that the most aggressive tumors over-produce HIF-1. If just 10% of malignant cells over-activate HIF-1 the tumor is more likely to resist radiation treatment. [Molecular Cancer Therapeutics 3: 647-54, 2004]

Cancer investigators believe HIF-1 inhibiting drugs may overcome the problems posed by fast-growing solid tumors. Researchers exclaim that *"the most exciting possibility would be the discovery of small-molecule inhibitors of HIF-1."* [Nature Medicine 9: 677-84, 2003] Small molecules would be able to penetrate inside the nucleus of tumor cells, to genetically inhibit the activity of HIF-1. [Current Cancer Drug Targets 3: 391-405, 2003]

Researchers now believe HIF-1 is a promising drug target, and that resveratrol, a red wine molecule, appears to be the small molecule they were searching for since it *"dramatically inhibits the stimulatory effects of hypoxia on invasive tumor cells."* [Molecular Cancer Therapeutics 4: 1465-74, October 2005] Once tumor cells no longer exhibit high HIF-1 activity, blood vessels that supply nutrients to these malignant cells begin to recede, the tumor cells begin to utilize oxygen once again, and these otherwise immortal cells begin to age and die off.

Infection and cancer

Infection is a cause of cancer, more so than published reports indicate.

There is infection by parasites, such as worm-like organisms, or by bacteria, viruses, fungi and amoeba.

Researchers in France estimate the worldwide proportion of cancers attributable to infection is 15.6% (1,450,000 cases in 1990). The primary infectious agents noted were the hepatitis B and C viruses (liver cancer), the human papillomaviruses (cervical cancer), Epstein Barr virus, human T-cell lymphotrophic virus I, HIV, the bacterium Helicobacter pylori (stomach cancer), schistosomes, or liver flukes. There would be 21% fewer cases of cancer in developing countries and 9% fewer cases in developed countries if these infectious diseases were prevented. The attributable fraction at the specific sites varies from 89% of cervix cancers attributable to the papillomaviruses to 1% of all leukemias attributable to human T-cell lymphotrophic virus I. [Cancer Epidemiology Biomarkers Prevention 6: 387-400, 1997]

It is interesting to note that countries with the warmest climates and the spiciest cuisines also have the lowest rates of cancer. [Quarterly Review of Biology 73:3-49, 1998] Certain spices have been found to have strong anti-bacterial properties. Garlic, onion, allspice and oregano, for example, were found to be the best all-around bacteria killers (they kill everything), followed by thyme, cinnamon, tarragon and cumin (any of which kill up to 80% of bacteria). Capsicums, including chilies and other hot peppers, are in the middle of the antimicrobial pack (killing or inhibiting up to 75% of bacteria), while pepper of the white or black variety inhibits 25% of bacteria, as do ginger, anise seed, celery seed and the juices of lemons and limes.

It just could be that the spices we add to our foods protect us from the eventual onset of cancer.

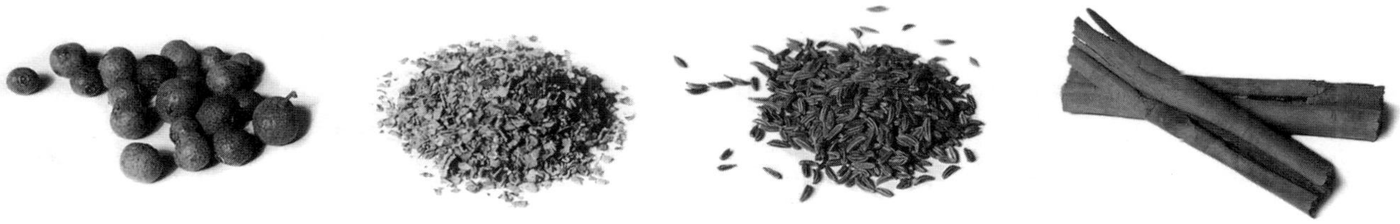

Top 30 Spices with Antimicrobial Properties

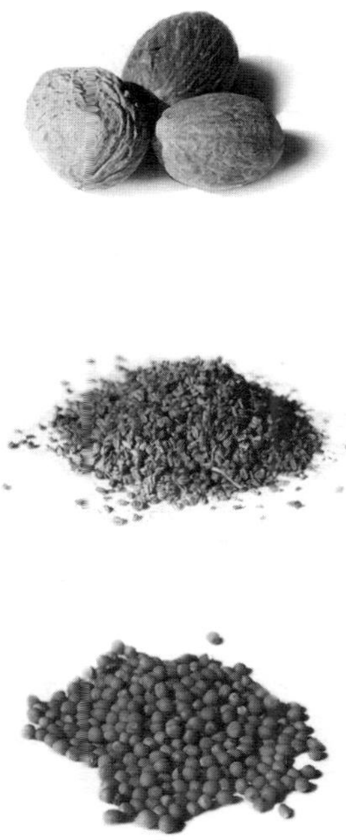

Listed from greatest to least inhibition of food-spoilage bacteria

Source: "Antimicrobial Functions of Spices: Why Some Like It Hot," Jennifer Billing and Paul W. Sherman, "The Quarterly Review of Biology", Vol. 73, No. 1, March 1998

1. Garlic
2. Onion
3. Allspice
4. Oregano
5. Thyme
6. Cinnamon
7. Tarragon
8. Cumin
9. Cloves
10. Lemon grass
11. Bay leaf
12. Capsicums
13. Rosemary
14. Marjoram
15. Mustard
16. Caraway
17. Mint
18. Sage
19. Fennel
20. Coriander
21. Dill
22. Nutmeg
23. Basil
24. Parsley
25. Cardamom
26. Pepper (white/black)
27. Ginger
28. Anise seed
29. Celery seed
30. Lemon/lime

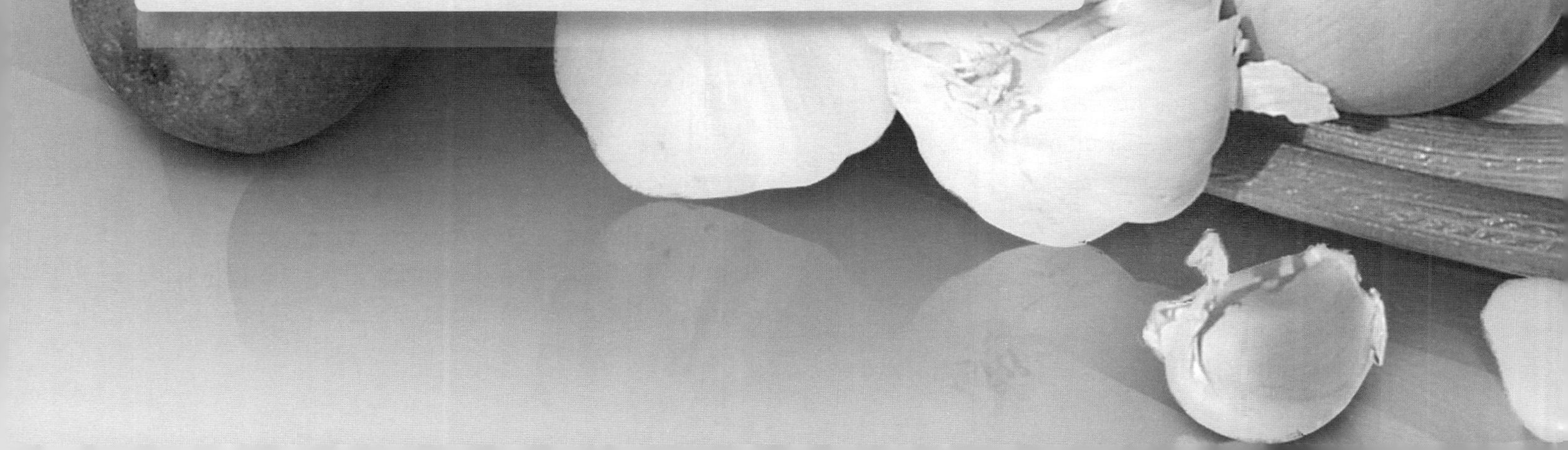

While cancer researchers estimate that about 15.6% of worldwide cases of cancer are attributable to infection, there is no prophylaxis in practice. Modern medicine only treats infection after it is diagnosed. For example, *Helicobacter pylori*, a parasitic bacterium, is known to be the primary cause of gastric cancer. In the cases of *H. pylori*, about 50% of Americans are infected and could potentially develop gastric cancer from this bacterium, but treatment in the form of antibiotics is not prescribed until gastric ulcers arise. [Epidemiology Reviews 22:283-97, 2000] The use of antibiotics induces germ-resistant forms of H. pylori which then prevail regardless of which therapy is utilized.

The saga of two Australian physicians is indicative of the commercial influence over the practice of medicine today. Gastric ulcers were long thought to be caused by excessive stomach acid. Antacids like Tums and Pepto-Bismol were often prescribed. But in 1982 Drs. Barry Marshall and Robin Warren, Australian physicians, discovered that a bacteria caused chronic gastritis and peptic ulcers. In 1984, Dr. Marshall intentionally infected himself, developed an ulcer and cured it with antibiotics to demonstrate his discovery. It is now firmly established that H. pylori causes more than 90% of duodenal ulcers and up to 80% of gastric ulcers.

In 1984, there was a lot at stake. Tagamet, a designer antacid, began to be prescribed by physicians from 1974 to 1977. Hundreds of millions of dollars worth of this drug were being sold. Prompted by the drug company that sold the antacid, physicians were slow to change from a prescription antacid to antibiotics. Doctors and pharmaceutical companies were profiting handsomely. The Tagamet patent ran out in 1994. That's exactly when a National Institutes of Health Consensus Development Conference panel concluded that *H pylori* plays a significant role in the development of ulcers and that their eradication with antibiotics can cure peptic ulcer disease. [Postgraduate Medicine 102: Nov. 1997] Health authorities had let the full term of the drug patent run its course while ulcer patients suffered.

How many people died of gastric cancer due to *H. pylori* infection while drug companies profited is unknown. Public health authorities and pharmaceutical interests are often in collusion without regard for public welfare.

Approximately two-thirds of the world's population is infected with *H. pylori*. Infected persons have a 2- to 6-fold increased risk of developing gastric cancer and mucosal-associated-lymphoid-type (MALT) lymphoma compared with their uninfected counterparts. The Centers for Disease Control says that because the source of *H. pylori* is not yet known, they have not issued any recommendations for avoiding infection. This is another example of how modern medicine lets cancer happen and then treats it incorrectly.

Is cancer a bacterial infection?

Dr. Alan Cantwell, a retired Los Angeles physician, faced a saga similar to that of Dr. Marshall. In his book, *The Cancer Microbe* (1990, Aries Rising Press, Los Angeles), Cantwell attempts to describe a stealth microbe that may be THE cause of cancer. He says it is universally found at the site of tumors, but its small size, ability to alter its shape, slow growth, and lack of a *"back bone,"* make it very difficult to detect. With the realization that many cancers are caused by germs, Cantwell's assertions demand re-evaluation. To recall, the American Cancer Society continues to assert that cancer is not contagious, yet there is little argument today that certain forms of cancer are caused by bacteria or viruses. Cancer researchers continue to claim the cause of cancer is unknown, or that there are so many causes or locations for cancer that it is hundreds of diseases and its origin cannot be determined.

Cantwell says the link between cancer and microbes escapes discovery because microbiologists like to classify germs by their shape, size, staining ability, etc. But he maintains that there is a stealth bacterium that is as small as a virus, has no cell wall, is amorphous (no typical shape), and can resemble a fungus, a spore or a virus. It is a mycoplasma, the tiniest of bacteria. Because it grows and replicates slowly, it cannot be detected by culturing it (accelerating its numbers) in a lab dish until at least a year or more.

Cantwell's notion about cancer being caused by germs is further substantiated by the meticulous investigation of Dr. Lawrence Broxmeyer, a New York physician who carefully outlined the history of the germ theory of cancer. [Medical Hypotheses 63:986-96, 2004]. Dr. Virginia Livingston, working with other investigators, could distinguish cancerous tissue from healthy tissue by the presence of one type of bacterium – mycobacterium. The American Medical Association muzzled the news press when Dr. Livingston created a live exhibit at their annual meeting in 1953. Dr. Broxmeyer even cites what may have been a cancer cure in 1926, known as *"Glover's Serum."* Dr. Joseph Glover developed a serum that came from horses inoculated with a Cryptococcus fungus, which was obtained from cancer patients. Dr. Glover observed the fungus caused *"tumors"* in experimental animals. The antibody-rich horse serum was given to many patients with reported success.

Later, Dr. Cornelius Rhoads, chief at Sloan Kettering Cancer Hospital in New York, sought to discredit the germ theory of cancer. Rhoads was head of chemical warfare during the Korean War and was deeply committed to using toxic chemicals to kill cancer cells.

Other investigators validated the link between mycobacteria and cancer. In 1965, Canadian researchers had confirmed the existence of bacterial-like organisms inside tumors. [Canadian Medical Assn Journal 92: 31-33, 1965] The germ was believed to be a variant of tuberculosis, a known mycobacterium. In 1970, a researcher in Japan convincingly showed that mycobacterium causes cancer. His report was published in the Annals of the New York Academy of Science [Annals NY Academy Science 174: 729-64, 1970]

Broxmeyer noted that a striking analogy between cancer and tuberculosis was noticed in the late 1800s. Even into modern times, Dr. Florence Siebert who standardized the present day tuberculin skin test, validated the existence of TB in cancer cells. The whole sordid coverup can be found in a 1994 issue of Medical Hypotheses, under the title *Is cancer just an incurable infectious disease?* by Dr. Lawrence Broxmeyer. [Medical Hypotheses 63:986-96, 2004]

The Trojan Horse Bacterium: Is cancer a tuberculosis infection?

"In the end, every man has a little tuberculosis."
Source: Sir William Osler 1892

Stealth chameleon bacterium

Mycobacteria, such as tuberculosis and para-tuberculosis, have been called a *"Trojan Horse."* [Trends in Cell Biology 15: No. 5, May 2005] They are stealth bacteria.

The outer shell of the TB bacterium is very fatty and repels staining by standard detection methods. Since it has an oily outer membrane, it resists drying and most disinfectants.

PARA-TB is almost invisible to the human immune system. It penetrates inside of other living cells and multiplies, thus averting detection by the immune system. PARA-TB actually uses germ-fighting cells called phagocytes to disseminate infection to other parts of the body. [Immunology Cell Biology 77: 364-72, 1999]

The main distinguishing feature of paratuberculosis is its slow growth. [Israel Veterinary Medical Association, 59: 2003] PARA-TB can reside in animals and humans for years without necessarily causing disease. Infected animals aren't apparent to cattle raisers.

Mycobacteria simulate and look like viruses in every way. [Medical Hypotheses 2003] They can fool the most seasoned bacteriologist.

Millions of people may have already been infected and don't know it. PARA-TB may not cause any symptoms for years. It is so difficult to detect (it eludes a TB skin test), that it has taken years for researchers to positively link PARA-TB with Crohn's disease (an inflammatory disease of the gastrointestinal tract, often affecting the small intestine and colon). Many Crohn's disease sufferers develop cancer.

Mycobacteria are notoriously resistant to conventional antibiotics. Only a select few antibiotics kill mycobacterial infections effectively. Chlorination of tap water doesn't reliably kill off mycobacterium.

PARA-TB resists pasteurization. At the first sign of heat it forms a spore, and when milk cools, it re-emerges into its original form. The walls of PARA-TB cells contain mycolic acid, which is found nowhere else. Mycolic acid helps PARA-TB resist antibiotics.

Tuberculosis

With such a vast percentage of Earth's human population infected with pulmonary (lung) tuberculosis (nearly 2 billion out of 6 billion humans), and possibly billions more infected with latent TB (asymptomatic or showing no symptoms) and

Family of Tubercular Mycobacteria	
Mycobacterium tuberculosis	→ Cause of tuberculosis in humans
Mycobacterium bovis	→ Cause of tuberculosis in cattle
Mycobacterium avium	→ Cause of tuberculosis in birds
Mycobacterium paratuberculosis	→ Cause of Johne's disease
Mycobacterium leprae	→ Cause of leprosy (Hansen's skin disease)

PARA-TB, this is a health disaster of unheard of proportions. What's more, in countries where TB is prevalent other maladies, such as lupus (skin TB), intestinal problems, and cervical lymphadenopathy are also common.

Milk appears to be a risk for tuberculosis as well. Lacto-vegetarians are at 8.5 times increased relative risk for lung tuberculosis compared with daily fish/meat eaters. [Thorax 50: 175-80, 1995]

Many Americans believe that tuberculosis is a disease that has been mainly conquered and is certainly under control. They couldn't be more wrong. TB is the most lethal infection due to a single germ, even surpassing malaria. Tuberculosis is an even greater health problem now than it was 100 years ago! While an estimated 2 million people die of lung TB annually on a global basis, another 8 million are diagnosed. There may be untold numbers who develop cancer from tuberculosis and its cousin, para-TB.

Each person with TB will infect up to 15 others. TB killed 1 billion people between 1850 and 1950. [Clinical Chest Med 10: 341-53, 1989] It is believed that the global incidence of TB is probably under-reported. [Emerging Infectious Diseases 4: 1998]

Mycobacterium tuberculosis is a very small rod-shaped bacterium, only 3 to 4 micrometers in length. TB resists common microbiological staining procedures for detection. It is slow growing, dividing only every 12-24 hours. Its impermeable cell wall makes it resistant to disinfectants and antibiotics. TB can be acquired from close person-to-person contact via airborne transmission. About 1.9 billion people on earth are already contaminated with TB. Only about 5% of people exposed to TB develop active disease within 2 years of exposure while twice as many may develop the disease sometime later in life. Weight loss, cough and night sweats are common symptoms. But you may harbor this bacterium in your body for years without exhibiting symptoms. Maybe billions more will some day suffer from this infectious disease which in addition to tuberculosis of the lung can also cause many different maladies depending on its anatomical location (lung, digestive tract, brain, etc.). Actually, it is one infection from a family of tubercular mycobacteria that produces many diseases.

INFECTION AND CANCER

What about TB testing?

Infectious agent		Target
Papillomavirus	→	Cervix
Helicobacter pylori	→	Gastric tract
Hepatitis B	→	Liver
HIV	→	Kaposi's sarcoma (bone)
Human T-lymphotropic viruses	→	T-cell leukemia, lymphoma
Epstein-Barr virus	→	Burkitt lymphoma

Dr. Lawrence Broxmeyer, who has exhaustively investigated the role of TB and PARA-TB in human disease, explains that the tuberculin skin test is flawed because it relies on an intact immune system to generate an antibody response. Most humans and animals that have had tuberculosis for any significant time are immunosuppressed by tuberculosis, which he calls *"the greatest immunosuppressor of all time."* So there is no noticeable reaction to the TB skin test. Therefore, a negative TB skin test does not mean that the person or animal does not have the disease. On the contrary, it could very well mean that the skin test recipient has too much of the disease. He says knowledgeable doctors know a negative TB skin test means nothing. X-rays to detect TB in the lung are also somewhat worthless since TB can reside outside the lung. Broxmeyer notes that a more sensitive TB skin test was removed from the market three years ago due to lack of use by clinicians. That test utilized 250 tuberculin units versus only 5 in the current test.

With a test that is not sensitive enough to detect many symptomless cases, current TB surveillance programs amount to *"practically nothing,"* says Broxmeyer. World health authorities agree there is a need for a more sensitive test to detect TB. [J National Medical Association 97: 394-96, 2005]. Broxmeyer implicates yet another bacterium in the TB-family,

Paratuberculosis bovis, as the primary culprit in meat that is linked with mad cow disease. Broxmeyer provides a list of authoritative reports on the link between bacteria and disease at http://www.medamericaresearch.org/

Reports are streaming in from across the globe of linkage between tuberculosis infection and cancer. Here are some of them:

- It is interesting to note that while 75-90% of people who develop lung cancer are smokers, a smaller proportion of smokers (25-33%) develop lung cancer. Researchers have explored the reasons why this is so. They found smokers were more likely to develop lung cancer if they had a prior history of tuberculosis. [Cancer Causes Control 15: 819-27, 2004]

- A case of lymphoma draws attention. A patient was diagnosed with lymphoma of the central nervous system associated with acquired immune deficiency syndrome (AIDS). After radiation treatment failed, doctors conducted a spinal cord biopsy. They found tuberculosis instead. [Journal Neurology Neurosurgery Psychiatry 75: 1636-38, 2004]

- Eye doctors have found tuberculosis masquerading as ocular tumors. [Survey Ophthalmology 49: 619-20, 2004]

- In Poland, researchers report the case of a 47-year-old man with Hodgkin's lymphoma and enlarged lymph nodes in his neck. After tests were conducted, no viruses could be found. The insertion of a scope into the patient's lungs to obtain a tissue sample resulted in the discovery of tubercular bacteria. [Leukemia Lymphoma 46: 471-75, 2005]

- Doctors in Serbia report that lung tuberculosis is associated with malignancies most frequently seen as leukemia, T-cell lymphoma and Hodgkin's lymphoma. [Medical Pregl 57: 65-68, 2004]

- Researchers at The Johns Hopkins Medical Institutions in Baltimore, Maryland report that tuberculosis of the pancreas and pancreatic lymph nodes is an extremely rare disorder that has been reported with increased frequency in the past several years. [Journal Gastrointestinal Surgery 9: 254-62, 2005]

- Researchers in France report that the diagnosis of tuberculoma is difficult because of its tumor-like aspects. A man with a suspected brain tumor was found to have a tubercular malignancy. [Southern Medical Journal 987: 489-91, 2005]

- Investigators in Korea report that tuberculosis can mimic a variety of abdominal disorders. The case of a 22-year old woman with abdominal tuberculosis was mistaken to have cancer. [Korean Journal Internal Medicine 20: 72-75, 2005]

- In Turkey, doctors examined hospital records of patients treated for lung cancer over the past 10 years who also had lymph gland swelling and found many also had a history of tuberculosis. [Acta Chir Belgium 105: 180-82, 2005]

- Doctors in Turkey have also documented a case of pelvic tuberculosis mimicking as ovarian cancer. The tuberculosis raised tumor markers (CA-125), giving doctors the misimpression the patient had a tumor. [International Journal Gynecology & Obstetrics 90: 76-77, 2005]

- Tuberculosis usually occurs as a lung infection. However, doctors at the MD Anderson Cancer Center in Houston report that tuberculosis outside the lung was relatively common in younger patients with active tuberculosis infection, and is often initially misdiagnosed as cancer. [Cancer 104: 2882-87, 2005]

- To show how confusing the appearance of tuberculosis and cancer is for diagnosticians, a woman in Japan was found to have an abnormal shadow on her chest x-ray film and was admitted to the hospital. She had a mass in her upper left lobe of her lung. A scan was performed and also revealed a mass in her ileum, part of her colon. When anti-TB drugs were administered, both masses disappeared. The doctors assume both were tuberculosis, but these masses could just as easily (and mistakenly) been diagnosed as cancer. [Nippon Shokakibyo Gakkai Zasshi 103:420-5, 2006]

Doctors in Korea report a case of gastric tuberculosis that physically appeared to be gastric cancer. Anti-TB drugs caused the tumor to disappear without surgery. There report said: *"Clinicians must bear in mind that, even in the absence of immunodeficiency, as in this case, tuberculosis can involve any site in the gastrointestinal tract and may present with a variety of characteristics,"* and appear to be cancer. [Korean Journal Internal Medicine 21:62-7, 2006]

These are just of few of the many cases being reporting worldwide in which tuberculosis of various organs has been misdiagnosed as cancer.

So it may be that cancer is just an infection. The stealth bacterium known as Mycobacterium tuberculosis may be the originator of all or many cancers.

Cancer vaccines

Will there ever be a cancer vaccine? The idea of a universal cancer vaccine that would immunize against all forms of cancer has certainly been toyed with for some time.

William B. Coley, a New York City surgeon in the early 1900s, used a vaccine that consisted of killed bacteria to prompt a tumor-killing response. It was the first reported attempt to boost immunity.

The idea of a cancer vaccine may not be clear to the public since vaccines are usually employed against viruses, such as influenza. However, not all cancer emanates from viral infection, though it is thought that 15% of malignancies have a viral origin. Some cancer vaccine technology seeks to make proteins within tumors antigenic (being able to induce an antibody response).

A vaccine against a major form of cancer is in the making. The papillomavirus is present in 99.7% of cervical cancer cases. Recently a papilloma vaccine was shown to prevent cervical abnormalities among a reported 100% of women.

Two vaccines against papillomavirus have now been shown to be almost totally effective against the two most prevalent strains of the virus that cause 70% of cervical cancers. [Lancet 364: 1757-65, 2004] However, the vaccine does not protect against all strains of the virus. Long-term, the vaccine may not reduce the incidence of cervical cancer because infection from less-common strains may eventually occur.

There has not been sufficient critical analysis of the vaccine. While the vaccine was shown to be 100% effective for women age 16-23 years over a 3.5 year period, this was only for the most common strain of papillomavirus. Buried in published reports was a measurement of the vaccine's effectiveness in preventing precancerous lesions (called cervical intraepithelial neoplasia) for any type of papillomavirus. It only reduced these lesions 52%. Furthermore, researchers observed no statistically significant difference in the incidence of abnormal Pap tests among placebo and vaccine recipients. [Obstetrics Gynecology 107: 18-27, 2006]

Moreover, since the papillomavirus is sexually transmitted, there has always been a way to prevent this type of cancer – to remain sexually monogamous.

Some worry that such a vaccine may contribute to women engaging in more unprotected sex. However, since most young women appear to be oblivious to the connection between sex and cervical cancer, the availability of a vaccine should not play a significant role in sexual behavior among women.

Four out of five women will contract the human papillomavirus during their lifetime, but only about 7% of infected women will develop cervical cancer. So there are other factors involved. It is estimated that Epstein-Barr, a herpes family virus that infects 90% of the world's population, is associated with lymphoma. But obviously this virus is only the first step in the development of cancer. [Clinical Cancer Research 10: 803-821, 2004]

The availability of a vaccine may not significantly reduce mortality from cervical cancer in developed countries where Pap smears frequently detect early stages of cancer. The major point here is that this type of cancer has always been preventable, and that Pap smears will still likely be performed regardless of vaccination rates, and early surgical treatment now serves as an effective way of reducing mortality rates. In 2002 only 5,000 American women died of cervical cancer, a 75% drop from 1950. [Science 308: 618-21, 2005]

Folic acid superior to vaccine

While the vaccine for human papillomavirus is promising, there is evidence that folic acid supplementation may be superior since it protects against all strains of the virus.

Every year, between 250,000 and 1 million women in the United States are diagnosed with cervical dysplasia (a precancerous condition). While it can occur at any age, the peak incidence is in women between the ages of 25 and 35. It can take 10 years or longer for cervical dysplasia to develop into cancer. Dysplasia can be detected from a Pap smear, the single most important step that a woman can take to prevent cervical cancer.

Mild dysplasia is the most common form, and up to 70% of these cases regress on their own (i.e., the cervical tissue returns to normal without treatment). This fact goes unexplained. Moderate and severe dysplasia are less likely to self-resolve and have a higher rate of progression to cancer.

Some research shows that women who use oral contraceptives may be at a higher risk for developing cervical dysplasia. One reason may be that oral contraceptives interfere with folic acid metabolism in the cells around the cervix, and folic acid may help prevent or reduce cervical dysplasia.

A study at the University of Alabama was the first to demonstrate the connection between folic acid deficiency and increased risk for papilloma viral infection of the cervix.

Researchers at the University of Alabama conducted a 24-month study involving folic acid and human papilloma virus infection. Their hypothesis was that high concentrations of folic acid are associated with the occurrence and duration of papillomavirus infection. Scientists measured blood concentration levels of folic acid from samples obtained from 345 women who were at risk for cervical neoplasia (cancer-like changes in the cervix). Tests were performed every 6 months. Women with higher folic acid levels experienced a 73% risk reduction for a positive test for cancerous changes of the cervix! The researchers concluded that increasing folic acid intake in women at risk of getting infected, or already infected, with high-risk papillomavirus, may have a beneficial impact in the prevention of cervical cancer. [Cancer Research 64: 8788-93, 2004]

Other viruses associated with cancer are: hepatitis B and C virus with liver cancer, human T cell leukemia virus associated with T cell leukemia, and Kaposi's sarcoma - associated herpes virus with sarcomas and more recently with a form of bone marrow cancer (myeloma). There is evidence that the Simian virus 40 is associated with a lung cancer called mesothelioma. Viruses seek to inactivate tumor-suppressing genes, which is what makes them so troublesome. [Journal Molecular Medicine 73: 529-38, 1995]

The aim of cancer vaccines is to teach the patient's own immune system to recognize tumor cells and develop antibodies against them, but not against normal tissues. Currently, there is only one vaccine, against hepatitis B-induced liver cancer, that is approved for human use.

There are drawbacks to cancer vaccines. Their mechanism – to alter the human immune system to selectively attack tumor cells – may disrupt normal immune surveillance against infection and may induce undesirable autoimmune reactions. Furthermore, vaccines are only expected to be efficient against small tumors and they may not shrink tumor size. Cancer vaccines may be more useful in the early stages of cancer. [Toxicology 214: 151-61, 2005]

Cancer vaccines are a fertile area for research, but currently are not a practical answer for most types of solid tumors. Hopefully, cancer researchers will be surprised by a breakthrough in cancer vaccines at some time in the future.

For the present time, given the prevalence of herpes viruses in humans, it would be wise to incorporate foods and dietary supplements that inhibit herpes family viruses. Quercetin, found in red onions and red apple skin, and also available as a dietary supplement, is the most studied plant molecule that inhibits viral growth. [Journal Medical Virology 15: 71-79, 1985] It has also been shown to inhibit the human papillomavirus. [Oncogene 22: 5504-14, 2003]

Inflammation and cancer

A strong association has been established between chronic inflammation and the eventual appearance of tumors. [Progress Drug Research 60: 59-92, 2003] Therefore, can we assume that the use of anti-inflammatory drugs like aspirin, ibuprofen, and COX-2 inhibitors like Vioxx and Bextra, will reduce the risk for cancer? A lot of doctors think so. But recent studies don't bear this out:

- A large study of 77,413 women could not find a preventive effect for aspirin or non-steroidal anti-inflammatory drugs against breast cancer. [Cancer Epidemiology Biomarkers Prevention 14: 261-64, 2005]

- The long-term (10-year) use of aspirin among nearly 20,000 women did not result in a lower risk for breast, colon-rectal or total number of cancers. [Journal American Medical Assn 294: 47-55, 2005]

- While anti-inflammatory drugs generally reduce the risk for cancer, acetaminophen (Tylenol) use appears to raise the risk for leukemia. [Leukemia Research, August 10, 2005]

- The long-term use of anti-inflammatory drugs only produces a modest drop in the risk for prostate cancer. [Journal National Cancer Institute 97: 975-80, 2005]

- Yes, aspirin reduces the risk for colon/rectal cancer. But a significant benefit doesn't appear until more than a decade of use, with maximal risk reduction at doses greater than 14 tablets per week. The risk for intestinal bleeding from aspirin use can offset risk reduction for cancer. [Journal American Medical Assn 294: 914-23, 2005]

- Furthermore, aspirin appears to increase the risk for bladder and brain cancer mortality among women. [Anticancer Research 24: 3177-84, 2004]

- Side effects from long-term aspirin use probably outnumber any tumor prevention benefits. Use of non-steroidal anti-inflammatory drugs resulted in 107,000 hospitalizations and 16,500 deaths in 1997 in the U.S. alone. [Current Topics Medicinal Chemistry 5: 517-25, 2005]

- Many aspirin users will claim they take a coated aspirin to prevent ulcers. A 325 mg coated aspirin tablet still produces very little increase in life expectancy (2 weeks), with approximately 1 in 15 aspirin users experiencing a side effect and 1 in 556 individuals premature death. [Annals Pharmacotherapy 39: 51-57, 2005]

- Additionally, one-third of gastric ulcers produced by non-steroidal drugs involve low-dose daily aspirin. [American Journal Gastroenterology 100: 1694-95, 2005]

- COX-2 inhibitor drugs like Vioxx and Bextra are widely promoted for potential cancer prevention, but they increase the risk for heart attacks and strokes. [Journal Association Physicians India 53: 623-27, 2005] There appear to be misdirected efforts to keep COX-2 inhibitor drugs on the market by combining them with fish oil to overcome their side effects. [Cancer Research 65: 8022-27, 2005]

COX-2 Inhibitors not living up to expectations

Inflammation is a key element in nearly all diseases including arthritis, cancer, diabetes, Crohn's and heart disease. Steroidal hormones (cortisone) reduce inflammation but reduce wound healing, may cause swelling and cataracts and deplete the body of many essential nutrients. Non-steroidal anti-inflammatory drugs (NSAIDs) are a common alternative to steroids. NSAIDs include aspirin, ibuprofen and naproxen. More recently, because NSAIDs can cause stomach irritation potentially leading to bleeding ulcers, a newer class of prescription non-steroidal anti-inflammatory drugs called COX-2 inhibitors (Celebrex, Vioxx) were approved which were widely touted to reduce these risks.

However, upon further examination, the benefits of COX-2 inhibitors with regard to stomach symptoms appear quite small. While there is a reduction in small ulcers compared to standard non-steroidal drugs, these small ulcers are not clinically important. Symptoms of indigestion and pain appear to be about the same in these two classes of drugs. [Gerontology, Nov. 1, 2002, Health and Age, and J Am Med Assn 282: 19611-63, 1999]

There is current concern that the non-steroidal anti-inflammatory drugs also may increase the risk of heart attacks and may interfere with blood-pressure-lowering drugs. [Amy Erickson, Pharmacy Today, *"Do COX-2 inhibitors compromise cardiovascular safety?"* www.pharmacist.com] Bleeding events have also been reported among users of blood- thinning drugs when combined with the COX-2 inhibitors. [Australian Ad Drug Reactions Bulletin 20: 2, 2001]

Healthy adults who use anti-inflammatory drugs like aspirin, Motrin or Vioxx to prevent cancer are more likely to die of a heart attack or stroke induced by these drugs than from cancer. [British Medical Journal 330:1366, 2005]

Before these drugs were taken off the market temporarily by the FDA, Celebrex and Vioxx generated $5 billion in annual sales to treat rheumatoid arthritis and osteoarthritis. A daily dose of Celebrex or Vioxx costs about $2.50 a day. Other non-steroidals like ibuprofen (Advil) and aspirin cost only about 10 cents per pill.

The next step in snuffing out inflammation

Pharmaceutical companies think they have come up with a master anti-inflammatory mechanism that may be useful in preventing cancer as well as treating inflammation and pain. Blockage of just one inflammatory enzyme, known as p38, can inhibit most all of the other inflammatory proteins produced in the body, which includes COX-2, TNF alpha, C-Reactive Protein, prostate specific antigen and Interleukin-1beta. [Current Medicinal Chemistry 5: 921-28, 2005; Clinical Cancer Research 7:1773-81, 2001]

Some time ago Johnson & Johnson announced acquisition of SCIOS Inc., the Sunnyvale, CA-based company that led a pack of pharmaceutical companies in introducing a new class of anti-inflammatory drugs called p38 blockers. The price of the acquisition was $2.4 billion and included a drug for congestive heart failure. [Reuters, Feb. 10, 2003]

If approved by the Food & Drug Administration, the p38 enzyme inhibitor would be a breakthrough oral anti-inflammatory drug, say SCIOS executives. SCIOS is in clinical trials of its SCIO-469 anti-inflammatory agent that blocks p38.

p38 kinase enzyme		
TNF Tumor necrosis factor	COX-2 Cyclooxygenase inhibitor	CRP C-Reactive protein

Currently, drugs like Enbrel (Amgen), Remicade (J&J) and Humira (Abbott Labs) that target TNF, must be injected. These drugs now generate $1 billion in annual sales. SCIOS indicates it develops *"novel treatments"* for inflammatory disease and that its SCIO-469 drug could be the first oral product that blocks TNF and other inflammatory proteins.

"An oral drug that shows the same effectiveness as an injectable would be a huge home run," says John McCamant, executive editor of the Medical Technology Stock Letter.

Four other pharmaceutical companies in early stages of development of p38 blockers include Vertex Pharmaceuticals,

Inc., GlaxoSmithKline, Sankyo and ArQule. The chief financial officer of SCIOS says: *"This is a very tight race. We don't intend to be second."* [Reuters, Jan 7, 2002]

Advancing age increases the production of the p38 kinase inflammatory enzymes. [Mechanics Ageing Dev 123: 881-90, 2002] Dietary salt also increases the production of p38 kinase enzymes. [FASEB Journal 16: 1683-84, 2002] Americans consume a very high amount of sodium, about 4,000 mg per day, which is linked with elevated risk for hypertension and now with inflammation. So the market is ripe for an alternative to the COX-2 inhibitors.

New market for p38 blockers

Wall Street analysts state that the p38 blocker is one that *"most of Wall Street hasn't woken up to yet."* This approach to controlling inflammation has been called *"one of the most exciting things going on in the pharmaceutical industry today."* [Reuters, Feb. 9, 2003] Sales of p38 blockers are expected to exceed $2 billion a year. One analyst predicts sales of $6 billion for this new class of drugs by 2009. [PR Newswire Oct. 28, 2002]

It's easy to see why Wall Street is so excited about the prospects of p38 blockers. The p38 kinase enzyme blockers are being hailed in medical reports as a *"new therapeutic option in the treatment of inflammatory diseases."* [J Immunology 168: 4070-77, 2002]

Just look at the applications:

> The stimulation of TNF is believed to initiate the development of pre-malignant cells. [Cancer Detection Prevention 24: 91-99, 2000] So a p38 blocker by virtue of its ability to block TNF would be a promising anti-cancer agent. Researchers say TNF is *"an important mediator of cancer development."* [Mechanics Aging Development 123: 1655-63, 2002]

One can readily recognize the potential here – one drug that would prevent or treat cancer, prevent cardiovascular disease, arthritis and inflammatory bowel disorders. The prospect of a p38 blocker, such as SCIO-469, would have enormous impact; it would be a multiple blockbuster drug.

But will SCIO-469 ever get approved?

The progress of these drugs has not been without failure. Vertex Pharmaceuticals announced on Sept. 24, 2001, suspension of its VX-745 oral drug that inhibits the p38 kinase inflammatory enzyme because of safety problems. Vertex switched to another p38 blocker. The decision to terminate the development of VX-745 was based upon adverse central nervous system reactions in animal experiments. Wall Street is hyping a drug that may never get to market. Even very small side effect rates can doom a drug that would be so widely used. Could other p38 blockers face the same fate?

Did nature beat the drug companies?

In the meantime, a review of the medical literature reveals that nature may have beaten the pharmaceutical companies to a p38 blocker. The following seven natural agents– four herbal extracts and three micronutrients – have demonstrated ability to inhibit the p38 kinase inflammatory enzyme. [Cytokine 18: 266-73, 2002]

1. Green tea

It has been estimated that a daily consumption of 10 Japanese-size cups of green tea results in delayed cancer onset. Even five cups of green tea a day has been shown to delay the onset of breast cancer. Researchers now suggest green tea, by virtue of its ability to inhibit TNF, could be used before the onset of cancer as well as during and after conventional cancer treatment. [J Cancer Res Clinical Oncology 125: 589-97, 1999]

Green tea extracts (0.1%) added to drinking water of animals has been shown to block TNF production in animals. [Biofactors 13: 67-72, 2000]

2. NAC

N-acetyl cysteine (NAC), a sulfur-based amino acid sold in health food stores, has been shown to reduce TNF. [FASEB Journal 16: 1931-33, 2002] NAC also inhibits all three classes (p38, JNK and P-extracellular) of what are called mitogen-activated protein enzymes (kinases) which are generated when there is tissue injury. [Molecular Cell Biochemistry 240: 19-29, 2002]

NAC has a demonstrated ability to block p38 kinase enzymes in brain cells. [Proc Soc Exp Biol Med 222: 236-45, 1999]

3. Carnosol

Carnosol, a naturally occurring antioxidant in rosemary, has been shown to inhibit the p38 kinase enzyme. [Carcinogenesis 23: 983-91, 2002] Carnosol accounts for about 90% of the antioxidant activity in rosemary extract. [Xenobiotica 22: 257-68, 1993] Carnosol also blocks COX-2 as well as p38. [Cancer Research 62: 2522-30, 2002]

4. Red wine extracts

Red wine extracts have been shown to inhibit the growth of colon cancer cells via their ability to block p38 kinase enzyme. [Journal Nutrition 133: 2814-88, 2002]

5. Quercetin

Quercetin, a natural substance found in red onions and the skin of red apples as well as Ginkgo biloba, inhibits the p38 kinase enzyme and improves the survival of cells in laboratory experiments. [Kidney International 58: 1078-87, 2000; J Endotoxin Research 7: 431-38, 2001] Quercetin and Ginkgo biloba both have been shown to inhibit the production of p38 kinase enzyme. [Biochem Pharmacology 62: 963-74, 2001]

6. Ginger

Ginger is a spice that possesses anti-inflammatory properties by virtue of its gingerol content. Ginger and its components are natural COX-2 inhibitors. [Food Chem Toxicology 40: 1091-97, 2002] Gingerol inhibits the spread of cancer cells. Pure gingerol was shown in one experiment to reduce cancer cell growth to the point where the cells could not be distinguished from normal healthy cells. [Cancer Research 61: 850-53, 2001] Gingerol is believed to be a safer form of *"aspirin"* since it blocks inflammation and thins the blood much like aspirin pills do. Researchers have suggested making synthetic gingerol-like molecules that could become patented drugs. [Thrombosis Research 103: 387-97, 2001]

7. Hyaluronic acid

Hyaluronic acid is a gel-like substance that is naturally produced in the human body. It is also available as a dietary supplement, frequently used to treat joint inflammation. Hyaluronic acid inhibits p38 inflammatory proteins and could help to delay cancer. [International Journal Molecular Medicine 14: 139-44, 2004]

Natural molecules appear to be better suited at reducing the risk for cancer by inhibiting chronic inflammation than are drugs, given that they produce fewer side effects.

Blood clots and metastatic cancer

Cancer has surely struck someone in your circle of family members and loved ones. People generally don't die of localized tumors, but rather succumb to tumors that spread, or what is called metastasis.

In the next few pages you will learn about a simple cancer cure that could save the lives of many. A reliable way to stop the spread of cancer is to thin the blood.

To repeat: most cancer patients don't succumb to localized tumors but rather to metastatic (spreading) tumors or the side effects of treatment. If tumors can be kept from spreading to other sites in the body, survival is greatly improved.
Tumor cells get into the blood circulation and look for a place to build a remote colony at another organ site. Roaming tumor cells may get stuck in blood capillaries and eventually begin to grow and migrate into surrounding tissues.

Circulating tumor cells usually get stuck in the first capillary bed (smallest blood vessels) that they encounter. This usually occurs in the lungs or the liver, the common sites of metastasis. Some tumor cells also produce chemical factors that cause blood platelets, the cells that initiate blood clotting, to accumulate. Tumor cells then stick to blood platelets like flies to fly paper. Blood platelets are rich in growth factors and iron that cause tumor cells to grow. More roaming cancer cells will arrive and harbor themselves within sticky blood clots which provide an environment for the growth of tumor cells. [Cancer Research 40:1212-6, 1980]

For a number of decades it has been known that cancer patients tend to have thick blood, or what is called sticky blood platelets. The relationship between tumors and blood clots was first described in 1865 when Armand Trousseau reported a high frequency of blood clots in the legs of patients with gastric cancer. [Clinique Medicale de l'Hotel-Dieu de Paris, 282-332, 1865] Tumor cells cause injury to the lining of blood vessels and may trigger blood clots. [British J Exp Pathology 153: 301-13, 1972; Blood Coagulation Fibrinolysis 1:71-8, 1990]

A recent review by doctors at the University of San Padua in Italy found that in about 10% of cancer of blood clots in veins (venous thrombosis), cancer is also subsequently diagnosed. [Current Opinion Hematology 13: 362-65, 2006] Any event that triggers blood clotting, such as an injury or a stroke, or even cancer surgery itself could increase the risk for the spread of cancer by as much as 300%. [New England J Med 342: 1953-58, 2000; Hematologic Complications of Cancer, Hematology/Oncology Clinics of North Am 10: 499-530, 1996; Emergency Medicine Sept. 85-86, 1998] To make matters worse, chemotherapy increases blood clotting and the risk of a spreading tumor. [Haemostasis 28: 50-60, 1998] The addition of estrogen or tamoxifen may further increase the risk of blood clotting and the spread of tumors. [J Clinical Oncology 9: 286-94, 1991]

> Chemotherapy for cancer increases blood clotting and the risk of a spreading tumor. The addition of estrogen or tamoxifen may further increase the risk of blood clotting and the spread of tumors.
> *[Haemostasis 28: 50-60, 1998]; Journal Clinical Oncology 9: 286-94, 1991*

The incidence of blood clots (venous thromboembolism) is not only directly life threatening if they enter the lungs or block circulation to the brain or heart but also portends a poor prognosis for cancer patients. Only 12% survive beyond a year if they develop clots. An estimated 11 to 20% of cancer patients on chemotherapy develop blood clots. [Thrombosis Research Dec. 30, 2005]

In 1964, Dr. L. Michaels of Manitoba, Canada, provided conclusive evidence that blood thinners will stop the spread of cancer. Among 540 of Dr. Michaels' patients who had been treated with anti-blood clotting drugs over a period of a decade or more, only 19 developed metastatic tumors and only one patient died instead of a predicted eight based on prior studies [Lancet, Oct. 17, 832-35, 1964]

Low-dose blood thinners are sometimes utilized during treatment of cancer. [Thrombosis Haemostasis 79: 23-27, 1998] The blood thinner warfarin (Coumadin) is often used to treat cancer but only a low percentage (~20%) of patients actually experience improvement. Heparin, another anti-clotting drug, is more effective in preventing clots than warfarin but certainly is not effective in all cases. [Cancer 80: 649-55, 1997]

Because clots can cause strokes or lung blockages, cancer doctors advise patients to avoid vitamin K supplements or vitamin K-rich foods (green leafy vegetables), since vitamin K is required for blood clotting. But vitamin K has been shown to actually be a potent inhibitor of tumor colony formation. [Cancer Treatment Reports 69: 527-32, 1985]

The anti-blood-clotting effect of aspirin may also inhibit the spread of cancer, though aspirin does pose a risk for hemorrhage, bleeding ulcers, and depletes the body of essential nutrients like folic acid and vitamin C which are needed to fight cancer. [Drug-Induced Nutrient Depletion Handbook 2nd edition, 2001]

A significant percentage of older adults harbor undetected cancer which may release tumor cells into the blood circulation. A healthy immune system will destroy most of these roaming tumor cells, but the development of blood clots will create an environment for the growth of a tumor at a distant site from the original tumor. If blood clotting is inhibited, through the use of natural blood thinners, then the spread of tumors is blocked and the immune system has an opportunity to destroy roaming tumor cells.

The use of blood-thinning dietary supplements throughout adulthood would be a safe way of preventing metastatic cancer, particularly after age 55 when more than 80% of cancers are detected. Four dietary supplements come to mind and the simultaneous consumption of all four will not over-thin the blood, whereas other blood thinners like aspirin will.

The four natural anti-blood clotting nutrients are magnesium [Southeast Asian J Trop Med Public Health. 33 Suppl 2:6-9, 2002; J Vet Med Sci 60: 837-42, 1998], vitamin E [Hormone Metab Res 334: 49-54, 2002; Platelets 12: 389-94, 2001], garlic [Prostaglandins Leukot Essent Fatty Acids. 63:217-21, 2000; Thombosis Res 32: 155-69, 1983] and omega-3 oils from fish or flaxseed. (Note: omega-6 oils from corn, safflower and sunflower, encourage blood clotting.) [Life Sci 73: 2083-90, 2003; Thrombosis Haemostasis 82: 1522-27, 1999]

The relationship between spreading tumors and cancer was first reported over a century ago, yet researchers are still calling for more studies. In 1999, researchers in Austria suggested that anticoagulants may hold promise for the prevention and treatment of metastatic tumors. [J National Cancer Institute 91: 22-36, 1999] A more recent report said that anticoagulant drugs (blood thinners) could *"alter the fundamental biology of cancer."* [Chest 124: 58-68S, 2003] However, a 1984 report called the use of blood thinners in the treatment of cancer *"controversial."* [Am J Hematology 16: 193-202, 1984] Some doctors continue to think clotting occurs as a general course of cancer and do not link it to being a cause of metastasis. Millions more people will likely die prematurely of cancer while the scientific community continues to debate the role of blood thinners in the prevention and treatment of metastatic cancer.

You don't have to wait for that dreaded phone call from the doctor that you had better get your affairs in order because your body is filled with tumors in many locations. You can use natural blood thinners to prolong your life and increase survivability before you have been diagnosed with cancer. The use of blood-thinning dietary supplements with prescription blood thinners (Coumadin, warfarin) should be discussed with a physician knowledgeable in the use of dietary supplements.

Does alkalinity cure cancer?

Many people believe the promotion of alkalinity in the body can prevent cancer. Is this true?

Widely promoted on the internet and elsewhere is a simple test of salivary acidity or alkalinity which is said to *"measure your susceptibility to cancer, heart disease, osteoporosis, arthritis and many other degenerative diseases."*

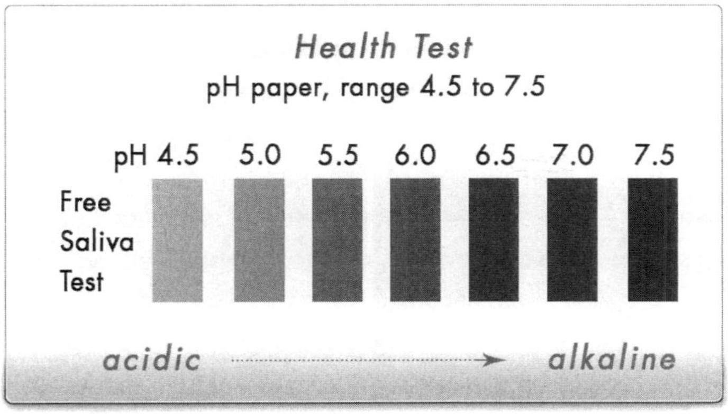

At one website visitors are invited to test the pH of their saliva. If your pH is 7.5 the website says *"you are healthy."* If your pH is below 6.0, then *"you have contracted at least one degenerative disease."* (pH of 7.0 is neutral, not acidic nor alkaline.) The website claims that salivary pH reflects cellular pH and the state of health. The website goes on to say that *"cancer needs an acid and low oxygen environment to survive and flourish within. Terminal cancer victims are around 1,000 times more acidic than normal healthy people."* Also, it states that *"cancer victims have extremely low* alkaline reserves."

Understanding pH

PH is a measure of the degree of the acidity or the alkalinity of a solution as measured on a scale of 0 to 14. The midpoint of 7.0 on the pH scale represents neutrality. A *"neutral"* solution is neither acid nor alkaline. pH below 7.0 indicate acidity; pH above 7.0 indicates alkalinity. pH stands for *"potential for hydrogen."* Actually hydrogen is responsible for acidity and alkalinity. The neutral point of 7.0 actually indicates the presence of equal concentrations of free hydrogen and hydroxide ions.

pH numbers are exponents of ten. The difference between 1.0 and 2.0 in pH is ten times. The body rids itself of acid daily to maintain pH balance. The normal pH varies in tissues throughout the body.

Living cells produce acidic waste products constantly. The body makes a massive and system-wide effort to control acidity. The urine and perspiration rid the body of excessive acid. Alkalosis (too akaline) is less common than acidosis (too acidic). The lungs and kidneys also help maintain pH, but organic minerals are the main alkalizing agents. Since carbon dioxide (CO2) has been found to contribute to acid states, it is now known that the expelling of CO2 via the lungs helps control acidity.

As the body's cells produce acidic waste products, alkaline buffers must be acquired from the diet or elsewhere from mineral pools to control pH.

Normal blood pH is 7.4 (slightly alkaline). A change in blood pH of 0.2 units in either direction is considered serious. The blood must be maintained at pH 7.4 – below 7.2 is considered a mortal state. It is said that pH below 6.8 is incompatible with survival but low pH (as low as 6.5) has been recorded with little physiological disturbance and complete recovery. [Causes, Diagnosis and Effects of Abnormal pH Status, M J Bookallil, University of Sydney, Australia] The ideal pH of the blood is 7.4 and if it drops below 6.8 or rises above 7.8, it may be lethal.

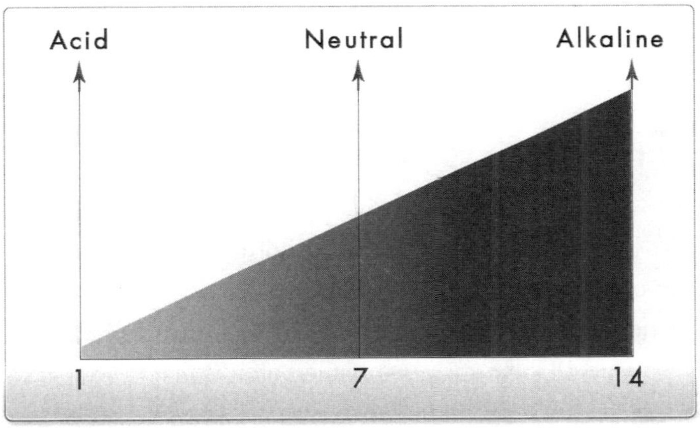

Most foods are on the acidic side, notable exceptions being bakery products, corn, eggs, and milk. As examples, lime has a pH of about 2 (very acidic), orange juice is about 4 (acidic), meats typically are about 6 (mildly acidic), and eggs about 7 to 8 (neutral to *"base"*). Base is another term for alkaline. Base foods tend to neutralize acidic foods. If consumption of alkaline foods is excessive, then appetite is suppressed.

Baking soda has a pH of about 8 and milk of magnesia a pH of over 10, which is why they are used as antacids. You can refer to this FDA website for information on the acidity of several foods:

http://vm.cfsan.fda.gov/~mow/app3a.html.

Alternative medicine practitioners often disseminate lists of alkaline foods. But there is a misconception over which foods help to control cancer. Yes, alkaline foods may be desired, but the contrary is not true, that acidic foods promote cancer. For example, citrus fruits are highly acidic, but there is no indication in the medical literature that they accelerate the growth of cancer cells. In fact, contrary evidence exists. [J Agriculture Food Chemistry 50: 7449-54, 2002] For example, one study ranked fruits which inhibit liver cancer in this order: cranberry, lemon, apple, strawberry, red grape, banana, grapefruit, and peach. [J Agriculture Food Chemistry 50:7449-54, 2002] The more acidic fruits were found to be more protective against cancer. Oddly, salt is alkaline, yet it has been found to increases the risk of stomach cancer. [International Journal Cancer 10: 34-36, 1997]

The Acid-Ash Theory

It's not whether a food is acidic or alkaline that determines its ability to control pH. It is its ash value. Ash is a chemical term referring to the inorganic portion of a food sample remaining after the sample is burned at 600°C for two hours. Ash is what's left over after digestion. Alkaline ash is rich in alkaline minerals such as calcium, phosphorus, sodium, potassium, magnesium and manganese.

The alkaline approach to health goes beyond just cancer. If calcium is needed to maintain an alkaline state in the body, then it will be pulled from the bones, which is a mineral repository. Thus, the continued need to maintain an alkaline state could lead to premature thinning of the bones (osteoporosis). The *"acid-ash"* hypothesis holds that high animal protein intake increases urinary calcium loss which is compensated for by increased calcium absorption in the digestive tract, given that there is sufficient calcium provided in the diet. This is where some doctors with an alternative bend began to develop a long list of diseases cured by calcium.

Cornell researchers say that limitation on meat consumption may do more to reduce the risk of osteoporosis than increasing calcium intake. Americans consume higher levels of dietary calcium than do Asians, but have higher rates of hip fracture than Asians. [Cornell University, News Release Nov. 6, 1996] While animal protein-rich diets have been associated with osteoporosis, it is the ratio of animal protein over vegetable consumption that is of concern, not necessarily the total amount of animal protein consumed. In other words, it may be better to increase vegetable consumption than to reduce meat intake. [Am J Clinical Nutrition 74: 411-12, 2001] Furthermore, a very recent study casts more doubt on the idea that a high-calcium diet reduces osteoporotic hip fracture. A recent study showed calcium did not reduce hip fracture rates, whereas 800 IU of vitamin D did. [Am J Clinical Nutrition 77: 504-11, 2003]

The debate continues

How did this craze for alkalinity and saliva testing start? It started decades ago with a German biochemist named Otto Warberg.

According to one website, *"the underlying cause of all cancer, no matter what type, may have been discovered by Otto Warberg, over 50 years ago. Summarized in a few words, the prime cause of cancer is the replacement of the respiration of oxygen in normal body cells by a fermentation of sugar."*

While Warburg published in scientific journals [Biochem Z 152: 309-44, 1924; Science, 123: 309-314., 1956], it was Dr. William Hay in 1933 who is most responsible for publicizing and expanded this theory with the publication of his book entitled A New Health Era. Basically, he asserted in this book that all disease is caused by acid accumulation in the body. In more recent times, Dr. Theodore Baroody, ND, DC, PhD, in his book Alkalize or Die, also maintained that *"countless diseases...come from the same root cause... too much tissue acid waste in the body."*

Alkaline theory of cancer continues

The alkaline theory of cancer continues to be widely promoted. It has been widely claimed on television infomercials that the low rate of cancer on the island of Okinawa is due to the inhabitants' intake of calcium from coral.

Alternative medical practitioners often claim cancer cells go into a dormant state if their pH is around 7.4. (7.0 is neutral and 7.4 is slightly alkaline.) They claim acidity prevents the production of A, C, G and T nucleotides, the steps on the spiral-shaped DNA ladder, that allow for normal DNA synthesis. Is all this true?

"Cancer authorities" claim that by consuming minerals such as salts of rubidium and cesium, which are heavy metallic minerals, cancer patients can raise their pH to as high as 8.5. It is said that under oxygen-rich, alkaline conditions, cancer cells die quickly, with no damage to the healthy cells, and therefore no serious side effects.

However, cesium is not without complication. It can initiate an irregular heart rhythm and is used in scientific experiments to induce an abnormal heart beat. Side effects have been reported. [Therapeutic Drug Monitor 25: 114-16, 2003]

The appearance of science

Here is what one advocate of alkaline therapy says:

> *"In his publication, Cesium Therapy in Cancer Patients, Sartori describes the 2-week treatment of 50 last-stage, metastasized, terminal cancer patients (13 comatose), with cesium chloride salts. All were expected to die within weeks, with the survival rate being less than one in ten million. After 2 weeks, 13 died with autopsies showing no presence of cancer. After 12 months, 12 more had died, but 25, or an astounding 50%, survived. Unfortunately, both cries of 'quackery' and persecution from the medical establishment have driven this caustic cancer therapy research, started by Nobel Prize winner Dr. Otto Warburg, underground."* [Pharmacology Biochemistry Behavior 21 Suppl 1:7-10, 1984; Pharmacology Biochemistry Behavior 21: 11-13, 1984]

However, Sartori's research, conducted nearly two decades ago, also included vitamins, chelating (mineral removing) agents, selenium and a special diet. So his results cannot be solely attributed to the effects of cesium.

Another alkaline therapy is called *"High pH Therapy for Cancer"* and was developed by A. Keith Brewer, PhD. [*"The High pH Therapy for Cancer, Tests on Mice and Humans,"* Pharmacology Biochemistry & Behavior, Supplement Q, v. 21: 1-5, 1984] Here is how it is described:

> *"Mass spectrographic and isotope studies have shown that potassium, rubidium, and especially cesium are most efficiently taken up by cancer cells. This uptake was enhanced by Vitamins A and C as well as salts of zinc and selenium. The quantity of cesium taken up was sufficient to raise the cell to the 8 pH range... Tests on mice fed cesium and rubidium showed marked shrinkage in the tumor masses within two weeks. In addition, the mice showed none of the side effects of cancer. Tests have been carried out on over 30 humans. In each case the tumor masses disappeared. Also all pains and effects associated with cancer disappeared within 12 to 36 hours; the more chemotherapy and morphine the patient had taken, the longer the withdrawal period."*

Again, vitamins and selenium were employed, so it is difficult to attribute the effects in Brewer's work to cesium therapy alone.

There is an appearance of scientific evidence here. Often cited are Nobel Prize winning scientists, and PhDs who have tested their alkalizing cures on mice and humans, and despite the drawbacks of their research, the popularity of high pH therapy for cancer continues.

Are these claims true?

Let's examine each claim for the pH therapy of cancer. I'll take these claims one by one and explain why they just doesn't hold water...or calcium!

1 The claim that pH therapy has been driven underground is unfounded. Oncologists (doctors who treat cancer) are experimenting with altered pH carriers to aid in the delivery of various cancer drugs. [J Pharm Pharmacol 53: 155-66, 2001] In fact, drugs like hydralazine, captopril, and nifedipine slightly alkalize the tumor area and have been shown to delay, but not prevent, tumor growth. [Oncology Research 11: 179085, 1999]

2 The claim that *"cancer is virtually unknown among the Hopi Indians of Arizona and the Hunzas of northern Pakistan,"* is also unsubstantiated. It is said these people maintain protection from cancer as long as they live in their native environment and drink water that is naturally high in alkaline minerals such as cesium. But Hopi Indian women who live on their reservation are known to develop breast cancer. [Prev Med. 27:135-43, 1998]

3 The claim that calcium may help prevent colon cancer is now widely accepted, but not necessarily because of the creation of an alkaline state in gastric tissue. The loss of an acid gastric tract permits the colonization by unfriendly bacteria and the formation of cancer-causing chemicals. [European J Gastroenterology Hepatology 12: 165-73, 2000] An increase in pH towards alkalinity in the gastric tract is associated with increasing severity of gastric lesions. [J National Cancer Institute 76: 621-27, 1986] Gastric cancer begins with hypochlorhydria, a state of low stomach acid. [Current Gastroenterology Reports 4:463-70, 2002] The acid-forming bacteria (Acidophilus, Bifidus) protect the gastric tract from invasion and colonization by H. pylori, the germ that causes stomach cancer. Furthermore, an acid stomach (about pH 4.0) is required for the proper absorption of many essential nutrients like folic acid, which is involved in cancer prevention.

A telling study conducted in the 1980s reveals the importance of stomach acid as protection against cancer throughout the body. British researchers examined data of patients who had undergone surgical removal of their stomach. The theory is that, without stomach acid to protect the remaining digestive tract from carcinogens in foods and water, that there may be an increased risk for cancer in other organs over time. Cancer in other organs didn't arise quickly, signs of cancer began appearing 20 years following surgery. But then significant increases in the risk for various types of cancer were noted.

SITE	Increased cancer risk
Biliary tract	9.1 times (910%)
Stomach (remaining)	4.5
Pancreas	4.0
Breast	4.0
Bladder	2.4
Esophagus	2.3

Source: Gut 28: 924-28, 1987

While alkalizing calcium may prevent colon cancer, this is not true for all other types of tumors. Recently, the American Journal of Clinical Nutrition published a report showing that high calcium intake (more than 600 mg per day from dairy products) ,among 21,000 men, resulted in a 32% higher risk of prostate cancer than among men who consumed no more than 150 mg per day over an 11-year period. [American Journal of Clinical Nutrition 74:549-554, 2001] To be fair, there are distinctions between dairy calcium and the widely promoted calcium carbonate obtained from coral reefs off Okinawa.

However, another study showed that the provision of 3,000 mg of supplemental calcium carbonate, providing 1,200 mg of elemental calcium, produced a moderate reduction in the occurrence of adenomas in the colon and rectum. [New England Journal Medicine 340: 101-07, 1999] So apparently any calcium supplement affords some protection from colon cancer.

4 If the claim is true that the body continually pulls calcium from the bones to maintain a state of alkalinity then why do drugs that impair the release of bone calcium into the blood circulation exhibit anti-tumor activity?

About 10 to 20% of cancer cases result in hypercalcemia. Hypercalcemia is characterized by high blood serum calcium levels. This condition generally occurs in the late stage of cancer and is a marker of early mortality. [J Pakistan Med Assoc 52: 361-64, 2002] At first glance this information would seem to back up claims by advocates of high pH therapy. The cells are attempting to release calcium in order to alkalize tissues, they just overdo it a bit.

Drugs that inhibit the loss of calcium from bones (bisphosphonates) are utilized to treat hypercalcemia in cases of cancer. [Expert Opinion Pharmacotherapy 3: 521-27, 2002; Seminars Oncology 29: 12-18, 2002] But oddly, not only do biophosphonates slow down the release of calcium and other bone minerals into blood, they also exhibit anti-tumor activity. [Seminars Oncology 29: 33-42, 2002] Biophosphonates induce tumor cells to mature and die off and prevent the spread (metastasis) of tumors. [Seminars Oncology 29: 43-49, 2002] The high pH theory is going out the window.

Furthermore, there appears to be an undesirable buildup of calcium inside tumor cells as well as in the blood circulation. As cell energy declines in tumor cells, the sodium/calcium pump, which normally maintains an alkaline balance of these minerals inside the cell, is weakened. Thus calcium begins to accumulate. [Novartis Found Symp 240: 169-81, 2001] Without sufficient energy, the calcium cannot be pumped out of the tumor cell.

Calcification is a common feature of tumor cells. Tumor calcification forms the basis of many diagnostic tests for cancer, most notably mammography. [Mol Med Today 6: 15-19, 2000] Cancer is a state where there is excessive calcium in the tumor cell, not a shortage of calcium!

5 If the body continually draws from its large pool of calcium in the bones to maintain an alkaline state, assuming the provision of calcium from the diet is insufficient, then it would be anticipated that the skeleton would collapse and fractures would result before tumors would appear. All that supplemental calcium would do is protect against loss of bone mineralization, since calcium and other alkaline minerals are relatively abundant in bones. Furthermore, one would expect cancer rates to be lower in countries where calcium consumption is higher. The Japanese have lower cancer rates than do Americans, but consume only about 400 mg of calcium daily compared to 800 mg by Americans.

6 The effectiveness of various cancer treatments such as hyperthermia (heat treatment) and drugs may be enhanced by decreasing tumor cell pH, not by alkalizing tumor cells. [Radiotherapy Oncology 2: 343-66, 1984] Hyperthermia treatment of tumors is more effective when cells have low or acidic pH (6.8). [Int J Radiation Oncology Biol Physics 49: 1391-98, 2001]

7 Another expected finding if the high pH theory was true, would be that women with cancer should be more prone to osteoporosis given that the body has been dumping calcium into the blood to prevent acidity and the spread of cancer. But to the contrary, women with cancer tend to have higher bone density. A study of 8,203 post-menopausal women for 3.7 years revealed an increased risk for breast cancer among women with higher bone mineral density. Women with the highest bone mineral density were almost twice as likely to develop breast cancer. [J Clin Epidemiol 54: 417-22, 2001] This is corroborated by other studies. Another study showed that bone mineral density was positively associated with uterine but not colorectal cancer. [BMC Cancer 2: 22, 2002] Yet in another study of 6,854 women over age 65 years, the risk of breast cancer was found to be about 30 to 50% higher for every measured increase in bone mineral density. [J Am Med Assoc 276: 1404-08, 1996]

8 While Brewer and others cite experiments which appear to show the remission of tumors in animals and humans with *high pH therapy*, a more recent study casts doubt on these early reports. The use of high pH therapy to treat cancer has already undergone more recent experimentation. Researchers hypothesized that an acid state in the body enhances the formation and growth of tumors, whereas an alkaline state may control tumor growth and induce regression. So researchers instilled a cancer-inducing chemical into the bladder of rats and tested both alkaline and acid diets on the rate of tumor progression. Ammonium chloride was introduced into test animals to induce an acidic state. Other animals were given sodium chloride to maintain an alkaline state in their body. Treatment with sodium chloride caused a high incidence of papillomas and carcinomas of the bladder. Yet a tumor protective effect with urinary acidification was not found. In fact, both acidification and alkalization tended to aggravate bladder tumors. [Food Chemistry Toxicology 37:1159-66, 1999]

Believe it or not, cancer cells aren't acidic

To reiterate, conventional medicine has not completely ignored Warburg as has been charged. In fact, there are a number of published reports which review Warberg's work and theorize how it can be utilized to treat cancer. Obviously advocates of the alkaline cures haven't read the latest science. Cancer cells exhibit a neutral pH. Cancer cells aren't acidic at all!

Researchers now have more precise tools to measure the pH of cancer cells. What they've found is that it's the environment surrounding cancer cells that is acidic, not the tumor cell itself. In fact, the pH inside tumor cells is more alkaline than normal, about pH 7.1 to 7.2. [J Theoretical Biology 196: 237-50, 1999] The fluid in the surrounding area of the tumor is more acidic, 6.5 to 6.8 pH. [Novartis Found Symposium 240: 46-62, 2001; Molecular Medicine Today 61: 15-19, 2000] Metastasis, the spread of tumors, appears to be accelerated when the lactic acid levels surrounding tumors are elevated. [Cancer Research 21: 4757-59, 1995]

In other words, those who espouse the alkaline cure for cancer simply haven't fully investigated the scientific literature and don't have a proper understanding of tumor dynamics.

All this makes sense. The tumor cell begins to utilize sugar instead of oxygen to produce energy, just as Warberg hypothesized, and the enzymatic breakdown of sugar (called glycolysis) produces lactic acid which is expelled outside the cell. Cancer cells produce about 40 times more lactic acid than do healthy cells.

What happens when tumor cells are infused with sugar (glucose)? The provision of more glucose to tumor cells produces more lactic acid which further reduces the pH in the area surrounding tumor cells. [Cancer Research 49: 4373-84, 1989] In another study, researchers grew tumor cells in rats and infused them with glucose. At normal sugar levels the pH ranged from 6.72 to 7.01. When glucose was instilled, the pH shifted to the acidic side, to pH 6.43 in the area around the tumor cells. [Br J Cancer 68:492-500, 1993]

Cancer cells exhibit abnormal energy production. Instead of generating ATP, the energy molecule, from respiration of oxygen, tumor cells use sugar (glucose) as their main energy source. The by-product of tumor cells is lactic acid, which in turn generates gluconeogenesis, the production of more sugar. Thus, cancer cells are assured a continuous supply of glucose for their growth. An enzyme, lactate dehydrogenase, catalyzes the production of lactic acid. With a prolonged fever, this process of feeding tumor cells with sugar can be interrupted, which in turn results in hypoglycemia and a resultant increase in blood pH which represses the enzyme, lactate dehydrogenase. [Medical Hypotheses 56: 693-94, 2001] Of interest are plant molecules that inhibit lactate dehydrogenase. For example resveratrol, a red wine molecule, markedly reduces lactate dehydrogenase levels. [Cardiovascular Research 47:549-55, 2000; Acta Pharmacology Sin 24:703-10, 2003] Diallyl trisulfide, a breakdown product of allicin from garlic, also inhibits lactate dehydrogenase. [Biofactors 21:171-4, 2004] Quercetin, a plant extract often obtained from onions, also inhibits production of lactic acid. [Xenobiotica 33:587-602, 2003; Physiology Chemistry Physics 7:473-5, 1975] This may be a primary reason for reported anti-cancer effects of these herbs.

While it is often said that bouts of fever kill off cancer cells, it is interesting to learn that fever comes and goes with malaria, which is a disease induced by a parasite that produces abundant amounts of lactate dehydrogenase. [Journal Biological Chemistry 279: 31429-31439, 2004] It is possible that remissions of cancer associated with fever actually establish competition for sugar in the body as a growth factor for tumor cells and the malaria parasite (plasmodium).

Lactic acid is not the only acidifier. Recently it has been found that CO2 also produces some of the acid surrounding tumor cells. [Clinical Cancer Research 8: 1284-91, 2002]

Hence the area surrounding the tumor cell becomes acidic and the tumor cell becomes immortal, that is, it is alkaline and has a distinct advantage over other cells and doesn't die off normally in a process called apoptosis. High intracellular pH (an alkaline state) gives a tumor cell an advantage over normal cells for growth. [Molecular Medicine Today 6: 15-19, 2000]

Warberg's theory

German chemist Otto Warberg was awarded two Nobel prizes for his achievements in cancer cell metabolism. Warberg accurately described how cancer cells begin to utilize sugar (glucose) for metabolism and energy production rather than oxygen. Warberg pointed out that an acid state develops in tumor cells, but he did not have the precision instruments at the time to make the more recent discovery that cancer cells are actually alkaline due to the lack of cellular energy to pump out alkaline minerals like calcium. The elimination of acidic byproducts (lactic acid) from the breakdown of glucose (sugar) produces an acidic state in the connective tissue outside cancer cells. This acidic state may be responsible for the observed resistance by cancer cells to the toxicity of certain cancer drugs.

Warberg also correctly noted that there is a disruption of normal cell metabolism in cancer cells. Researchers now understand that low antioxidant levels in the mitochondria of tumor cells reduce cellular energy levels (ATP) and the cell begins to utilize sugar instead of oxygen, a change that is facilitated by low coenzyme Q10 levels.

Those parties who continue to mistakenly aggrandize the health benefits of coral calcium and other alkalizing agents have failed to fully investigate the work of Otto Warberg. Cancer cells are more alkaline than surrounding tissues which results in their immortality. Furthermore, tumor cells are overloaded with calcium, which is why they are so alkaline. High pH therapy is a false cure which distracts many who suffer with cancer, or who wish to prevent cancer. Millions of dollars of coral calcium continue to be sold as a cure all for cancers and other diseases when credible evidence points in the direction of antioxidants such as coenzyme Q10, acetyl L-carnitine, alpha lipoic acid, selenium, IP6 rice bran extract, vitamin C, vitamin D and vitamin E.

What did Warberg really say?

Cancer Research recently published a lengthy report confirming Otto Warberg's findings and noted that in 1956, Warberg talked about the mitochondria being impaired in cancer cells. The mitochondria are cell bodies that produce ATP or cellular energy. Hundreds of mitochondria can be viewed within live cells under a microscope. [Cancer Research 62: 6674-81, 2002] Alkalinity advocates don't talk about the mitochondria.

It has been mistakenly believed that oxygen insufficiency causes cancer cells to produce large amounts of lactic acid. Actually, a defective mechanism in the mitochondria is the problem. [Mol Cancer 1:9, 2002] Acidity surrounding the tumor cell is caused by metabolism within the cell, and not by lack of oxygen. [Neoplasia 5:135-45, 2003]

Mitochondria produce up to 80% of the energy needs of a cell. Mitochondrial dysfunction is related to a diverse number of adult-onset diseases including cancer, diabetes, deafness, stroke and other maladies.

The DNA in mitochondria is more vulnerable to mutations than the DNA in the nucleus of the cell. [Mutation Research 488: 119-33, 2001] Mitochondrial DNA mutations *"can initiate a cascade of events leading to a continuous increase in the production of reactive oxygen species (rusting agents), a condition that probably favors tumor development."* [Cancer Investigation 20: 557-69, 2002]

Most of the rusting (oxidation) in the body occurs inside the mitochondria of cells, which are very small cell bodies next to the cell nucleus that can be observed through a microscope. The mitochondria are the steam engines or atomic power plants of living cells, where cell energy is produced in the form of adenotriphosphate, or ATP.

The production of ATP is repressed in human cancer cells (carcinomas). [Cancer Research 62: 6674-81, 2002]

Think of how much cell energy is needed for all the cellular functions of the body. Just the energy needed to replace old cells with new ones (about 2 trillion cell divisions in an adult human every 24 hours or about 25 million a second) requires lots of ATP.

In a state of low cell energy the cells cannot perform normal housekeeping functions. Cellular debris accumulates and DNA mutations may result, leading to precancerous and cancerous cells.

Says Donald J. Reed, PhD, Distinguished Professor of Biochemistry, Director, Environmental Health Sciences Center, of the Linus Pauling Institute, *"ATP carries chemical energy in cells. In diseased mitochondria ATP energy is not put to useful work but is released instead as heat. Examples of adverse heat production in biological systems are inflammation associated with arthritis and fever stimulated by infection. Antioxidants such as vitamin C, vitamin E, lipoic acid, carnitine and coenzyme Q10 work inside the mitochondria to help maintain its proper function."*

Dietary supplementation with antioxidants may protect the mitochondria against respiration-linked oxygen stress, with preservation of the genetic and structural integrity of these energy-producing cell bodies.

To quote another recent report: *"Mitochondrial damage caused by reactive oxygen species and concomitant decline in ATP synthesis seem to play a key role not only in aging, but also in the fundamental cellular process of apoptosis (cell death). Although dietary supplementation with antioxidants has not been able to increase consistently the species-characteristic maximum life span, it results in significant extension of the mean life span of laboratory animals. Presently, the focus of age-related antioxidant research is on compounds, such as coenzyme Q10, alpha-lipoic acid, and the glutathione-precursors like N-acetylcysteine, which may be able to neutralize undesirable reactive oxygen species at their sites of production in the mitochondria."* [Ann NY Acad Sci 959:508-16, 2002]

The Mitochondria and coenzyme Q10 get overlooked

A key mitochondrial antioxidant produced naturally in the body which can be taken in supplemental form is coenzyme Q10. CoQ10 is essential for the transport of electrons inside the mitochondria. [Clin Investig 71: S55-9, 1993] CoQ10 increases mitochondrial respiration and production of ATP cell energy. [Cell Mol Biol 43:741-9, 1997]

Mutations in mitochondrial DNA may lead to reduced ATP energy levels in living cells which can sometimes be corrected with supplemental CoQ10. [Ann Clin Lab Sci 31:25-67, 2001]

When living cells are deprived of oxygen (hypoxia), as seen in tumor cells, then ATP cell energy levels decline rapidly. The provision of supplemental CoQ 10 has been shown to facilitate resynthesis of ATP in functionally impaired mitochondria. [Arch Int Pharmacodyn Ther 287: 96-108, 1987; Surgery 91:631-7, 1982]

A deficiency of CoQ10 has been described in aging and cancer and when statin cholesterol-lowering drugs are employed. [J Am Coll Nutr 20: 591-98, 2001]

For example, CoQ10 levels in tissue of breast cancer patients are significantly decreased compared to surrounding tissues. [Clinical Biochemistry 33: 279-84, 2000] Breast cancer patients are more likely to exhibit low CoQ10 levels than are healthy people. [Biochemical Biophysical Research Communications 234: 296-99, 1997]

The provision of supplemental CoQ10 (390 mg) to breast cancer patients has been shown to induce complete regression in some cases. [Biochemical Biophysical Research Communications 199: 1504-08, 1994; 212: 172-77, 1995] One small group study showed that the provision of an array of antioxidant supplements including coenzyme Q10 to high-risk breast cancer patients was beneficial in reducing the spread of cancer and increasing quality of life. [Mol Aspects Med 15: 231-40S, 1994]

Statin cholesterol-lowering drugs are known to deplete the body of CoQ10. Thus, it would be of interest to investigate whether cancer rates are higher among statin drug users. Surprisingly, some studies champion statin drugs as novel anti-cancer agents. [Clin Cancer Res 7:2067-75, 2001] Over a five-year period, one study did not confirm any association between statin drugs and the risk of cancer. [American Journal Medicine 15;110: 716-23, 2001] But other disturbing studies do confirm a relationship between statin drug use and breast and prostate cancer. [Epidemiology 13: 262-67, 2002] More studies are underway.

Electrical and magnetic fields

Wherever electricity flows, electric and magnetic fields are present. Laboratory experiments show that magnetic fields can cause changes in living cells. For comparison, humans are commonly exposed to solar ultraviolet radiation which can damage tissue, but the body's repair mechanisms usually prevail. Still, the public is often concerned about undue health risks, especially for small children. Increasing distance from electrical sources is the most practical way of reducing exposure.

While there have been inconclusive and conflicting studies involving the health impact of electromagnetic fields (EMFs) in the range of household appliances there has been a small but significant increased risk of leukemia noted among children exposed to EMFs. There have also been reports of an increased risk of solid tumors among electrical workers. [Cad Saude Publica 18:221-33, 2002] Consistent epidemiologic evidence of an association between childhood leukemia and exposure to extremely low frequency magnetic fields has led to their classification by the International Agency for Research on Cancer as a *"possible human carcinogen."* [Pediatrics 116:e303-13, 2005]

In regard to EMF exposure from cell phones, most of the animal studies show negative results. [Bulletin Cancer 92:637-43, 2005] However, another analysis concludes there may be a relationship between EMF exposure from cell phones and cancer, but because the studies used to draw these conclusions have some flaws, the issue is deemed inconclusive. [J Toxicology Environmental Health B Critical Review 7:351-84, 2004].

A study in Britain now shows there is a relationship of some sort between childhood cancer and proximity of home address at birth to high voltage power lines. [British Medical Journal 330:1290, 2005] But this may only be an association, not a causal relationship as EMFs lose their strength with increasing distance from their source, in this case, distant power lines. Childhood exposure to EMFs is near zero from power lines. [British Medical Journal 331:634-635, 2005]

Magnetic fields- exposure measured in milligauss

Electrical source of magnetic fields	1.2 inches away	12 inches away
Microwave oven	750 to 2000	40 to 80
Clothes washer	8 to 400	2 to 50
Electric range	60 to 2000	4 to 40
Fluorescent lamp	400 to 4000	5 to 20
Hair dryer	60 to 20,000	1 to 70
Television	25 to 500	0.4 to 20

Source: Cancer Causes & Control 7: S49-54, 1996

Possibly the risk for cancer from EMFs doesn't emanate until later in life. A study was conducted in Israel over a period of more than 13 years among women over age 60. An increased risk for breast cancer was found among women who had greater exposure to EMFs (three hours or more of use of computers, mobile telephones, television sets, or household appliances). [In Vivo 19:563-6, 2005]

There may be obscure or hidden factors that make risk analysis from EMFs difficult. For example, it is difficult to sort out one type of close exposure (for example, cell phones or computers) from another distant source (power lines).

A vigorous scientific debate exists as to whether there is or isn't a health risk from EMFs. [J Experimental Clinical Cancer Research 23:353-64, 2004]. Some investigations yield positive findings, others negative findings. [Bioelectromagnetics. 6: S74-100, 2003] One report says electromagnetic field exposure could hypothetically contribute to tamoxifen drug resistance observed in breast cancer after long-term treatment. [Biochem Biophys Res Communications Sep 13, 2005] But do EMFs, in fact, interfere with tamoxifen treatment in a normal household environment? Nobody really knows.

Since 1991, 15 population studies have associated male breast cancer with exposure to electromagnetic fields. One published report involving EMFs and male breast cancer warrants analysis. Three cases of male breast cancer were diagnosed among a small group of men who worked in a basement office of an office building. This office was adjacent to an electrical switchgear room which generated high magnetic fields in the work space. The risk of male breast cancer in this group was increased about 100-fold (observed three cases, expected 0.03 cases). [American Journal Industrial Medicine 46:86-7, 2004]. However, it is curious that researchers overlooked an obvious yet unapparent risk factor. Indoor work, particularly a basement workplace, would deprive workers of sunlight exposure. Sunlight produces vitamin D in humans. A deficiency of vitamin D is linked with breast cancer. Was the increase in male breast cancer caused by magnetic fields or by lack of vitamin D? These are the types of questions that make it difficult to ascertain if there is a link between EMF exposure and cancer.

To make matters worse, a cell biologist doing work on EMFs for the Department of Energy, faked data linking cancer to electromagnetic fields in order to gain $3.3 million worth of grants for scientific research. [New York Times, July 24, 1999] This casts a shadow on the existing scientific base for analysis.

To conclude, the scientific literature concerning EMFs and cancer is confusing, whatever risk that may exist is small, and scientists don't look like they are going to be able to unravel this issue anytime soon. Just prepare yourself for tomorrow's news headlines, that another study found a slight risk for cancer from exposure to some kind of electromagnetic energy. The next day, there will be a contrary news report. Until there is sufficient evidence to draw conclusions, it's probably best to limit exposure to EMFs by keeping electrical appliances or cell phones, a measured distance away.

GERMS CAUSE CANCER Biological (Germs) Considered To Be Carcinogenic *Source: European Journal Epidemiology 20: 565-74, 2005*	
Germ	Cancer site
Helicobacter pylori	Stomach
Schistosoma hematobium	Urinary bladder
Human papilloma virus (HPV)	Cervical or anal cancer
Herpes simplex virus 8	Kaposi's sarcoma
HIV-1	Non-Hodgkins lymphoma, Kaposi sarcoma
Epstein-Barr virus (herpes family)	Lymphoproliferative diseases, nasopharynx
Aspergillus flavus (aflatoxins)	Liver
Hepatitis B virus, hepatitis C virus	Liver

Important Occupational Carcinogens *Source: European Journal Epidemiology 20: 565-74, 2005*			
Occupational exposure	Cancer site	Population exposure	Main professions exposed
Arsenic	Lung, skin	Rare	Insecticide sprayers
Asbestos	Mesothelioma, lung	Uncommon	Brake lining, demolition
Benzene	Leukemia	Common	Painters, petroleum workers
Diesel exhaust	Lung	Common	Railroad, bus, truck workers
Formaldehyde	Nose	Rare	Laboratory, wood, paper workers
Hair dyes	Bladder	Uncommon	Hairdressers and barbers
Pesticides	Lung	Common	Sprayers, agricultural workers

Lifestyle and Environmental Factors That Promote Cancer	
Factor	Cancer sites
Smoking	Lung, urinary bladder, esophagus, oral cavity, larynx, kidney, pancreas, liver, other,
Alcohol	Esophagus, larynx, oral cavity, pharynx, liver, breast
Ionizing radiation (x-rays, gamma rays)	Bone marrow, breast
Solar UV radiation	Skin, lip
Chlorinated water	Bladder, kidneys, rectum

Medicines That Cause Cancer *Source: European Journal Epidemiology 20: 565-74, 2005*	
Factor	Cancer site
Cancer chemotherapy drugs	Bone marrow
Immune suppressing drugs	Reticuloendothelial system
Hormone pills	
- Estrogen (hormone replacement)	Endometrial, breast
- Anabolic steroids	Liver
- Oral contraceptives	Liver, breast
Tamoxifen	Endometrial, breast
Phenacetin	Kidney

Cases of Cancer per 100,000 population

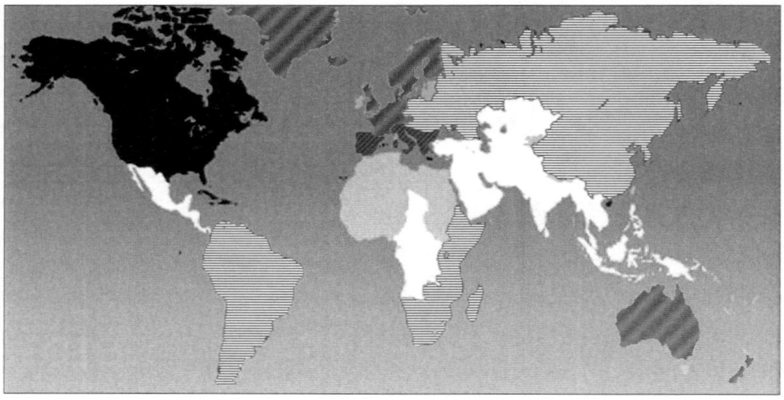

Under 100
100 - 150
151 - 200
201 - 250
251 - 300
301and above

Does radon gas cause lung cancer?

Radon is another environmental presence that has been cited as a cause of cancer. The Environmental Protection Agency (EPA) says that *"everyone should test their homes for one of the leading causes of lung cancer in the country: indoor radon gas."* Yet most of us have never heard of anyone who came down with lung cancer due to radon gas.

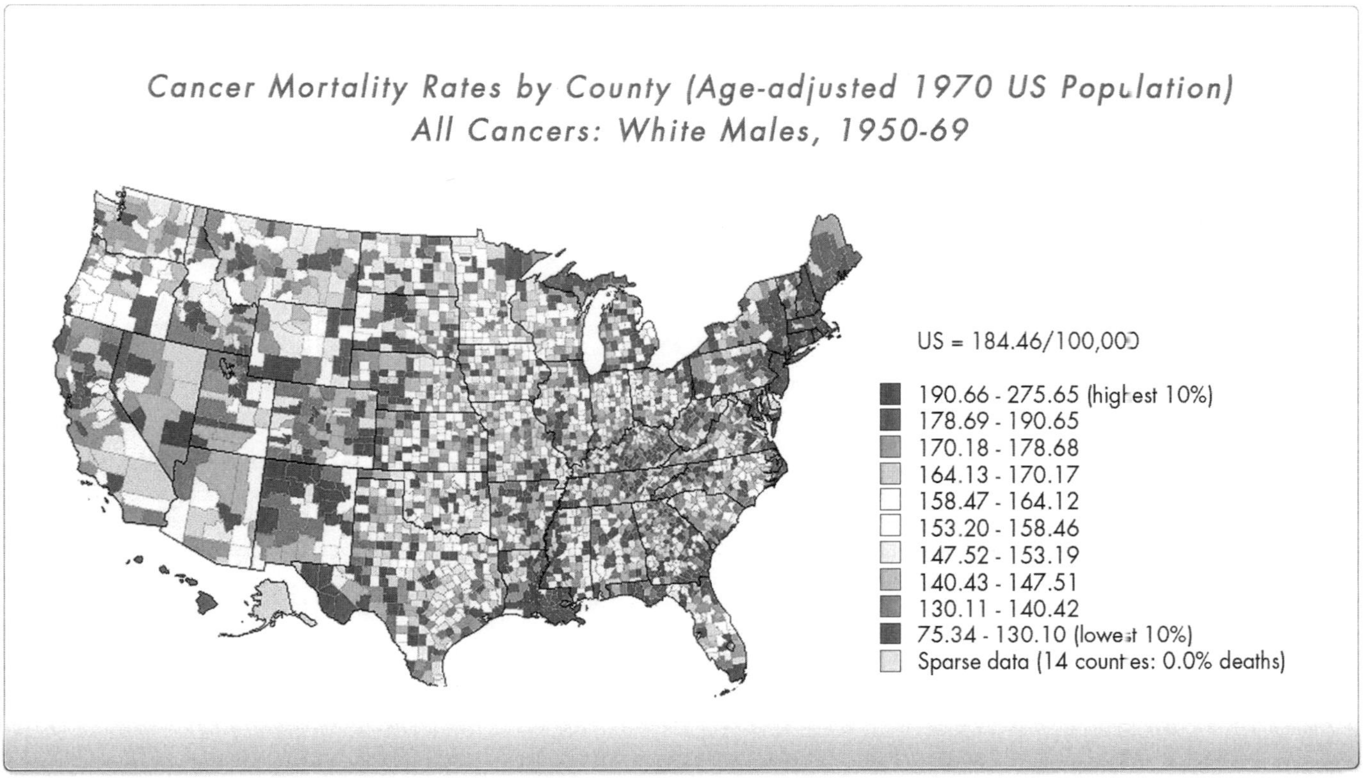

Darker areas in map above display counties with low cancer rates among U.S. males, which coincide with the areas of high radon gas exposure.

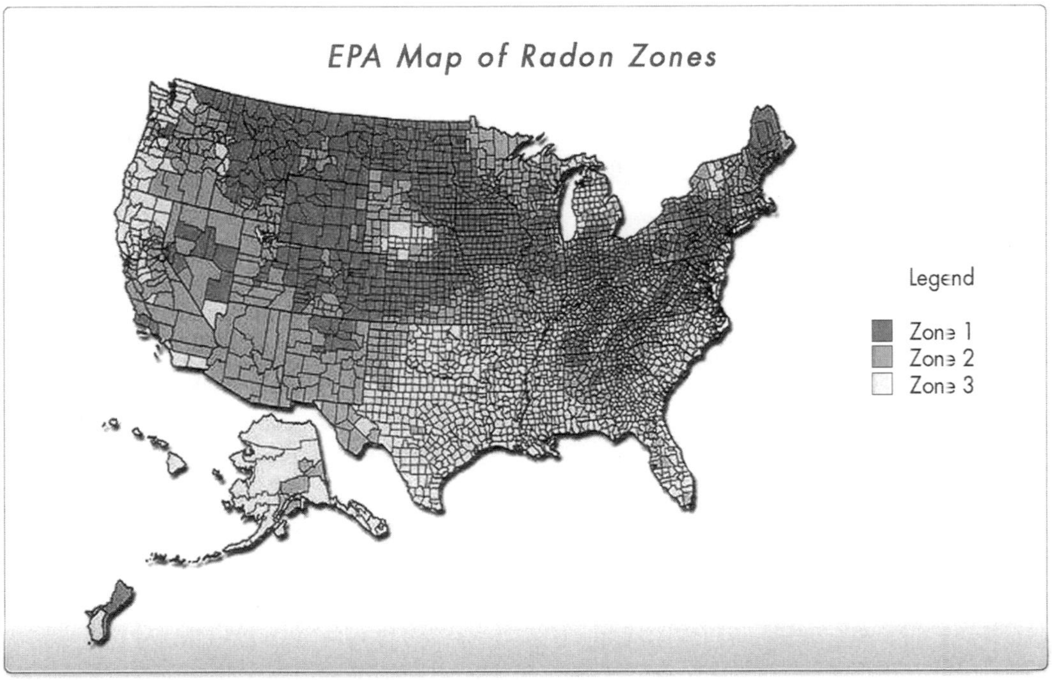

Dark areas on map above display counties with high radon gas levels.

When non-smokers develop lung cancer, health authorities don't go running down to the deceased person's home to check for radon gas exposure.

Radon is a naturally occurring radioactive gas that is emitted from soils and rocks and is in some water sources. The EPA promotes radon monitoring and sealing of homes to prevent an indoor radon gas hazard. The range of radon gas in U.S. homes varies by a factor of over 1,000. The EPA says *"there is no safe level of radon – any exposure poses some risk of cancer."* The EPA bases its claim on studies published by the National Academy of Sciences in 1999 which said radon gas is the second leading cause of lung cancer in the United States after cigarette smoking. Radon in drinking water causes an additional 180 deaths a year, estimates the EPA. The EPA offers a videotape about radon and has produced several publications about radon for homeowners.

But before you buy into the EPA's propaganda on radon, you might want to examine the following information.

Two maps are reproduced to help you analyze this issue for yourself. One displays the areas of high radon gas emission. The other is a map displaying areas with high and low cancer rates. It's obvious from the maps that high radon gas areas have low rates of cancer.

There are other obvious inconsistencies with the alleged radon gas health threat. First, there is Misasa, Japan. Japanese doctors report that people who live in the Misasa villages in Japan, where there are high radon levels in drinking water, exhibit far lower rates of cancers than do people in adjacent villages. [Journal Japanese Cancer Research 83: 1, 1992]

Evacuate Ramsar, Iran?

Another compelling study is that of the people in Ramsar, Iran, who receive an annual dose of radiation from environmental sources that is 25 times higher than in the U.S. and 13 times higher than what is permitted for radiation workers in health care and industry. Some health authorities prematurely called for the government of Iran to evacuate Ramsar because of the potential hazard posed by natural radiation exposure.

Ramsar has areas with some of the highest recorded levels of natural radiation measured on the earth. The radioactivity is brought to the surface of the earth by hot water springs. The concentrations of radium in these hot springs are 18 times higher than found in other water sources in the same country. [Health Physics 77: 150–3, 1999]

People in Ramsar consume 12 times more radium from vegetables grown in their area than what is considered to be a toxic dose of radiation. [Journal Environmental Radioactivity 66: 215–25, 2003] Yet there is no increased incidence of leukemia or cancer in Ramsar. [Health Physics 82: 87–93, 2002]

The fact that Iranians in Ramsar appear to have lived for generations in relatively good health despite living in an area of high radiation, poor nutrition, lack of availability of physicians and low-population density compared to developed nations, all point to some possible protective effect from low-dose radium and radon gas. The opposite of what you would expect to find.

B.L. Cohen of the University of Pittsburgh says that despite extensive investigation, the idea that inhalation of low-dose radon products poses a cancer risk appears to be without solid scientific substantiation. [Health Physics 68: 157–74, 1995]

Cohen's conclusions were recently backed by another study which showed no association between radon gas exposure and the risk of leukemia. [Health Physics 81:272–88, 2001]

With all of the warnings about radon gas issued from the Environmental Protection Agency, where are the dead bodies, the cancer clusters, the ill families in areas of high radon exposure? Following are more reports providing evidence that runs contrary to the EPA's warnings about radon gas.

- Radon exposure causes lower cancer risk among women younger than 61 years. [Pathology Oncology Research 4: 125–29, 1998]

- A study of white females, living in 2,821 counties in the U.S., found radon gas exposure actually decreases the risk for lung cancer. [Human Experimental Toxicology 17: 691–96, 1998]

- A suspicion arose among geneticists over mutations on a particular gene in persons exposed to radon, which could potentially lead to leukemia. But subsequent studies have not found a relationship between this gene mutation and radon exposure, nor any elevated rates of leukemia. [Environment Molecular Mutagen 37: 7–16, 2001]

- Yet another study compared the amount of natural radiation in Rocky Mountain States which is 3.2 times greater than in Gulf Coast states. Data from the American Cancer Society reveals the overall cancer death rate in Gulf Coast states is actually somewhat higher than in Rocky Mountain States. [Health Physics 75: 428–30, 1998]

> The EPA says: *"Although some scientists dispute the precise number of deaths due to radon, all the major health organizations (like the Centers for Disease Control and Prevention, the American Lung Association and the American Medical Association) agree with estimates that radon causes thousands of preventable lung cancer deaths every year. This is especially true among smokers, since the risk to smokers is much greater than to non-smokers."*

While the EPA continues to warn the public of the potential dangers posed by radon gas, in fact, low-dose radiation appears to be beneficial to human health, stimulating the immune system. [Natl Medical Journal India 7: 169–72, 1994].

> *Radon gas enters the lungs and should, theoretically, increase the risk of lung disease.*
> *Environmental Protection Agency.*

This is exactly what people who regularly bathe in radium spring water spas contend.

The Iowa Story

Iowa has the highest radon exposure anywhere in the U.S. A study of females in Iowa, conducted by the University of Iowa, College of Public Health, found that 60% of the radon readings in basements of people who developed lung cancer, along with others who did not, were above the U.S. Environmental Protection Agency's action level for radon. There were hardly any differences in radiation exposure between healthy women and women with lung cancer. But researchers incredulously concluded that *"this indicates that residential radon exposure is a significant cause of lung cancer."* Maybe that's because the politically correct answer preserves everybody's job and keeps grant money flowing for more radon risk studies.

The presumed link between radon and lung cancer was initially based upon a study in Sweden, but subsequent studies elsewhere have not shown a consistent link. Flaws were also found in many radon studies. Few of the studies actually even measured radon exposure. Where radon levels were measured, a relatively small percentage of studies found a statistically significant positive association with lung cancer. Oddly, while some studies report a link between radon and lung cancer, there was no association for lung cancer among houses located near uranium or radium processing waste sites. At best, the association between radon gas and lung cancer is considered weak. [Cancer Detection Prevention 15: 435–43, 1991]

Researchers concede that the health risks posed by low-dose radiation exposure have been *"highly politicized."* There is an exaggerated perception of a threat to public health. There is no question that miners exposed to radon experience health risks, but this involves high-dose exposure. The EPA admits it primarily relies upon data from miners in regard to radon hazards. For low doses, the risk estimates are all hypothetical, calculated from data involving high-dose exposure. [Radiation Environment Biophysics 39: 17–24, 2000]

The problem with the EPA's radon gas mortality numbers is that they aren't a count of dead bodies, they are mathematical extrapolations. If X number of people die from exposure to high-dose radiation, then how many would die from chronic exposure to low-dose radiation? The assumption is that low-dose radiation would pose an accumulated risk.

Oddly, higher levels of lung disorders have never been reported among pets living in homes where radon levels are high.
Environ Health Perspectives 105:1312–9, 1997

EPA's Disclaimer

If you wade through the EPA website carefully you finally find their disclaimer. Says the EPA: *"The probability of a radiation-caused cancer or genetic effects is related to the total amount of radiation accumulated by an individual... Based upon current scientific evidence, any exposure to radiation can be harmful or can increase the risk of cancer, however, at very low exposures, the estimated increased in risk is very small."* [Ionizing Radiation Fact Sheet Series No. 2, EPA, Oct. 21, 2002]

There you have it. How small a risk? Radon gas is an imaginary risk at best. Remember what the EPA is doing for you, and your family. Says the EPA, the cost of sealing a home from radon gas buildup generally ranges from $800 to $2,500 (with an average cost of $1,200). And according to the EPA, *"hundreds of thousands of people have reduced radon levels in their homes."*

Cancer and aspartame

Aspartame, the artificial sweetener, was approved by the U.S. Food & Drug Administration without adequate testing. It was approved for use in soft drinks in 1983, but it has made virtually no impact upon the growing problem of obesity and diabetes, both which are risk factors for cancer.

Now, decades after its introduction into foods as a non-caloric sweetener, researchers in at the Cesare Maltoni Cancer Research Center in Bologna, Italy, report that aspartame (Nutrasweet) provokes tumors in animals at doses less than what is considered acceptable for daily human intake. The daily intake level is 50 mg per kilogram (2.2 lbs) of body weight in the U.S. and 40 mg in Europe. This would be about 3,500 mg in the United States or 2,800 mg in Europe for a 160-pound adult. The Italian researcher found aspartame increased cancer risk at 20 mg per pound of body weight. The researchers say: *"On the basis of these results, a reevaluation of the present guidelines on the use and consumption of aspartame is urgent and cannot be delayed."* [Environmental Health Perspectives 114: 379-85, 2006]

Spontaneous remissions

Cancer researchers spend too much time studying disease and too little studying health. Too much time is spent trying to kill cancer cells rather than healing the body. Too many resources are spent attempting to treat cancer once it occurs rather than understanding the dynamics of how the human body keeps cancer in check.

Studies reveal there are many more mutated cells produced that can initiate cancer than actual number of tumors that develop. The initiation of cancer appears to be a far more frequent event than the cases of cancer that develop. [Cancer Research 60: 1254-60, 2000]

Spontaneous remission of cancer is defined as the disappearance of the malignancy without any treatment or obviously inadequate treatment. The validity of these remissions often demands confirmation. Doctors want to see evidence, x-rays, or preferable pathology slides showing no malignant cells remain. Yet such evidence exists.

It could be argued that only early-stage cancer has been observed to disappear. But in 1989 a case of malignant lymphoma, which had appeared in eight different locations during a seven-year follow-up period following initial diagnosis, was found to have completely disappeared 22 years later. [Missouri Medicine 86: 275-77, 1989]

It could be said that remissions aren't observed in solid tumors, but German researchers report the case of a 61-year-old man *"with extensive metastatic disease"* from lung cancer. A large metastatic tumor was also found in the abdominal wall as well as in the liver. These tumors were all confirmed by biopsy. Eight months after diagnosis the patient was operated on for a hernia and the surgeon noted the complete remission of the abdominal tumor. Five month later there was no evidence of liver or lung tumors on x-ray pictures. Complete remission persisted for more than five years. [Annals Oncology 8: 1031-39, 1997] Other cases of inexplicable remission from lung cancer among elderly subjects have been reported in the modern literature. [Lung Cancer 45: 263-66, 2004]

In 1996, cancer surgeons in Germany reported that seven patients who underwent partial removal of tissue for rectal cancer were completely free of the disease 10 years later even though they did not undergo radiation or chemotherapy following surgery. [Langenbecks Archives Chir 113: 133-35, 1996]

In 1996, investigators in the Netherlands reported that a 59-year-old man who had undergone surgical prostate removal nine years earlier, developed a metastatic tumor in his pelvis as confirmed by a bone scan. Two years later radiation treatment was applied to the area. Subsequently his PSA test dropped to a low of 0.4 mcg per liter and the bone tumor completely disappeared. The spontaneous remission of a bony tumor secondary to prostate cancer is extremely rare. [Journal Urology 155: 653-54, 1996]

Even in bladder cancer, which has a low survival factor, four of 20 cases examined disappeared spontaneously without treatment according to a study conducted in Spain. [Ch Espana Urology 43: 643-45, 1990]

From 1900 to 1976, reviewers have recorded 176 cases of spontaneous, unexplainable remissions from cancer in the medical literature. [National Cancer Institute Monograph 44: 5-9, 1976]

There may be more spontaneous remissions from cancer than reported. One physician reported four such cases in his office practice alone. [Hawaiian Medical Journal 59: 379-87, 2000]

These mysterious spontaneous remissions prompt a question. How many cancers would go into remission if never treated with radiation, chemotherapy and surgery?

Cancer doctors have, for some time, been reluctant to accept the existence of spontaneous remissions in cancer disease. Researchers M. Heim and R. Schwarz in Germany state that examination of cancer remissions *"could serve as a kind of natural experiment that would lead to more efficient therapy."* [Z Psychosomatic Medicine Psychotherapy 46: 57-70, 2000]

Scientists speculate that exposure to cancer-causing chemicals, hormones, radiation or infection, may be behind these puzzling cancer remissions. Following are some intriguing reports to corroborate these suspicions.

Cancer remissions and sex hormones

High hormone levels are linked to increased cancer risk. Researchers in England report of a case of metastatic breast cancer that resolved on its own with cessation of hormone replacement therapy. [Clinical Oncology 13: 200-01, 2001] Many cases of cancer that arise during pregnancy, when sex hormone levels are highest, resolve with birth or the termination of pregnancy. For example, a 28-year-old woman in the third trimester of her pregnancy was found to have acute myelocytic leukemia. The baby was delivered early by Cesarean section and her leukemia disappeared for a short time, only to reappear as her hormone levels rose again. [Cancer 63: 1621-23, 1989] A 47-year-old man who happened to be supplementing with progestagen (progesterone) developed a secondary tumor in his lung after his right kidney had been removed due to cancer. The removal of the hormonal supplement caused the long tumor to disappear, which was confirmed by x-rays. The remission was reported to persist for at least 3.5 years. [Dutch Medical Wochenschr 114: 420-23, 1989]

Cancer remissions and immunity

Another case is that of a 69-year-old woman who suffered from rheumatoid arthritis since the age of 40. Rheumatoid arthritis is considered an autoimmune disease where the immune system attacks the body, in this case, the joints. The patient had been undergoing treatment with an immune-suppressing drug, methotrexate, for three years. She reported swollen glands in her neck to her doctors which was diagnosed as non-Hodgkins lymphoma. The tumor resolved completely 14 months after withdrawal of the immune-suppressing drug. [British Journal Hematology 118: 567-68, 2002]

Doctors in Canada report six cases of non-small-cell lung cancer that were in long-standing remission (7-14 years) until the patients took immune-suppressing drugs. [Medicina, Buenos Aires 56: 74-82, 1996] The immune system was keeping these tumors at bay for over a decade.

Cancer remissions and thyroid hormone

In 1993, the reported remission from metastatic lung cancer by a patient who had extreme thyroid hormone deficiency alerted researchers there may be some relationship. [Journal National Cancer Institute 85: 1342-43, 1993] Lab dish studies show that thyroid hormone deficiency may interfere with the activity of the p53 tumor suppressor gene. [Anticancer Research 18: 289-93, 1998] Thyroid hormones are the major glandular controller of growth, metabolism and cellular maturation. Thyroid hormones also help to control the production of growth hormones (insulin growth factor, or IGF-1) that may accelerate tumor growth. Low thyroid levels (hypothyroidism) are associated with prolonged remission from diagnosed cancer. [In Vivo 10: 235-47, 1996]

The use of a drug that inhibits thyroid gland hormone production was employed among 22 patients with recurrent brain (glioma) cancer along with tamoxifen, an estrogen-blocking, anti-cancer drug. The group of patients that developed low thyroid levels survived three times longer (10.1 versus 3.1 months) than did patients on tamoxifen with normal or high thyroid levels. [Anticancer Research 23: 617-26, 2003]

An analysis of patients treated in England for a high thyroid condition (hyperthyroidism), found a reduced risk for lung cancer, along with a small decreased risk for cancer of the pancreas, bladder and other sites, thus concluding that there was a link between low-thyroid and increased ability to fend off cancer growth and subsequent mortality. [The Lancet 353: 2111-15, 1999] This wasn't an absolute cure. Researchers expected to find 761 cancers in the group of 7,417 patients treated for high-thyroid and detected only 634 cases.

Magnetic resonance imaging (MRI) confirms that low thyroid cancer patients exhibit tumors that are half the size of patients with high thyroid. [Aleck A. Hercbergs, M.D., 93rd Annual Meeting of the American Association of Cancer Research, San Francisco, April 6 – 10, 2002] There is a *"growing body of evidence that suppressing thyroid function alone may improve response to cancer treatment,"* says Aleck A. Hercbergs, MD, of the Cleveland Clinic. Subsequent research shows that small-cell lung cancer patients who have a low thyroid condition are diagnosed 4.3 years later than normal thyroid patients (70.73 vs 66.43 years). Also significant is the finding that hypothyroid cancer patients live longer than normal thyroid patients (mean 14.5 vs. 11.1 months).

It is interesting to note that foods such as soybeans, turnips, cauliflower, rutabagas, cabbage, peaches, peanuts, mustard, broccoli and spinach contain substances called glycosinolates which interfere with the absorption of iodine and inhibit normal thyroid gland function. These foods are also reported to protect against cancer. Indole 3-carbinol, a type of glycosinate found commonly in cruciferous vegetables is reported to reduce cancer risk. [Journal Agriculture Food Chemistry 53:5164-9, 2005]

It is also reported that molecules in soy inhibit cancer. It is also frequently claimed that soy is a food that can interfere with thyroid function. However, this has been disproven in a controlled study. [Journal Medicinal Food 6:309-16, 2003] Asian women who emigrate to the United States and alter their traditional diet are more likely to develop thyroid cancer. The majority of these cases of thyroid cancer are explained by a decline in the consumption of soy. [Cancer Epidemiology Biomarkers Prevention 12:144-50, 2003] One of the reasons why there has been so much confusion regarding the role of soy in the thyroid function is that animals studies have shown that soy interferes with thyroid gland function in animals. [Environmental Health Perspectives 110:349-53, 2002] But this has not been shown in humans.

Also, there is intriguing evidence that vitamin D should be explored since it has been shown to inhibit hyperthyroid conditions. [Metabolism 46:1184-8, 1997] This may be one of the reasons why vitamin D is considered a strong anti-cancer molecule.

Glucosinolate Content of Selected Cruciferous Vegetables

Food (raw)	Serving	Total Glucosinolates (mg)
Brussels sprouts	½ cup (44 g)	104
Garden cress	½ cup (25 g)	97
Mustard greens	½ cup, chopped (28 g)	79
Turnip	½ cup, cubes (65 g)	60
Cabbage	½ cup, chopped (45 g)	35
Kale	1 cup, chopped (67 g)	34
Watercress	1 cup, chopped (34 g)	32
Cabbage, red	½ cup, chopped (45 g)	29
Broccoli	½ cup, chopped (44 g)	27
Horseradish	1 tablespoon (15 g)	24
Cauliflower	½ cup, chopped (50 g)	22
Bok choy	½ cup, chopped (35 g)	19

Cancer remissions and infection

The idea that infections are an underlying cause of cancer is worthy of study, particularly after examination of some reported cancer remissions. A 57-year-old woman in Japan with adult T-cell leukemia experienced a spontaneous remission after an antibiotic was given for lung and bladder infections. [Blut 61: 346-49, 1990] A 31-year-old leukemia patient with accompanying severe bacterial infection (Group G streptococci), was initially treated with antibiotics and the leukemia went into remission within six weeks. [Annals Hematology 83: 189-94, 2004]

It is known that spontaneous remissions from cancer are often preceded by a severe infection accompanied by a high fever. [Cancer Biotherapy Radiopharmacology 13: 209-10, 1998]

Infection that is accompanied by fever is reportedly involved in some cancer remissions. [Neuroimmunomodulation 9: 55-64, 2001] The application of whole body high-temperature therapy (hyperthermia) is now employed as a secondary cancer treatment. It is said that many cancer patients claim they were never ill before the onset of cancer. Some researchers believe there may be a link between the lack of illness (fever) and cancer. One study found an increased risk for cancer among who had no history of former infectious diseases (5.7 times increased risk), no history of common colds or fever (15.1 times increased risk). [Med Klin 78: 95-98, 1983] However, this is not conclusive.

In another converse study, 21 of 353 individuals who had a history of measles developed cancer versus only 1 in 230 who had a negative history of measles. [Cancer 1-5, 1985]

There is evidence that cancer risk increases when a person receives an organ transplant. Immune-suppressing drugs may be responsible. [Annals Surgery 202:9-20, 1985] Oddly, when doctors at Wayne State University School of Medicine studied a rare case of spontaneous remission from kidney cancer, they found no enhancement of natural killer cells or other white blood cell activity. [Journal Urology 152: 156-57, 1994]

It is possible that prescription or non-prescription drugs, used for conditions other than cancer, may induce tumors. The case of a woman who experienced a spontaneous remission from cancer when she withdrew from taking a decongestant drug is an example. [Canadian Medical Assn Journal 153: 561-66, 1995]

These spontaneous remissions from cancer point to natural mechanisms that are so powerful as to cause tumors, even metastatic cancer, to disappear. If only we could learn how to tap into these mechanisms!

Can some people be genetically resistant to cancer?

The current thinking is that it is possible that some human beings may be genetically resistant to developing cancer. At least this has been demonstrated in animals. Zheng Cui, of the Department of Pathology at Wake Forest University School of Medicine, Winston-Salem, North Carolina, discovered a mouse that resisted cancer even when large doses of cancer cells were injected into its body.

At first, Cui thought he had made a mistake. Maybe he hadn't injected the mouse with cancer cells after all. So he called a colleague and asked what he should do with this mouse, dispose of him? His colleague thought better and suggested he re-inject the mouse, this time with twice the normal test load of cancer cells, 400,000 cancer cells.

Normally, lab mice, after injection of tumor cells, will develop an accumulation of fluid in their belly and appear puffed up (a condition called ascites). Not this mouse. He withstood the assault by tumor cells. Two million cancer cells were injected – still no tumors. Then two hundred million cancer cells were injected – same result.

Eventually mice were bred from this original *"super mouse"* and they repeatedly resisted a great number of cancer cells, a thousand or even a million times the lethal dose. Cui found that the innate immune system, the one mammals are born with, not any acquired immunity, was responsible for the cancer resistance in the mouse. Cui actually observed cancer cells, taken from this mouse, rupture and die off. As the special bred mice aged, their immune system began to falter. They would begin to show puffed up bellies, and then this condition would disappear. Cancer would develop, but then subside. Now if only humans could be bred in the same manner! [Cancer Immunity 3:14, 2003]

CHAPTER 3

Treatment

p 78 - 108

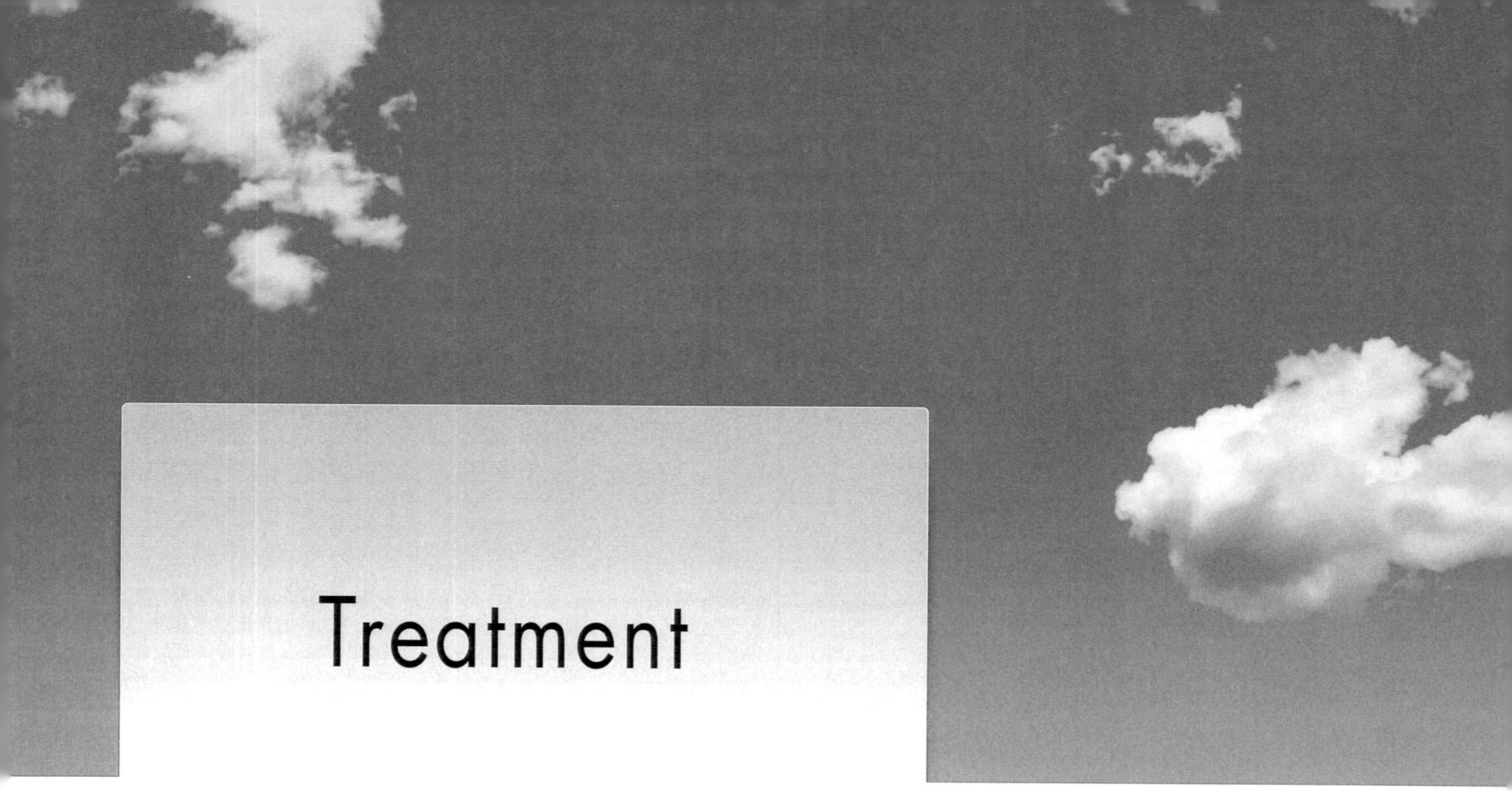

Treatment

Is there no balm in Gilead? Is there no physician there?
Why then has not the health of the daughter of my people been restored?

- Holy Bible, Book of Jeremiah 8:22

Modern cancer treatment: surgery, chemotherapy, radiation treatment

This chapter reviews in detail the pros and cons of conventional cancer care – surgery, chemotherapy and radiation therapy. This chapter is for the serious reader who wants to find out whether modern cancer treatments work. The current state of cancer care is rather dismal. So reading this chapter is not for the faint of heart.

The dilemma is that patients make decisions about treatment in a state of fear and urgency. Regardless of how ineffective and problematic cancer treatment may be, patients and their families often elect to trade side effects for the possibility of prolonged survival, even if it is a marginal extension of life.

This book advocates natural home-based therapies for cancer. To that end, patients need to fully comprehend what they are getting into when they consent to cancer treatment. Only when patients recognize there is little chance that modern cancer treatment will work are they likely to consider the alternatives presented in this book.

Surgery for cancer

Certainly there is a place and time for surgery to remove expanding tumors that are robbing the body of blood supply and nutrients, pressing on nerves and causing pain, and causing weight loss and physical wasting.

But there is the common misconception, often promoted by surgeons themselves, that surgery *"got all of the tumor."*

One study reveals most patients would prefer surgery over medication due to their desire to get all of the cancer out of their body. [Medical Decision Making 25: 614-19, 2005]

Imagine that a particular tumor weighs about 100 grams (3.5 ounces). Consider the following:

100 gm of tumor = 100 billion cells (approx.)

If a tumor can double in volume in a matter of weeks, it would make sense to decrease the size of the mass of the tumor right away. Otherwise, a patient could not make it through a treatment course.

Surgery is the way to radically reduce the volume of a tumor, removing anywhere from 80 to 99% of the tumor mass. Recent advances in surgical technologies have aided in the removal of brain tumor tissue with a newer, higher net percentage tumor reduction of 90-99%. These include computer assisted stereotactic surgery, laser instrumentation (carbon dioxide, argon, and Yag), ultrasonic aspiration, operative phototherapy, etc.

However, consider the following:

* 90% removal of tumor (100,000,000,000 cells), leaves 10 billion cells
* 99% removal of tumor (100,000,000,000 cells), leaves 1 billion cells

Thus, no matter how good the local surgical therapy is, the patient is still left with at least 1 billion tumor cells!

There now remains the combination of therapies: follow up the initial volume reduction therapy with something else. The usual choices are radiation or chemotherapy. In the best of circumstances, one could expect another 90-99% reduction in tumor cell number. Another 90-99.9 % cell reduction still leaves 1 million to 100 million cells.

The logical procedure now would be to hit the tumor again with yet something else, (usually radiation or chemotherapy) that might attack the remaining cell population.

If left without treatment a third time, it is possible that the tumor could return to its original size in as few as 6 weeks, factoring in the numbers mentioned above.

Tumor	Doubling time (Days)
Testicular Carcinoma	21
Ewing's Sarcoma	22
Non-Hodgkin's Lymphoma	25
Osteogenic Sarcoma	34
Hodgkin's Disease	36
Fibrosarcoma	48
Colonic Adenocarcinoma	95
Pulmonary Adenocarcinoma	154

Source: New England Journal Medicine 336: 1569-74, 1997

If a one-millimeter ball of tumor cells remain after surgery that means 1 million malignant cells remain. Surgery never addresses the cause of cancer. Neither does chemotherapy or radiation therapy. Physically remove or destroy every cancer cell and new ones will likely arise. Modern cancer treatment is an effort in futility.

If billions of cancer cells could be killed off at one time, this would create an enormous mass of cellular debris that would clog lymph glands, create inflammation and infection. This would be counterproductive.

Does surgery accelerate the progression of cancer?

Researchers report that tumor removal is followed by accelerated growth of recurrent tumors and metastases. This is likely due to growth factors that are promoted during the wound-healing process. [Annals Thoracic Surgery 80: 1046-50, 2005]

Cancer researchers are attempting to find ways for cancer cells to die off slowly, without the need for surgery, by a process called apoptosis (normal die off), or programmed cell death. A few cells in our body die off and are replaced by new ones every day. Cancer cells, however, are immortal. They resist apoptosis. They remain like young cells that never grow up and mature.

Radiation therapy

Radiation causes cancer. There are different forms of radiation. The invisible solar ultraviolet rays can induce DNA damage that eventually results in skin cancer. X-ray radiation from medical imaging and CT scans are also believed to increase the risk for cancer. A report issued by the Food & Drug Administration now suggests the risk for cancer from medical x-rays may be as much as 1 in 1,000. There are over 3 billion x-ray images taken annually in the world. Dr. Richard C. Semelka, MD, says patients receiving multiple CT scans today are being exposed to doses of radiation comparable to those given off by the x-ray machines used in the 1930s and 1940s. Cancers do not emanate from x-rays till years later. This makes it difficult to attribute radiation exposure to the onset of cancer. [The Lancet 367: 1712-14, 2006]

In 1976, Drs. Irwin Bross and Leslie Blumenson of Buffalo's Roswell Park Memorial Laboratory estimated that, based on radiation dosage exposure, twice as many deaths as cures could result from mammographic screenings of mostly healthy women. [Journal Surgical Oncology 8: 437-45, 1976] Makers of mammography equipment quickly reduced the dosage patients were exposed to and digital imaging was also employed. But millions of women exposed to higher-dose radiation during mammography years ago when they were in their early 40s are likely at higher risk to develop breast cancer in their 60s and 70s.

Risks for cancer from medical x-ray radiation are real and usually are never discussed with patients. Repeated exposure is the problem. Patients undergoing x-ray filming should take supplemental antioxidants, such as vitamins C and E, since they have been shown to limit the damage caused by medical radiation. [Biology Trace Element Research 94:149-56, 2003] Such advice is rarely shared by doctors with patients.

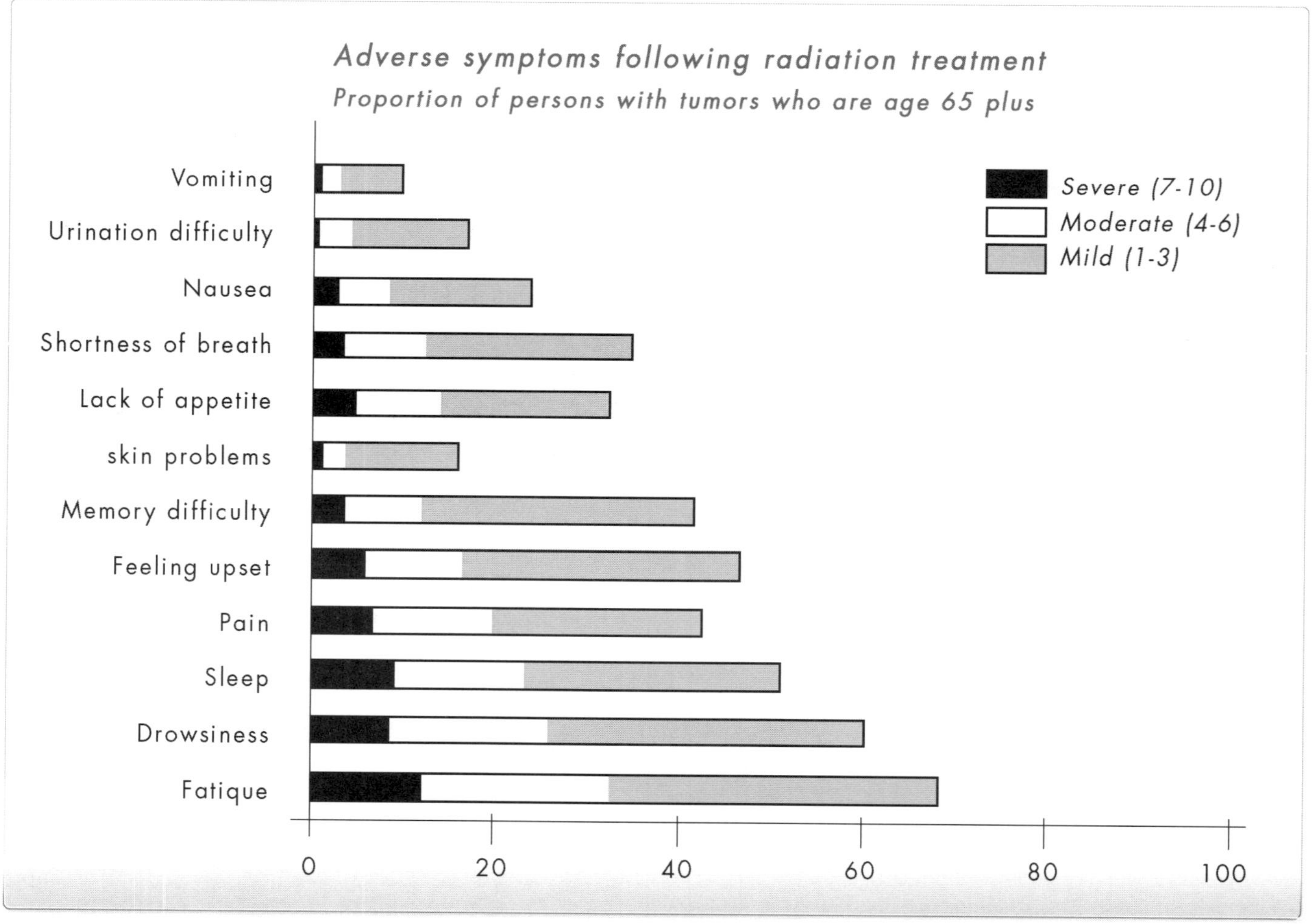

Frequency of adverse symptoms, reported by intensity, following radiation treatment
Source: Journal Pain Symptom Management 30: 433-42, 2005

Chemotherapy

In pain shalt thou use many medicines; for thou shalt not be cured.
- Holy Bible, Book of Jeremiah 46:11

Year	Cancer Mortality per 100,000 (age adjusted)
1994	200.9
1991	203.1
1982	185.1
1970	189.6

Source: New England Journal Medicine 336: 1569-74, 1997

- *"There are 1.2 million cancer cases diagnosed each year, and current treatments only cure 5-10% of patients."*
  - CNN Report, Feb. 23, 2000
- *"Sure, it's poison, but all chemotherapy agents are."*
  - CEO of a pharmaceutical company
- *It remains a fact, that for most common cancers, there is no effective treatment.*
  – Garth Powis, DPh, The Toxicity of Anticancer Drugs, Pergamon Press, 1991.
- *A panel that advises the Food and Drug Administration recommended approval yesterday of the cancer drug Iressa, despite concerns by the agency's staff about the drug's effectiveness. Iressa shrank tumors in 10% of non-small lung cancer patients who had not responded to two previous drug treatments.*
  – New York Times, Sept. 25, 2002

The longstanding statement that cancer treatment consists of "*slash, burn and poison*" only serves to create unwelcome anxiety that patients are likely to dismiss. What else have cancer patients to cling to but what their cancer doctor recommends? The certificate on the wall at the oncologist's office says "*Mayo Clinic.*" Why should cancer patients mistrust their oncologist?

It is not even a surety when cancer patients are confronted with the harsh facts and realities of chemotherapy that they will resign from treatment. Family pressure is often exerted. Patients are frequently too ill to be able to evaluate contrary information. There is no time to make a mistake.

Only cancer patients know how dreaded chemotherapy really is. Even family members cannot really fathom the suffering and irreversible physical damage caused by chemotherapy. It is said that more cancer patients succumb from the side effects of treatment than from cancer itself.

Sleight of hand

One of the deceitful methods employed to justify chemotherapy is the removal of *"all-cause mortality"* from the scientific studies. This means, if chemotherapy causes a cancer patient to succumb to the side effects of the drug, and let's say the patient experiences heart or kidney failure, as many cancer victims commonly do, these mortality figures are often not calculated into survival figures.

Frequently it is said that the gravity of the growth and spread of cancer must be weighed in favor of toxic treatment over prevention of side effects. But this dismisses the importance of side effect control. Side effects may prevent up to one in five breast cancer patients from getting full-dose chemotherapy. Furthermore, frequently cancer patients succumb to heart failure or a heart attack during the course of treatment. This leads the cancer doctor to announce to the patient's relative, "*we shrank the tumor, but unfortunately, the patient succumbed to a weak heart.*"

The doctor is not leveling with the family here. The weak heart was likely induced by toxic treatment. A survey at MD Anderson Cancer Center in Houston, published in the journal *Circulation* (June 29, 2001) found that there is no class of cancer drug that is free of potential damage to the heart. Even the targeted therapies like Avastin and Erbitux cause heart problems. Side effects must be addressed. Patients often take antioxidant supplements to reduce unnecessary side effects, but their use is often discouraged by oncologists. They say it interferes with treatment.

Chemotherapy: over-promoted

One of the problems in sorting out the effectiveness of cancer therapies is ascertaining exactly how much treatment itself contributes to survival. There are now approximately 10 million Americans living with cancer. The very term "*cancer survivor*" is used loosely in the cancer industry and is often misused to imply patients have survived due to the care they have received. Many of these patients are in remission and many are not. The debate over the term has prompted the suggestion that a more accurate term might be "*people living with cancer.*" [Journal National Cancer Institute 96: 1414, 2004]

The Pharmaceutical Research and Manufacturers of America (PhRMA), which represents the country's leading pharmaceutical research and biotechnology companies, says "*medicines dramatically increase the survival rate for cancer.*" PhRMA claims the 5-year survival rate for cancer has increased from 50.0% in 1979 to 62.7% in 1995, a 25% relative increase in survival. [PhRMA website, April 22, 2004] But is this due to chemotherapy?

A group of doctors at the Northern Sydney Cancer Centre in Sydney, Australia, sought to determine the effectiveness of cancer chemotherapy. The evaluators did not tabulate whether chemotherapy improved numbers like white blood cell count, or hormone levels, or antibodies, or even if they shrank tumors. All they wanted to know was, how much chemotherapy actually contributes to the overall 5-year survival of cancer patients? They evaluated 22 types of cancer. Chart below shows results of that study for Australia and the United States (1998 data).

The 5-year relative survival rate for cancer in Australia is now over 60%. In the United States, the 5-year survival rate is about 64%. It is clear that chemotherapy only makes a

Impact of chemotherapy upon 5-year survival of Australian and U.S. adults, 1998
Clinical Oncology 16: 549-60, 2004

	United States 1998			Australia 1998		
Location of cancer	Number of cancers evaluated	Absolute number 5-year survivors due to chemotherapy	Percent 5-year survival due to chemotherapy	Number of cancers evaluated	Absolute number 5-year survivors due to chemotherapy	Percent 5-year survival due to chemotherapy
Stomach	3001	20	0.7%	1904	13	0.7%
Rectum	5533	189	3.4%	4036	218	5.4%
Colon	13,936	146	1.0%	7243	128	1.8%
Lung	20,741	410	2.0%	7792	118	1.5%
Breast	31,133	446	1.4%	10,661	164	1.5%
Total 22 cancer sites	154,971	3306	2.1%	72,903	1690	2.3%

minor contribution to cancer survival. [Clinical Oncology 16: 549-60, 2004] A review published in 1986 reported that the overall contribution of chemotherapy to 5-year survival was 4.3%. [British Medical Journal 293: 871-876, 1986] So these dismal numbers are not improving. An editorial in the Australian Prescriber wonders if chemotherapy can survive in its present form. [Australian Prescriber 29 2-3, 2006]

Most cancers do not respond to chemotherapy. Measured responses to cancer therapy (such as tumor markers) often do not translate into improvements in overall survival.
Source: M.V. Blagosklonny, Ordway Research Institute, Albany, New York Cell Cycle 4: Dec. 15, 2005

Chemotherapy studies may be misleading

There are so many reasons why the published results from cancer trials must be regarded with suspicion. First, cancer is a disease of advanced age, yet studies show that far fewer senior Americans (over age 65) are enrolled in cancer studies (25%) than the estimated proportion of the United States population with cancer (63%). [New England Journal Medicine 341: 2061-67, 1999] The studies may not be relevant to the senior population that incurs most cases of cancer. Older patients do not respond as well to treatments such as chemotherapy.

> *Investigators have found that 30% of the volunteer patients in clinical trials report that they took their medication when they did not, which raises questions over the accuracy of conclusions drawn from published studies.*
> - Chest 118:290-5, 2000

Definition of a successful cancer drug

Contrary to what you may believe, pharmaceutical companies don't have to submit data to the FDA that their anti-cancer drugs improve survival. They only need to show what percentage of patients experience a 50% reduction in tumor size for one month or more, not whether patients live any longer. [Food & Drug Administration] Cancer chemotherapy today is about slowing down the disease and handling symptoms and side effects, not about curing cancer. The problem is that tumor shrinkage is not correlated with survival. Of the 66 drugs approved by the FDA between 1990 and 2001, 48 did not prolong survival.

> *Many oncologists take it for granted that response to therapy prolongs survival, an opinion which is based on a fallacy and which is not supported by clinical studies.*
> U Abel, Biomedicine & Pharmacotherapy 46: 439, 1992

Many of the headlines concerning newly approved cancer chemotherapy drugs report on the drug's ability to shrink the size of tumors, not survival. Or a news reports will claim survival was prolonged by 45%. But compared to what? When you read the fine print, you'll then find out that the addition of a new cancer drug to other chemotherapy regimens may improve survival by just one month over the other chemotherapy drugs alone. That's what the blockbuster headline that says "*45% increase in survival*" really means.

If survival for a particular type of advanced cancer is just six months, and treatment prolongs survival by just another three months, the doctor will say treatment improves survival by 50%. So will the newspaper headlines, and spokespersons for the American Cancer Society. So survival, in terms of hard (not relative) numbers is three months.

Cancer repair shop

Imagine you take your car to the repair shop. The mechanic flushes the carburetor, replaces the muffler and some exhaust valves, and charges the battery. But when you place the key in the ignition, the car doesn't start. This is pretty much what the cancer industry is doing. Replacing parts, treating the body, and showing some numbers improved. That is all. Would you pay for repairs that don't work? Insurance companies keep paying for these ineffective treatments because patients keep demanding them. Withhold treatment and patients will be interviewed by news reporters, who will demand to know why patients were denied treatment.

Cancer care in the news

Most of the positive news stories surrounding new cancer drugs today are intended to impress investors in drug stocks, not to deliver promising news to patients. If an existing cancer drug is prescribed to 250,000 patients in a year, and a new drug will replace it or be used in combination, and the new drug costs $1,000 for a one-month course, investors gleefully can calculate a $250 million bonanza for every month the drug is used by cancer patients.

When it was announced that the new anti-cancer drug Avastin, when combined with chemotherapy, resulted in lung cancer patients living four months longer, Genentech's stock rose dramatically and nearly $17 billion was pumped into the company. [Associated Press, March 29, 2005]

Commercial interests dominate the cancer industry today. Most cancer patients are oblivious to how they have become pawns for Wall Street. If a real cure for cancer was discovered, Wall Street would collapse. Drug stocks prop up the entire stock market.

New Cancer Drugs

Forbes Magazine publishes reviews of cancer drugs mainly from a financial viewpoint. Which upcoming drugs are likely to obtain FDA approval and significantly increase a drug company's stock price? A recent Forbes review of cancer drugs undergoing human trials is revealing. [Forbes Magazine, August 3, 2005] Most new drugs are evaluated by their ability to shrink tumors, not increase survival. Here is how *Forbes Magazine* described some of these new cancer drugs, with my own interpretation in parentheses:

"Produced dramatic tumor shrinkage in at least some patients" (failed to work)

"This colon cancer drug is somewhat similar to..." (nothing new)

"A more potent version of......." (nothing novel, likely more toxic)

"A trial of cancer patients showed the drug slowed the disease's progression" (they still died)

"7 of 92 patients saw tumors shrink by more than 20 %" (would you take this drug?)

"Three of sixteen patients saw their cancer vanish, at least for the moment" (for a moment? would you even buy this company's stock?)

Doctors say terminal cancers overtreated

As evidence of the trend to treat rather than cure, doctors recently expressed concern over the disturbing trend for terminal cancer patients to receive chemotherapy and other aggressive but futile treatment in the last days of their lives. Dr. Roy Herbst of the MD Anderson Cancer Center in Houston aptly says: *"Patients don't like to give up."* A survey shows nearly 12 % of cancer patients who succumbed to their disease received chemotherapy in the last two weeks of life. *"Overly aggressive treatment gives false hope and puts people through grueling and costly ordeals when there is no chance of a cure,"* say cancer specialists." [Dr. Craig Earle of the Dana-Farber Cancer Institute and Harvard Medical School, American Society of Clinical Oncology, Atlanta, June 2006; Associated Press, June 2, 2006]

Chemotherapy cannot penetrate solid tumors

The vast majority of tumors are of the solid variety, producing malignant masses in the lungs, colon, breast and prostate, compared to cancer of the blood (leukemia) or lymph system, for example. But cancer researchers admit chemotherapy drugs do not efficiently penetrate solid tumors. [Nature Reviews Cancer 6: 583-92, 2006]

Overdiagnosis and overtreatment

Overdiagnosis refers to the detection by screening (mammograms, PSA tests) of cancers that would not have become apparent to a doctor or produce symptoms detectable to the patient before an individual died of other causes. Cancer is prevalent, far beyond the number diagnosed in human populations, and most adults will die with, but not of, their cancer. Treatment and invasive or toxic screening methods (radiation from x-rays, mammograms, needle biopsies) for tumors that may never progress to cause symptoms or death in an individual's lifetime would represent overdiagnosis and needless treatment.

Autopsy studies reveal how many people incidentally had cancer on the day they died, which did not contribute to their death. For example, autopsy reports of 24,708 individuals found 167 cases of lung cancer, 47 being incidental (didn't contribute to death). [Respiratory Medicine 99: 501-07, 2005]

There are other similar studies:

> In a series of 20,000 autopsies over a 25-year period, 11% (700) of cancers found were undetected during the person's life and over half were of no importance to the patient. [Acta Pathologica Microbiologica Immunologica Scandinavia 98: 496-500, 1990]

In a series of 1,014 autopsies in Singapore, 18 incidental colon/rectal cancers were found. If unsuspected and undiagnosed colon/rectal cancer existed in the general population to the extent found in this group then an additional 146 cancer cases would be added to the total colon-rectal cancers that year and represent nearly 47.9% of the colon/rectal cancer cases. [Cancer 61: 1059-64, 1988]

An elderly man in Michigan who died suddenly was found to have three incidental malignant tumors diagnosed at autopsy. [American Journal Forensic Medical Pathology 12: 265-71, 1991]

In a study reported by the University of Iowa, only 1.2% of 2,938 autopsies on males conducted between 1991-2001 exhibited invasive prostate tumors (35 cases), none however were found to significantly extend beyond the prostate. [Journal Urology 174: 1785-86, 2005]

An analysis of 852 autopsies of women not known to have breast cancer during their lifetime found a prevalence of 1.3% for invasive breast cancer and 8.9% for ductal cancer. If these figures are calculated for the population of females in the United States, then about 2 million would have ductal cancer. In 1992, an estimated 24,000 women in the U.S. were diagnosed with ductal cancer and 10,000 underwent breast removal (mastectomy). If all of the 2 million women estimated to have ductal breast cancer were diagnosed and the same percentage elected to undergo mastectomy, then 832,000 women would undergo surgical breast removal. [Annals Internal Medicine 127: 1023-28, 1997] This is astounding, given that all of the autopsy cases studied produced no known symptoms during their lifetime. This would mean virtually all ductal cancer treatment is needless.

In a study conducted in Germany, among 400 autopsies of subjects that were found to have colon-rectal cancer, 32% (126) remained undetected during the patients' lifetime. In 22 of the 126 undetected tumors, colon/rectal cancer was only incidental and not a cause of death. [Gastroenterology Journal 47: 293-3000, 1989]

Among 571 autopsies of gastric cancer cases evaluated in Norway, 165 (29%) were incidental and not a cause of death or symptoms. [European Journal Surgical Oncology 16: 417-22 1990]

Among autopsies of adults over age 95 that were reviewed, cancer as a cause of death was underestimated by nearly 50%. [Clinical Geriatric Medicine 13: 55-68, 1997] This means many were living with symptom-less cancer till their dying day.

Among 139 autopsies of males reviewed in Hungary, 38.8% had incidental prostate cancer detected only at autopsy. Cancer cells were detected as early as the third decade of life. [European Urology 48: 739-44, 2005]

In a study conducted in Scotland, of 28 deaths occurring among women who had been diagnosed with breast cancer, only 9 (32%) were attributed directly to breast cancer. [British Journal Cancer 67: 1086-89, 1993] This either speaks for a high rate of needless diagnosis and treatment, or mortality from the treatment itself.

Rates of incidental cancer represent the rate of unnecessary screening and treatment. One conclusion is that the immune system keeps many cancers from producing symptoms or threatening life and not all cancers require treatment. This runs contrary to the widely practiced program of mass cancer screening and early detection.

Do chemotherapy drugs cause cancer?

The answer is yes. Chemotherapy drugs are carcinogens. They are toxic to cancer cells and healthy cells. Researchers have also found that chemotherapy drugs meant to kill existing malignant cells can cause breaks in chromosomes of healthy cells which sets the stage for future cancer growth. [Cancer Cell 1: 89-97, 2002]

A startling fact is that second tumors often occur with greater frequency years after treatment with chemotherapy drugs than without chemotherapy. Sometimes various research studies reveal higher-dose chemotherapy may improve survival. But these studies often do not evaluate the long-term effects of increased radiation or chemotherapy.

Charles B. Pratt MD and Ching-Hon Pui MD state that *"as the cure rates for primary cancer have improved with the use of intensive treatment, the number of therapy-related second tumors has also increased."* Anti-cancer drugs have been used to treat organ transplant recipients by suppressing their immune system to prevent organ rejection. The development of lymphomas in kidney transplant patients were first reported in the 1970s.

Many patients succumb to their primary tumor so it makes it difficult to assess the risk for secondary tumors. Among 6,514 patients treated with chemo or radiation therapy for Hodgkin's disease, their risk for solid tumors after treatment more than doubled. [American Cancer Society August 1, 2000]

Survivors of breast, ovarian, brain and lung cancer are now recognized to be at increased risk for leukemia (cancer of the blood). The mean latency period for secondary tumors to arise is about 44 to 62 months following initial treatment.

Men treated successfully for testicular cancer with radiation or the drug cisplatin may develop leukemia 5 to 10 years following treatment. The increased risk may be small or large.

For every 10,000 patients treated for testicular cancer, there may be an additional 25 cases of leukemia. [American Cancer Society August 1, 2000]

For ovarian cancer, among 10,000 patients treated with cisplatin, 21 may develop leukemia. [New England Journal Medicine 340: 351-57, 1999]

Chemotherapy facilitates the spread of cancer

Most roaming cancer cells are eliminated by the immune system. For cancer to spread to a distant location from its site of origin, it must stop in the blood circulation for about 20 minutes so it can replicate, create a tumor and invade surrounding tissues. Blood clots facilitate the stoppage of circulation in small blood vessels, usually in the lungs or liver, where new tumors begin to grow and invade tissues, a process called metastasis. It is metastasis that is the primary cause of mortality among cancer patients.

Chemotherapy for cancer increases blood clotting and the risk of a spreading tumor. [Haemostasis 28: 50-60, 1998] The addition of estrogen or tamoxifen may further increase the risk of blood clotting and the spread of tumors. [J Clinical Oncology 9: 286-94, 1991] Avastin, the newly introduced anti-angiogenesis drug, carries a serious risk of blood clots, its manufacturer has warned. [American Cancer Society News Center, August 17, 2004]

The annual incidence of blood clots (venous thromboembolism) is not only directly life threatening if they enter the lungs or block circulation to the brain or heart, but they also portend a poor prognosis for cancer patients. Only 12% survive beyond a year if they develop clots. An estimated 11-20% of cancer patients on chemotherapy develop blood clots. [Thrombosis Research Dec. 30, 2005] It's a wonder any cancer patients survive chemotherapy at all.

Insanity of chemotherapy

The general consensus of oncologists is that chemotherapy toxicity is necessary to produce shrinkage of tumors. Yet studies show that patients who experience toxic effects from chemotherapy do not respond any better to treatment than patients without drug-induced toxicity. [Cancer 19: 1785-95, 1966]

Sulfur mustard, used in World War I as a weapon, became the first chemotherapy drug used to fight cancer when two young pharmacologists at Yale University, Alfred Gilmand and Louis S. Goodman, showed in animal tests that it could produce temporary remission from lymphoma. Early in 1942, sulfur mustard was used to treat human lymphoma. The era of toxic modern cancer chemotherapy was born.

> Eradicating every ominous cell from a cancer patient's body is a difficult goal – and in many cases, it may not be possible or even necessary.
> *Source: Scientific American, Sep 1996*

The side effects and hazards of anticancer drug therapy are tolerated because of the belief that the higher the dose of anticancer drugs, the greater the likelihood of a favorable response. It didn't dawn upon cancer researchers to employ less toxic therapies, such as immune boosters (so-called biological response modifiers), until much later, in the late 1980s. Drugs like interferon and interleukin-2 arose, but these too led to disappointment.

It would be too confusing to review each and every chemotherapy drug, or even all the classes of drugs, since the doctor chooses the appropriate drugs and dosage for each patient. There are about 50 drugs commonly used for cancer chemotherapy. The most commonly used drugs in cancer treatment are vinca alkaloids (vinblastine), anthracyclines (doxorubicin) which are iron chelators, epipodophyllotoxins (etoposide), cisplatin, and paclitaxel (generic name for Taxol), and 5-FU (5-Fluorouracil).

> Ultimately, by a variety of mechanisms, a multi-drug-resistant tumor evolves. At this point, additional chemotherapy only induces toxic effects in the patient without reducing the tumor.
> *Source: Chemtech 28, 31-36, 1998*

Chemotherapy effectiveness is often impossible

Researchers in Japan report that it is necessary to preserve the blood vessels that feed tumors so that chemotherapy drugs can get into the tumor site. Surgical removal of a cancerous tumor often involves removal of the blood vessels that feed the tumor area. Therefore, post-surgical application of chemotherapy may be less effective. [Gan To Kagaku Ryoho 32:1315-7, 2005] This means that only pre-operative chemotherapy may be of value in many cases.

Side effects not reported in published studies

Only recently have cancer doctors come to realize that chemotherapy produces serious side effects that generally are unreported in published studies. Chemotherapy patients are more likely to be hospitalized or visit emergency rooms for side effects related to chemotherapy, such as fever, infection, nausea, diarrhea, malnutrition, dehydration or low white blood cell or low platelet count. [J National Cancer Institute 98:1108-17, 2006]

Chemo brain

Most cancer drugs cannot discriminate between healthy and cancerous cells. They damage both. Patients can never get back to a state of wellness during chemotherapy. Brain tissues are particularly vulnerable. During and following chemotherapy, some patients experience difficulties with memory, attention, and other aspects of cognitive function. This constellation of deficits is commonly referred to as *"chemo brain fog."* [Annual Review Medicine 34:35-46, 1983]

It is said that up to 25% of chemotherapy patients are affected by symptoms of mental confusion caused by treatment. A more recent study says 8 in 10 patients experience adverse effects to the frontal cortex of the brain as an aftermath of chemotherapy. Adverse effects are apparent even 10 years following treatment. [Breast Cancer Research Treatment, Sept. 29, 2006 online]

Women undergoing chemotherapy for breast cancer often experience decreased memory, concentration and recall. Nausea, vomiting, fatigue and hair loss are among the most commonly reported side effects of treatment. But more recently, functional brain impairments have also been noted. The effect may last years after treatment. [Associated Press, March 28, 2000] The problem here is that this may impair patient compliance (ability to take medicines at home), or impair judgment for future treatment decisions. [J Clinical Oncology 20: 485-93, 2002]

When you treat with conventional chemotherapy, all the mice end up dead, either because the tumors become drug-resistant or you kill them with the higher dose of chemo.
Source: Judah Folkman, noted cancer researcher

One probable cause of diminished working memory may be that chemotherapy significantly reduces vitamin B12 absorption. [Z Gastroenterology 27: 606-10 1989] Impaired B12 absorption is so prevalent following chemotherapy one wonders why doctors don't routinely prescribe supplemental B12 after treatment.

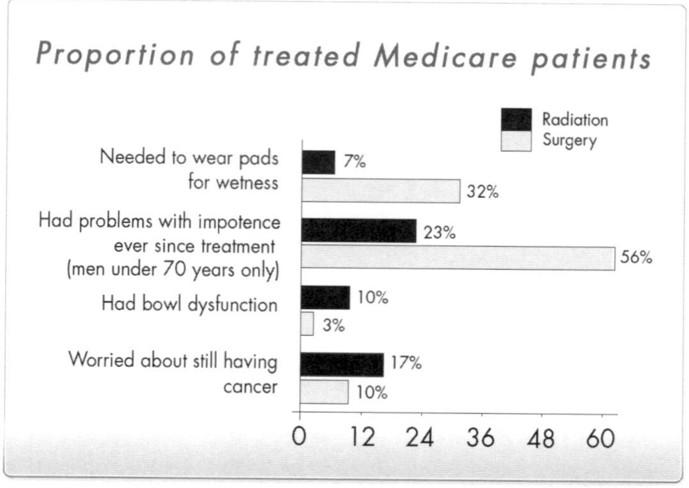

Source: Journal of Clinical Oncology 14:2258-65, 1996

Multi-drug therapy

Drug(s)	Dose-limiting toxicity	% Full Dose	% Complete Remission
Methotrexate (MTX)	Marrow	100	21
Mercaptopurine (MP)	Marrow	100	27
Vincristine (VCR)	Neuropathy	100	47
Prednisone (Pred)	Steroid	100	57
MTX + MP		50 + 50	45
PRED + MP		100 + 100	86
PRED + VCR		100 + 100	92

Drug(s)	Toxicity	% Full dose	% Remission
Nitrog. Mustard	Marrow	100	10
VCR	Neuropathy	100	5
PRED	Steroid	100	5
Procarbazine	Marrow	100	15
MOPP		60/100/100/60	70 (50% cure)

Most of the time multiple drugs are employed to treat cancer. The following charts reveal the ineffectiveness of single drugs against acute lymphocytic leukemia and Hodgkin's lymphoma. However, while multi-drug therapy is more effective, it is also more toxic.

Dose-limiting toxicity is the toxicity that limits the dosage. What the charts above show is that more than one drug is required, and this increases toxicity.

Chemotherapy doesn't work once cancer has spread

There is no cancer treatment that is 100% effective against cancer that has already spread to distant sites from their origin. Almost half of all cancers have already spread to distant organs on the day of diagnosis. Yet for various reasons, including the demands of the patients and their families, useless chemotherapy is still employed.
[Annual Review Medicine 53:615-27, 2002]

> All existing therapies fail in some patients because their tumors evolve into a resistant strain.
> *- Scientific American, June 9, 2003*

It is difficult to conceive how chemotherapy drugs could ever be effective. They are toxic both to healthy and cancerous cells thus resulting in severe side effects and life-threatening toxicity, and the human body perceives chemotherapy agents as toxins and puts up a strong defense against them. This is called drug resistance.

Typically, the first course of chemotherapy proves highly beneficial, nearly annihilating a tumor. But a few drug-resistant cancer cells often survive and begin to multiply. Too often, despite more aggressive second and third courses of chemotherapy, the remaining drug-defiant cells thrive, display increased resistance to drug therapy and eventually become invulnerable to chemotherapy. It's at this point, when chemotherapy begins to fail, that patients should begin to search for alternatives.

Chemotherapy drugs are detected as toxins by the body, to be detoxified immediately by enzymes in the liver (cytochrome P450 enzymes), or actually expelled from cancer cells (P-glycoprotein). [Oncogene 25:1679-91, 2006; Current Drug Metabolism 7: 23-37, 2006]

Resistance to chemotherapy is believed to cause treatment failure in over 90% of patients with metastatic cancer. [Drug Resistance Laboratory, Centre for Cancer Research and Cell Biology, Queen's University Belfast, Belfast, N Ireland, UK Journal Pathology 205: 275-92, 2005]

Reduction of drug resistance has been extensively studied. However, several clinical trials have failed to show any important benefits in terms of response to chemotherapy or the length of survival using drug-resistance reversing agents. [Current Medical Chemistry Anticancer Agents 2:387-401, 2002]

Nanotechnology

What drug companies are attempting to do now is create more stealth chemotherapy molecules that don't trigger drug resistance. By coating their molecules with fats (liposomes) or making them ultra-small (nanotechnology), they can possibly improve the effectiveness of treatment.

The current director of the National Cancer Institute has announced, if we can all just wait a few years, nanotechnology will detect or cure all cancers when they are still miniscule and beyond detection with today's methods.

These particles are colloidal structures with a diameter smaller than 1,000 nanometers and therefore can penetrate through diminutive capillaries into the cell's internal machinery. [Journal Cellular Biochemistry 97:1184-90, 2006]

A nanometer equals one billionth of a meter. A human hair is about the thickness of 80,000 nanometers. Nano-sized particles can easily enter cells and are being explored to diagnose and treat cancer.

> Resistance to chemotherapy is believed to cause treatment failure in over 90% of patients with metastatic cancer.
> *Source: Drug Resistance Laboratory, Centre for Cancer Research and Cell Biology, Queen's University Belfast, Belfast, N Ireland, UK Journal Pathology 205: 275-92, 2005*

Surprisingly, nanotechnology may not be needed. We already have nano-tech available in the form of small molecules found in nature, such as resveratrol from grapes, quercetin from onions, and allicin from garlic, that can penetrate into the nucleus of cells and favorably influence genes. There are numerous research reports that indicate a simple off-the-shelf molecule known as phosphatidylcholine, (lecithin), enhances the absorption and passage of molecules into cells. This simple emulsifier has been shown to improve the biological action of natural herbal products such as quercetin, ginkgo biloba and silybin, the active ingredient in milk thistle. [Planta Medica 67: 326-30, 2001; European Journal Cancer 39: 2403-10, 2003; Bioscience Biotechnology Biochemistry 67: 2548-55, 2003]

Anemia: Erythropoietin

Iron deficiency anemia resulting in low red blood cell count is common among cancer patients. Cancer activates inflammatory molecules that destroy red blood cells. [European Journal Haematology 64: 353-58, 2000] Furthermore, when cancer occurs, the body binds up all the iron to proteins produced in the liver (ferritin, transferrin, lactoferrin, albumin) to withhold iron from tumors since iron is a growth factor for cancer cells. This is a survival mechanism.

So anemia, paleness and fatigue are commonly experienced by cancer patients. One study shows that 26% of cancer patients being treated with chemotherapy were anemic. [Value Health 8: 149-56, 2005] Another study indicates up to 63% of patients undergoing chemotherapy were anemic. [Oncology 68: 3-11, 2005]

The modern remedy to this problem has been to use a hormone-like drug to stimulate red blood cell production. Drugs such as Procrit, Epogen and Aranesp are frequently used. These drugs represent over $8 billion in annual sales and have been in use for over 15 years.

However, because of lax oversight by the Food & Drug Administration, these drugs were allowed to be marketed without studies to prove their safety. Only now has it come to light that while these drugs may improve the quality of life of cancer patients, they may lead to their earlier demise.

An alarming report in the *Journal of the National Cancer Institute* says one study using a red-blood cell boosting drug was halted when it was found that patients with metastatic breast cancer had higher mortality rates (76%) than patients not receiving the drug (70%). The drug apparently increased the risk for blood clotting, stroke and metastasis. Another study showed this type of drug increased tumor progression and mortality. Lab dish, experiments show that these drug molecules actually cause prostate and ovarian tumor cells to grow and spread. These findings were called *"disturbing."* [Journal National Cancer Institute 95: 1820-21, 2003]

These red-blood cell boosters are indicative of a cancer treatment industry that has lost its compass. The gold standard to evaluate treatment is survival. Even the claim of improved quality of life attributed to these drugs is more modest than originally hoped for. [Journal Clinical Oncology 23: 5865-68, 2005] Over time, there is a gradual decrease in the effectiveness of these drugs. [Current Medical Research Opinion 21: S16-18, 2005] This evidence is further confirmation of the claim that cancer treatments are often worse than the disease.

Worse yet, there is evidence that only a few cancer patients can clearly benefit from red-blood cell boosting drugs. [Current Opinion Hematology 5: 103-08, 1998] It might be better to use drugs or nutraceuticals that reduce the inflammatory proteins that destroy red blood cells, than to use drugs that boost red blood cell production.

One of the reasons these drugs don't work is because of a shortage of available iron. Regardless of the hormonal stimulation of red blood cell production, red blood cell production requires iron. However, the provision of iron may paradoxically promote the growth of tumor cells. When hemoglobin levels drop very low, below 6-8, then the immune system is compromised, so some supplemental iron may need to be given. [Anticancer Research 25: 3495-500, 2005] If supplemental vitamin C is given with these drugs, there is better utilization of iron and the dosage of the drugs can be reduced. [Kidney International 67: 1161-70, 2005; Nephrology Dialysis Transplantation 16: 35-39, 2001] There is other evidence that erythropoietin works better when supplemental folic acid, vitamin D and carnitine is provided to anemic patients. [Nephrology Dialysis Transplantation Sept. 6 2005; Current Opinion Hematology 6: 121-26, 1999]

Health authorities have stopped short of halting the use of red blood cell boosting drugs during cancer treatment. If they did so, three major pharmaceutical companies would fail financially.

There is evidence that there are more natural, non-drug approaches to raising erythropoietin hormone levels in the kidneys to elevate red blood cell production. In an experimental study, an iron chelator (remover) and vitamin A were shown to raise synthesis of erythropoietin. [Endocrinology 140: 641-45, 1999] Such approaches go unused.

Cancer Immunotherapy

Once tumor cells escape from their primary source and enter the blood circulation, they are subject to identification by the human immune system. Generally, the immune system kills off most (99.9%) of the escaping tumor cells. A small number of tumor cells escape death and may begin a colony elsewhere.

Boosting the immune system is a relatively new concept in cancer treatment. Drugs- - like interferon, Interleukin-2, Filgrastim, Levamisole, monoclonal antibodies - attempt to raise the numbers of natural killer cells, phagocytes, lymphocytes, macrophages, all types of cells that comprise the human immune system. Of course, natural molecules, such as beta glucan, resveratrol, vitamin D, and selenium, that attempt to do the same thing, are ignored in favor of the exotic, prescription drugs that produce many side effects.

Natural killer cells are of importance because they represent the first line of defense against cancer. Natural killer cells represent about 5-16% of white blood cells. They literally target cancer cells and destroy them.

Healthy natural killer cell activity is essential in controlling micrometastases, small undetectable cancer populations that have escaped and spread from the original diagnosed tumor.

Cancer surgery, chemo and radiation therapy impair the immune system, making micrometastases more of a threat. [Cancer 43: 945-51, 1979; Cancer 68: 482-88, 1991; Journal Immunology Letters 80:55-66, 2002; Journal Veterinary Internal Medicine 20:342-7, 2006] Anesthetics used during cancer surgery suppress natural killer cell activity. [Anesthesia Analgesia 97: 1331-39, 2003] Partial sleep deprivation, often experienced while patients are undergoing cancer treatment, also impairs natural killer cell activity. [Psychosomatic Medicine 56: 493-98, 1994] Chemotherapy attempts to treat the primary tumor by its toxic effects and in so doing impairs immunity and facilitates the occurrence of micrometastases. It is a wonder that patients survive these treatments.

Weight loss and wasting

To fight the tumor the body burns more calories and there is a breakdown of proteins and body fat stores. The sense of taste and smell are diminished, which results in appetite loss. Food doesn't attract any longer. Cancer patients who experience wasting often exhibit shiny skin and bony prominences are accentuated. With diminished food intake, less vitamin B1 is consumed, which can result in heart failure and nerve irritation in feet and hands. Vitamin B2 (riboflavin) deficiency often results in cracked skin around the lips. Shortages of niacin (vitamin B3) are often manifested by skin changes (dermatitis) in the extremities, face and neck. Folic acid (vitamin B9) shortage impairs the ability to repair broken strands of DNA. Vitamin K deficiency may lead to pronounced bleeding and often results from overuse of antibiotics, or malnutrition. More than 8 in 10 cancer patients have reduced serum albumin, a protein that often dictates survival time. Insufficient protein intake results in swelling (pitting edema of legs). This often signals a stage where the tumor must be removed or whittled down to size by other treatments. It is important to re-nourish the body with the proper form and dosage of vitamins and minerals during cancer treatment, say doctors at the MD Anderson Hospital and Tumor Institute. [Postgraduate Medicine 87: 164-70, 1990]

Do nutrients interfere with or enhance chemotherapy?

The prevailing thought is that antioxidants, herbal ingredients and other dietary supplements interfere with chemotherapy. Chemo and radiation therapy induce free radicals to destroy cancer cells, and antioxidants, by virtue of their ability to prevent free radicals, theoretically could interfere with treatment. But the evidence points in a different direction.

Actually, oxidation impairs chemotherapy by degrading the anti-cancer molecules themselves. Furthermore, oxidation may kill cancer cells in a manner that results in masses of dead cells that produce inflammation and toxic response. The idea is to gently provoke cancer cells to die off in a natural manner, a process called apoptosis. Cancer cells that die off due to apoptosis are literally digested and removed by immune cells called phagocytes, thus preventing the inflammatory response. A by-product of oxidation, hydrogen peroxide, inhibits the ability of some anti-cancer drugs to induce apoptosis. When antioxidants are added to the mixture, the anti-cancer drugs work better at inducing apoptosis. [Blood 96: 307-13, 2000] The important lesson here is that it is how you kill off cancer cells which determines whether treatment is successful or problematic.

Kenneth A. Conklin, of the Department of Anesthesiology at UCLA Center for Health Sciences, reports that antioxidant supplements taken during chemotherapy enhance treatment and prevent side effects. Conklin maintains excessive oxidation in cancer tissues interferes with the anti-cancer drugs. Anti-cancer drugs damage DNA in an attempt to cause cell death. Tumor cells often go into a state of dormancy where they are not actively dividing and becoming new cells. In this state, chemotherapy is far less effective. Anti-cancer drugs are only effective when tumor cells are rapidly increasing in number.

Cancer cells have unique properties. Compared to healthy cells, they exhibit much higher levels of vitamin E, which retards spoilage of fats and oils (peroxidation) within cells. Tumor cells have sophisticated antioxidant systems that overcome the stresses in the environment. Conklin writes that antioxidants, alleged to interfere with anti-cancer drug therapy, are often maligned by oncologists. But most anti-cancer drugs don't kill off cancer cells by creating free radicals (oxidation).

Often not mentioned is that chemotherapy often induces latent tumors or leukemia, four or five years after treatment. These latent tumors are more resistant to treatment. The generation of free radicals during chemotherapy can cause DNA mutations that produce the latent tumors. Antioxidants go beyond preventing chemotherapy side effects. They actually enhance treatment and survival, says Conklin.

Antioxidants overcome side effects

- **Vitamin E** has been shown to enhance the desirable type of tumor cell death, apoptosis, and counter the side effects of cisplatin without interfering with treatment. Vitamin E also protects the heart against drug toxicity during treatment.

- Daily administration of supplemental **vitamin C**, 1,000 mg, when taken two weeks before and after bleomycin need definition-drug therapy, prevents damage to chromosomes.

- Supplemental **coenzyme Q10** restores levels of this antioxidant after doxorubicin (anti-cancer drug) treatment and thus protects against cardiac toxicity. Beta carotene has been shown to enhance the action of various anti-cancer drugs.

- Intravenous **glutathione**, another antioxidant, also protects against drug side effects, especially if administered immediately before or after chemotherapy.

- **Selenium** exhibits properties similar to the above-mentioned antioxidants. Quercetin also enhances the activity of various anti-cancer drugs.

If supplemental antioxidants do nothing more than improve the quality of a cancer patient's life, they are worth prescribing. [Nutrition and Cancer 37: 1-18, 2000]

False assertions

False assertions have been made that antioxidants interfere with chemotherapy. An experiment conducted by Rudolph I Salganik, MD, at the University of North Carolina, mischaracterized the role of antioxidant therapy in cancer treatment. Salganik bred a strain of mice so they produced an excess of free radicals, and then depleted their diet of antioxidants. He claimed more oxidation occurred within tumor cells when the antioxidants were withheld and tumors were half their normal size. The claim was made that, by withholding antioxidants, more cancer cells died off by the desirable process of apoptosis. But the published study only indicated about 3% of the cancer cells died via apoptosis. [Annual Meeting American Society Cell Biology, 1999; Carcinogenesis 21: 909-14, 2000] Was this misleading? Salganik then extrapolated his mouse study into advice for cancer patients by saying *"vitamins may prevent cancer cells from self-destructing."* The harm had been done. Salganik's experiment made headlines. Cancer patients were misled.

To add fuel to the argument against antioxidants, David Golde, MD, of Memorial Sloan-Kettering Cancer Center, New York, published papers claiming that vitamin C as an antioxidant counters the action of cancer treatment and may impair therapy. It was as if cancer patients were being told essential nutrients for life actually caused cancer. None of this was true, but the headlines confused the public.

An example of how antioxidants enhance cancer treatment was demonstrated in a scientific experiment conducted by researchers at the University of Colorado. In a lab dish, prostate cancer cells were subjected to an anti-cancer drug (adriamycin), and typical inhibition of cancer cell growth was noted. Then vitamin E was added to the anti-cancer drug and instilled into the lab dish, and prostate cancer cell growth was inhibited even further. Researchers concluded that *"vitamin E could improve the effectiveness of this drug while having a protective effect against side effects caused by the drug, such as heart problems."* [Journal Urology 136: 529-31, 1996]

One of the most toxic cancer drugs is cisplatin. In a laboratory study, mice were administered vitamin E concurrently with cisplatin. Survival was not affected. In mice who had melanoma cancer cells implanted and were then given high-dose cisplatin, vitamin E prolonged survival. While cisplatin alone produces death in about 70% of mice, the combination of vitamin E and cisplatin reduced this figure to 30%. Thus, vitamin E was found to protect against the toxicity of cisplatin without affecting survival. [International Journal Cancer 104: 243-450, 2003]

> Today there is a tendency to associate with cancer the disease -- wasting, hair loss, infection and bleeding -- that is, in fact, caused by the drugs used to treat the disease.
>
> *Source: Garth Powis, DPh, The Toxicity of Anticancer Drugs, Pergamon Press, 1991*

Does cancer or chemotherapy cause the side effects?

Cisplatin induces a depletion of magnesium in up to 90% of treated patients. Symptoms caused by magnesium shortage are often indistinguishable from cancer itself.

- → Muscle spasms
- → Seizures
- → Muscle weakness
- → Twitching eyes
- → Psychiatric manifestations
- → Heart rhythm irregularities
- → Depression
- → Anorexia
- → Irritability
- → Constipation

[Cancer Treatment Reviews 25: 47-58, 1999]

Kenneth A. Conklin, MD, PhD, of the University of California Los Angeles, writes that antioxidants are needed to boost the number and activity of phagocytes that digest and remove cancer cells. [Nutrition Cancer 37: 1-18, 2000] *"Nuking"* cancer cells abruptly stops the cell cycle and slows down apoptosis, the slow but methodical process of cell die-off. Cancer cells must devide rapidly to be killed off effectively by chemotherapy. Antioxidants prevent cancer cells from changing into a state of dormant slow growth that makes them less vulnerable to anti-cancer drugs. Despite a plethora of scientific reports that antioxidants actually enhance cancer chemotherapy, oncologists doggedly maintain antioxidants interfere with treatment. Science does not rule here, professional opinion does.

Folic acid, a B family vitamin, is rapidly used up by cancer cells for growth. Anti-folic acid drugs, such as methotrexate, are utilized in cancer treatment. But now there are second thoughts about anti-folate drugs. Folic acid enters cells through the folate receptor. By coupling anti-cancer drugs with folic acid, the drugs can enter cells more readily. Since cancer cells have a voracious appetite for folic acid, 500,000 times greater than healthy cells, this kind of treatment becomes more targeted than standard chemotherapy. [Reuters, Sept. 14, 2000]

Methotrexate

Methotrexate is a folic-acid blocking drug used to treat cancer. Folic acid is required for DNA repair. It has been documented that methotrexate induces genetic injury and that the co-administration of folic acid with methotrexate protects against drug-induced genetic damage. [Z Rheumatology 60: 63-68, 2001] Methotrexate causes side effects that commonly cause cancer patients to withdraw from the drug. Folic acid supplementation minimizes drug toxicity and discontinuation. [Z Rheumatology 64: 353-58, 2005]

Cisplatin

Cisplatin (Platinol) is a widely used anti-cancer drug. Cisplatin is toxic to the kidney and may impair hearing. Alpha lipoic acid, an antioxidant, has been shown to prevent loss of hearing by cisplatin. [Laryngoscope 109: 1740-44, 1999] Supplemental vitamin E and the amino acid cysteine may partially prevent some of this drug's toxicity. [J Pharm Belgium 53: 87-93, 1998] Silibin, an extract from milk thistle, protects against cisplatin toxicity to the kidneys. [Nephrology Dialysis Transplantation 11: 55-62, 1996] A lab dish study indicates quercetin may inhibit cisplatin toxicity. [Archives Toxicology 72: 536-40, 1998] Vitamin C is another anti-toxin to cisplatin. [Acta Biochim Poland 48: 233-40, 2001] Patients taking vitamin E and cisplatin experience a decrease in nerve damage. [Journal Clinical Oncology 21: 927-31, 2003]

Adriamycin

Adriamycin is an anti-cancer drug that can produce life-threatening side effects. Adriamycin (doxorubicin) is used to treat a wide variety of cancers of the blood, lymph system, bladder and breast. The heart tissue is vulnerable to toxicity from adriamycin, which can cause a profound decrease in blood pressure, a markedly increased heart rate, and a decrease in the volume of blood the heart pumps. This is often accompanied by fatigue and sometimes depression. This drug has also been shown to deplete cancer patients of vitamin C. [Free Radical Biology Medicine 21: 383-90, 1996]

Adriamycin is a mycin antibiotic and, cancer cells develop resistance to them over time. What's more, adriamycin works only for a short time.

Among children and young adults treated with adriamycin, adverse effects upon the heart have now been found up to 22 years following treatment. [International Journal Cardiology July 21, 2006 online]

Adriamycin often induces heart failure among cancer patients. It has even been found to induce late onset heart failure, five years or more after completion of treatment. Taxol, another anti-cancer drug, may cause a slowed heart rate (bradycardia) in up to 29% of patients treated. The combination of Adriamycin and Taxol can produce heart failure in up to 18% of treated patients. 5-FU also produces toxicity to the heart. Radiation therapy can also be cardiotoxic. [Cancer Investigation 17: 408-22, 1999] The heart is at great risk during chemo and radiation therapy.

A key antioxidant that alleviates some of the cardiac risks posed by cancer drugs is coenzyme Q10 (CoQ10). This supplemental antioxidant prevents changes in the electrocardiogram of adriamycin patients. [Research Communications Chemical Pathology Pharmacology 23: 199-202, 1979] Intravenous CoQ10 has been shown to significantly reduce abnormalities in the cardiogram (from 92 to 64%) of human cancer patients. [Gan To Kagaku Ryoho 11: 1420-27, 1984] CoQ10 protects heart tissues without interfering with the anti-tumor effect of adriamycin. [Research Communication Chemical Pathology Pharmacology 29: 309-15, 1980] In an animal study more mice survived adriamycin treatment when given coenzyme Q10 (80% vs 40%). [Research Communications Chemical Pathology Pharmacology 24: 401-04, 1979] No side effects have been reported from CoQ10 supplementation of up to 200 mg. [Ureskr Kaeger 159: 7309-15, 1997]

Drug versus natural therapy: same mechanism

An interesting comparison is the mechanism of the anti-cancer drug Adriamycin (doxorubicin) and the mechanism of vitamin C. Both Adriamycin and intravenous vitamin C destroy tumors by generating hydrogen peroxide inside cancer cells. The difference is that Adriamycin is a very toxic drug. Even one dose can cause blindness. And, it harms healthy cells as well as cancer cells. On the other hand, intravenous vitamin C selectively kills cancer cells without toxicity.

A study conducted by researchers at the University of Iowa Carver College of Medicine and Holden Comprehensive Cancer Center, Iowa City, Iowa, found that intravenous Adriamycin exerts its cancer-killing effect by increasing hydrogen peroxide (H2O2) inside tumor cells. Hydrogen peroxide levels rise by 4-fold in prostate cancer cells when Adriamycin is employed. [Archives Biochemistry Biophysics 440: 181-90, 2005]

Now researchers clearly show high-dose vitamin C, when administered intravenously, can increase hydrogen peroxide (H2O2) levels within cancer cells and selectively kill them. I.V. vitamin C has also been demonstrated to kill germs and may be an effective therapy for infectious disease. [Proceedings National Academy Sciences 102: 13604-09, 2005]

Unlike cancer drugs, I.V. vitamin C selectively kills cancer cells, but not healthy cells, and shows no toxicity. The ability of intravenous vitamin C to kill lymphoma cells is remarkable – almost 100% at easily achievable blood serum concentrations.

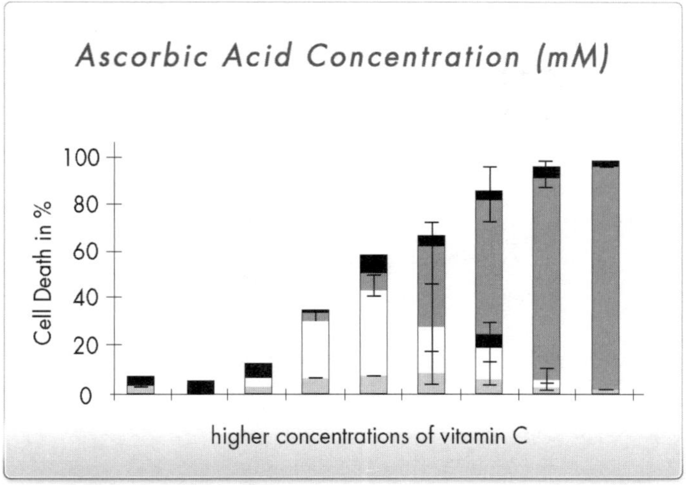

Chart Shows High-Dose Intravenous Vitamin C Killed Almost All Lymphoma Cancer Cells

It has now been shown that intravenous vitamin C can produce 140-times greater concentration of vitamin C in blood serum, a sufficient concentration to kill cancer cells. [Annals Internal Medicine 140:533-7, 2004] This revelation vindicates the work of Dr. Linus Pauling who conducted studies years ago and demonstrated that intravenous vitamin C can prolong the life of terminal cancer patients.

A national commitment to the prevention of cancer, largely replacing reliance on hopes for universal cures, is now the way to go.
Source: John C. Bailar III, MD, PhD in Cancer Undefeated, New England Journal Medicine 336: 1569, 1997

Some anti-cancer drugs are synthetic versions of natural molecules that can be mimicked with less problematic and less costly natural molecules. For example, the anti-cancer drug oltipraz is a synthetic version of the molecules found in cruciferous vegetables like cauliflower, brussels sprouts and cabbage.

Business Week magazine says there are now 402 cancer drugs in development, compared to 126 a decade ago. The American public is going to have these drugs literally shoved down their throat.

Reasons why chemotherapy doesn't work

- Drug resistance produced by enzymes in the liver (cytochrome p450 enzymes).
- State of the tissue (native untreated tissue, chemotherapy is up to 90% effective, but in previously treated tissues, this drops to 20-30%)
- Detoxification antioxidants in tissues (glutathione) that nullify toxic drugs
- Physical barriers (blood/brain barriers)
- Poor movement of anti-cancer drugs toward the tumor
- pH surrounding the tumor: acidity repels and destroys drug before it enters cancer cells
- Length of chemotherapy (prolonged treatment increases drug resistance)
- Inability to enter cell nucleus
- Activation of DNA repair enzymes that counter toxic drug effects
- Synthesis of P-glycoprotein on the surface of cells (pumps anti-cancer drugs out of cells)

Despite promising discoveries and multibillion dollar investments, cancer research is quietly undergoing a crisis. Initiatives will be soon introduced in hopes they will help salvage the field.
- Gardiner Harris, New York Times, Dec. 21, 2005

Most tumors are not sensitive to the drugs

Suffering through chemotherapy is worth it — when it helps patients live longer. But many patients end up with no benefit from chemotherapy as a secondary treatment after cancer surgery. A shocking study shows that just 4% of patients undergoing chemotherapy for non-small cell lung cancer experienced prolonged survival. In fact, the 5-year survival for patients who elected not to undergo chemotherapy was 39%. [New England Journal Medicine 355: 983-91, 2006]

5-Fluorouracil (5-FU) is the most commonly used drug to treat colon cancer. Virtually every colon cancer patient receives a course of 5-FU. It has been used for decades. However it only works in about 20-25% of patients. [Tumori 78: 258-61, 1992; Cancer 76: 1709-14, 1995; Nature Medicine 3: 1233-41, 1997] For most patients receiving 5-FU, there is little chance it will work and the patient may experience side effects.

Drug resistance

Drug resistance is a major obstacle in the treatment of cancer. [Nature 390: 404-07, 1997] Multi-drug resistance has remained a major issue for over a decade. The mechanisms behind drug resistance are known. Various chemicals can effectively inhibit drug resistance, but most are toxic themselves.

The intricate defense-mechanisms in living cells are intriguing. A substance produced inside gastric cells, called P-glycoprotein, literally pumps toxic anti-cancer drugs out of cells and inhibits their absorption. So now drug researchers are attempting to place their cancer drugs inside liposomes or nanospheres, to hide them from cellular detoxification systems. [Journal Medicinal Chemistry 46: 4805-17, 2003]

Some drugs, like verpamil, cyclosporine, nifedipine, quinidine and reserpine, inhibit P-glycoprotein. However, these drugs are weak inhibitors of P-glycoprotein and drug resistance still develops.

Natural agents like hypericum in St. John's wort and grapefruit juice can decrease levels of drugs by increasing the action of P-glycoprotein. The very introduction of toxic anti-cancer drugs activates more P-glycoprotein that makes cancer cells even more resistant to treatment. Chemotherapy then proceeds in a backwards fashion. There is little wonder that chemotherapy often fails.

Overcoming cancer resistance

There also may be genetic resistance to anti-cancer drugs. Dr. Robert Nagourney, a hematologist/oncologist, established Rational Therapeutics, Inc., in 1993 in Long Beach, California, in order to bring some sense of intelligent use of anti-cancer drugs as opposed to the seemingly haphazard methods employed by most oncologists. Oncologists admit their drugs often don't work, and even if they do initially, over time tumor cells begin to resist the drugs and they become ineffective. Patients may have pre-existing resistance to cancer drugs. Then, since tumor cells have been subjected to prior treatment, they may exhibit more resistance to other subsequent drugs that may be prescribed. Dr. Nagourney recognized that the loss of tumor cell membrane integrity correlated with survival.

Once Dr. Nagourney's laboratory receives a fresh sample of diseased tissue that has not been exposed to chemotherapy or radiation in the past four weeks, it can be analyzed to see how it would respond to various anti-cancer drugs. A published study of 27 cancer patients with ovarian cancer who were treated with two drugs, found when tissue samples were assayed for effectiveness of anti-cancer drugs, there were 26% complete and 44% partial responses to treatment, or an overall response rate of 70%. [Gynecologic Oncology 88: 35-39, 2003] Dr. Nagourney's idea is to start with drug therapy that is more likely to work than not in an individual patient. It is dismaying that there is no rational method to select anti-cancer drugs for individual patients after more than 50 years of their use. There are many testimonies from patients who underwent unsuccessful chemotherapy and then after tissue assay and appropriate drug selection, they survived cancer treatment.

[www.rational-t.com] Rational Therapeutics is located at 750 East 29th Street, Long Beach, CA 90806. Telephone (562) 989-6455.

Glutathione

Glutathione is another detoxifying agent in the body that causes drug resistance. The content of glutathione in living tissues dictates its resistance to anti-cancer drug treatment.

Glutathione Content Among Normal Human Tissues		
Tissue	Minimum	Maximum
Breast	0.72	29.53
Colon	0.54	21.95
Rectal	2.15	35.08
GI	3.96	18.84
Melanoma	0.29	18.75

Source: Cancer Research 54: 5351-56, 1994

High levels of glutathione also inhibit radiation treatment for cancer. [International Journal Cancer 67: 661-67, 1996] Buthionine sulfoximine is a drug used to lower glutathione levels in cells. This drug has been shown to enhance the cancer-fighting activity of various drugs. [Journal Radiation Oncology Biological Physics 16: 1289-95, 1989]

A study of uterine cancer patients correlated the concentration of glutathione in cancer cells with response from chemotherapy. A greater than 50% reduction in tumor size was produced by chemotherapy among 7 of 10 patients whose tumor glutathione levels were low compared to only 3 of 10 patients whose glutathione tumor levels were high. However, it should be noted that there must be other factors involved to explain why 3 of 10 patients with high glutathione tumor levels did in fact experience reduction in tumor size. [Cancer 79: 521-27, 1997]

Glutathione is a natural detoxifier and antioxidant in the body. Efforts to reduce glutathione to increase drug effectiveness only result in greater side effects, and the patient never gets well.

Natural inhibition of drug resistance

In laboratory dish studies, essential fatty acids, omega-3s from fish or flax (EPA and DHA), and GLA oils from primrose, borage or black currant seed, have been shown to reverse resistance for selected drugs like vincristine, cis-platinum and doxorubicin. [Prostaglandins Leukotrienes Essential Fatty Acids 58: 39-54, 1998]

Natural Inhibitors of P-glycoprotein

(Listed from greatest to least inhibition of food-spoilage bacteria)

Source: FEBS Letters 272: 4725-40, 2005; Biochemistry Biophysical Research Communications 327: 866-70, 2005 Cancer Chemotherapy Pharmacology 34: 459-64, 1994

- Silymarin from milk thistle
- Gensenosides from ginseng
- Piperine from black pepper
- Curcumin from Turmeric
- Resveratrol from red grapes
- Gingerol from ginger
- Capsaicin from cayenne pepper
- Quercetin from red onions
- Diallyl sulfide from garlic

Garlic and chemotherapy drug resistance

Diallyl sulfide from garlic inhibits P-glycoprotein production to normal levels in tumor cells. [Carcinogenesis 25: 941-49, 2004] Diallyl sulfide is able to increase the programmed cell death (apoptosis) of tumor cells. [Nutrition & Cancer 44: 89-94, 2002]

After 24 hours, tumor cells made resistant to an anti-cancer drug, then treated with diallyl sulfide from garlic became 23% less able to produce P-glycoprotein, the protein that pumps toxic cancer drugs out of tumor cells. After 72 hours, this inhibition of drug resistant protein was 79%. Researchers claim that their experiment reveals that a garlic molecule is *"a novel, selective and highly potent inhibitor of drug resistance... that exhibits little or virtually no side effects without any increase in medication burden on the patient."* [Cancinogenesis 25: 941-49, 2004]

Electric pulses

Studies show that electrical pulses can weaken cellular barriers that prevent the entry of anti-cancer drugs. The ability to kill cancer cells by one anti-cancer drug was increased by 95 times when tumor cells were exposed to electrical pulses. [Urology Research 28: 391-97, 2000] In another study, electric impulses plus chemo and radiation produced up to a six-fold more delay in tumor growth than chemo and radiation alone. [Radiation Research 162:185-93, 2004] How often electric impulses are employed to overcome drug resistance is unknown. Hopefully, further studies will reveal whether this additive therapy increases survival.

The future of chemotherapy

New cancer drug shrinks tumors, doesn't extend life.
Source: Headline, USA Today, November 2002

Gene targeted drugs

Gene-targeted drugs have been the latest drugs to be heralded as the answer to cancer.

The drugs are here, said the article by the Associated Press, 2003, but so is cancer. "*Even though some of these drugs have received FDA approval, lasting results are rare,*" said Daniel Y. Haney, Associated Press reporter. Haney is talking about the new gene-targeted anti-cancer drugs like Iressa, Herceptin and Erbitux. The drug that caused the initial euphoria, Herceptin, was later found to only delay the progression of breast cancer by a few months among patients with a specific genetic profile. Slight progress like this "*is sometimes breathlessly reported,*" said Haney. "*Right now, in the short run, we can bring an occasional miracle and have an overall small benefit,*" Dr. John Glaspy, medical director of the UCLA surgical oncology center was reported to have said.

"*They haven't panned out they way we thought they would,*" said oncologist David Decker of William Beaumonth Hospital outside Detroit about the gene-targeted drugs. One striking success, Gleevec, which works only on rare forms of blood cancer and digestive cancer, wears off over time.

> *Avastin, Erbitux, Gleevec... The new wonder drugs might make you think we're finally beating this dreaded scourge. We're not.*
> - Clifton Leaf Fortune Magazine, March 9, 2004

Yet, the gene targeted drugs go on being extolled. *"Stunning," "revolutionary," "jaw-dropping," "wonder drug," "cuts disease recurrence in half,"* are the words used to describe the three reports published in the New England Journal of Medicine involving Herceptin (trastuzumab). But if the published results are so "*jaw-dropping,*" why weren't they heralded earlier, when they were first reported at the American Society of Clinical Oncology meeting?

Women battling breast cancer are never going to hear the details of these studies. They are already rushing to line up for treatment. One woman in India was reported to be selling her house to pay for Herceptin. [London Times Oct. 20, 2005] It costs $48,000 (wholesale price) for a 12-month course of intravenous therapy. Herceptin isn't a stand-alone drug either. It was administered to women who had already undergone surgery and chemo and radiation therapy.

> *"Cancer doctors facing waiting rooms full of dying cancer patients, with little to offer but easing misery and perhaps a few extra months of survival, clearly had wished for more."*
> *Source: Daniel Q. Haney, Associated Press, 2003, speaking of the failure of targeted cancer drugs to cure cancer.*

Drowned out in the front-page publicity over Herceptin is the fact the Food & Drug Administration just issued a warning to doctors about the increased risk for heart failure when Herceptin is used with another chemotherapy drug, like the one used in the *New England Journal of Medicine* report. The incidence of heart failure rose over 500% (from 0.8% to 4.1%) among women receiving Herceptin and chemotherapy. [FDA Bulletin] [FDA Patient Safety News: #45, November 2005]

The news media, in typical fashion, unquestionably heralds Herceptin as a cure for breast cancer. Associated Press says 200,000 women are diagnosed with breast cancer each year in the United States and 40,000 die. But only 20% of these patients have the type of cancer influenced by the HER2 gene, the type of cancer that is targeted by Herceptin.

It is anticipated 30,000 American women may be taking Herceptin intravenously for at least a year following initial treatment. That's another $1.4 billion added to the healthcare bill for a year of treatment for these women. Bottom line, after deaths caused by Herceptin itself (due to heart failure) are deducted from the lives saved from breast cancer, there remains only about 1,500 more American women who will live at least another four years compared to women who don't take Herceptin.

Herceptin did seem to do an excellent job of preventing the spread of cancer to other organs (metastasis). However, Herceptin was not used on women who already had experienced a metastasis. Nor did Herceptin appear to do a good job of preventing the spread of cancer to the brain. In one of the three studies reported by the New England Journal of Medicine, 143 of 1,694 patients receiving Herceptin dropped out of the study because of adverse events. This may have skewed the results. Researchers acknowledge that "*we only have an incomplete picture of the risks associated with Herceptin. The risk of heart failure was low, but this could change over time.*" [New England Journal of Medicine 353: 1659-72, 2005]

Another unreported drawback is that Herceptin when combined with Taxol (Paciltaxel), another anti-cancer drug, may produce photosensitivity. Patients should be warned about sun exposure when taking these drugs. [Journal Dermatological Treatment 16: 19-21, 2005]

Given the high price of Herceptin, it should be noted that components found in olive oil (oleic acid) have been found to inhibit the HER2 proteins by 36%, while Herceptin inhibits them by 48%. [Journal Annals of Oncology, Jan. 10, 2005]

The reports extolling Herceptin in the *New England Journal of Medicine* were preceded by another report in *Nature Magazine* that said single-gene targeted drugs like Herceptin should be abandoned in favor of drugs that control many genes. [Nature 437: 942-943, 13 October 2005]

Herceptin

Trastuzumab

anti-HER2 monoclonal antibody

WARNINGS:
CARDIOMYOPATHY

HERCEPTIN administration can result in the development of ventricular dysfunction and congestive heart failure. Left ventricular function should be evaluated in all patients prior to and during treatment with HERCEPTIN. discontinuation of HERCEPTIN treatment should be strongly considered in patients who develop a clinically significant decrease in left ventricular function. The incidence and severity of cardiac dysfunction was particularly high in patients who received HERCEPTIN in combination with anthracyclines and cyclophosphamide. (See WARNINGS.)

HYPERSENSITIVITY REACTIONS INCLUDING ANAPHYLAXIS
INFUSION REACTIONS
PULMONARY EVENTS

HERCEPTIN administration can result in severe hypersensitivity reactions (including anaphylaxis), infusion reactions, and pulmonary events. Rarely, these have been fatal. In most cases, symptoms occured during or within 24 hours of administration of HERCEPTIN. HERCEPTIN infusion should be interrupted for patients experiencing dyspnea or clinically significant hypotension. Patients should be monitored until signs and symptoms completely resolve. Discontinuation of HERCEPTIN treatment should be stronly considered for patients who develop anaphylaxis, angioedema, or acute respiratory distress syndrom. (See WARNINGS.)

Herceptin Breast Cancer Statistics
Source: New England Journal Medicine 353: 1673-84, 2005

Herceptin/ breast cancer (only represents 20% of breast cancer patients)	Surgery + radiation + chemotherapy + Herceptin	Surgery + radiation + chemotherapy	Difference
Disease-free survival			
3 years	87.1%	75.4%	11.7%
4 years	85.3%	67.1%	18.2%
Distant cancers (metastases)			
3 years	90.4%	81.5%	8.9%
4 years	89.7%	73.7%	16.0%
Absolute survival	Because Herceptin causes heart failure in conjunction with chemotherapy, the net number of women still living (not just free of breast cancer) must be considered.		
Absolute survival at 3 years	94.3%	91.7%	2.6% (of 100 women who get Herceptin, only about 6 will die versus 8 who don't get the drug)
Absolute survival at 4 years	91.4%	86.6%	4.8% (of 100 women who get Herceptin, only about 8 will die versus 13 who don't get the drug)

The outrageous cost of gene-targeted drugs

Patients have a different view of the costs of cancer treatment. They feel they are facing a disease that poses a mortal risk, they paid for their health insurance or Medicare, and the insurers need to do battle over costs, not the patient. But patients are now paying considerable amounts of money out of their pockets because the newer types of drugs are not covered, or only partially covered by insurance.

A report written by Jeff Donn of the Associated Press says modern anti-cancer drugs produce an unanticipated side effect: acute sticker shock. He cites the case of a cancer patient who was told she would have to come up with $18,000 in cash to pay for one of these drugs because insurance didn't pay for it. The patient evaluated the few months of extended life against the cost and elected to forgo the treatment. *"It wasn't worth it,"* said the patient's husband.

The Associated Press reporter asks: *"Is the chance for several months of life – maybe a year or more with luck – precious enough to spend a small fortune?"* But up to a third of Americans want *"everything possible"* done to save their lives, according to a poll conducted by the Pew Research Center for the People and the Press. [Expensive Treatments force patients to choose, Jeff Dunn, Associated Press, August 27, 2006] What a situation to place patients in.

Selective chemotherapy

One cancer researcher states: *"For us, the Holy Grail would be finding a way to selectively kill cancer cells and not damage healthy ones."*

The goal of chemotherapy is the elimination of tumor cells from the host. This is achieved by the use of therapeutic agents that are often more harmful to normal tissues than to the targeted tumor.
- Therapeutic Drug Monitoring 26:231-5, 2004

The ideal anti-cancer drug would selectively kill cancer cells while leaving healthy cells intact. Unfortunately, most modern chemotherapy drugs are indiscriminate. However, allicin from garlic, resveratrol from red grapes, IP6 from rice bran, all selectively kill cancer cells without harming healthy ones, but go unnoticed and unused by modern medicine.

With over 300 drugs in the pharmaceutical pipeline, each designed to address cancer at a specific site, what would happen if an anti-cancer molecule were developed that prevents or treats cancer in all organs and tissues? That is precisely what resveratrol does.

When treatment is over, now what?

It is estimated that there are more than 10 million Americans living with cancer. [Journal National Cancer Institute 96: 1412, 2004] An embarrassing, if not distressing, report reveals that many cancer patients are not provided adequate follow-up care after treatment. The problem, says a report from the National Cancer Policy Board of the Institute of Medicine, is that cancer survivors mostly *"go it on their own."* After treatment, patients are sent back to their primary care physicians, often without a plan for follow-up care. The big problem is that doctors aren't reimbursed for follow-up care, so it gets neglected. [CA Cancer Journal Clinicians 56: 65-67, 2006] This is puzzling since a list of good health habits, dietary measures and dietary supplement regimens would suffice. A pre-printed sheet of paper with after-care instructions would go a long way. Once all the billing codes have been utilized for insurance claims, physicians virtually abandon patients.

We may look back on this period as the dark ages of cancer treatment, when our ignorance of the basic causes of cancer and the biology of the cancer cell led us to use toxic mixtures of randomly selected chemicals, more in the hope than in the expectation of a cure for the disease.
– Garth Powis, DPh, The Toxicity of Anticancer Drugs, Pergamon Press, 1991.

Which Model of Cancer Care Is Best?

Conventional Cancer Treatment	Alternative Cancer Treatment	Nutritional Cancer Care
■ Chemotherapy ■ Radiation therapy ■ Surgery	■ Herbal therapy example: Essiac tea ■ Diet therapy example: Gerson diet ■ Chelation therapy ■ Vitamin therapy ■ Alkaline therapies ■ Vitamin B17 apricot pits: laetrile	■ Natural enzyme inhibitors: quercetin, resveratrol ■ Natural blood thinners: flax/fish oil, vitamin E, garlic (allicin), magnesium, resveratrol ■ Natural chelators: IP6 rice bran extract ■ Natural cell regulators: curcumin, resveratrol ■ Natural anti-inflammatory agents: flax/fish oil, pomegranate, resveratrol ■ Natural gene suppressors: resveratrol

A man fights for the life of his wife

Following is an example of what a friend of mine wrote me when his wife was diagnosed with cancer:

Some months ago I told you my wife had stage four lung cancer. I read about IP6 rice bran extract. The problem at the time was that my wife only wanted what the hospital and her oncologists were offering. I can't say that I blame her. This is life or death for her.

After chemo and several radiations, and the many horrific side effects, she developed another tumor in her brain. She has refused radiation and is now going to another doctor, an alternative MD. She is taking many nutrients three times daily, including IP6 and many I never heard of. She is following the approach of a European doctor.

Anna has gone back to work. She looks and says she feels great. Am I hoping for a miracle?

Second communication:

I am so naive and stupid. Having just bought and read, "*Cancer cures and what they don't want you to know.*" I should have realized that the author is right on. "*It is all about the money.*" There is much info on the web about the European doctor's work I mentioned earlier. I am just trying to save my dear wife from an early death, but the money comes first.

Third communication:

I won't email you after this, but I must tell you that when my wife went to the oncologist, and asked about vitamins, he said take *"a major multivitamin intended for use by children"*. After months of chemo the tumor in her lung got larger. When I asked the oncologist if acupuncture could help the terrible pain my wife was suffering, in the groin, even with large doses of morphine drugs, he said acupuncture does not work with cancer. The very next day at the alternative doctor's clinic she got an hour of acupuncture, and went to work the following day, pain free.

My wife's life is hanging by a thread, and I don't know who the hell to believe anymore. Please give me some advice.

Acts of desperation: when all else fails

Word of an overlooked and unpatentable cancer drug began to spread like wildfire in early 2007 when a Canadian researcher begged for research funds to study the drug. [Cancer Cell 11: 37-51, 2007] The drug, dichloroacetate, or DCA, works by restoring energy to energy compartments within cancer cells, making them self-destruct. While unproven, terminal cancer patients heard something different – hope.

Knowing they have limited time and that their doctors have run out of treatments to prescribe, an online effort began to educate the public about DCA, and another sister website to sell DCA (though no claims about a cancer cure are made there). These unprecedented events went so far as setting up an online database to collect results from cancer patients, a kind of unofficial way of alerting the public to DCAs effectiveness and safety, or lack thereof. The battle between dying patients who want immediate access to unapproved drugs and health plans is ongoing. [Nature 446: 474-75, 2007; New Scientist March 31, 2007] DCA is just another example.

God knows, humanity needs a treatment for cancer that works and doesn't kill the patients before it cures. So a University of Alberta press release says a *"small molecule offers big hope against cancer."* DCA is an odorless, colorless, inexpensive, and *"relatively non-toxic"* drug that has already been used in humans to treat a condition called lactic acidosis.

OK, lactic acidosis is the common state of metabolism in cancer cells. Cancer cells, lacking the ability to produce energy from within their own cellular machinery (mitochondria), revert to producing sugar for cell energy, which produces lactic acid as a by-product. The lactic acid dumps outside the cell, repelling anti-cancer agents and making the cancer cell immortal. Dammit, these tumor cells won't die off like normal cells.

So the researchers found that dichloroacetate (DCA) revives the energy-producing compartments (mitochondria) within cancer cells, eventually resulting in cancer cell death (what researchers called apoptosis). DCA did no harm to surrounding healthy cells, so it might be non-toxic.

Modern medicine is desperately searching for anti-cancer molecules that kill cancer cells and leave healthy cells alone. Unfortunately, chemotherapy today is very toxic to tumor and healthy cells alike, and the patient often succumbs to the treatment rather than their disease. Furthermore, cells don't like the toxic drugs, they develop a resistance to them, so chemotherapy usually only works for a short time.

The University of Alberta researchers note that DCA has already been used in humans to treat mitochondrial disease with *"relative"* non-toxicity. But they lament that DCA is unpatentable so it is not likely to receive any attention, or research funding, from a pharmaceutical company.

Now there is the rub. The admission there may be a cure for cancer out there, but it's gotta make a big profit for a drug company or they won't pay attention to it. This is commercially understandable. However, this serves to say, simpler remedies may exist, but patients are going to have to go on a scavenger hunt to find them on their own.

The university-based researchers sought widespread publicity for DCA hoping a private source would provide research funds. [Small molecule offers big hope against cancer, University of Alberta press release, Jan. 17, 2007]

But treating mice in the laboratory is a long way from proving a cancer drug not only kills cancer cells, but actually improves survival. There are a lot of drugs that shrink tumors, but don't improve survival. When DCA was used in humans in 1983, it effectively reduced lactic acidosis and normalized blood pressure. The drug itself produced no known toxicity, but 12 of 13 DCA-treated patients still died. [New England Journal Medicine 309: 390-96, 1983]

In animals, DCA induces liver toxicity and neoplasia (yep, cancer!). DCA is actually a by-product of water chlorination, chlorine being one of the most toxic molecules on the planet. [Environmental Health Perspectives 106 (Suppl 4): 989-994, 1998]

Of interest, the toxic side effects of DCA may emanate from inducement of a vitamin B 1 (thiamine) deficiency. The chronic use of dichloroacetate (DCA) for diabetes has been compromised by nerve and other forms of toxicity. DCA is metabolized to glyoxylate, which is converted to oxalate and, in the presence of adequate thiamine levels, to other metabolites. Nerve toxicity from DCA administration appears to result from depletion of body thiamine stores and abnormal metabolism of oxalate, a known nerve toxin. The co-administration of vitamin B1 with DCA reduces urinary oxalate levels from 86% above normal to only 28% above normal. [Toxicological Sciences 14: 327-37, 1990] Maybe this tips off how DCA actually works, by depriving cells of an essential nutrient.

The flurry of interest in DCA will continue just as Rife machines, laetrile and alkaline therapy for cancer has persisted for decades with no real observable cures. Once these cures become urban legends, they are perpetuated by the desperate and the naïve. Resveratrol, known as a red wine molecule, has similar biological action to DCA without known toxicity, and should be investigated by cancer patients before racing to the internet to purchase DCA.

5-Year Cancer Survival			
Type	1974-76 %	1977-80 %	1981-87 %
All types	49	49	51
Oral cavity and pharynx	53	52	51
Esophagus	5	5	8
Colon	50	53	57
Rectum	48	50	54
Liver	4	3	5
Pancreas	3	3	3
Larynx	65	66	66
Lung	12	13	13
Melanoma of skin	79	81	82
Breast (female)	74	74	77
Cervical/uterus	68	67	66
Ovary	36	38	39
Prostate gland	67	71	74
Testes	78	88	93
Urinary bladder	72	75	78
Kidney	51	52	53
Brain & nervous system	22	24	25
Thyroid gland	92	93	94
Hodgkin's disease	71	73	78
Non-Hodgkins' lymphoma	47	48	51
Multiple myeloma	24	26	27
Leukemia	34	36	35

Cancer Survival Time, in years, by Age at diagnosis 1960-73 data *Source: Carcinogenesis and Aging Volume II CRC Press 1987*					
Tumor site	Under 45	45-54	55-64	65-74	75 and over
Colon	4.5	3.4	3.2	2.6	1.2
Lung	6.3	6.6	5.7	5	3.5
Breast	10	10	7.3	5.9	3.3
Prostate	1.9	6.7	5.8	4	2.1

Common Drugs Used to Treat Cancer, by Location	
Organ	Drug
Heart	Doxorubicin (Adriamycin), daunomycin
Kidney	Cisplatin, methotrexate, nitrosourea
Peripheral nervous system	Vincristine, cisplatin
Ears (hearing)	Cisplatin
Gastrointestinal - Nausea/vomiting - Mucositis	Most drugs, esp. cisplatin Methotrexate, 5-fluorouracil Vincristine, 5-fluorouracil
Liver	Methotrexate, 6-mercaptopurine, sytosine arabinoside, nitrosoureas, L-asparaginase
Bladder	Cyclophosphamide
Colon	5-FU, levamisole, interferon
Lung	Bleomycin, busulfan, carmustine, methotrexate
Testes	Alkylating agents
Ovary	Busulfan, chlorambucil, cyclphosphamide, vinblastine
Bone	Methotrexate, 6-mercaptopurine
Bone marrow	Most drugs except vincristine, bleomycin, cisplatin
Skin and blood vessels - Hair loss	Doxorubicin, cyclphoosphamide, nitrosoureas, 5-fluorouracil Nitrogen mustard, anthracyclines, actinomycin D, vinblastine, mitomycin C

CHAPTER 4

Alternatives

p 110 - 124

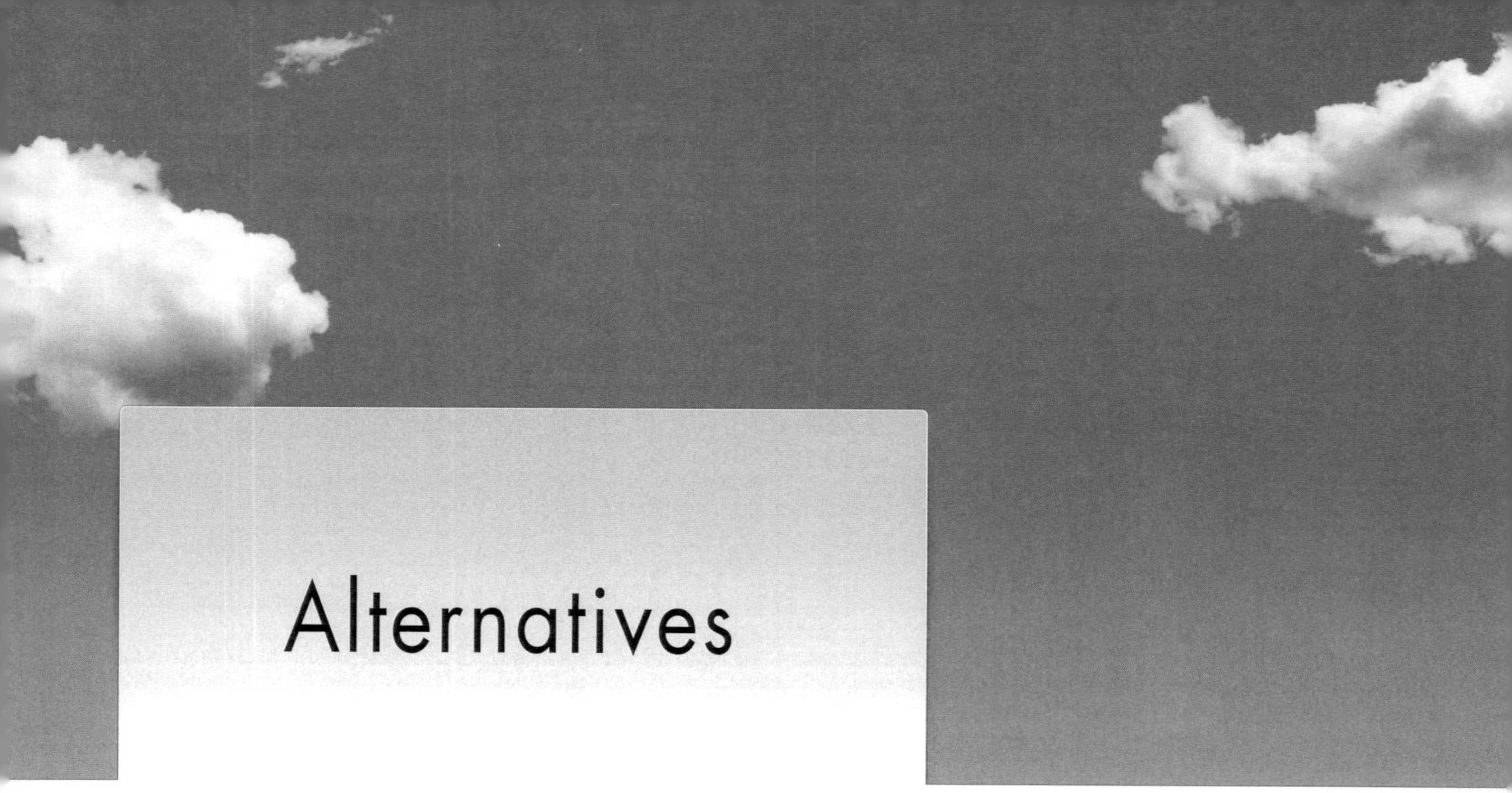

Alternatives

Alternative cures for cancer

The primary theme of this chapter is that alternative remedies for cancer, many spawned in past eras on nothing more than a hunch that they would work, need to be abandoned in favor of more promising alternatives that are now backed by hard science.

Many alternative therapies for cancer are so entrenched that they are not likely to disappear. For instance, even though shark cartilage was not found to produce remissions from cancer, patients still ask about it. Vitamin B17-laetrile, which may be an effective cancer treatment in the hands of a doctor who can administer it intravenously, may be ineffective, or even toxic when given by an incompetent doctor.

Time line of alternative cancer therapies

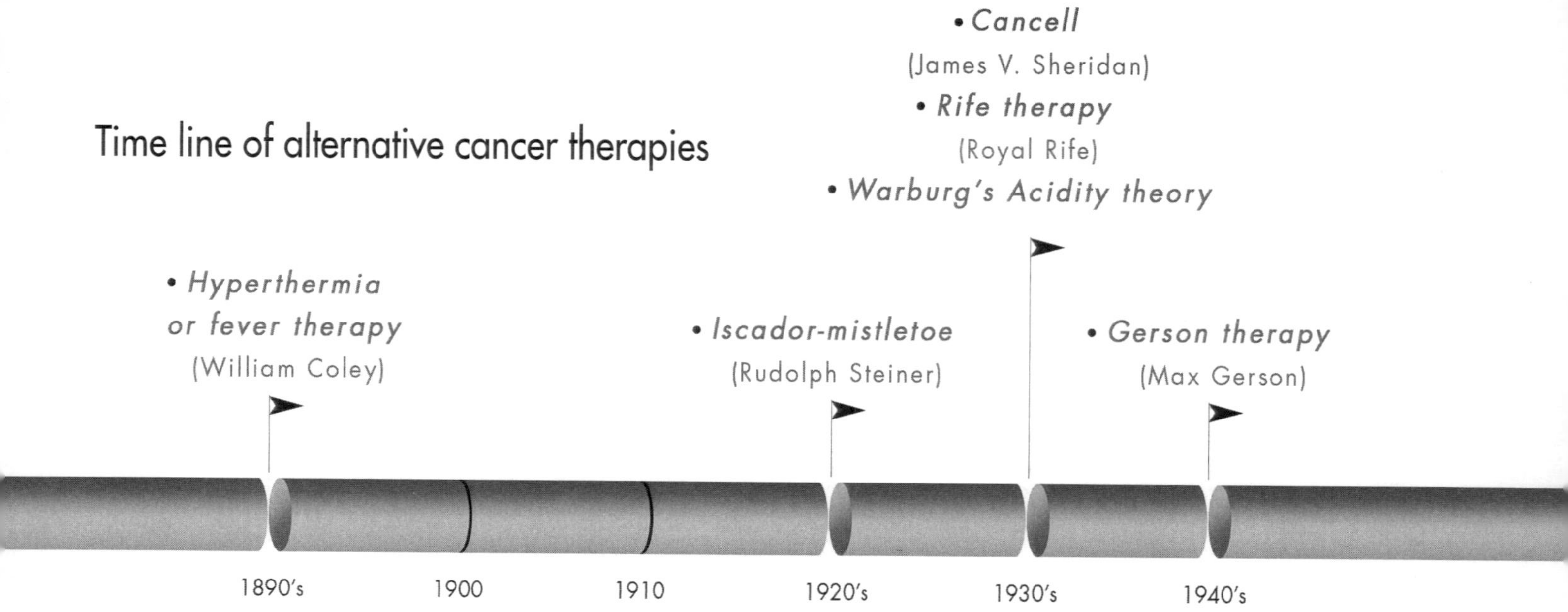

The good news is that there are scientifically valid alternatives to harsh chemo and radiation treatments that are available to cancer patients today. But to find them, cancer patients may need to abandon the traditional remedies of the past.

Cancer patients cannot be faulted for trying every possible means to cure this disease. What are cancer patients to do? The 30-year, $30+ billion (actually $200 billion) campaign to cure cancer has failed. Survival rates have not improved and many cancer patients are told, after undergoing numerous rounds of harsh radiation and chemotherapy, that there is nothing more that can be done. So the search for alternatives is often begun when the cancer has spread and there is even less hope for remission. Desperation prevails.

Cancer patients search for alternatives because they are aware that modern treatment is harsh and many have friends and family members for whom cancer treatment was ineffective. A report in a cancer journal concedes: *"A major reason for today's massive public and professional interest in alternatives is dissatisfaction with the technologic and impersonal nature of modern medicine."* [Cancer 77: 1026, 1996]

A published paper suggests that *"alternative therapies may mislead patients away from potentially helpful treatments to unproven therapies."* [Cancer 77: 1026, 1996] Yet a 1984 study found that 51% of doctors providing alternative therapies were MDs themselves.

Much of modern cancer treatment has been disproven, while many alternative therapies are unproven. So we find doctors practicing what doesn't work over what hasn't been fully investigated as yet. It's all part of the insanity in cancer care today.

Andrew Vickers, PhD, a research methodologist at the Memorial Sloan-Kettering Cancer Center in New York, asserts that alternative cancer cures are not just unproven, they have been disproven. [CA Cancer Journal Clinicians 54: 110-18, 2004] Dr. Vickers, like many others, has blinders on. The failings of modern cancer therapy are readily apparent. Conventional cancer treatment has been disproven as well. This is the depressing state of affairs in cancer treatment today. Nothing works, and some treatments are toxic.

Alternative treatments for cancer often are nothing more than a grab-bag of outdated traditional remedies or outright

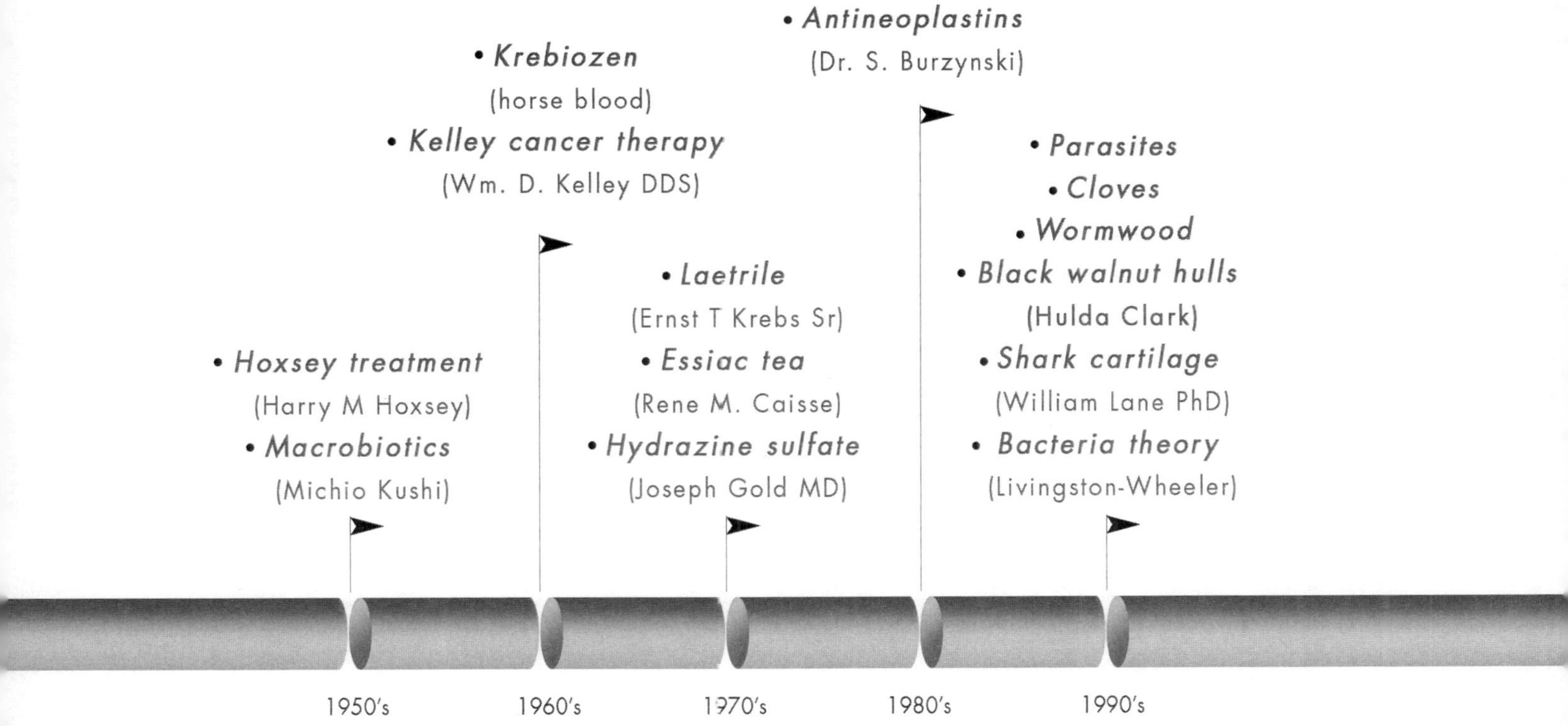

fraudulent cures that have little chance of prolonging survival. The main advantage of conventional cancer care is that the patient receives guidance from his or her doctors and sometimes the support of a staff, whereas the cancer patient opting for alternative therapies will often be on an unguided tour of myriads of so-called cancer cures and may not have the support of family and friends. Also, let's not forget that insurance covers conventional care, whereas patients are on their own financially when it comes to unconventional treatments.

Does alternative cancer therapy work?

In 1992, researchers in Norway surveyed 1,000 cancer patients about alternative treatments. Their study did not find that alternative treatments produced longer survival time than did conventional treatments, though it is likely that many cancer patients may have resorted to using alternative therapies when their tumors were beyond treatment, which would produce an unfair comparison. [European Journal Cancer 31: 1785-89, 1995] Still, alternative therapies, with the exception of high-dose vitamin C, have yet to clearly demonstrate any advantage over conventional treatment.

Readers may wonder why there is such a brief mention of many widely promoted alternative cancer therapies in this book. The reason is that many of these therapies are not based upon sound theory, are outdated, and are frankly ineffective. This may disappoint readers who have their own pet anti-cancer therapies. There will surely be those whose personal experience runs contrary to what has just been stated. But unless alternative anti-cancer treatments are solely utilized, the effectiveness of any one product or treatment method would be difficult to prove. Most people use a combination of treatments.

There are some who believe that proven anti-cancer remedies have been withheld from the public by pharmaceutical companies. There may be some truth to this, but many of the possible cures that have been withheld are not found in most of the widely utilized alternative therapies in vogue today.

The new alternatives

The alternative medicine community should be trumpeting the charge towards the new molecular therapy for cancer. Instead, it is mired in the meager treatments of the past.

The mapping of the human genome and the ability to conduct gene array tests to determine which molecules switch genes *"on or off"* is revolutionizing the approach to prevention and treatment of disease. Small molecules, such as found in grapes, olives, garlic, pomegranates and cherries, are able to pass through cell walls and the nucleus of cells to switch genes on or off. Small molecules like allicin from garlic, resveratrol from grapes, quercetin from onions, hydroxytyrosol from olives, influence so many genes they are being heralded as the drugs of the future.

Many people falsely believe that to concede that alternative cancer therapies are ineffective gives tacit credence to often despised toxic conventional treatments. Advocates of alternative cancer therapies are going to have to let go of their favorite remedies in favor of the new generation of anti-cancer molecules that are being revealed in scientific studies almost on a daily basis.

The growing evidence that nutrients such as folic acid, rice bran extract (IP6), vitamin D, vitamin C, and resveratrol, to name a few, and not patentable man-made molecules, are the most potent weapons we have against cancer. This should bring embarrassment, if not shame, upon the entire cancer research and treatment community. Molecules that cannot be improved upon, that are safe and economical, that have existed in nature for centuries, have been grossly overlooked by cancer doctors. Millions of people have died prematurely because of this oversight.

Conventional cancer treatment is entrenched because it is delivered by entities that exert control over insurance and research funding. The prevailing pharmaceutical and physician groups will attempt to prolong their sources of income as long as possible. Pharmaceutical companies have already infiltrated the FDA, the National Cancer Institute and the Memorial Sloan Kettering Cancer Center, in order to maintain their income stream. Alternative medicine advocates only facilitate the status quo and the domination of toxic cancer therapies when they continue to embarrass themselves by embracing marginal therapies. Just show the public ANY alternative treatment that works, and the whole counterfeit cancer treatment system will collapse.

While Rife Technology, laetrile, shark cartilage, and many other alternative cancer treatments have not withstood scientific scrutiny over the course of time, the hallowed research laboratories sponsored by the National Cancer Institute are now validating natural molecules as far more effective than the re-arranged pharmaceutical molecules that comprise most cancer drugs in use today. Resveratrol, curcumin, indole 3 carbinol, IP6 rice bran extract, vitamin D, and flax lignans, are being widely extolled in scientific journals such as *Science and Nature Magazine, Carcinogenesis, Cancer Research*, and many other journals. Why not begin to use them, in measured doses and concentrations that are known to work?

Status quo

One of the reasons why alternative medicine is not ready to break away from its past is that its practitioners, just like doctors who practice conventional cancer treatment, are financially dependent upon their therapies. This is why this book promotes the idea of self care. Cancer prevention and therapy can be practiced at home, without harm. Only a patient-driven movement will revolutionize cancer treatment and improve survival rates. Doctors, whether conventional or alternative, are not likely to offer treatments that put themselves out of business. If effective cancer prevention is practiced, the growing number of baby boomers who face an increased risk for cancer as they pass the age of 50, may be able to avoid or delay the onset of cancer. As previously explained in this book, once cancer is detected it is usually too large (more than a billion cells) or has spread (metastasized) to the point where any treatment would be ineffective. As they say, an ounce of prevention is better than a pound of cure.

Prevailing over poor health habits

Another glaring weakness in modern cancer treatment is that patients who successfully endure treatment are not seriously encouraged to follow any preventive measures beyond the advice to eat more plant foods and stop smoking. Recurrence rates are high because virtually nothing is being done to effectively prevent cancer's return. As previously mentioned, most people aren't able to successfully withdraw from tobacco, nor implement an unfamiliar diet.

The new anti-cancer molecules, now widely available as food supplements, have the potential to overcome poor health habits and prevent recurrence. While taking them doesn't give license for people to continue to smoke or to eat damaging foods, the fact is, people don't find it easy to give up their habits.

While this book emphasizes that the "*gold standard*" used to compare cancer treatments is survival, other important aspects of cancer care are degree of pain and side effects. Family members don't want their loved ones to be in pain, or to experience constant diarrhea, nausea, or fatigue, which are common side effects experienced during and after conventional cancer treatment. While there has been a greater emphasis on pain management during end-stage cancer treatment in recent times, other issues that may seem trivial to cancer doctors, such as nausea and constipation, are aggravating and often unremitting to the cancer patient. The quality of life for a cancer patient is equally important during the course of treatment. A recent survey conducted among patients with breast, colon and lung cancer, found 73 percent took dietary supplements with some improvement in symptoms of constipation, appetite loss, and fatigue. [Supportive Care Cancer July 30, 2005]

Should You Shun Conventional Medicine and Embrace Alternative Therapies?

Should cancer patients shun conventional medicine and embrace alternative therapies? Michael Gearin-Tosh, an eminent scholar in English literature at Oxford, faced this question head on when he was diagnosed with early stage multiple myeloma in 1994 at the age of 54. He wrote a book about his experience, *Living Proof, A Medical Mutiny* [Scribner, 2002] Turmoil and terror gripped Gearin-Tosh as he looked at the depressing survival data in the textbooks. Guerin-Tosh asked: *"if there is no cure, then what was the purpose of being rushed into treatment?"*

His friends aided in him in his research about this form of cancer. A friend consulted with Professor Ernst Wynder, formerly of Sloan-Kettering Cancer Research Center in New York. Wynder said: *"If your friend touches chemotherapy, he's a goner."* When asked by another friend if he had cancer, he said, *"yes."* She responded by saying: *"For God's sake, don't let the doctors kill you."* That was enough for him. Yet his colleagues were alarmed that he would even consider alternative therapies and reject chemotherapy.

Despite a host of experts from the cancer world who lined up to recommend chemotherapy, Guerin-Tosh opted for a mixed bag of alternative therapies including Gerson therapy, dietary measures such as a low-iron diet, high dose vitamin D and vitamin C, selenium, acupuncture, breathing exercises, and juicing, to name a few. It was not a popular decision. Even Wynder said *"I would not put my dog on Gerson therapy."*

Among the many substances and practices he followed, the only alternative measures likely to have been beneficial would be his low-iron diet and high vitamin D therapy. Guerin-Tosh, like many millions who live in northern climates, most likely did not produce enough vitamin D from sun exposure due to the angle of the sun at that latitude. The cancer belt in the world runs around the globe in northern latitudes. Guerin-Tosh's advisors gave him enough information to avoid toxic treatment which carries the risk of death. On the other hand, the advice he received on alternatives was only marginally helpful. Guerin-Tosh succumbed to cancer in 1965, nine years following his diagnosis. His quality of life during that period was better than most patients with the same type of cancer.

Acidity and Cancer

Acidity is an undesirable state, say many alternative health practitioners. The idea sounds plausible. The theory that an alkaline state is biologically beneficial began in the 1930s when two-time Nobel Prize winner Otto Warburg discovered that cancer cells are acidic. In reality, modern testing reveals cancer cells are slightly more alkaline than acidic, which is why they cannot ward off cancer-causing toxins or germs. Cancer cells are energetically weak and must produce energy via fermentation. A byproduct of fermentation is lactic acid which is expressed outside the cell, and which prevents cancer drugs or natural therapies from reaching the cancer cell. This is called drug resistance.

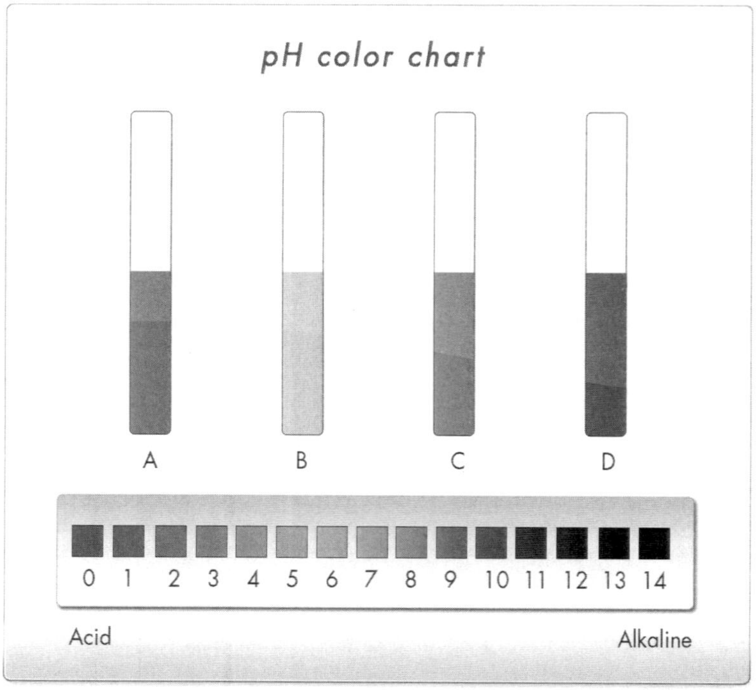

Acidity required for health

The human body utilizes acidity to protect itself from germs. The stomach is acid. Without stomach acid, germs like H. pylori can grow which can result in stomach cancer. An acid state is required to absorb many nutrients from foods and supplements, such as iron, calcium, zinc, vitamin C and B vitamins. Frequent use of antacids often results in a vitamin B12 deficiency. The bladder must maintain acidity or bacteria will adhere to the bladder wall, resulting in bladder infection.

The only exception to the rule is in the oral cavity where acid-forming streptococcus bacteria reside. The acidity of Streptococcus then eats through the enamel in teeth, resulting in dental cavities. But alternative health practitioners frequently advise their patients to test their pH orally with test strips. Overgrowth of the Streptococcus bacteria, or even reflux of stomach acid into the oral cavity, can result in an acidic state in the mouth. The pH in the mouth, however, does not reflect the pH level in other organs in the body.

A neutral pH is automatically maintained through blood circulation. If pH were dependent upon what humans eat, a state of acidosis or alkalosis would likely be common and require frequent trips to the hospital. In fact, the body continually maintains pH in the blood within a very tight range (7.35–7.45).

Cancer researchers confirm that there is an acidic shift in untreated tumors. However, there is a notable shift toward alkalinity in animal breast tissues following Adriamycin drug treatment. In one study, human brain tumors did not significantly differ in pH from healthy brain cells. But in another study involving bone tumors, the pH was more alkaline. Tumors that are larger may be easier to treat with radiation, which in turn generates more acidity. The greater the blood flow to a tumor (angiogenesis), the greater the alkalinity. This alkaline shift may be due to better blood flow removing lactic acid away from the tumor site, or decreased lactic acid production itself. [Cancer Research 48: 4075-85, 1989]

The area surrounding the tumor cells becomes acidic, not the tumor cell itself.

Warburg's findings led some astray. Warburg conducted research in the 1930s. By the 1980s researchers found that cancer cells in humans were neutral or slightly alkaline.

The connective tissue surrounding solid tumors is significantly more acidic compared to normal tissues, which reduces the uptake of some chemotherapy drugs and negates their effectiveness. [British Journal Cancer 80: 1005-11, 1999]

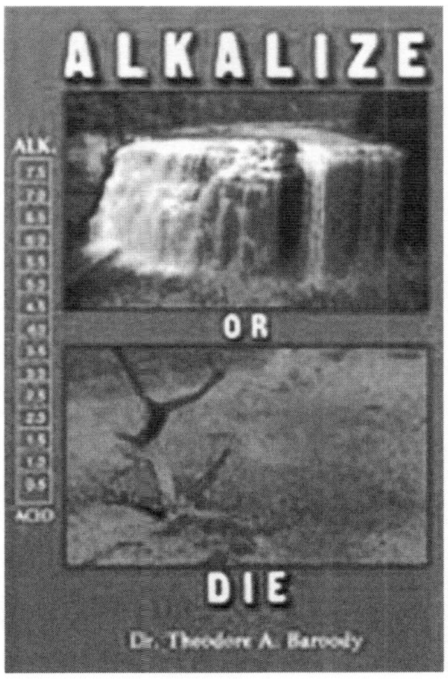

Alkalize Or Die
Dr. Theodore A. Baroody

University of Mississippi researchers reveal how health habits, like alcohol consumption, are involved in triggering metastatic cancer and the production of lactic acid. As alcohol enters cells, cells attempt to eliminate it. Because alcohol is difficult to break down, cells must increase metabolic activity which requires oxygen. The cells become oxygen deprived in their attempt to break down alcohol, a condition known as hypoxia. Oxygen- deprived cells then rely on fermentation for production of cellular energy, which results in the excretion of lactic acid from the cells. As previously explained, the acidity occurs outside the tumor cell.

Hypoxia, in turn, activates growth factors to produce new blood vessels (angiogenesis) to deliver more oxygen to the cells. New blood vessels then deliver more nutrients to cells and the tumor cells grow. [National Institutes of Health, American Physiology Society, April 4, 2006]

Even moderate consumption of alcohol can heighten the problem of angiogenesis and the growth and spread of tumors.

Antineoplastin therapy

Stanislaw Burzynski, MD, has gained considerable public attention for his antineoplastin cancer treatment in Houston, Texas. The therapy utilizes mixtures of amino acids and other simple organic substances that are said to promote the body's natural defenses. The public outrage over sanctions against alternative medical practitioners has caused authorities to back away from banning antineoplastin therapy outright. The treatment costs around $20,000 per patient and is not available outside of Texas. Because of its high cost and lack of affordability, and because there are many potentially more efficacious therapies at hand, this therapy is not promoted in this book. Its inventor claims antineoplastin therapy activates a system within the body that kills cancer cells that does not involve the human immune system. Burzynski has adequately defended antineoplastin therapy. [Townsend Letter for Doctors, March 1993] He now markets an affordable oral version of his therapy featuring amino acids, called Aminocare A10.

Bacterial theory

Virginia Livingston-Wheeler, MD, postulated in the 1990s that cancer is caused by a sole bacterium which she called *Progenitor cryptocides*. Her therapy included vaccines derived from urine, enemas, digestive enzymes, vegetarian diet, mineral supplements, and stress reduction. Livingston-Wheeler came close, but fell short of a cancer cure. Bacteria, viruses and other germs are believed to cause 10 percent of all cancer. Her remedies should have been antibiotics and proven immune boosters. Her hit-and-miss approach was ineffective. Livingston-Wheeler was acting on the hunch there may be a hidden bacterium that initiates most tumors. However, she could never accurately identify that bacterium. It may be a stealth germ called paratuberculosis. To learn more, read the section in this book on Para TB.

Cancell, also known as Entelev, Cantron and Quantrol

A secretive cancer cure was designed by James Vincent Sheridan in the 1930s to reduce the voltage of living cells. Cancell is reported to contain inositol, nitric oxide, sodium sulfite, potassium hydroxide, sulfuric acid and catechol.

Essiac tea

An herbal remedy developed by Rene M. Caisse, a Canadian nurse,contains burdock root, Indian rhubarb, sorrel, and slippery elm. Essiac was named for Caisse by spelling her last name backwards.

Evidence of anticancer activity for Essiac tea, is limited to anecdotal reports recorded for some 40 years in Canada. Individuals report Essiac tea improves quality of life, alleviates pain, and in some cases, impacts cancer progression. Experimental studies confirm the individual herbs used in this tea mixture have antioxidant, anti-estrogenic, immune-stimulating, and anti-tumor effects. However, enthusiasm for Essiac has not been found in the research community. No clinical studies of Essiac have been published to date. [Phytotherapy Research 14: 1-14, 2000]

It must be remembered that Essiac tea came into use in an era prior to Tamoxifen and other anti-estrogen drugs for breast cancer, which was its first intended use.

A lab dish study suggests Essiac stimulates growth of tumor cells. [Breast Cancer Research Treatment, March 16, 2006 online], but another study indicates the opposite. [Journal Alternative Complementary Medicine 10: 687-91, 2004] Given the penchant of cancer researchers to create pseudoscience to disprove traditional cancer remedies, the effectiveness of Essiac becomes confusing.

Whatever the effectiveness of Essiac may be, this combination herbal tea is probably more appropriate for sex-hormone related breast and prostate tumors than for other types of tumors because of its anti-estrogenic action. While the public awaits clinical trials to validate the use of Essiac, doctors at the University of Toronto report the case of a 64-year old man whose hormone-resistant prostate cancer disappeared while taking Essiac. [Canadian Journal Urology 12: 2841-42, 2005]

Gerson therapy

Max Gerson became known in the 1950s. Gerson's therapy cured Dr. Albert Schweitzer of his diabetes at the age of 75 and Schweitzer went on to win a Nobel Peace prize and work past the age of 90 at his mission station in Africa. The Gerson Method for cancer consisted of detoxification methods (coffee enemas), organically-grown plant foods and dietary supplements. Gerson advocated consumption of 13 glasses of fresh juices a day. The National Cancer Institute evaluated just 10 cases of Gerson's cancer patients and could not draw a conclusion as to the effectiveness of his treatment because the patients were also receiving conventional cancer treatments. [CA Cancer Journal Clinicians 40: 252-56, 1990]

Gerson Therapy has not been adequately reviewed by cancer authorities. A more recent review of melanoma patients found Gerson Therapy improved survival of small groups of patients compared to other selected studies. For instance, of 14 patients with stages I and II (localized) melanoma, 100% survived for 5 years, compared with 79% in a large study. Of 17 patients with stage III-A melanoma, 82% were alive at 5 years, in contrast to 39% in another study. Remarkably, of 18 patients with stage IV-A melanoma, 39% were alive at 5 years, compared with only 6% in another widely compared study. [Alternative Therapies Health Medicine 1:29-37, 1995] A naturopathic doctor tracked 21 cancer patients on Gerson therapy and found only one had survived past the 5-year mark. [Townsend Letter for Doctors, August 1995]

Gerson therapy touches on a mechanism of cancer control, that of depriving tumors of iron. Fasting and vegetarian diets deliver low amounts of iron, which may explain any reported successes. [Townsend Letter for Doctors, April 1996] But Gerson therapists have little understanding of how iron controls cancer. It is just intuitively practiced.

Fluke Worm Theory

One of the most outrageous and damaging claims made by alternative medical practitioners is one that spawned a book entitled *The Cure For All Cancers byHulda Clark.* The unfounded claim put forth in the book was that the largest of all intestinal parasites, a fluke (worm) called *Fasciolopsis buskii*, is responsible for all the cancer in the world. This parasite lays eggs in the human digestive tract and often causes anemia because it utilizes most of the iron in foods that are eaten. Anemia would reduce, not increase, the risk for cancer. Flukes are a cause of cancer in the liver and bladder, and more uncommonly in breast, prostate and other tissues. The geographic distribution of liver cancer worldwide coincides with endemic areas of the liver flukes, Opisthorchis viverrini and Clonorchis sinensis. Parasitic fluke infection is responsible for more than 60% of liver tumors in northeastern Thailand. [Asian Pac J Cancer Prevention 5:118-25, 2004] There is little question that parasitic worms may induce cancer of the liver and bladder. [Indian Journal Medical Microbiology 23:74-9, 2005] Liver flukes represent just 1.3% of the infections among immigrants to the United States. [Journal Travel Medicine 11:157-9, 2004] Hulda Clark would have everyone undergo herbal therapy to rid their body of flukes. Clark disseminates half truths. Liver flukes don't cause all cancers. If so, cancer would arise at any age with parasitic infection. Instead, cancer is largely an age-related phenomenon.

Hoxsey treatment

In the 1920s naturopathic doctor Harry Hoxsey promoted a therapy passed down to him by his father and great grandfather. It consists of red clover, licorice, burdock root, stillingia root, Berberis root, pokeroot, cascara, prickly ash bar and buckthorn bark plus potassium iodide, but the actual formula varies from patient to patient. Hoxsey therapy should be abandoned for more authoritative herbal remedies. Recall, Hoxsey was working with limited tools and only had limited number of herbs to use.

Hydrazine sulfate

Developed in the 1970s by Joseph Gold MD to treat weight loss that accompanies advanced cancer. The sulfur component of this cancer medicine yielded some benefit.

Hyperthermia (Coley's toxins)

The inclusion of "*fever therapy*" in this section of the book may mischaracterize it by association with less credible therapies. Hyperthermia cancer treatment began with a theory by William Coley, a surgeon at Sloan-Kettering Cancer hospital in New York during the 1890s. Coley found that advanced cancer patients suffering simultaneous bacterial infections showed tumor shrinkage, and in a few cases, complete remission for extended periods of time. Dr. Coley used a mixture of germs to "*inoculate*" cancer patients, with mixed success. His treatment caused high fever and chills. His success rate was reported to be 22%. Later studies conducted in the 1940s and 1970s could not verify that this was a reliable treatment. It was shown, however, that infection stimulates the production of tumor necrosis factor (TNF), an inflammatory protein that is toxic to some, but not all, cancer cells. Administration of TNF itself into tumor sites has also not been fruitful. [Cell Molecular Life Science 54: 291-98, 1998]

There is little doubt that serious infections can retard and even halt tumor growth, which blocks the formation of new blood vessels that nourish tumors. [Journal Immunology, May 15, 2001] Infections may also compete for iron and copper, which are growth factors for tumors and germs, thus limiting the available supply of growth factors to the tumor.

In the modern era of cancer research, there are numerous reports which validate hyperthermia in cancer treatment. Hyperthermia or heat treatment (greater than 42 degrees Centigrade) is based upon the sound rationale that heat affects malignant cells more than it does healthy ones. [J Environmental Pathology Toxicology Oncology 15: 289-97, 1996] Researchers in England say that hyperthermia, when combined with radiation therapy, "*appears to have an important role in the clinical management of breast cancer, and there should be no doubt that further studies of the use of hyperthermia are warranted.*" [International Journal Radiation Oncology Biology Physics 35: 731-44, 1996]

Heat treatment also potentiates chemotherapy. This was demonstrated in an animal study of liver cancer where chemotherapy alone resulted in 12% of animals surviving 2 years, whereas chemotherapy plus heat treatment resulted in 35% of the animals surviving 2 years. [Seminars Oncology 24 S6, 1997]

Some Japanese researchers even advocate total-body heat, or sauna therapy, as the sole treatment for cancer. [Rinsho Kyobu Geka 9: 540-44, 1989] One has to wonder if sauna therapy is an applicable companion to cancer treatment. In an animal experiment, a single whole-body heat treatment for 6-8 hours caused a temporary reduction in tumor size and a delay in tumor growth among animals with breast tumors. [J Cell Physiology 177: 137-47, 1998]

Another intriguing combination cancer treatment was investigated in Japan. Researchers there used heat treatment combined with omega-3 oils. The oils were used to induce cancer cells to become more vulnerable to the heat treatment. The combination of the two induced higher levels of free radicals (oxidation) to kill off cancer cells in an animal experiment. [Cancer Research 57: 2200-02, 1997]

Iscador

An extract of mistletoe, this cancer treatment was introduced by Rudolph Steiner, a Swiss physician. A recent study shows that mistletoe can induce a condition known as eosinophilia (an increase in the number of eosinophils, a type of white blood cell) in healthy adults. [Journal Society Integrative Oncology 4: 3-7, 2006] Mistletoe extract has been shown to reduce adverse effects of radiotherapy and chemotherapy on the microcirculation and the immune system of cancer patients. [Anticancer Research 25:601-10, 2005] Iscador is popular in Germany where it was recently shown to improve survival (slightly) among malignant melanoma patients. [Arzneimittelforschung 55:38-49, 2005] Iscador has also been shown to prolong survival among breast cancer patients. [Arzneimittelforschung 54:456-66, 2004]

In a study of 10,226 cancer patients in Germany, survival for patients treated with Iscador was longer for all types of cancer studied. Among the 10,226 patients studied, 396 pairs of cancer patients were matched for age, type and stage of cancer. The mean survival time in this subgroup was 4.23 years for Iscador users compared to 3.05 years for cancer patients who did not use Iscador (a 40% improvement). [Alternative Therapy Health Medicine 7:57-66, 2001] This is comparable with many so-called new *"blockbuster"* anti-cancer drugs that have been widely promoted.

However, while safe, it is not without side effects. So cancer patients should not fly to Germany for Iscador (mistletoe extract) treatment as it is not generally regarded as a cure for cancer.

Kelley metabolic therapy

Promoted by William Donald Kelley, DDS, in the 1960s, Kelley therapy involves dietary supplements, dietary measures, enzymes, and other recommendations. Dr. Kelley's treatments were helpful, but not a cure for cancer.

Laetrile

According to the entrenched cancer treatment establishment, laetrile is a *"toxic drug that is not effective as a cancer treatment."* But according to its advocates, laetrile B17 is a natural remedy that has a high cure rate against cancer. Who should the public believe?

Also known as amygdalin and vitamin B17, laetrile is derived from apricot pits. It contains cyanide which is naturally produced within apricot pits. Advocates of natural cancer therapy were able to prevail in court rulings that dying cancer patients have the right to choose their own therapy. Between 1976 and 1981 twenty-four states in the US passed legislation *"legalizing"* laetrile.

In the 1920s and 30s travelers to the Hunza Valley in Pakistan claimed they couldn't find a single case of cancer among the people who lived there and attributed it to the apricot kernals that contained laetrile B17 in the Hunza diet.

Laetrile continues to be promoted, often buoyed by the book *World Without Cancer* by G. Edward Griffin, who claimed the Hunza people who live in remote parts of Pakistan don't get cancer because they chew apricot pits. Actually, the Hunza lifespan is not long and they do get cancer.

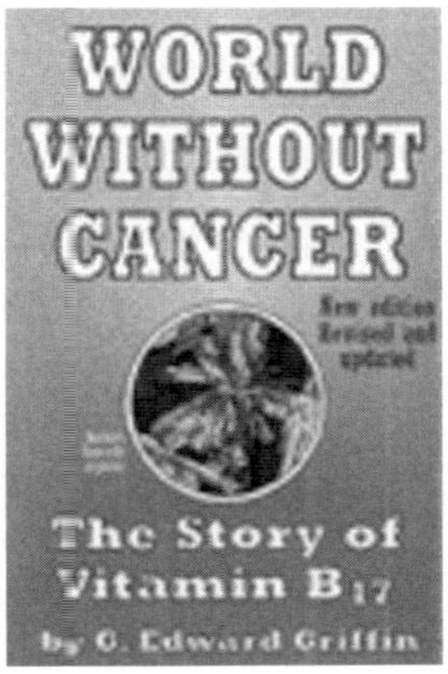

World Without Cancer
G. Edward Griffin

One of the common problems in evaluating alternative therapies is that they are rarely employed alone. For example, a book touting laetrile advocates changes in diet, avoidance of alcohol and tobacco, pancreatic enzymes, vitamin C, amino acid tablets, and mineral pills, along with intravenous laetrile injections. These may contribute greatly to successful treatment. [Laetrile Case Histories, John A. Richardson MD, Patricia Griffin RN, American Media, Westlake Village, CA, 1977] A pro-laetrile article in the Townsend Letter for Doctors states that *"laetrile, as part of a total metabolic program, might lead to the lifelong control of cancer."* [Townsend Letter for Doctors, June 1995]

It is the cyanide component of laetrile B17 that kills cancer cells. Laetrile was used as a cancer treatment long before the modern controversy erupted over its use. As early as 1845, doctors were using purified amygdalin (laetrile) to treat cancer patients.

In controlled studies, rats with cancer appear to live longer when given laetrile B17. Most of the human studies have employed purified oral or intravenous laetrile B17, not the apricot pits which are widely sold as a cancer remedy. The renowned Dr. Hans Nieper of Germany later endorsed laetrile B17 for prevention of cancer, but not as therapy for existing tumors.

One secret of the laetrile B17 cancer therapy is the described ability of an enzyme called glucuronidase to liberate cyanide from its carrier molecules and deliver it to tumor sites. Glucuronidase is more abundant where inflammation, infection and tumors occur. Therefore, the carrier molecules (nitrilosides) render laetrile B17 relatively harmless until it is unzipped by glucuronidase. When removed from its carrier, cyanide is delivered at the right place, at the right time.

A report in the Journal of the *American Medical Association* even attests to the lack of toxicity when intravenous laetrile B17 is employed. [Journal American Medical Assn 245: 591-94, 1981]

What modern medicine did to discredit laetrile B17 was to conduct a study using dogs in which the unzipping enzyme (glucuronidase) was prematurely produced by combining B17 with almond paste. The dogs developed nerve damage from the prematurely released cyanide. [referenceJournal American Medical Assn 239:943-7, 1978] Even those who advocate the use of laetrile B17 say it should not be used in combination with apricot kernels that may pre-release cyanide, but it should be purified and administered orally or intravenously, where it is subsequently attached to carrier molecules (glucuronidated) in the liver and transported to cancerous tissues.

In 1998, researchers in London attempted to activate laetrile B17 specifically at tumor sites without toxicity to healthy cells by conjoining to cloned antibodies that would direct the drug to the cancer site. This experiment increased the cancer-destroying properties of amygdalin (laetrile) 36 fold and practically eliminated toxicity! [International Journal Cancer 78: 712-19, 1998]

So the advice offered by cancer doctors, that *"laetrile B17 should not be used to treat cancer,"* apparently is correct only if you are referring to apricot pits. [CA Cancer J Clin 41: 187-92, 1991] Apricot pits themselves can cause potentially fatal cyanide poisoning. [Annals Emergency Medicine 32:742-4, 1998] In fact, there is a reported case where a 68-year old cancer patient, after taking 3,000 milligrams of amygdalin (laetrile), needed emergency care due to seizures and severe acidity. She had also been taking high-dose vitamin C which is known to increase the conversion of amygdalin to cyanide. [Annals Pharmacotherapy 39: 1566-69, 2005] Laetrile B17 treatment, administered either intravenously or orally as a purified product by a physician, may be an effective cancer treatment.

A criticism of laetrile is that it does not preferentially kill cancer cells. [The Journal of School Health 48:409-16, 1978] However, neither do conventional modern-day anti-cancer drugs.

The Macrobiotic Diet

The macrobiotic diet was developed in the 1930s by an educator in Japan, who moved to the United States where it was championed by one of his understudies. Macrobiotics is a quasi philosophical/therapeutic system of health that advocates a semi-vegetarian diet, with an emphasis on whole grains, soy beans, miso soup, raw foods and herbal teas. The strictest of macrobiotic diet consists of just brown rice and water. The standard macrobiotic diets are low in calories and fat and high in fiber from whole grains.

The macrobiotic diet is also rich in plant estrogens (phytoestrogens). These elements speak for why the macrobiotic diet became popular among cancer patients. It provides natural sources of IP6 from bran and seeds that control iron, which is a growth factor for cancer. Furthermore the vegetarian diet is low in iron. Phytoestrogens also contain anti-growth factors that inhibit tumor growth and calm sex hormones that stimulate tumor growth.

The American Cancer Society says it has found no evidence that macrobiotic diet is useful as a cure for cancer in humans and strongly urges cancer patients to avoid dietary programs as the sole treatment for cancer. [CA Cancer Journal Clinicians 43:309-19, 1993] This is an odd statement because the National Cancer Institute backed a dietary regimen of 5 servings of fruits and vegetables. It is surprising that the American Cancer Society has not conducted any research to determine the effectiveness of the macrobiotic diet.

A report in the Journal of Nutrition indicates a macrobiotic diet lowers estrogen levels in females which may be beneficial in reducing the risk for breast cancer, and that overall, *"on the basis of available evidence and its similarity to dietary recommendations for chronic disease prevention, the macrobiotic diet probably carries a reduced cancer risk."* [Journal Nutrition 131: 3056-64S, 2001]

Bloodroot

An Associated Press news story cited a South Georgia preacher for practicing medicine without a license. [Associated Press August 29, 2005] FDA agents raided his business after he dispensed bloodroot, a traditional remedy for treatment of skin cancer. The preacher appeared before the medical board with before-and-after photos of patients and the board never filed charges against him. The preacher's son smeared bloodroot paste on his own nose and stated it encourages a process called apoptosis that causes cancer cells to die off slowly.

Bloodroot (sanguinarine extract) has been shown to be non-toxic to animals after oral intake. [Journal Toxicology Environmental Health 20: 199-208, 1987] It does indeed induce a process called cellular apoptosis. [Molecular Cancer Therapies 3: 933-40, 2004] It also has antiseptic properties. [Journal Canadian Dental Association 5: 7-12, 1990]

Dermatologists report that this escharotic (caustic) paste is a traditional remedy for abnormal skin growths that works in a manner similar to zinc chloride. Dermatologists reported on four patients who used bloodroot paste to treat their skin cancers, and while they denounced its use and branded it as harmful, their report in the Archives of Dermatology admits that one patient experienced a complete disappearance of a skin tumor that later returned. A second patient had eradicated all tumors, but experienced severe scarring. A third patient was healed of a skin tumor that recurred more than 7 years later. [Archives Dermatology 138: 1593-96, 2002]

While bloodroot paste may be inconsistent from brand to brand, it has a long history of use. The preacher who sold bloodroot paste was a retired farmer plagued with skin cancer that doctors surgically removed from his face and arms. When a 3-inch tumor later grew on the side of his neck, he tried the bloodroot paste. He cited relatives who had died of skin cancer after conventional treatment and said: *"I knew there was a better way."* Bloodroot has been proposed as an oral therapy for prostate cancer as well. [Molecular Cancer Therapies 3: 933-40, 2004]

Oxygen therapies

Various forms of oxygen (O_2), delivered as hydrogen peroxide (H_2O_2), or ozone (H_2O_3) have been used as therapy for cancer. In 1993, *CA-The Cancer Journal for Clinicians* reviewed these therapies and found them to be ineffective, if not sometimes toxic. The idea of using forms of oxygen to treat cancer emanated from early use of peroxide to treat infections by I.N. Love MD in 1888. This was in an era prior to the availability of antibiotic drugs. In the 1930s, two-time Nobel Prize winner Otto Warburg observed that cancer cells do not operate on aerobic (oxygen rich) respiration as do healthy cells and in fact grow better in oxygen-deprived tissues. In reality, cancer cells lose energy and revert to fermentation of sugars for cellular energy, which produces acidic waste product (lactic acid). The idea is to re-supply cancer cells with oxygen to cause tumors to shrink. Actually, this treatment would be more appropriate to treat infection, not cancer. Germanium, an herbal product is used in oxygen therapies since it is purported to be an *"oxygenator."*

It is interesting to read the critical comments by the cancer establishment regarding oxygen therapies. They state that ozone and hydrogen peroxide produce *"highly reactive oxygen containing radicals"* that are toxic. [CA-Cancer Journal for Clinicians, 43: 47-62, 1993] That is exactly how chemo and radiation therapy kill cancer cells! It is amazing how two-faced these arguments are. Both oxygen therapies and chemo and radiation therapy generate free radicals that indiscriminately kill living cells, both healthy and cancerous. This is why modern cancer treatment produces so many side effects. The trick is to find therapies that are toxic to cancer cells, but not to healthy cells. There are some natural therapies that do this, such as IP6 rice bran treatment and resveratrol.

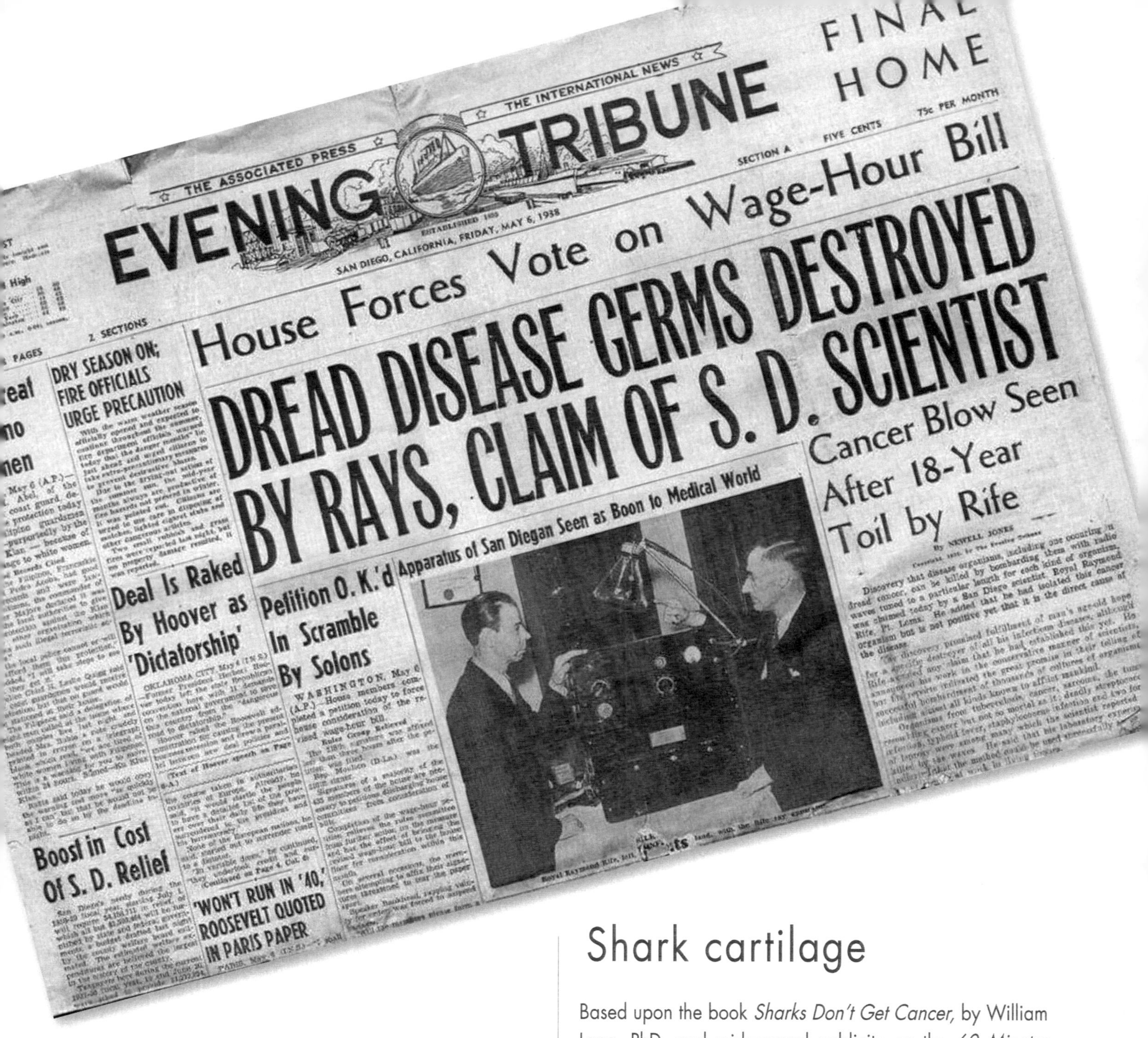

THE ASSOCIATED PRESS — THE INTERNATIONAL NEWS

EVENING TRIBUNE

FINAL HOME

SECTION A — FIVE CENTS — 75c PER MONTH

SAN DIEGO, CALIFORNIA, FRIDAY, MAY 6, 1938

2 SECTIONS

House Forces Vote on Wage-Hour Bill

DREAD DISEASE GERMS DESTROYED BY RAYS, CLAIM OF S. D. SCIENTIST

Cancer Blow Seen After 18-Year Toil by Rife

By NEWELL JONES

Apparatus of San Diegan Seen as Boon to Medical World

DRY SEASON ON; FIRE OFFICIALS URGE PRECAUTION

Deal Is Raked By Hoover as 'Dictatorship'

Petition O. K.'d In Scramble By Solons

Boost in Cost Of S. D. Relief

'WON'T RUN IN '40,' ROOSEVELT QUOTED IN PARIS PAPER

Shark cartilage

Based upon the book *Sharks Don't Get Cancer,* by William Lane, PhD, and widespread publicity on the *60 Minutes* television program, shark cartilage became the rage in the 1990s. The theory is that cartilage is a bloodless tissue and cannot grow tumors. Sharks, being largely cartilaginous creatures, were claimed to be free from cancer. Actually, marine veterinarians indicate sharks do get cancer. Adding more cartilage to the human body doesn't block cancer. The body produces its own cartilage from vitamin C and amino acids. But desperate cancer patients were misled for a time. The use of shark cartilage has waned in recent times.

Rife therapy

Developed by Dr. Royal Rife in the 1930s, this therapy utilizes a sound and light frequency generator to kill cancer cells. Still widely promoted in underground cancer

A story

Raul was a young, newly married man, who developed testicular cancer. A diet of southern fried foods didn't help his condition. But testicular cancer has a fairly high rate of survival if for no other reason than it often occurs among young men like Raul who have an intact immune system. Raul opted for alternative therapies. Vitamins, herbs, various natural therapies appeared to have thrown his cancer into remission.

Then, one day, at a health fair with his wife, he decided to undergo a session of iridology. An iridologist believes that various signs of disease are evident in the coloration, folds and patterns of the iris of the human eye. Though no careful study has ever validated its claims, iridology is still practiced. Raul told the iridologist that despite having cancer, which he believed he had overcome, he still planned to have a family. The iridologist suggested he take DHEA, a hormonal supplement that helps to elevate levels of testosterone, to improve virility. Though the iridologist was well intentioned, his suggestion to Raul produced unwanted side effects – the roaring return of testicular cancer.

Raul and his wife were stunned to learn that DHEA should never have been suggested to a cancer patient in remission from a hormonally-driven cancer. Raul was flown by family members to the M.D. Anderson Cancer Hospital in Houston for aggressive chemo and radiation therapy. All things alternative are not necessarily harmless.

Raul's last hope was a cancer treatment hospital in Mexico. He and his family felt "*the presence of God*" there. The all-vegetarian diet the hospital recommended will take some getting used to for Raul, yet no cancer doctor had previously suggested it to him. He is getting heavy doses of intravenous laetrile, vitamin C and ozone and UV therapies. Raul was surprised that the doctors in Mexico suggested the same chemotherapy drugs used at the MD Anderson Cancer Hospital. Alternative medicine has its surprises too. Raul later succumbed to his cancer.

Conventional vs. Alternative Cancer Therapy

Shari Roan, an accomplished health writer for the *Los Angeles Times*, related the one-sided story of a man who developed kidney cancer that had spread to his brain, and how he and his wife were fleeced by practitioners of alternative medicine. [LA Times, Feb. 4, 2006]

The patient, a 60-year old man who had withered from 155 to 95 pounds, was in dire condition. He had spent thousands of dollars on alternative treatments, such as Rife machine treatment, intravenous vitamin drips, and herbal pills, all in lieu of surgery to remove a cancerous kidney. Gamma knife radiation treatment was consented to, given that the patient was experiencing twitching on his left side from the brain tumor. But that treatment was so horrific that the patient and his wife turned to less invasive treatment from alternative practitioners.

His wife had already paid one herbal healer $18,000 and was now confronted with a bill for $120,000 for more herbal cures, according to the article When the patient's wife asked the herbalist for a social security number, which he couldn't provide, she was quoted to have said: *"At that point it all hit me. I knew this guy was a fake and that I'd never see him again. At that moment, it all made sense."* She never paid the herbalist the bill for $120,000 and dismissed him from her home.

The LA Times article when on to say: *"The therapies for which he and his wife had paid so dearly — using up much of their savings and forsaking traditional cancer treatments that might have prolonged his life — were useless, doctors say."* That they were, but so are most of the treatments offered by cancer doctors.

Roan argued that alternative medicine practitioners have been given some level of credibility by their integration with doctors who provide conventional care. *"So-called complementary and alternative medicine has gained a foothold in today's medical world, garnering grudging respect from many mainstream physicians and researchers... But with this measure of legitimacy has come a rise in unprofessional, even fraudulent, practitioners,"* wrote Roan.

But conventional cancer care, prescribed by trained oncologists from prestigious university medical centers, often have no greater legitimacy than treatments provided by alternative practitioners. Conventional cancer care only has the appearance of legitimacy.

Back to the LA Times, article, the patient's wife explained that the herbalist they employed *"was guaranteeing that he could cure my husband... Here's Western medicine with its horrible side effects and here's this holistic, gentle nutritionist who acts so concerned."*.

"It wasn't just the money they took," she said, *"It was the time. He (my husband) may have lived longer — or achieved a remission — had he chosen conventional medical care."*

But the cancer doctor quoted in the article conceded that *"our track record with this kind of tumor is pretty dismal."* There is little evidence that conventional treatment would have offered this patient more than a couple of extra months of life, and at what cost? The cost of conventional cancer care went unmentioned in the newspaper report. Caught between one seemingly credible cancer care system and the over-promised cures of alternative therapists, it seems patients are victims from both sides.

CHAPTER 5

Prevention

p 126 - 136

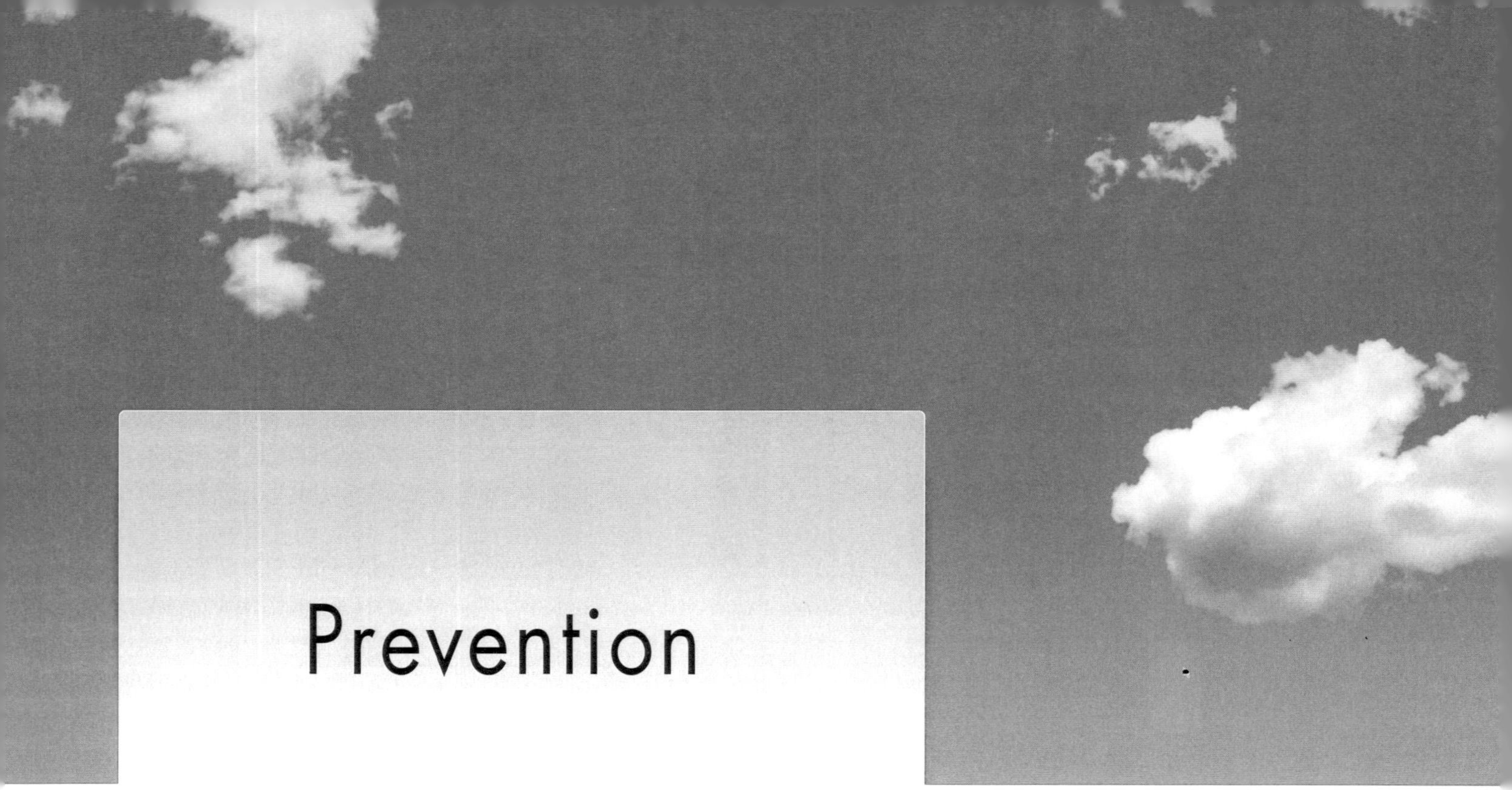

Prevention

Cancer prevention

No matter how efficient we may become at delivering health care, we must also seek to reduce demand by keeping people from developing diseases in the first place.
Devar Lee Davis, Calum Muir, Environmental Health Perspectives, November, 1995

> *"In the long run, if we want to reduce cancer [risk] we're going to have to look at other things and not put too much hope in fruits and vegetables."*
> *– Walter Willett, Harvard Medical School*

A worldwide study estimates, of the 7 million deaths from cancer worldwide (2001 figures), 35 percent were attributed to preventable factors. Smoking, tobacco, over-consumption of alcohol, diet, obesity, infection, are all modifiable factors. [Lancet 366: 1784-93, 2005]

Cancer prevention encompasses the use of dietary measures (5 servings of fruits and vegetables), drugs, chemicals or nutraceuticals (called chemoprevention), avoidance of carcinogens (smoking, excessive solar radiation, toxic chemicals like chlorine), and screening for early-stage cancer (pap smears, colonoscopy, PSA prostate tests, skin exams, etc.)

It's disheartening to realize all the efforts to encourage plant food diets, smoking cessation and early screening have been met with disappointment.

By the time most tumors are discovered, they have spread to other organs and tissues. In the US, 72 percent of lung cancers, 57 percent of colon/rectal cancer and 34 percent of breast cancer has metastasized by the time they are diagnosed.
Scientific American, June 9, 2003

Cancer Prevention	
Approach	**Examples**
Dietary measures	5-a-day fruits and vegetables
Health habits, avoidance of carcinogens	Smoking cessation, alcohol in moderation, avoid toxic chemicals, avoid sunlight
Early detection	Pap smear, colonoscopy, PSA test, mammography, skin exams
Chemoprevention (drugs, nutraceuticals, etc)	Aspirin, anti-inflammatory agents, calcium, nutraceuticals like resveratrol, curcumin, others

Cancer screening: more treatment, not longer survival

Cancer screening programs are effective at finding more disease to treat, but work on the assumption that treatment is effective at improving survival, which it isn't. The public doesn't recognize this.

By detecting cancer at earlier stages, all that has been accomplished is to give the statistical false impression that treatment is improving survival time. For example, if a theoretical person would normally have more advanced-stage colon cancer detected at age 64 and stool blood testing or colonoscopy detects cancer at age 59, then it would falsely appear treatment extends life by an additional 5 years. In fact, the patient would succumb to cancer at about the same age, at age 65.

Plant food diets disappoint

The results "*were astonishing*" said one reviewer. The recent issue of the Journal of the National Cancer Institute concludes "*fruit and vegetable intake is unrelated to cancer incidence.*" Yikes! After nearly a decade and $40 million the National Cancer Institute (NCI) spent on the 5-A-Day program, it is an abject failure. The World Cancer Research Fund examined 4500 published reports in 1994 and concluded that *"if everyone ate at least five servings of fruits and vegetables a day, cancer rates could be reduce by more than 20 percent."* Now, the latest study doesn't support this notion. Plant food diets marginally help reduce the risk for heart disease, but not cancer. [Journal National Cancer Institute 97: 1307, 2005]

The National Cancer Institute (NCI) program to promote 5 servings of fruits and vegetables is another disappointment. The NCI didn't want to take it on the chin for this misdirection, so it quietly conceded its 5-a-day program didn't reduce mortality rates for cancer, then suggested 9-13 servings of plant foods a day, something only 2 percent of the population currently achieves. [Journal National Cancer Institute 96:1577-84, 2004]

Yet again, with no supporting studies, the NCI has now altered their dietary recommendation - 9 to 13 servings of plant foods a day to ward off cancer. Just what Americans need - advice to eat more food.

Cancer authorities reacted quickly to the negative study. One commentator said plant foods contain variable amounts of anti-cancer molecules, so this might sway the results of the study. (Exactly what we've been saying all along, dietary supplements would provide reliable amounts of active ingredients.) Others said it might make a difference if people consumed raw or cooked vegetables. (Yes, exactly, again this is why we say dietary supplements would be advised.)

Challenges to the prevailing wisdom of aggressive treatment with surgery, radiation and chemotherapy are becoming more common, as a result of discouraging results with these therapies. A few novel approaches offer hope, but the failure of many such approaches does not bode well. Hence, calls for cancer prevention are becoming increasingly vocal, though not yet sufficiently heeded.

Ralf G Rabwan, BPharm, PhD, Ohio State University

+

Cancer Preventive Agent	Comment
Vitamin A	Synthetic vitamin A is being promoted over natural vitamin A
Aspirin	Anti-inflammatory; aspirin resistance in 40% of users; causes gastric bleeding and anemia; depletes tissues of vitamin C and folic acid; causes esophageal narrowing; causes irreversible asthma; causes bleeding gastric ulcers and sometimes death
Bexarotene	Synthetic vitamin A, promoted to prevent cancer
Calcium	May work by detoxifying action on saturated fats; American diet is over-sufficient in calcium; dairy products that provide calcium may be contaminated with stealth cancer-causing bacterium (paratuberculosis); excessive calcium causes constipation, muscle spasm, heart spasm, migraine, back aches, leg cramps, calcifications.
Celecoxib (Celebrex)	COX-2 inhibitors have been linked to increased risk of heart attacks; inexplicably placed on chemoprevention list
Curcumin	Natural anti-inflammatory from turmeric
DHEA	Pre-cursor for testosterone and estrogen; may increase risk for hormonal tumors
Fenretinide	Synthetic form of vitamin A
Finasteride (Propecia)	Shrinks prostate; slight reduces risk for prostate cancer
Indole-3-carbinol	Commonly found in broccoli, Brussels' sprouts
l-Perillyl alcohol	Found in citrus peel oil (D-limonene)
Lycopene	Red pigment found in tomatoes, watermelon; extensively studied as prostate cancer inhibitor
Selenium	Trace mineral; compelling study show daily use as a supplement reduces risk for nearly all forms of cancer
Soy isoflavones	Provides anti-growth factors, hormone inhibitors
Tamoxifen citrate	Fraught with side effects; inexplicably included in chemoprevention list; causes cancer after 5 years use
Tea polyphenols	Binds to iron; inhibits tumor growth
Vitamin D (hormone)	Immune normalizer; reduces risk for colon, uterine, breast and prostate cancer

Promising Chemopreventive Agents Not On National Institutes of Health List	
Resveratrol	Most striking anti-cancer molecule found; inhibits initiation, growth and spread of tumors; natural COX-2 inhibitor; accelerates DNA repair
Quercetin	Anti-inflammatory, anti-histamine, anti-viral action; binds to iron
IP6 rice bran extract	Metal chelator (remover); major antioxidant; facilitates DNA repair
Vitamin C	Inhibits spread of tumors (metastasis) by maintaining integrity of endothelial cells lining blood vessels; in high-IV dose, able to create hydrogen peroxide that selectively kills cancer cells
Flaxseed lignans	Inhibits action of estrogen; natural aromatase inhibitor; applicable for prostate and breast tumor inhibition
Omega-3 oil (flaxseed/ fish oil)	Facilitates death of cancer cells; inhibits growth of cancer cells; possible companion to cancer drugs
Folic acid	Required for DNA repair and inhibition of homocysteine (methylation); depleted by some anti-cancer drugs
Coenzyme Q10	Depleted by most anti-cancer drugs; supplemental CoQ10 elevates cellular energy (ATP) levels

Chemoprevention

Chemoprevention is defined as the use of chemical compounds to prevent, inhibit or reverse cancer. These can be drugs or natural chemicals. Because chemopreventive agents would be given to healthy patients for long periods of time, these agents must have minimal or no toxicity.

The above list of compounds have shown some evidence they may be able to prevent cancer and are under study by or of interest to the public and researchers (list by the National Cancer Institute)

Cancer researchers are beginning to suggest it's now time to consider chemoprevention. But they can't seem to find safe alternatives to the problematic drugs. A report entitled "*Chemoprevention of colorectal cancer: ready for routine use?*" notes that this type of cancer is believed to take 15-20 years to develop, providing a window of opportunity for prevention. Adenomas (polyps) usually precede cancer, but not always. The report says "*chemoprevention is a new emerging science, means the use of agents to inhibit, delay or reverse cancer.*" But the report dwells on the use of anti-inflammatory drugs which cause 107,000 hospitalizations and 16,500 deaths annually due to side effects. [Current Topics Medical Chemistry 5: 517-25, 2005]

Two long-term studies fail to show that aspirin use significantly thwarts cancer. A 10-year study of 39,876 women taking a low-dose 100 milligram aspirin tablet found no risk reduction for cancer at any site except for a slight reduction in lung cancer risk. Nor was there any reduction in cancer mortality. [J American Medical Assn 294: 47-55, 2005] A higher-dose aspirin tablet (325 mg) taken twice a day significantly reduces the risk for colon cancer, but the preventive benefit did not become apparent until more than a decade of use and the risk of gastric bleeding would discourage the use of high-dose aspirin. [J American Medical Assn 294: 914-23, 2005]

COX-2 inhibitors like Vioxx, Celebrex ibuprofen, are much too problematic to suggest their widespread use for cancer prevention in millions of people. The masses would be trading cancer prevention for heart toxicity. [New England Journal Medicine 352: 1092-1102, 2005]

First, identify high-risk patients

The current idea is to identify high-risk patients and then implement chemoprevention. For example, esophageal (throat) cancer is common and pre-cancerous changes (squamous dysplasia) precedes cancer (carcinoma). In one study conducted in China, researchers found that 200 mcg of daily selenium (as selenomethionine) inhibited the progression of pre-cancerous cells to cancer whereas an anti-inflammatory drug (COX-2 inhibitor) did not. [Gastroenterology 129: 863-73, 2005] Folic acid supplements may also play an important role in prevention of squamous cell cancers. Folic acid deficiency can result in the loss of activity of certain tumor suppressor genes. [Cancer Detection Prevention 29: 46-53, 2005]

Sometimes modern medicine buys into an idea that may be useless. The prevailing concept to prevent colon cancer, the second leading cause of cancer-related death, is to detect adenomas (polyps) via colonoscopy, surgically remove them, and utilize any dietary, drug or dietary supplement to prevent recurrence.

The problem here is, while polyps are prevalent in 70-90 percent of colon/rectal cancer patients, what of the 10-30 percent who develop this form of cancer without evidence of polyps? Even after removal, their recurrence rate is 40-50 percent, almost making surgical removal a fruitless effort.

The use of calcium supplements is often suggested, based upon population studies which appear to show decreased risk for colon cancer among persons who consume more calcium. However, researchers critically examined 24 studies and could only find three that met proper criteria for analysis. Patients ranging in age from 35-76 years were involved in the three studies and were followed for periods ranging from 3-4 years. Colonoscopy was used to identify the existence and recurrence of adenomas. Calcium supplementation ranged from 1200 to 2000 mg in the three pooled studies. Dietary calcium consumption ranged from 940 to 1600 milligrams which would be additional to the supplemental calcium.

Here are the results of the study:

→ Recurrence rate of adenomas (polyps) in groups that took calcium supplements:
176 of 627 developed recurrent polyps for a rate of 28%

→ Recurrence rate of adenomas (polyps) in groups that did not take calcium supplements:
231 of 652 developed recurrent polyps for a rate of 35%

So the result of high-dose calcium intake produced a 7% reduction (7 in 100) in the recurrence rate of polyps. This is not a big difference. Many patients with polyps will take extra calcium and receive no benefit. [American Journal Gastroenterology 100: 390-94, 2005] Furthermore, researchers remain ignorant of any side effects from high-dose calcium. Some common side effects are constipation, heart flutter, muscle spasm, and long-term, possible calcifications in tissues throughout the body. Researchers claim *"it would be unfortunate if patients were falsely reassured by taking calcium and neglected their surveillance colonoscopies."* [American Journal Gastroenterology 100: 395-96, 2005] But this falsely assumes that adenoma reduction will prevent cancer and that early treatment will prolong life. There is no evidence for either.

Furthermore, a 4-year diet modification trail failed to reduce adenoma (polyp) recurrence. [New England Journal Medicine 342: 1149-55, 2000] A fiber diet also failed to reduce adenoma recurrence. [New England J Medicine 342: 1156-62, 2000 alberts]

Chemoprevention of stomach and colon cancer

An opportunity exists to prevent gastric cancer (and ulcers) by eradication of a bacterium called Helicobacter pylori. About 60 to 90 percent of all gastric cancer is attributed to this bacterium which infects up to 50 percent of the US population. However, repeated use of antibiotics would induce antibiotic resistant strains of this germ. [American Journal Gastroenterology 100: 2100-15, 2005] However, cancer doctors can't fathom the use of non-prescription antibiotics that do not induce antibiotic resistance, such as allicin from garlic and carvacrol from oregano. The use of acid-forming bacteria supplements (acidophilus), garlic preparations, or resveratrol, are comparable to the use of antibiotics to kill off H. pylori. [Molecular Cell Biochemistry 243: 29-35, 2003]

Folic acid supplementation may serve to prevent pre-cancerous changes in the digestive tract. Chromosomes (groups of genes) become unstable and genes that present cancer become inactive when folic acid levels are low. [Experimental Biology Medicine 229: 988-95, 2004] It has been demonstrated that 400 micrograms (mcg) of folic acid may decrease the risk for colon cancer. [Gut 54: 648-53, 2005]

Chemoprevention of breast cancer

Women aren't buying into the idea of taking Tamoxifen to prevent breast cancer. [Journal National Cancer Institute 96: 1410-12, 2004]

When women at risk for breast cancer were offered Tamoxifen, only 43% elected to take it, mostly out of fear of side effects. [Annals Surgical Oncology 2004]

In another study, out of 51 women eligible for Tamoxifen breast cancer prevention, only 12% chose the drug and another 12% said they were uncertain. [Breast Cancer Research Treatment 94:153-9, 2005]

In yet another study, only 1 of 89 at-risk women elected to take Tamoxifen for prevention of breast cancer and 42% of the women made their decision based upon a negative recommendation from their family doctors. [Annals Family Medicine 3:242-7, 2005]

In a survey of 250 women deemed to be at higher risk for breast cancer (2.8% over 5 years), only about 18% of these women chose to take Tamoxifen even though 32% of them felt a high self-perceived risk of developing breast cancer. [Cancer 103:1996-2005, 2005]

While Tamoxifen increases the risk for blood clots in the legs from 5/10th to 8/10ths of one percent, that is still a 63% increase. [British Journal Clinical Pharmacology 45:608-12, 1998]

New aromatase inhibitors reduce enzyme activity needed to produce estrogen by 97-99%. [Expert Opinion Emerging Drugs 7: 303-19, 2002] Little is said that such harsh reduction of estrogen will throw most women into mental depression, promote rapid withering of bones and cause women to show rapid signs of aging (wrinkles, thinning hair). Most women on these drugs will have to take bone hardening and anti-depressant medications. The inclusion of flaxseed in the diet has been shown to inhibit the occurrence and growth of breast tumors in humans. [Clinical Cancer Research 11: 3828-35, 2005] Flaxseed is rarely mentioned as a preventive measure. Yet populations that consume high levels of lignans found in flax, rye and other grains, exhibit low rates of breast cancer.

An unheralded breast cancer weapon is the trace mineral selenium. Women with hereditary mutations in the BRCA1 gene are at increased risk for breast and uterine cancer. The BRCA1 gene is responsible for producing a protein that repair double-stranded breaks in DNA that increase the risk for cancer. White blood cells were obtained from women who are carriers of the CRCA1 gene mutation and subjected to a chemotherapy drug (bleomycin). There were more DNA breaks among mutated BRCA1 samples than healthy controls. After 1-3 months of supplementation with selenium, the frequency of breaks in chromosomes were significantly reduced to the point they compared to subjects who did not have the BRCA1 mutation! Canadian researchers conclude that *"oral selenium is a good candidate for chemopreven-*

tion in women who carry a mutation in the BRCA1 gene." [Cancer Epidemiology Biomarkers Prevention 14: 1302-06, 2005] Will most women with this gene mutation hear about this discovery?

Chemoprevention of prostate cancer

If there is a type of cancer that shows considerable evidence for response from chemoprevention it would be prostate cancer. Various researchers are now asking, *"is chemoprevention for prostate cancer ready for prime time?"* Wow, researchers believe they are on the cusp of discovery – prostate cancer could be prevented!

However, some researchers still cling to the drug model, claiming finasteride (Propecia, Proscar) is the drug of choice to prevent prostate cancer. [Canadian Journal Urology 2: 2-4, 2005]

It is estimated that widespread use of finasteride by adult males would add 300,000 years of life over a 10-year period. [Urological Oncology 22: 362-68, 2004]

However, for a hypothetical group of one thousand 62-year-old men treated with finasteride, an increased survival of 140 life-years is forecasted, an increase in survival of about a month (0.14 years per individual). [Journal Urology 175:934-8, 2006]

For males, finasteride (Propecia), a drug often used to treatment prostate inflammation, has been shown to reduce risk for prostate cancer by about 25%. But finasteride decreases male sex drive and may induce higher-grade tumors.

The landmark finasteride prevention study involved 9060 men. Among the men taking finasteride, 18.4% developed prostate tumors versus 24% in the placebo group, for a real difference of about 6 in 100 men. This means, over a 7-year period, for every 100 men taking the drug, 94 would experience no benefit while 6 would. But most men will develop cancerous cells in their prostate gland if they live long enough and few die from it.

In the finasteride study, only 10 men died of prostate cancer, five in each group taking finasteride or placebo. Men taking finasteride who were found to have prostate cancer were more likely to have a fast growing kind, which would be expected to be more deadly. So finasteride may slightly reduce the risk of prostate cancer, but not dying of prostate cancer. Men taking finasteride had more erectile dysfunction and loss of interest in sex, but also had fewer urinary problems. [New England Journal of Medicine 349:215-224, 2003]

Finasteride would cost about $3.4 billion per year for US men age 55-80. [Journal National Cancer Institute 96: 1410-12, 2004]

Researchers in Belgium paint a different picture. They note that extracts from saw palmetto berry (serenoa repens) are as effective at inhibiting the enzyme inhibiting drugs (5 alpha-reductase inhibitors) and don't interfere with PSA testing as does the drug. The Belgian doctors state that *"In addition to saw palmetto berry extracts, a combination of selenium, lycopene, natural vitamin E and fish oil, seems warranted."* [Aging Male 7: 155-69, 2004]

A study that employed supplemental vitamin C, vitamin E, beta carotene, selenium and zinc daily for 8 years found a measurable reduction in prostate cancer risk among men with normal PSA counts. There was no effect among men with high PSA counts. [International Journal Cancer 116: 182-86, 2005]

Some doctors are dubious of finasteride and note that weight control, dietary changes, lycopene, soy beans, omega 3 oil, selenium, vitamin E and avoidance of tobacco are without risks, efficient and commendable. [Review Med Suisse 2: 163-65, 2006]

Cancer Preventive Chemicals, By Tumor Site	
Breast	D-limonene, lignans, vitamin D, vitamin E, resveratrol
Colon	Curcumin, pomegranate, vitamin D, folic acid, resveratrol, selenium
Lung	Vitamin A, selenium, resveratrol
Prostate	Lycopene, soy, flaxseed lignans, soy, vitamin D, selenium, resveratrol
Skin	Green tea molecules, resveratrol
Cervix	Vitamin A, folic acid, quercetin, resveratrol, flaxseed lignans
Liver	IP6 rice bran extract, NAC (N-acetyl cysteine)

Chemoprevention of skin cancer

Skin cancer has to be the most frequent occurring form of cancer. Non-melanoma skin cancer is diagnosed in more than a million people every year in the US. Researchers have already documented that folic acid, selenium and silibin (a component of milk thistle), inhibit squamous cell cancer. Researchers at the University of Colorado (Denver), report that *"silibin's use against skin cancer is supported by sound rational in animal and cell dish studies and suggests its potential use for humans."* [European J Cancer 41: 1969-79, 2005]

Melanoma, the most dreaded of skin cancers, is thought to be caused by sun exposure. But studies show sun exposure actually is associated with increased survival, suggesting vitamin D may be an antidote since it is produced in the skin by solar ultraviolet rays. [J National Cancer Institute 97: 195-99, 2005] Diets low in alcohol intake and consist of vitamin D and carotenes (beta carotene, lycopene, lutein) which are skin antioxidants, may reduce the risk for melanoma. [Cancer Epidemiology Biomarkers Prevention 13: 1042-51, 2004]

Why not prevent them all?

There are so many types of cancer to prevent. Should adults take one pill to prevent "*this*" type of cancer, and another pill for "*that*" type of cancer? There are chemopreventive molecules that have widespread anti-cancer action.

The most remarkable of all chemopreventive agents is resveratrol, a molecule concentrated in red wine and also derived from dietary sources such as mulberries, peanuts and grapes. Resveratrol is receiving great attention because of its widespread chemical action. [Mutation Research 523: 145-50, 2003]

Here is what researchers at the University of Wisconsin Medical Science Center had to say about resveratrol and chemoprevention:

"Conventional therapeutic and surgical approaches have not been able to control the incidence of most of the cancer types. Therefore, there is an urgent need to develop approaches for the management of cancer. Chemoprevention via non-toxic agents could be one such approach. Many naturally occurring agents have shown cancer chemopreventive potential. An effective chemopreventive agent should have certain properties: (a) little or no toxic effects in normal and healthy

cells; (b) high effectivness against cancer in different locations; (c) capability of oral consumption; (d) known mechanism of action; (e) low cost, and (f) acceptance by humans. Resveratrol is one such agent." [International Journal Oncology 23: 17-28, 2003]

Greater dietary consumption of resveratrol decreases the risk for cancer. [European Journal Cancer Prevention 14: 139-42, 2005] Though the decreased risk was not observed for resveratrol-rich wine, which may mean the alcohol content of wine negates from of the protective effect of resveratrol. Researchers note that resveratrol blocks the three major stages of cancer (initiation, growth and progression), something no drug can claim. [Molecular Nutrition Food Research 49: 462-71, 2005] While some natural chemopreventive agents like selenium do not exhibit preventive benefit for skin cancer, resveratrol does. [FASEB Journal 19: 1193-95, 2005] As a mild plant estrogen, its use to prevent hormone-related cancers of the prostate and breast *"is warranted."* [Urology Oncology 7: 223-27, 2002; European J Cancer Prevention 14: 139-42, 2005]

Both curcumin and resveratrol inhibit COX-2 inflammatory enzymes and inhibit cancer in animal studies. [Anticancer Research 24: 2783-840, 2004; Current Medical Chem Anti Cancer Agents 2: 357-70, 2002] While curcumin and resveratrol are widely documented to inhibit cancer, and are deemed safer than COX-2 inhibitors, they are not in widespread use nor have they gained significant public attention. [Journal Chemotherapy 16: 3-6, 2004]

Curcumin has biological action similar to the drug etoposide. It inhibits topoisomerase II and encourages cancer cell death. [Journal Enzyme Inhibition Med Chemistry 18: 505-09, 2003]

Herbs and spices, and their extracted active ingredients, are being overlooked as potent chemopreventive agents. [Current Medical Chemistry 11: 1451-60, 2004]

Folic acid supplementation has widespread application as a cancer preventive agent, and is safe and economical.

Herbs and spices, and their extracted active ingredients, are being overlooked as potent chemopreventive agents.
Source: Current Medical Chemistry 11: 1451-60, 2004

Today we possess a plethora of mechanistic insights into how dietary constituents such as resveratrol (from red grapes), epigallocatechin gallate (from tea) and curcumin (from turmeric) can interfere with oncogenic events germane to differentiation, death and survival.
Andreas Gescher and William P. Steward July 2005

Agent	Agent type	Cancer prevention/treatment
Vitamin A + other retinoids	vitamin	skin, head + neck, & lung
Vitamin C	vitamin	colon & stomach
Vitamin D	vitamin	colon, breast, prostate, uterine
Vitamin E	vitamin	lung, head + neck, colon, & stomach
Folic Acid	vitamin	precancerous cells of the cervix
Selenium	mineral	all but skin cancer
Calcium	mineral	colon
Beta-Carotene	phytochemical	lung, head + neck, colon & stomach
D-limonene	phytochemical	breast

Case report

Tom is 71 years old, diagnosed with mild chronic lymphocytic leukemia. This is cancer of white blood cells (lymphocytes). It type of cancer is usually slow to progress. There is an increase in white blood cells in the blood and bone marrow. Tom thinks his doctor detected the problem three years ago, but only told him about it a year ago. He has no symptoms, but he was sent to an oncologist (cancer doctor) for a review. His doctors, like most, have nothing to recommend for Tom, other than wait for the disease to get worse. In addition to many dietary supplements he has taken over the years (multivitamin, fish oil, garlic pill, vitamin E, lutein, calcium and magnesium), he takes IP6 rice bran extract and mushroom extract over the past year. He has recently begun taking resveratrol pills. He is left on his own to prevent or delay leukemia. Modern medicine has no preventive remedies.

Anticancer Ingredients In Food

Allicin	• Garlic
Bioflavonoids	• Citrus peel, berries, cherries, grapes
Catechins	• Green tea
Curcumin	• Turmeric
Genistein	• Soy
Indoles	• Cruciferous vegetables
Isoflavones	• Soy
Lycopene	• Tomato, watermelon
D-limonene	• Orange peel oil
Omega-3 oils	• Flax, fish
Phenols	• Resveratrol, quercetin
Lignans	• Flax, rye

Geographical Location Dictates Cancer Rates

Locality	Age adjusted cancer incidence rates per 100,000 population
Nigeria	91
Israeli Arabs	96
Bombay India	135
Denmark	222
U.S. (Connecticut)	239
U.S. (Harlingen, Texas)	403

Source: Cancer Bulletin 25: 33, 1973

Antioxidant Activity of Common Plant Extracts, Based Upon Their Ability To Bind To Iron (reduce iron-generated free radicals, per 100 grams)	
Walnut	20.97
Pomegranate	11.33
Bilberry	8.23
Elderberry	4.31
Grape	1.45
Spinach	0.98
Onion	0.67
Wholemeal flour	0.33
Apple	0.29
Carrot	0.04

Source: Halvorsen BL, Systematic screening of total antioxidants, Journal Nutrition 1323: 461-71, 2001]

CHAPTER 6

Lung Cancer

p 138 - 162

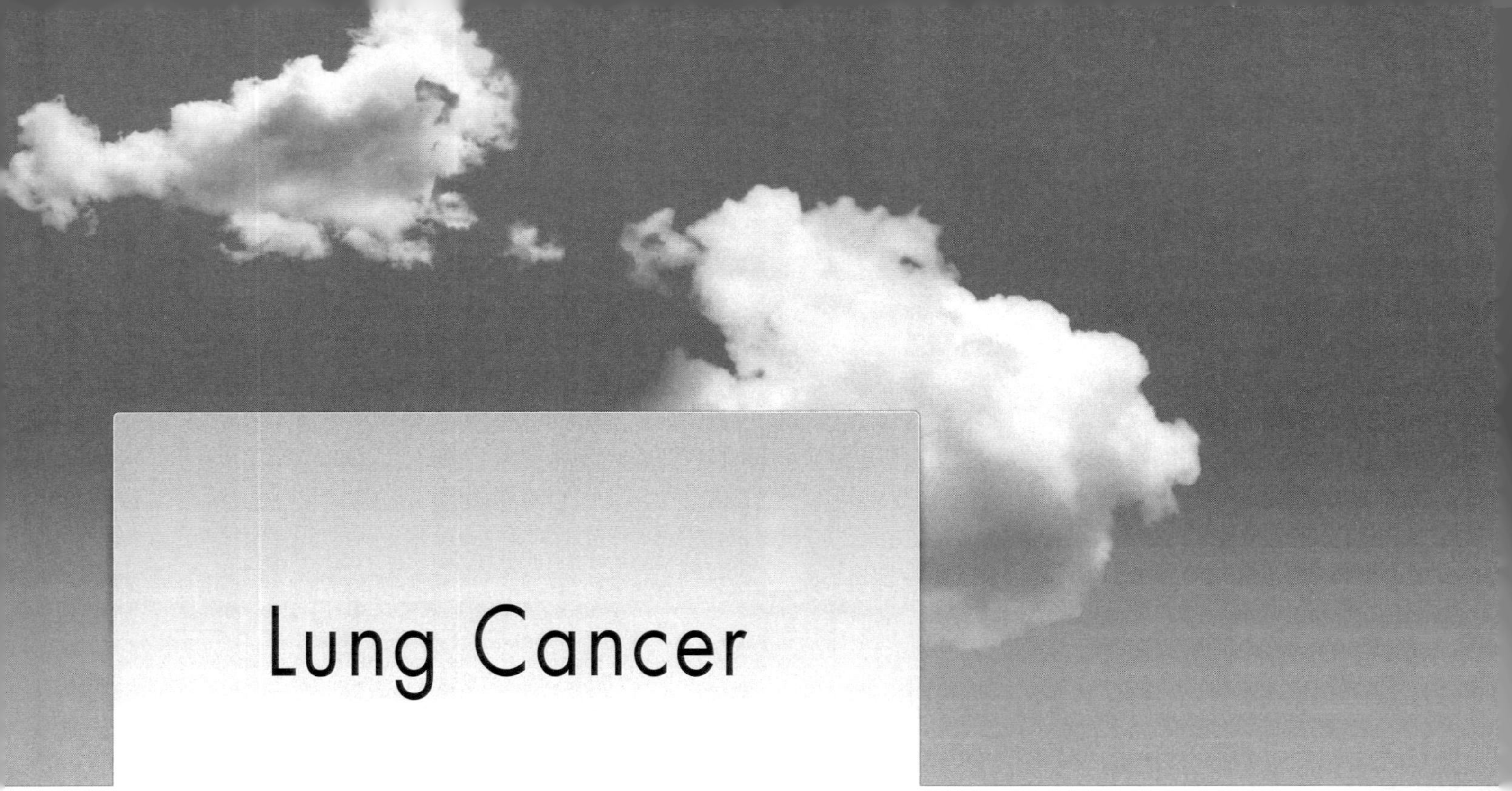

Lung Cancer

"Because conventional cancer therapies have failed to make a major impact on survival, newer approaches are necessary in the battle against lung cancer."
Source: Clinical Lung Cancer 7: 92-99, 2005

If you have lung cancer, you may be visiting this chapter hoping to find a cure. Despite a dismally low cure rate for lung cancer, there are unexplored options that patients and their families need to investigate.

If you are a current or past smoker and want to reduce your risk of ever developing lung cancer, many reports suggest that your cancer risk can be significantly reduced by employing simple measures in your diet and with dietary supplements.

Sadly, running to your doctor's office to inquire about these measures is not likely to be fruitful. Doctors generally advise conventional treatment only, even though it has already been disproven. Lung cancer prevention – doctors say this, too, is unproven.

It's a sad state of affairs today that doctors know of nothing that prevents lung cancer and can only recommend ineffective treatments.

This author is tempted to glibly state to readers, *"stop smoking, end of chapter."* However, with smoking cessation programs largely being ineffective, other life-saving options must be investigated.

And, not all lung cancer cases are caused by smoking. Chronic and sometimes undetectable infection in the lung can also cause lung cancer. But the vast majority of cases, and 87% of lung cancer deaths, occur among smokers.

But you probably already know all this. You may be reading this to find out if there is any new advice on how to avoid, treat or prevent recurrence of lung cancer.

You may wonder if there isn't something better than what modern medicine has to offer. There is.

If you are a smoker, you should be outraged by the time you reach the end of this chapter. Many promising avenues for prevention and treatment have gone overlooked or underutilized, and governments along with tobacco companies have covertly conspired to only give the appearance that they have been trying to stop lung cancer.

How to begin to explain all this in a convincing manner?

1billion people on Earth are smokers. A 5% reduction in the number of smokers by 2020 would save 100 miullion lives.

The psyche of smokers

There is a strange psyche involved among smokers. Anti-smoking ads can be measured for effectiveness. The most effective anti-tobacco TV ad ever aired was the one showing tobacco company executives testifying before Congress. The event occurred on April 14, 1994. The Congressional hearings discovered that tobacco industry scientists knew that the nicotine in cigarettes was addictive in 1963. The tobacco executives, under oath, claimed otherwise. That TV ad caused more smokers to back away from cigarettes than the tooth rot, facial wrinkles, cataracts, chronic cough and poor circulation caused by cigarettes. Smokers somehow felt conned. Health advice to avoid smoking didn't cause smokers to back away from their habit, x-ray pictures of scarred lungs didn't frighten them away from their habit, nor did the testimony of the "*Marlboro man*" who developed lung cancer, but only when smokers realized they were being lied to, did many throw away their stash of tobacco.

Actual and perceived relative risk of lung cancer (smoker's risk compared to non-smoker's risk)

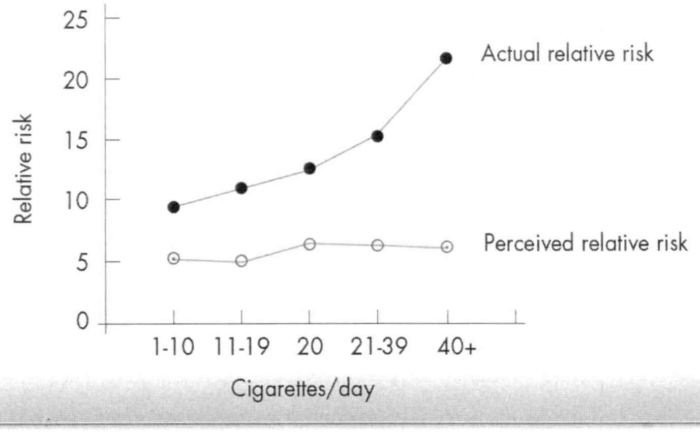

Not only do smokers vastly underestimate their risk for developing lung cancer, but surveys indicate more than half of smokers falsely believe exercise undoes most of the adverse effects of smoking. [Tobacco Control 14: 55-59, 2005]

With all of the grade school tobacco education programs, it has taken a long time to convince smokers of the link between their habit and lung cancer. That's because smoking habits usually begin during youth and lung cancer isn't diagnosed till decades later. The number of people who think cigarette smoking is one of the causes of lung cancer has changed over time:

Year	Believe smoking causes lung cancer
1954	41%
1999	92%

Survival rates

Lung cancer is such a large portion of all cancers that it skews all the other combined statistics regarding cancer rates and therapy. Most lung cancer cases involve smokers, and since early detection is difficult, treatment is largely ineffective.

The five-year survival rates are dismally low – about 14% in the United States. About 6 out of 10 people with lung cancer die within one year of being diagnosed with the disease. Between seven and eight out of ten will die within two years.

Your doctor is not likely to inform you that most of the treatments you will receive for lung cancer are ineffective and in fact have been disproven. The latest heralded treatments are costly and only add a month or two to life expectancy. Despite this, most people with lung cancer accept whatever the doctor has to offer, and hope for a miracle. There are miracles, aren't there? Yes, even a few people who purchase lottery tickets do win.

Doctors examine smokers in their offices, and keep a watchful eye for signs and symptoms of lung cancer, but practically speaking, when the patient begins coughing up blood, when there is chest pain, shortness of breath, bouts of pneumonia or hoarseness that lasts weeks, it is likely to be too late to significantly alter the progress of the disease.

Why it's so difficult to quit

Smokers are harangued to stop smoking. If it were only that easy to just quit.

Most smokers begin inhaling tobacco smoke when they are young, when the stimulation of this herb turned on biological reward switches in the brain, the same pleasure center involved in sexual satisfaction. Say, this isn't an easy habit to break!

American Indians smoked the Peace Pipe before pow-wows to think more clearly. While nicotine in tobacco leaves is believed to be one of the culprits that induces lung cancer, it is also an agent that inhibits formation of brain plaques and stimulates production of acetycholine, the memory molecule of the brain.

Believe it or not, nicotine is being considered as therapy for brain disease. Nicotine can improve working memory function, learning, and attention. [Psychopharmacology 184: 523-39, 2006] Nicotine is also being considered as treatment for brain disorders such as Parkinson's and Alzheimer's. [Expert Opinion Investigational Drugs 8: 747-60, 1999]

The tobacco industry has somehow created the idea that nicotine is the chief cancer-causing agent in cigarettes. This is misleading. Nicotine is actually the habit-forming component of tobacco. Lowering nicotine levels in cigarettes appears to be counterproductive. When low nicotine cigarettes were introduced, it only caused smokers to puff more to get the same amount of nicotine, and thus expose themselves to more cancer-causing chemicals like smoke, tar, nitrosamines and hidden additives. [Journal Toxicology Environmental Health 50: 307-64, 1997] In the past few years the level of nicotine in cigarettes has risen about 10 percent, making it more difficult to quit and easier to develop addiction. Only three states in the U.S. require tobacco companies to submit information on nicotine content in cigarettes. [British Medical Journal 333:566, 2006]

Why do most smokers never develop lung cancer?

While over 80% of lung cancers are attributed to smoking, 85% of heavy smokers never develop lung cancer.

Surprisingly, even heavy smokers usually don't develop lung cancer until after age 45. Fewer than 5% of smokers develop lung cancer before age 40. Lung cancer rates rise more sharply after age 65. But nobody explains why.

Another important fact is that about 64% of lung cancer cases are among men. Age and gender are important factors. Men begin to accumulate iron after full growth is achieved, while women delay iron overload until they stop menstruating. Dietary iron has been found to increase lung cancer risk, particularly among smokers. [Epidemiology 16:772-9, 2005] Male iron foundry workers have a particularly high rate of lung cancer. [American Journal Industrial Medicine 43:295-305, 2003] If you are a smoker, you may have been asked about your exposure to asbestos fibers that can enter the lungs and induce cancer. But you have probably never heard about the risk posed by iron.

The fact the iron chelators (molecules that removes iron) are employed with some anti-cancer drugs is a veiled admission that iron is an undesirable agent in lung cancer progression. [Cancer Biotherapy Radiopharm 20:467-78, 2005]

There is more to learn. Black men develop lung cancer at a higher rate than do Caucasian men. The reason for this is obvious, but for some reason escapes the attention of cancer doctors. Dark-skinned people have low levels of vitamin D due to melanin in their skin, and that's why they require far more sunshine to produce the same amount of vitamin D as do Caucasians.

There is yet another intriguing link to lung cancer. Smokers comprise most cases, and smoking depletes the body of vitamin C and carotenoids such as beta carotene, lycopene and lutein.

Few smokers ever learn the above facts, which certainly hint at the possibility of prevention or even a cure.

Doctors have overlooked reams of data that indicate that smokers who can't kick their habit could use dietary supplements to delay or even treat lung cancer.

There is great promise for nutritional therapy in regard to lung cancer. But when facts about nutrition and lung cancer are revealed, most people respond by asking: *"Why share this information with smokers when they need to stop smoking? This will now give them a license to continue smoking."*

But the fact is, most smoking cessation programs fail. That doesn't mean they should be abandoned. Millions attempt to quit, but only a few succeed. According to a National Institutes of Health panel, 70% of smokers want to quit, 40% make a serious attempt to quit each year, but fewer than 5 % succeed in any given year. [Reuters June 14, 2006] But by and large, we allow smokers to die early by not giving them life-saving information about nutritional therapy because we don't want to condone smoking. Do smokers really deserve to die prematurely because they got hooked on cigarettes?

Even when a tobacco habit is successfully abandoned, the risk for lung cancer remains elevated for years. There must be something that can be done to reduce risk.

The above facts should begin to raise the eyebrows of smokers at risk of developing lung cancer, those who are currently battling lung cancer, and others who wish to prevent its recurrence. There is strong evidence that nutrition may cure existing cases of lung cancer. But modern medicine is so wedded to expensive treatments, surgery, and drugs, that it does not consider any alternatives.

Beta carotene: good or bad?

Cancer doctors are quick to say beta carotene increases the risk of lung cancer among smokers. But the study they refer to only found that beta carotene was ineffective in smokers. [Journal National Cancer Institute 88: 1560-70, 1996] It didn't significantly raise the risk for lung cancer, despite what you may read or hear elsewhere. Inexplicably, cancer researchers now suggest a derivative of beta carotene may be helpful in treating or preventing lung cancer, but claim that beta carotene itself is toxic!

This author accuses cancer doctors of stonewalling patients over these issues. When the rare cancer patient comes into their office who has experienced dramatic improvement unexplained by conventional treatment, and the patient discloses he or she has employed nutritional therapy, the doctor will listen in silence and then goes on as if nothing was said. Doctors encounter patients like these from time to time, and dismiss them with no inquisitiveness as to why they fared so well. It's all part of the silent treatment that oncology gives to nutritional therapy.

Confront your doctor about these issues and he/she is likely to start talking about new treatments that are now available. Any decline in lung cancer mortality is likely to be attributed to improved treatment.

However, smoking in the United States is at an all-time low, with the lowest number of cigarettes (378 billion) reportedly sold since 1951, even though the population has doubled in size since then. [British Medical Journal 332: 687, 2006] Since there are more lung cancer deaths in the United States than there are breast, prostate, colon, or rectal cancer deaths combined, the decline in smoking is likely to result in a drop in the overall rate of cancer. For example, the greater decline in cancer death rates is due in large part to the substantial decrease in tobacco use among males. [Cancer 107: published online Sept. 6, 2006]

Do they really want you to stop smoking?

One wonders why smoking is still popular in the United States. There are social and governmental influences that stand in the way of its eradication. Recognize, political parties receive a great deal of their donations from the tobacco industry.

Worldwide, however, more than 1 out of 6 people on the planet smoke cigarettes. Harvard School of Public Health authorities estimate 4.83 million premature deaths in the world in the year 2000 were attributed to smoking. [Lancet 362: 847-52, 2003] Do health authorities really want to reduce smoking related deaths?

Health authorities are appointed by politicians, many of whom receive a great deal of funding from the tobacco lobby. A ruse is created that government has an anti-smoking campaign. In fact, it took years for tobacco advertising to be banned, and television networks had no moral hesitance to air tobacco ads prior to this.

Over a period of many years, the tobacco industry has placed its products in movies and television shows, associating their use with fun, excitement, sex and wealth and power. [Tobacco Control 11: I81-91, 2002] There are more than 1.2 billion smokers worldwide.

WebMD even published the Philip Morris website as an information source for people who wish to quit smoking. Do you think they really want you to stop smoking?

It's difficult to imagine that the lung cancer rate in 1930 in the U.S. was only 4.9 per 100,000 compared to 75.6 per 100,000 in 1990. [Morbidity Mortality Weekly Reports 48: 986-93, 1999] This is because it takes decades for smokers to develop lung cancer, so the high rates of cancer today reflect heavy cigarette use in the 60s, 70s, and 80s. Promotion of cigarette smoking is a worldwide problem. The European Union is paying tobacco farmers $1.1 billion in subsidies annually, which is 50 times more than the amount allotted to funds for reducing cigarette smoking. The subsidies are handed out to about 135,000 farmers, mostly in Greece, [Journal National Cancer Institute 95: 1187-88, 2003]

Tax and smoke

The government claims it invokes taxes on cigarettes to inhibit smoking. But an evaluation of state cigarette tax increases on cigarette sales in the 50 states for the years 1955 to 1988 found the average decline in cigarette consumption was a paltry three cigarette packs per capita (about 2.4%). [American Journal Public Health 82: 94-96, 1992]

Larger tax increases are associated with larger declines in consumption. [American Journal Public Health 82: 94-96, 1992] But tobacco taxes appear to be raised to reach a point where consumption begins to decline slightly, and then the taxes are fixed at that point.

The School of Public Health at the University of California, Berkeley, estimates taxes and anti-smoking advertising reduced cigarette sales by 819 million and 232 million packs of cigarettes respectively over a 12-year period in California. [American Journal Public Health 85: 1218-22, 1995] These numbers may sound big, but they are trivial.

The rise in cigarette taxes has reduced consumption by only 5% to 7%. [American Journal Public Health 82: 867-69, 1992]

In the U.S., states adjust their tobacco taxes to be lower than surrounding states so that consumers will cross state lines to purchase cigarettes in their state. Cigarette taxes are all about swiping money out of smokers pockets, not smoking cessation!

Tobacco taxes are pledged to be used to conduct anti-smoking advertisements. Exposure to anti-tobacco TV ads is said to increase the rate for quitting smoking by 10%, but this happens only after 5,000 TV spots are aired. [Health Education Research Nov. 14, 2005] These aren't tobacco eradication programs, they are public charades and excuses to tax citizenry.

How much of the tax on tobacco is actually spent on anti-tobacco advertising? From 1999 to 2002, the State of California imposed a per pack tax increase that was intended to reduce consumption by a miniscule 2.4 packs per capita per quarter and increase state revenues by $2.1 billion. [American Journal Public Health 95: 1030-35, 2005] California spends about $21 million annually on anti-smoking ads. That's a paltry amount compared to the financial take.

One authority estimates, as taxes are raised, many smokers opt to obtain tobacco via the internet or through other smuggled sources, skirting around taxation. So there is hidden tobacco consumption that doesn't get listed in the number of tobacco packs sold. States must implement anti-smuggling programs if their anti-smoking campaigns and taxes are to be effective. [Journal Health Economics 24: 277-97, 2005]

It was estimated that the deterrent effect caused by cigarette taxes implemented in 1983 would increase the number of people living to the age of 65 by 100,000 persons. [British Journal Addiction 84: 1217-34, 1989] But over two decades later, 160,000 Americans still die every year from lung cancer, with most of the deaths occurring among adults over age 65. Since lung cancer has a about a 20-year incubation period, any large decline in smoking will take years to produce a significant drop in mortality rates.

New smokers needed

Society keeps selling cancer sticks to kids. Every day 1,200 smokers die and another 3,500 stop smoking, so the tobacco industry needs fresh new candidates for their products. Since very few people start smoking after they reach adulthood, the tobacco industry must recruit children. Fortunately for the tobacco companies, 3,000 kids light up for the first time every day. Despite laws that forbid sales to children, 60-90 % of new smokers report they buy their own cigarettes. Laws, taxes, and anti-smoking ads aren't stopping the tobacco industry. [Journal American Medical Assn 2698: 793-94, 1993]

A study conducted by Stanford University School of Medicine finds that industry sponsored anti-smoking ads do more to promote corporate image than to prevent youth from smoking. *"By cultivating public opinion that is more sympathetic toward tobacco companies, the effect of such advertising is likely to be more harmful than helpful to youth,"* said their report. [Tobacco Control 15: 13-18, 2006]

A survey of the effectiveness of anti-smoking advertising shows these ads have little or no impact upon teenagers' intent to smoke unless the ads show young people suffering with disease. [American Journal Public Health 96: 906-13, 2006] The ads are designed to delay smoking till later in life, not to deliver a message that smoking should never become a habit.

A University of Maryland report says: *"Despite their public pledge, the tobacco companies routinely violate a variety of aspects of the Cigarette Advertising and Promotion Code."* This includes use of young-aged models in TV ads, building upon the image that cigarettes increase sexual attractiveness. [Journal Health Communications 10: 419-31, 2005] While cigarette manufacturers have adopted a code not to advertise to youth in the United States, at the very same time it is conducting youth-targeted advertising overseas.

Recognize that the local pharmacy where you go to purchase medicines and nicotine patches to help you stop smoking, also sells cigarettes.

There you have it – an American culture that only pretends to implement smoking cessation programs while preying upon youth who are moving away from parental authority and into the age of influence as they enter their teens. All that counts is making money off these kids.

The tobacco industry

"If we had any thought or knowledge that in any way we were selling a product harmful to consumers, we would stop business tomorrow."
Source: George Weissman, president, Philip Morris, 1954

"There is not one shred of conclusive evidence to support the link between cigarette smoking and lung cancer."
George Weissman, president, Philip Morris, 1957

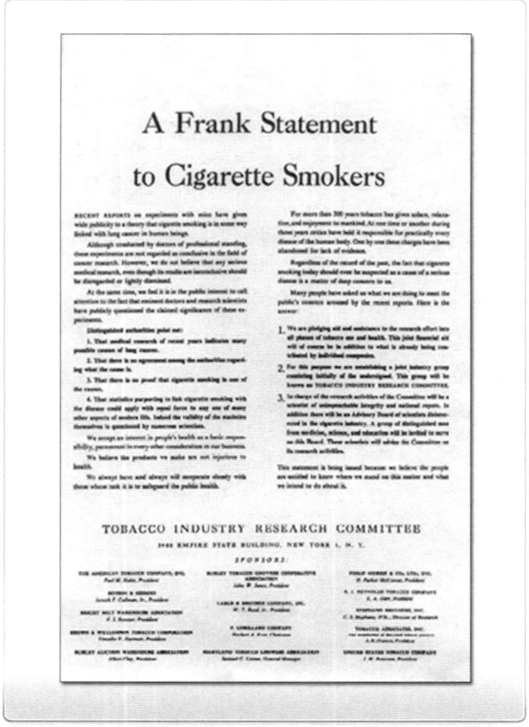
A Frank Statement

to Cigarette Smokers

TOBACCO INDUSTRY RESEARCH COMMITTEE

A Frank Statement
to Cigarette Smokers

The *"Frank Statement to Cigarette Smokers,"* an advertisement placed in 448 newspapers in 258 American cities in 1954 by U.S. tobacco manufacturers, questioned research which implicated tobacco as a cause of cancer. This ad promised that cigarettes were safe and pledged to support impartial research to investigate allegations that smoking was harmful to human health. Examination of internal records of tobacco companies shows some of their scientists acknowledged cigarettes were unsafe as early as 1940. [Tobacco Control 11: I110-17, 2002]

Cigarette smoking	→	670% increased risk
Rheumatoid arthritis	→	420% increased risk
Yogurt consumption	→	310% increased risk
Vegetable consumption	→	60% reduced risk

A Frank Statement to Cigarette Smokers

RECENT REPORTS on experiments with mice have given wide publicity to a theory that cigarette smoking is in some way linked with lung cancer in human beings.

Although conducted by doctors of professional standing, these experiments are not regarded as conclusive in the field of cancer research. However, we do not believe results are inconclusive, should be disregarded or lightly dismissed. At the same time, we feel it is in the public interest to call attention to the fact that eminent doctors and research scientists have publicly questioned the claimed significance of these experiments.

Distinguished authorities point out:

That medical research of recent years indicates many possible causes of lung cancer.

That there is no agreement among the authorities regarding what the cause is.

That there is no proof that cigarette smoking is one of the causes.

That statistics purporting to link cigarette smoking with the disease could apply with equal force to any one of many other aspects of modern life. Indeed the validity of the statistics themselves is questioned by numerous scientists.

We accept an interest in people's health as a basic responsibility, paramount to every other consideration in our business

We believe the products we make are not injurious to health.

We always have and always will cooperate closely with those whose task it is to safeguard the public health.

For more than 300 years tobacco has given solace, relaxation, and enjoyment to mankind. At one time or another during those years critics have held it responsible for practically every disease of the human body. One by one these charges have been abandoned for lack of evidence.

Regardless of the record of the past, the fact that cigarette smoking today should even be suspected as a cause of a serious disease is a matter of deep concern to us.

Many people have asked us what we are doing to meet the public's concern aroused by the recent reports. Here is the answer:

We are pledging aid and assistance to the research effort into all phases of tobacco use and health. This joint financial aid will of course be in addition to what is already being contributed by individual companies.

For this purpose we are establishing a joint industry group consisting initially of the undersigned. This group will be known as TOBACCO INDUSTRY RESEARCH COMMITTEE.

In charge of the research activities of the Committee will be a scientist of unimpeachable integrity and national repute. In addition there will be an Advisory Board of scientists disinterested in the cigarette industry. A group of distinguished men from medicine, science, and education will be invited to serve on this Board. These scientists will advise the Committee on its research activities.

This statement is being issued because we believe the people are entitled to know where we stand on this matter and what we intend to do about it.

The Tobacco Industry Research Committee
5400 Empire State Building New York 1, NY

Sponsors:

THE AMERICAN TOBACCO COMPANY
Paul M. Hahn, President

BENSON & HEDGES
Joseph Cullman, Jr., President

BRIGHT BELT WAREHOUSE ASSOCIATION
F.S. Royster, President

BROWN & WILLIAMSON TOBACCO CORPORATION
Timothy V. Hartnett, President

BURLEY AUCTION WAREHOUSE ASSOCIATION
Albert Clay, President

BURLEY TOBACCO GROWERS CO-OPERATIVE
John W. Jones, President

LARUS & BROTHER COMPANY, INC.
W.T. Reed, Jr., President

P. LORILLARD COMPANY
Kerbert A. Kent, Chairman

MARYLAND TOBACCO GROWERS ASSOCIATION
Samuel C. Linton, General Manager

PHILIP MORRIS & CO. LTD., INC.
O. Parker McComas, President

R.J. REYNOLDS TOBACCO COMPANY
E. A. Darr, President

STEPHANO BROTHERS, INC.
C.S. Stephano, D.Sc., Director of Research

TOBACCO ASSOCIATES, INC.
(An organization of flue-cured tobacco growers)
J.B. Hudson, President

UNITED STATES TOBACCO COMPANY
J.W. Peterson, President

Are you a Marlboro man? About 4 in 10 cigarettes sold in the U.S.A. are Marlboro's. It's the most popular cigarette sold. Just so you know, the families of an estimated 143,000 Americans who smoke Marlboro's will be scheduling funerals this year. Philip Morris, maker of Marlboro's, actually celebrated the demise of its customers on the occasion of the 50th anniversary of its Marlboro brand. The *"birthday party"* for Marlboro was an invitation-only affair with parties held in 49 U.S. cities featuring popular entertainers. Philip Morris is the only company that makes a product that kills its customers and throws a party! [Tobacco Control 15: 75-77, 2006]

Tobacco additives

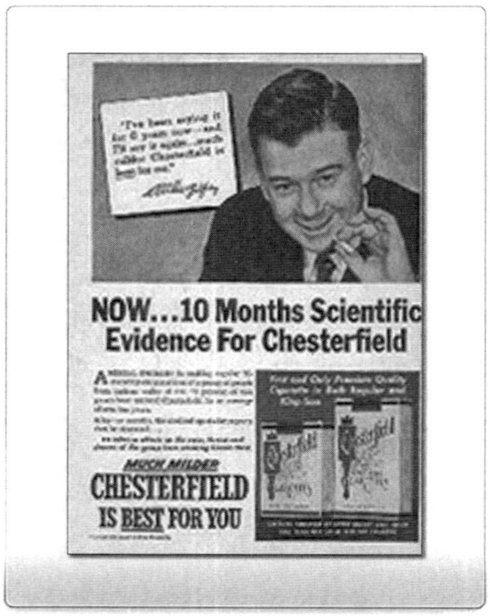

There are scientists working in laboratories today who are attempting to make cigarettes that are less irritating, tastier, and more habit forming. They have no qualms about what they do for a living.

There are many additives covertly added to cigarettes by tobacco companies. One report reveals 450 ingredients added to tobacco as flavorings, solvents, preservatives and binders. [Food Chemistry Toxicology 42: S3-37, 2004] Tobacco companies have added levulinic acid to cigarettes to enhance the habit-forming effect of nicotine. Levulinic acid reduces the pH of tobacco smoke, making it easier for smokers to inhale cigarette smoke deeper into the lungs. [Nicotine Tobacco Research 7: 761-71, 2005] Cigarette manufacturers may even be able to skirt around laws that limit nicotine content by using nicotine analogs (nicotine-like molecules). [Addiction 100: 701-12, 2005]

In Europe, authorities have debated whether to mandate that the top 10 additives in cigarettes be listed on product labels. The German Cancer Research Centre demanded that certain tobacco additives be banned because they increase the risk for cancer and tobacco addiction. German health authorities allege certain substances were added to cigarettes to make them more palatable to children and young people. Menthol was added as an anesthetic to dull the harsh effects of tobacco among first-time smokers. Even sugar and aromatics were added to make cigarettes taste better. Over a period of decades, cigarette makers added cocoa, ammonia and other agents to their products. By law, these additives can represent up to 10% of the total weight of one cigarette. These changes have been made without informing health authorities. [British Medical Journal 330: 690, 2005]

From 1954 to 1993, the tobacco industry reduced the amount of tar and nicotine smoke yield from its products by 60%. This made it appear that the tobacco industry was making cigarettes that were less habit forming and safer overall. However, large reductions in lung cancer incidence have not been observed since the introduction of these low-yield cigarettes. The tobacco industry knew what it was doing by reducing tar and nicotine. By reducing tar and nicotine levels, smokers inhaled deeper puffs of smoke into their lungs and smoked more cigarettes in a day. [Journal National Cancer Institute 92: 106, 2000]

The Federal Trade Commission utilized machines to rate cigarettes by the amount of tar and nicotine they produced in tobacco smoke. These machines underestimated the amount of tar and nicotine actually delivered to the lungs because they didn't calculate for the deeper puffs smokers took when using reduced tar and nicotine cigarettes. Government was in on the ruse. [Journal National Cancer Institute 92: 106, 2000]

Tobacco companies have also conducted extensive studies into reducing, masking or altering the visibility, odor, irritation and emission of tobacco smoke. [Tobacco Control 9: 283-91, 2000]

There is no difference in lung cancer risk for smokers who use reduced tar cigarettes compared to those who smoke regular cigarettes. [Cancer Epidemiology Biomarkers Prevention 14: 693-98, 2005] Tobacco companies marketed low-tar cigarettes to more health conscious smokers all the while knowing they didn't lower cancer risk. [Journal American Medical Assn 280: 1173-81, 1998]

Most cigarettes produced in the world have a filter, but it has been shown that the cellulose acetate fibers from the filter are released during puffing and can enter the lungs. [Tobacco Control 11: 151-61, 2002]

Filtered tobacco smoke, devoid of nitrosamines and hydrocarbons, produces lung tumors as effectively as does unfiltered smoke, which casts doubt on whether these chemicals are the primary causes of lung cancer. [Chest 125: 128S, 2004]

Tobacco companies have made half-hearted attempts to produce cigarettes that reduce exposure to cancer-causing chemicals, producing brands such as Eclipse, Omni, Advance Lights, Accord, and Ariva, but most established smokers don't like them. [Tobacco Control 15: 39-44, 2006]

One cigarette manufacturer wants to introduce what it calls a *"safe cigarette"* that reduces cancer risk by 90%. These are specially treated cigarettes with a new type of filter that supposedly looks and tastes like normal cigarettes. [London Times, Nov. 6, 2005] However, health authorities remind us that there are no safe cigarettes. [Tobacco Control Suppl 2:ii3-7, 2005] One cancer researcher likened these new cigarettes to *"jumping off the 15th floor instead of the 20th floor."*

Lung cancer rates, Japan

The odds of developing lung cancer in the United States are 40 times greater among smokers compared to non-smokers. However, although Japanese are avid smokers, the rates of lung cancer in American men have greatly exceeded that of Japanese men for a number of decades. In Japan, smokers only have a 3.5 times increased risk of developing lung cancer versus nonsmokers. [Cancer Epidemiology Biomarkers Prevention 10: 1193-99, 2001]

Mortality rates for lung cancer dramatically increased in both countries since 1950. However, the rates for lung cancer mortality in Japan remain about 47% lower than in the United States.

Mortality rates* lung cancer	1950	1985
Japan	3.3	38.2
United States	21.9	72.2

*Per 100,000

Source: Japanese Journal Cancer Research 83: 418-23, 1992

There are some differences between Japanese and American smokers that would account for this disparity in rates of lung cancer. Americans, on average, begin smoking about 2.5 years earlier than do Japanese. From 1955 to 1985, there was a decline in the prevalence of smoking (54 to 44%) in U.S. men, whereas the percentage of Japanese men who smoked increased over the same period (from 76 to 82%).

Why do Japanese smokers have far lower mortality rates from lung cancer than do Americans? Cancer researchers believe American cigarettes deliver a *"more toxic cigarette formulation"* as evidenced by higher concentrations of tobacco-specific nitrosamines in tobacco smoke. [Cancer Epidemiology Biomarkers Prevention 10: 1193-99, 2001]

Mortality rates from smoking are rising in Japan. The United States insisted that Japan open its markets to foreign trade, and one of those markets was tobacco. The introduction of U.S. brand cigarettes in Japan is responsible for much of the rise in smoking in Japan in recent years. [Tobacco Control 9: 193-200, 2000] The leading manufacturer of cigarettes in Japan, Japan Tobacco, of which the government holds two-thirds ownership, continues to question whether tobacco is a major cause of disease and death. Philip Morris has assisted Japan Tobacco, which is evidence of global collaboration. [Lancet 363: 1820-24, 2004]

Smokers as pawns to industry: screening programs

Smokers also find themselves as pawns to the medical profession. Many smokers know that early detection is their only hope for successful treatment. Smokers are eager to hear of any new technology that can detect lung tumors when they are still only a few million cells in size, small enough to remove surgically before they spread.

A so-called consumer group that represents smokers is suing Philip Morris to pay for yearly cancer screening. The group wants the tobacco company to pay for low-dose CT scanning of the chest. But the funding for this group is undisclosed. The head of this consumer group was formerly employed by an unnamed Fortune 500 company and had worked for various Congressional leaders. Has she been planted to head this consumer group? How would this leader represent smokers?

CT scanning has gained widespread attention, especially by ex-smokers who are fearful they will develop lung cancer and know that most diagnoses are usually made too late to effectively treat the disease. The annual scans cost about $500 each.

The CT scanning picks up lung scars and benign lumps better than it does tumors. So, most smokers who undergo the scans will be subject to needless medical care. So far, CT scanning has not been shown to reduce mortality rates among smokers.

One study showed that it took 1,520 prospective lung cancer patients to be screened to find 22,444 lung nodules in 1,000 individuals (or an average of 22.4 nodules per person) but only 25 lung cancers were detected. Twenty two patients underwent subsequent surgery, but seven of these cases were found to be benign nodules in the lung. [American Journal Respiratory Critical Care Medicine 165: 508-13, 2002]

Smokers are being duped into thinking CT scanning offers an advancement in tumor detection. When a radiology center in Oregon advertised a new screening test for early detection of lung cancer using the powerful spiral CT scanner, 300 smokers called in one day to schedule the $295 test. That would generate about $90,000 in revenue. [New York Times June 21, 2000] About 23% of those screened by the new test will have suspicious nodules and only 2.7% will actually have lung cancer. This is another test that is good for cancer centers, but not necessarily for patients.

An interesting fact surfaces in the cancer screening game. If adult smokers are screened annually for five years, there is a 75% chance of finding a lung abnormality. [European Journal Radiology 45: 2-7, 2003] But is that because of the radiation from the CT screening or the long-lasting effects of smoking?

If a 50-year-old female smoker undergoes annual CT lung screening until age 75, she would incur an estimated radiation-related lung cancer risk of 0.85%, in addition to her otherwise expected lung cancer risk of approximately 17%. If 50% of all current and former smokers in the U.S. population aged 50-75 years received annual CT screening, the estimated number of lung cancers associated with radiation from screening would be approximately 36,000, a 1.8% increase over the otherwise expected number. Given the theoretical upper limit of a 5.5% increase in lung cancer risk attributable to annual CT-related radiation exposure, a mortality benefit of considerably more than 5% may be necessary to outweigh the potential radiation risks. [Radiology 23: 440-45, 2004] Think twice before electing to undergo CT scanning on a regular basis.

Treatment for lung cancer

So let's assume you've got lung cancer. Here's what you face. About 75% of lung cancer cases are categorized as non-small cell lung cancer, and the other 25% are small cell lung cancer. Lung cancer often spreads quickly and forms large tumors, which can spread to lymph nodes and other organs.

If you have time to investigate, you may not be able to easily find out the true survival rates for lung cancer in the U.S. compared to other countries. Health authorities continue to publish misleading statistics regarding survival rates for lung cancer which makes it appear that treatment is better in the U.S. than in other countries. [Journal National Cancer Institute 97: 18: 1985]

The overall five-year survival rate is quoted at 14-15%, but when lung cancer is detected when it is small and confined to the lung, nearly half of the patients can be successfully treated by surgery. But only about 15% of lung cancer cases are detected this early. For non-small-cell lung cancer, only 10% of untreated patients are alive one year after initial diagnosis.

Small advancements in treatment are not what patients and their families are hoping for. With advanced forms of lung cancer, surgery plus chemo and radiation therapy can now increase two-year survival from 10 % to 48 %. [Reuters May 23, 2000] That's all the cancer industry has to offer – a couple of extra years of life or less for most patients.

Widely touted gene-targeted drugs, like Iressa, have failed to improve survival rates and may even harm some patients. Iressa costs $1,800 per month and is still being prescribed for non-small-cell lung cancer, the most prevalent form of lung cancer. [Boston Globe April 5, 2005] Public Citizen, the Ralph Nader organization, has petitioned the FDA to remove Iressa from the market because it does not improve survival rates and has been linked to deaths in Japan and the United States. Iressa actually increases your risk of dying from causes other than cancer, yet it is still considered a breakthrough.

The FDA recently approved three therapies to treat non-small cell lung cancer: Photofrin (porfimer sodium), Taxol (paclitaxel) in combination with the commonly used cancer drug cisplatin, and Gemzar (gemcitabine hydrochloride) in combination with cisplatin. Knowing of the public dismay over ineffective lung cancer treatments, these advancements were widely publicized by the FDA.

Photofrin, a light-activated drug, was approved in January 1998 for patients with early stage, non-small cell lung cancer who were unable to undergo surgery or radiotherapy due to other medical conditions. Administered intravenously, Photofrin accumulates in the tumor cells. A laser, directed toward the cancerous tissue, then activates the drug. A significant side effect is extreme photosensitivity, making it necessary for patients to stay out of the sun *"almost completely for about a month,"* says Grant Williams, M.D., a medical team leader in the division of oncology drug products in FDA's Center for Drug Evaluation and Research.

Williams admits that the number of patients with early stage lung cancer who will be helped by Photofrin will be quite limited. *"We're talking about a very small number of patients compared to the number of lung cancer patients who have extensive cancers that can't be operated on,"* he says.

Taxol and Gemzar may only give patients an additional month or two to live. *"There are not a lot of effective treatments for advanced stage non-small cell lung cancer,"* says Isagani Chico, M.D., a medical officer in FDA's division of oncology drug products.

The most notable advancement in cancer treatment of late is a non-surgical treatment called thermoablation. A radiologist advances a small needle into the lung and heat energy *"cooks"* the tumor. The treatment can be performed without need for overnight hospitalization. About 57% of patients with non-small cell lung cancer who underwent thermoablation lived about 3 years, two years beyond the average life expectancy. [Journal Vascular Interventional Radiology 17:1117-24, 2006] It's not a cure, but it will buy some time.

Chemotherapy and antioxidants

Most doctors advise their cancer patients to avoid antioxidant supplements because they are alleged to interfere with treatment. Nothing could be further from the truth. Examine the evidence presented below.

Antioxidant supplements appear to improve survival rates when given with chemotherapy for non-small cell lung cancer. One study found that the combination of 1,050 mg of vitamin E, 6,100 mg vitamin C and 60 mg beta carotene improved two-year survival from 11.1 to 15.6%. While this improvement is miniscule, and the overall survival rate remains very poor, it is equivalent to what many high-priced cancer drugs accomplish. [Journal American College Nutrition 24: 16-21, 2005] Even the use of unspecified multivitamins by patients with small cell lung cancer was found to improve survival by about five months. [Nutrition & Cancer 51: 7-12, 2005] Another study showed that lung cancer patients (non-small cell) who take multivitamins survive 4.3 years compared to two years for non-multivitamin users. [Lung Cancer 49: 77-84, 2005]

A small study of 18 patients with small-cell lung cancer reveals the importance of antioxidant supplementation when undergoing chemo and radiation therapy.

	Typical Survival 2-years	Survival with dietary supplements*
Small-cell lung cancer	15%	33%**

Source: Anticancer Research 12: 599-606, 1992

*Nutritional supplement regimen: Vitamin A 15,000-40,000 IU; beta carotene 10,000-20,000 IU; vitamin E 300-800 IU; Vitamin B1 150-750 mg; riboflavin 15-50 mg; vitamin B6 200-1,140 mg; vitamin B12 300-1,600 mcg; Niacinamide 150-400 mg; vitamin D 400-1,000 IU; vitamin C 2,000-5,000 mg; vitamin B5 50-300 mg; biotin 50-300 mcg; omega-3 oils 5,000-6,000 mg; magnesium 250-500 mg; calcium 500 mg; zinc 27 mg; copper 3 mg; selenium 856 mcg; chromium 780 mcg.
**1 patient survived 74 months (6+ years)

A study involving patients with non-small cell lung cancer also shows that survival is improved among users of vitamin supplements.

	Survival non-supplement users	Survival supplement users
Non-small cell lung cancer	11 months	41 months

* Supplements included vitamin E, vitamin C, selenium, folic acid, beta carotene

Source: Journal Surgical Oncology 68: 231-35, 1998

A remarkable study conducted by the Linus Pauling Institute showed that 1,000 mg of vitamin C per day, which is more than 10 times the Daily Value suggested intake level, protects smokers from the loss of vitamin C in their lungs. Smokers who took vitamin C and vitamin E supplements had about the same level of antioxidant protection as did non-smokers. Vitamin E is one of the first lines of defense in lung tissues against the toxicity of cigarette smoke. [Free Radical Biology Medicine 40: 689-97, 2006]

Antioxidants from fruits and vegetables are helpful, too, but only yield modest results. A study of 27,111 male smokers in Finland showed those smokers who consumed the most antioxidants from foods exhibited a small decreased risk for lung cancer (about 16% reduction). [American Journal Epidemiology 160: 68-76, 2005]

Prevention

Imagine walking into a store to buy cigarettes and there is a bottle of antioxidant vitamins on display right next to the cigarettes. That would only happen in a fictional world.

Cancer doctors keep talking about *"chemoprevention"* for lung cancer. It certainly makes sense for the most common type of cancer for which treatment is largely ineffective. But prevention programs never seem to materialize.

If you are a smoker or ex-smoker, you can't wait for research studies that take decades to complete. You will have to rely upon the best information now available.

So the question arises,

what are you going to do to prevent lung cancer ?

Don't let statistics discourage your efforts to stop smoking. The National Institutes of Health target to reduce smoking will not be reached. Smoking cessation programs are modestly successful (success rates ~25%). For example, a 10-week smoking cessation program that included physician participation, group sessions and nicotine gum, achieved a 21.7% success rate over a five-year period. For comparison, only 5.4% of smokers stopped smoking who weren't enrolled in the program. [Annals Internal Medicine 142: 233-39, 2005]

Even ex-smokers have an elevated risk for lung cancer years after they have stopped smoking. [Journal National Cancer Institute 97: 1634-35, 2005] In a study of women in Iowa, the risk for lung cancer remained elevated for up to 25 years after smoking cessation. [Cancer Detection Prevention March 30, 2006] Yet nothing is recommended beyond a sound diet to prevent lung cancer.

Cancer researchers continue to maintain that a healthy diet is all that can be done to counter the adverse effects of smoking. Yes, plant food diets are helpful. But smokers generally consume fewer fruits and vegetables than do non-smokers. [Journal American Dietetic Assn 94: 287-92, 1994]

A diet rich in fruits and vegetables is known to reduce lung cancer incidence by 25% and the reduction is the same magnitude among smokers, ex-smokers and never smokers. [Monaldi Archives Chest Disease 59: 207-11, 2003] Cruciferous vegetables (Brussels sprouts, broccoli, cauliflower) produce a strong risk reduction for lung cancer. [Lancet 366: 1558-60, 2005]

But there is much more that can be done to prevent lung cancer beyond a healthy diet, as outlined below.

Vitamin D and lung cancer

Why are lung cancer researchers missing the obvious?

An article in the *Washington Post* reveals the blinders that cancer researchers wear. In the report, entitled *"Race may be factor in lung cancer,"* it says Black smokers and native Hawaiians who smoked less than a pack of cigarettes a day are much more likely than Caucasians who smoke the same amount to get lung cancer. In fact, Blacks are 55% more likely than are whites to develop lung cancer from a tobacco habit. The racial differences disappear for heavy smokers. What's more, the differences persist even after researchers consider factors such as diet, socioeconomic status and occupation. [Washington Post, January 26, 2006; New England J Medicine 354:333-42, 2006]

"We observed quite striking differences," said Christopher A. Haiman of the University of Southern California, who led the study. Another researcher said: *"The biggest danger here is ideology on both sides getting in the way of trying to understand this phenomenon."*

What ideology? Blacks and darkly pigmented people don't make as much vitamin D from sun exposure. Vitamin D shortage is a strong factor in the development of cancer, particularly lung cancer.

Examine the lung cancer mortality rates for the 23 countries displayed on **map Nr. 1** in this chapter. The countries are divided by Northern climate (less vitamin D from sunlight exposure) and equatorial countries (more sunlight and higher

Age-standardized mortality rate (per100 000 person years) from lung cancer in males in 23 countries, 1971–1995	
Country	**1971–1995**
Northern Nations (lower vitamin D levels)	
Hungary	180.91
Poland	158.34
Belgium	144.87
Netherlands	129.4
Canada	107.71
USA	115.23
Denmark	103.74
England and Wales	101.21
Finland	90.2
Norway	67.36
Sweden	48.21
Equatorial Nations (higher vitamin D levels)	
Taiwan	58.44
Portugal	59.48
Japan	59.44
Cuba	72.9
New Zealand	79.31
Australia	80.86
Singapore	91.47
Spain	101.49
France	100.08
Greece	105.44
Hong Kong	110.13
Italy	117.1

vitamin D exposure). The Northern countries generally exhibit higher rates of mortality.

Let's see if cancer mapping is consistent with the hypothesis that vitamin D is a prominent factor in lung cancer. The following map shows that U.S. lung cancer mortality rates are highest in the east and south. If a shortage of vitamin D is a risk factor.

However, **map Nr. 2** shows that there is a high concentration of Blacks in the southeastern part of the country, exactly where the risk for lung cancer is highest.

Maps Nr. 3 and 4 display concentrations of adults who smoke, again centered in the South but also in northeastern states.

The highest concentration of Black smokers is in the northeastern United States followed by the southeastern area. Weaker solar ultraviolet light intensity in the northern states would be consistent with the theory that the lack of vitamin D is linked to lung cancer.

Let's examine more evidence. A study has found that patients who underwent lung cancer surgery for non-small cell cancer during summer months, when vitamin D production is highest from exposure to the sun, had better recurrence-free survival by far, compared to patients who underwent surgery in winter months. The five-year survival rates for patients operated on in summer was 56% compared to just 23% among patients operated on in winter. [Cancer Epidemiology Biomarkers Prevention 14: 2303-09, 2005]

In an animal study, it has been found that vitamin D strongly inhibits the spread of lung cancer. [Carcinogenesis 26: 429-40, 2005]

A research study suggests the minimum amount of vitamin D needed to effectively reduce cancer mortality rates is 1,500 IU. Most dietary supplements provide only 400 .I.U. [Journal National Cancer Institute 98:451-9, 2006]

Why do cancer researchers overlook this strikingly convincing data?

map 1

Cancer mortality rates by state (age-adjusted 1970 US population)
Lung, trachea, bronchus, pleura: white males, 1950 to 1994, all ages

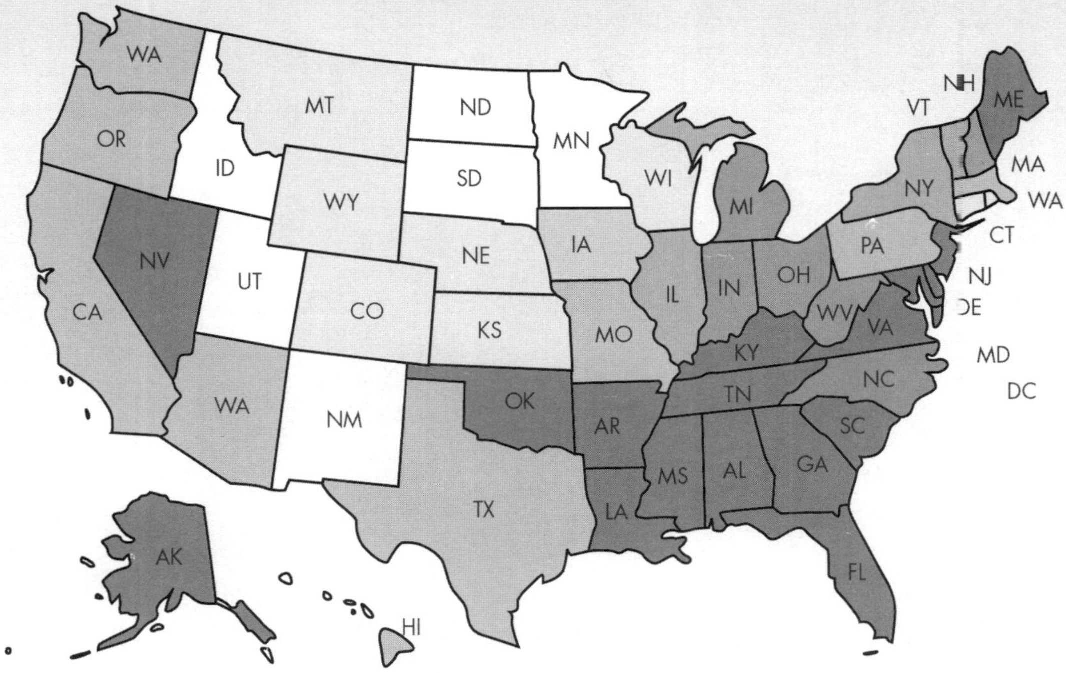

Rates per 100,000 person-years 1950 to 1994

- 68.83 - 76.25 (5; 9.8%)
- 66.58 - 68.86 (5; 9.8%)
- 63.62 - 66.58 (5; 9.8%)
- 31.42 - 63.62 (5; 9.8%)
- 60.46 - 61.42 (5; 9.8%)
- 57.32 - 60.46 (5; 9.8%)
- 56.15 - 57.32 (5; 9.8%)
- 50.16 - 56.15 (5; 9.8%)
- 43.73 - 50.16 (5; 9.8%)
- 30.36 - 43.73 (5; 11.8%)
- Sparse data (0)

Mortality rate	Confidence interval	No. of deaths
US 58.66	58.58 - 58.73	2,261,359

Does beta carotene really increase the risk for lung cancer among smokers?

In 1994, researchers heading a beta carotene study in Finland stopped the study when it was observed that current and former smokers taking beta carotene and vitamin A supplements were developing lung cancer at a higher rate than study participants taking an inactive placebo tablet. The study was halted just prior to a vote in Congress over the Dietary Supplement Health and Education Act. Was the study stopped for publicity effect? There was no explanation why there was an 18% relative increased risk for mortality among users of beta carotene supplements. Oddly, it was found the elevated mortality risk remained higher even 4 years after the end of the trial when no beta carotene supplements were in use. [New England Journal of Medicine 330:1029-35, 1994]

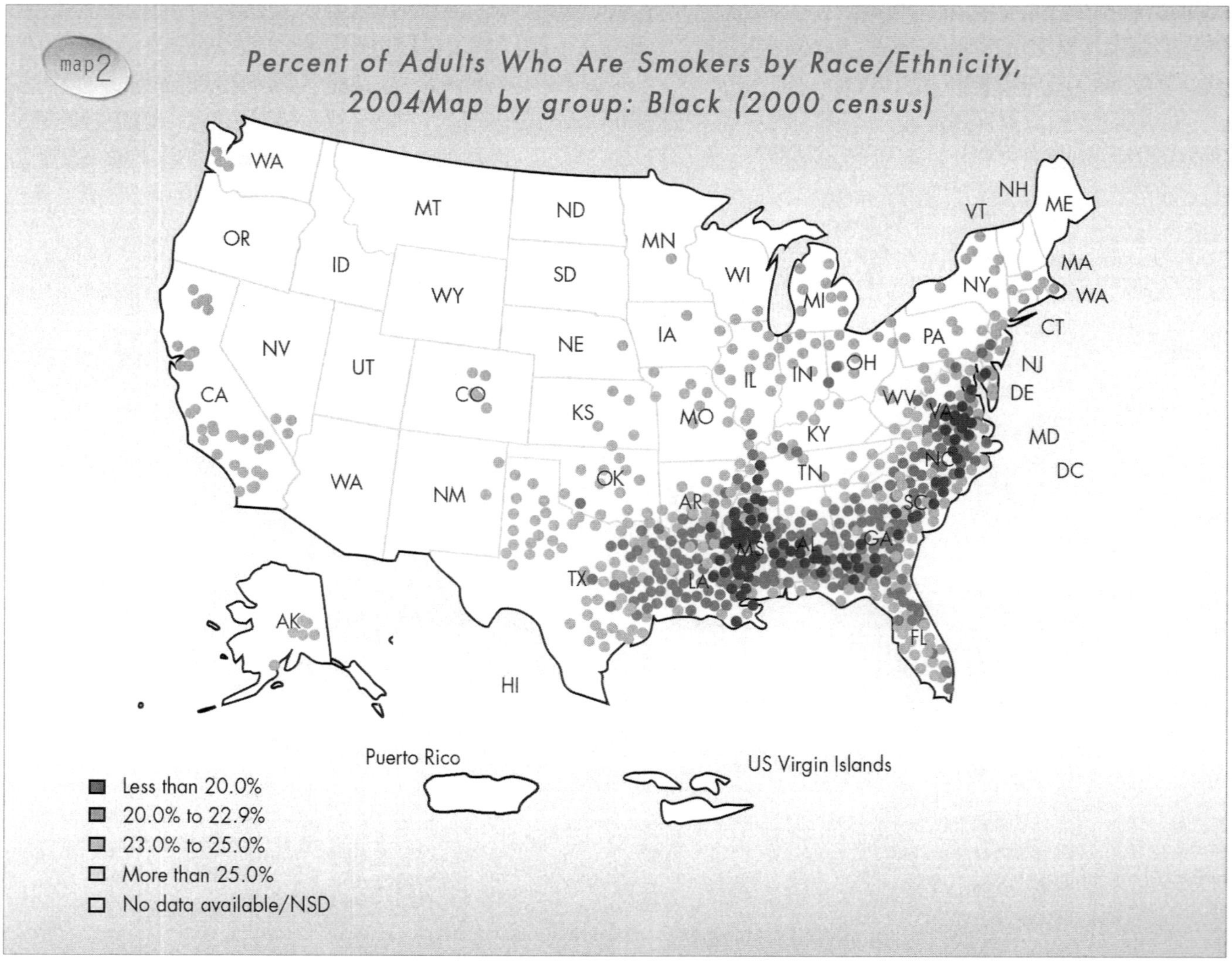

The beta carotene lung cancer study has now been etched into the minds of many misled doctors, researchers and the public. Smokers in Finland given 20 mg of supplemental beta carotene (the diet provides about 3-6 mg of beta carotene) experienced a reported 18% relative increased risk for lung cancer. In hard numbers, among 14,573 participants, 2.76% taking a placebo and 3.26% taking high-dose beta carotene, developed lung cancer. This is less than a 1% difference, but the news reports made it sound like it was 18 out of 100 increased cases of lung cancer. The difference was not statistically significant.

Furthermore, the slight increased risk for lung cancer was only observed among men who smoked 20 or more cigarettes per day. [J Natl Cancer Institute 97: 1319-20, 2005]

Another oddity of the Finnish study was that about a third of the smokers in the study developed yellow skin, a sign that beta carotene was being stored in their skin rather than being transported to tissues. It is widely known that smoking also impairs zinc levels. Zinc is required to produce a carrier protein that transports vitamin A (made from beta carotene) out of the liver to tissues. [British Journal Cancer 40: 927-31, 1979]

In 1991, researchers in Italy provided high doses of vitamin A (300,000 IU) to patients who had undergone lung cancer surgery, and reported no side effects or increased mortality. [Oncology 48: 131-37, 1991]

While beta carotene is considered a lung toxin for smokers, somehow a patentable derivative of beta carotene isn't. Researchers at Washington University School of Medicine in St. Louis now report that a compound related to vitamin A shows promise in preventing or slowing tumor growth in

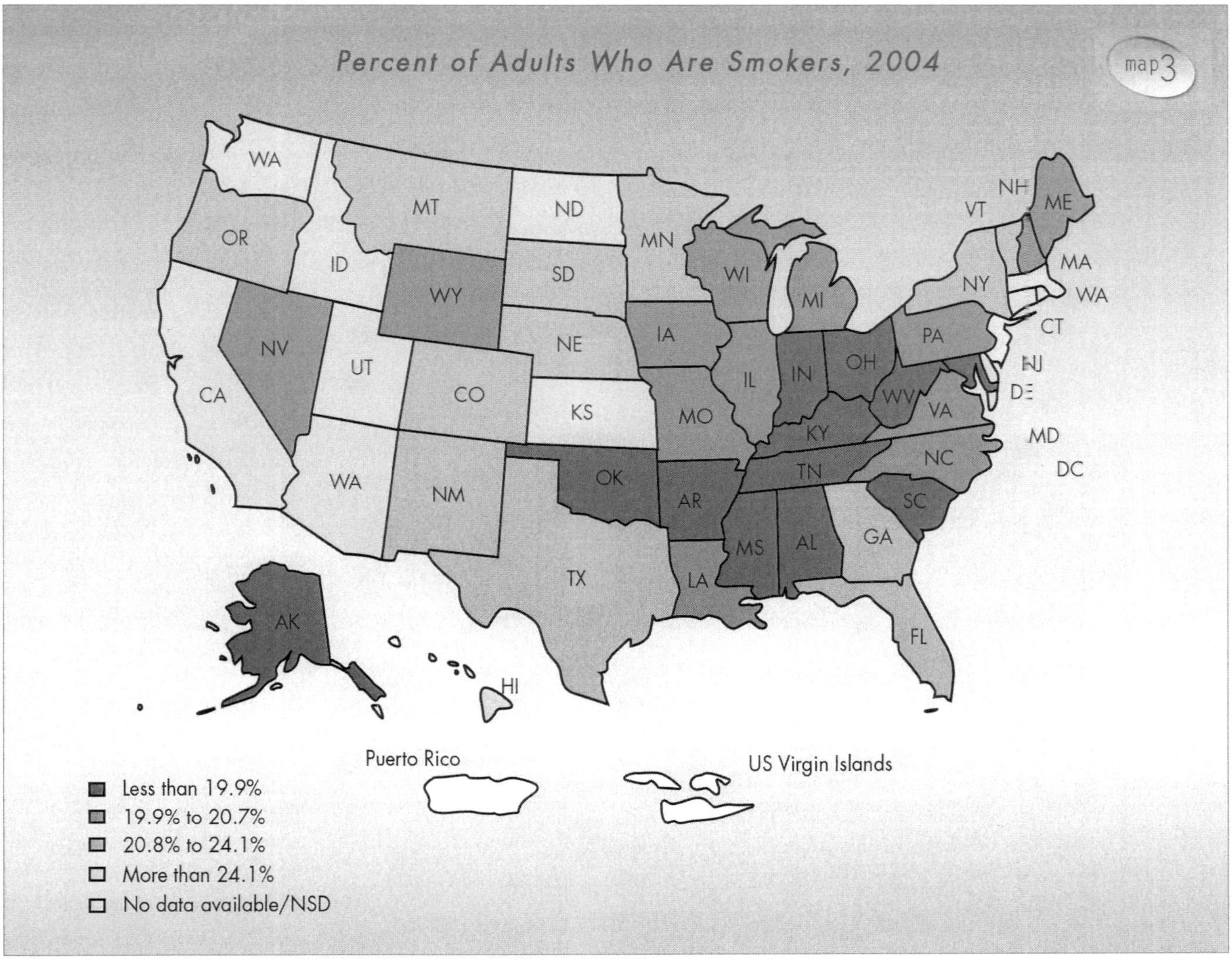

mice prone to develop lung cancer. The compound, bexarotene, is now considered a tumor blocker. [Oncogene 25: 1320-29, 2006] But the studies have only been performed in animals. Bexarotene used in humans for other types of cancer has been fraught with serious side effects.

Oddly, the controlled studies that have used beta carotene supplements have not only produced unexpected negative results, but they are in conflict with most population studies. Male smokers in Finland who consume more beta carotene-rich fruits and vegetables do have lower rates of lung cancer. Possibly the entire array of carotenoids provided in plant foods (lycopene, lutein, beta carotene) explains this phenomenon. [American Journal Epidemiology 156: 536-47, 2002] But smokers generally don't consume much plant food.

No corroboration

So are beta carotene supplements risky for smokers?

When researchers pooled the results of seven studies, no relationship could be found between beta carotene intake and lung cancer among smokers or non-smokers. [Cancer Epidemiology Prevention 13: 40-48, 2004]

Another subsequent study, the Physicians' Health Study, showed no adverse effects from beta carotene use among smokers and non-smokers. Two smaller studies also did not reveal any adverse effects from high-dose beta carotene on mortality. [Journal National Cancer Institute 96: 1729-31, 2004]

Even when researchers used an animal model (mice), they could not find an increased risk for lung cancer among map4

Percent of Adults Who Are Smokers by Race/Ethnicity, 2004Map by group: Black (2000 census)

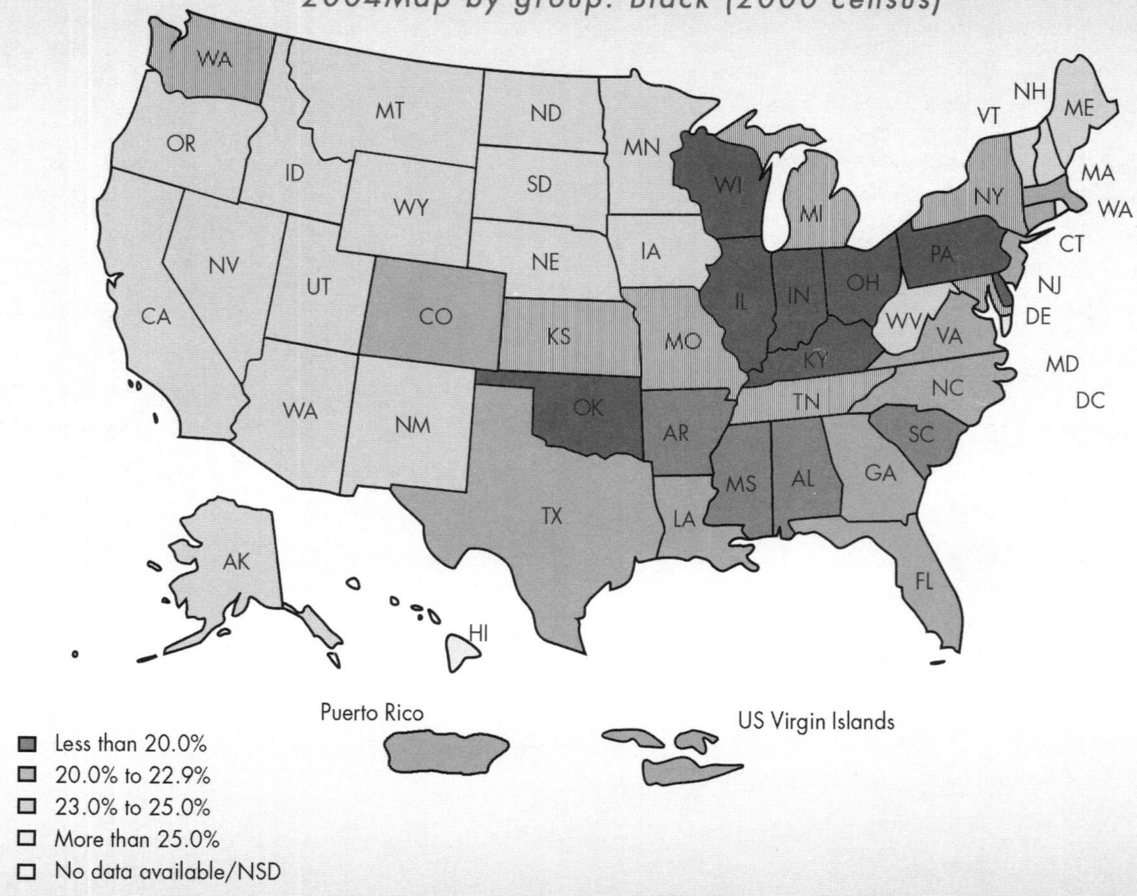

animals given beta carotene and then exposed to tobacco smoke. [Toxicology Science 69: 23-29, 2002]

A recent study of females concluded that high intake of beta carotene reduced the overall risk for lung cancer but more than doubled the risk for lung cancer among women who smoked. However, the dosage of beta carotene in supplements was only estimated, and in fact, it is difficult to imagine supplements being hazardous to smokers given they were only estimated to provide 2.1 mg of beta carotene, which is far less than the diet provides and magnitudes less than the infamous beta carotene trial in Finland which employed 20 mg of beta carotene.

When the women's beta carotene lung cancer study was analyzed, lung cancer occurred in only 5 non-smokers and 12 smokers out of a group of 59,910 women, 700 of whom developed smoking-related cancer other than lung cancer. [Journal Natl Cancer Institute 97: 1339-44, 2005] Conclusions made from comparisons from such small groups appear to be premature. Yet, this study produced news headlines across the globe. The experts continue to urge smokers to stay away from beta carotene supplements. Yet consumption of 9-13 servings of fruits and vegetables, as recommended by the National Cancer Institute, could result in higher intake of beta carotene from foods than is provided in most supplements (a carrot, for example, provides about 4 mg of beta carotene).

Oddly, researchers in France recently examined aging factors in the lungs (how much air is expelled when a person exhales). The volume of air exhaled declines with advancing age and this decline is significantly reduced among adults who consume relatively high amounts of beta carotene. Heavy smokers who consumed the lowest amounts of beta carotene experienced the greatest decline in lung function with advancing age. [Thorax 61: 320-26, 2006] This was not a study about cancer, but it does say beta carotene promotes healthy aging of the lungs, even among smokers!

In the Japan Collaborative Cohort Study, it was found that the greater the intake of carotenoids (lycopene, beta carotene, lutein) from the diet, the less the risk of death from lung cancer. [Journal Epidemiology 15: S140-49, 2005]

A more recent analysis shows the increased risk for lung cancer among beta carotene supplement users persisted even after supplement use was stopped, and that over time this increase was no longer statistically significant! [Journal National Cancer Institute 96: 1743-50, 2004] The cancer industry has started a myth it cannot erase.

Rethinking beta carotene

Just how could beta carotene, even in high doses, pose an increased risk for lung cancer among smokers when tobacco destroys beta carotene in blood plasma? Some researchers began to ponder if the widely reported risk was real.

The infamous beta carotene study relied upon smokers to accurately report on the number of cigarettes smoked per day. Previous studies show that there is a poor correlation between the reported number and true number of cigarettes smoked. [American Journal Epidemiology 155: 622-28, 2002]

Some researchers now believe high-dose beta carotene only correlated with increased lung cancer rates among male smokers because beta carotene served as a truer marker of smoking levels than did the levels reported by smokers themselves. [Journal National Cancer Institute 95: E4, 2003] Researchers scratched their heads and reconsidered the fact that smoking degrades beta carotene in blood plasma. Therefore, a decline in levels of beta carotene in blood plasma may be a marker of the true number of cigarettes smoked by individuals. But the research community isn't ready to come out and admit this.

If high-dose beta carotene does produce adverse effects, it isn't apparent by testing or urine samples among smokers. Even when given at high doses for many years, beta carotene does not promote oxidation in smokers or non-smokers, as measured by urine samples. [Nutrition Cancer 49: 1-6, 2004]

Exposure of blood plasma to cigarette smoke destroys carotenoids (lycopene, lutein, beta carotene) and vitamin E. [American Journal Clinical Nutrition 63: 559-65, 1996]
A study conducted in 1997 showed that the amount of carotenoids inside white blood cells of lung cancer patients is decreased considerably. [International Journal Cancer 74: 20-25, 1997] How can beta carotene be toxic when it is degraded by tobacco? Smokers need more, not less, beta carotene to make up for losses caused by tobacco itself.

An interesting study was conducted over a decade ago. The incidence of lung cancer on South Pacific island countries is far lower despite similar rates of smoking. The intake of beta carotene and lutein in these countries ranges from 2,500-8,000 mcg of beta carotene and 3,200-7,100 mcg of lutein (Hawaii, Tahiti, New Caledonia), but in Fiji dietary intake of beta carotene is ~14,000 mcg for beta carotene

Females	Hawaii	Tahiti	Cook Islands	New Calendonia	Fiji
Intake beta carotene in mcg	6,475	3,612	26,957	7,775	14,548
Intake lutein in mcg	5,993	3,979	7,216	3,869	23,647
Lung cancer incidence	37.5%	41.0%	24.8%	17.4%	1.8%
Ever smokers	63.6%	52.4%	33.7%	49.1%	40.9%
# cigarettes/day	19.6	16.1	11.5	8.6	4.1

International Journal Cancer 63: 18-23, 1995

and 25,000 mcg for lutein. For the lung cancer incidence for these countries see the table above.

Vitamin C and lung cancer

The argument for the use of antioxidant supplements for smokers is always countered by saying *"the safest course is to stop smoking."* Yet the damage caused by smoking may result in lung cancer many years later, even when a tobacco habit was shed years prior. Then the infamous beta carotene study, where smokers in Finland were claimed to have incurred higher rates of lung cancer after beta carotene supplementation, is brought up. So the scientific literature is always laced with reports suggesting *"caution"* for smokers who intend to use high-dose antioxidant supplements. [Nutrition Reviews 55: 369-70, 1997] It is never mentioned that smoking depletes antioxidants from the body. So replacement is never considered.

At the Second Conference on Vitamin C, published in the Annals of the New York Academy of Sciences in 1975, it was clearly documented that one cigarette destroys at least 25 mg of vitamin C in the body. Vitamin C, partially washed out of the body in urine, is virtually absent from urine in the pack-a-day habitual smoker. [Annals New York Academy Sciences 258: 156-67, 1975]

So to make up for the depletion of antioxidants from the body, health authorities raised the recommendation for vitamin C from 60 to 100 mg per day for smokers. [American Journal Clinical Nutrition 53: 1466-70, 1991] Why, that isn't even enough to replace what two cigarettes deplete from the body! Not even 500 mg of supplemental vitamin C per day is adequate for smokers. [European Journal Clinical Nutrition 51: 154-63, 1997]

It is interesting to observe what happens to guinea pigs exposed to tobacco smoke. Guinea pigs are different from most other animals. They do not produce their own vitamin C in their body as do animals like cows, dogs, cats and horses. Humans are in the same predicament. So the guinea pig model is ideal for examining the effects of smoking on humans. Complete protection against damage caused by tobacco smoke is not achieved till guinea pigs are given 15 mg of vitamin C. For a 1-2 pound (~0.5-1.0 kilogram) animal, this is equivalent to 1,050-2,100 mg for a 160-pound adult human. [Free Radical Biology Medicine 29: 115-24, 2000]

Smoking impairs the ability of arteries to widen by depleting vitamin C. Blood vessels are not static in size. They widen (dilate) or narrow (constrict) to maintain adequate blood pressure. Infusions of vitamin C correct this deficiency. [Circulation 94: 6-9, 1996]

Supplemental vitamin C (3,000 mg per day) has been shown to protect non-smoking individuals from the harmful effects of second-hand smoke. [Free Radical Biology Medicine 28: 428-36, 2000] Imagine what it would do for active smokers!

It is interesting to examine what happens inside the lungs of smokers from a chemical standpoint. The three times greater risk for lung cancer among current smokers is associated with chemicals that attach to sections of DNA (called adducts). Smoking increases the level of benzo(a) pyrene DNA adducts, which is believed to be responsible for the increased risk of lung cancer. When 500 mg of vitamin C and 400 units of vitamin E are given to female smokers, their DNA adduct levels decline by 31%. [Cancer Epidemiology Biomarkers Prevention 14: 237-42, 2005] Yet cancer authorities continue to maintain antioxidant vitamins are worthless in the fight against lung cancer.

Folic acid and lung cancer

Smoking also depletes the body of folic acid, an essential B vitamin necessary for DNA repair. [Journal American College Nutrition 13: 68-72, 1994]

Higher dietary intake of folic acid has been found to protect against lung cancer, more so among alcohol drinkers and heavy smokers. [Cancer Epidemiology Biomarkers Prevention 12: 980-96, 2003] Folic acid is found in dark-green leafy vegetables like spinach, kale, and Romaine lettuce. However, folic acid from supplements is much better absorbed.

Other nutrients and lung cancer

Selenium appears to be a protective agent against lung cancer only among populations that do not consume adequate amounts of selenium in their diet. [Cancer Epidemiology Biomarkers Prevention 13: 771-78, 2004]

Calcium-D glucarate, a nutrient found in fruits, may be a preventive agent against lung cancer. [Chest 125: 149-50S, 2004]

Mentha piperita

What about adding something directly to cigarettes that would render them harmless? *Mentha piperita*, or peppermint, is an intriguing therapeutic agent for lung cancer. It is often used to alleviate nausea, flatulence and vomiting in traditional medicine. Mentha extract has antioxidant properties. Mentha and Mentha oil have antibacterial and antifungal properties.

The provision of menthe extract reduces the number of lung tumors in chemically induced lung cancer in animals (from 61% to 26%). [Mutagenesis 21: 61-66, 2006] Very high oral doses of menthe extract (human equivalent of 56,000 mg) have been shown to protect again skin cancer. [Biofactors 22: 87-91, 2004] Mentha oil given to animals exposed to high-dose gamma radiation reduces 30-day death rate from 100% to 17%. [Phytotherapy Research 18: 546-50, 2004] If the human equivalent of 70,000 mg of mentha is given orally to mice prior to exposure to radiation, it protects against bone marrow damage. [Indian Journal Experimental Biology 41: 229-37, 2003]

A chewing tobacco mixture known as shamma, that contains ash, oils, spices, tobacco and other additives, has been shown to produce oral cancer. However, one variety of shamma that contained mint leaves (mentha) does not cause cancer. An experiment with hamsters also shows that tobacco chew placed against the cheek of animals will induce cancer, but not if it contains peppermint leaves. [Carcinogenesis 19: 1975-1801, 1995]

Russian doctors have experimented with menthe oil and believe inhalation of mentha oil can aid in the treatment of tuberculosis, a lung infection. [Probl Tuberk 4: 36-39, 2002]

> Mentha may inhibit cancer by its ability to bind to iron.
> *Source: Toxicology Industrial Health 20 :119-22, 2004*

Mentha piperita (peppermint) is available in pills, granules and liquid from various sources. Modest doses should be consumed. Excessive oral dosage may cause side effects (heartburn, muscle cramping, rash, slowed heart rate).

Berberine

Berberine, found in herbs such as goldenseal, Oregon grape and barberry, has been found to possess anti-metastatic (anti cancer-spreading) properties by inhibition of collagen degradation surrounding lung tumors. [Toxicology Applied Pharmacology 214: 8-15, 2006]

Resveratrol

Resveratrol is the most profound anti-cancer agent ever identified. It is known as a red wine molecule, though it can be consumed as a dietary supplement. A lower risk for lung cancer among wine drinkers compared to consumers of other alcoholic beverages has been observed, which may partly be explained by its resveratrol content. Resveratrol prevents lung cancer via its ability to control the action of genes. [International Journal Cancer 92: 18-25, 2001] Pre-treatment with resveratrol enhances the effect of radiation treatment of the lung. [Journal Radiation Research 46: 387-93, 2005]

Startling remissions from lung cancer documented

Researchers at the University of Nevada report on the case of a 78-year-old man who was diagnosed with tumors in both lungs on July 31, 2000. He began taking high-dose omega-3 fish oil (~10,000 mg) and most of his tumors began shrinking or showed no growth except for one large tumor. He increased his intake of omega-3 fish oil to ~15,000 mg, and the remaining tumor began to shrink. By April of 2004 he was without symptoms and the lung tumors had dramatically shrunk to from 5.0 x 3.6 centimeters to 2.2 x 1.2 centimeters. [Nutrition & Cancer 52: 121-29, 2005]

There is also a startling case of complete long-standing (42-month) remission from spindle cell lung cancer after taking oral germanium. [Chest 117: 591-93, 2000]

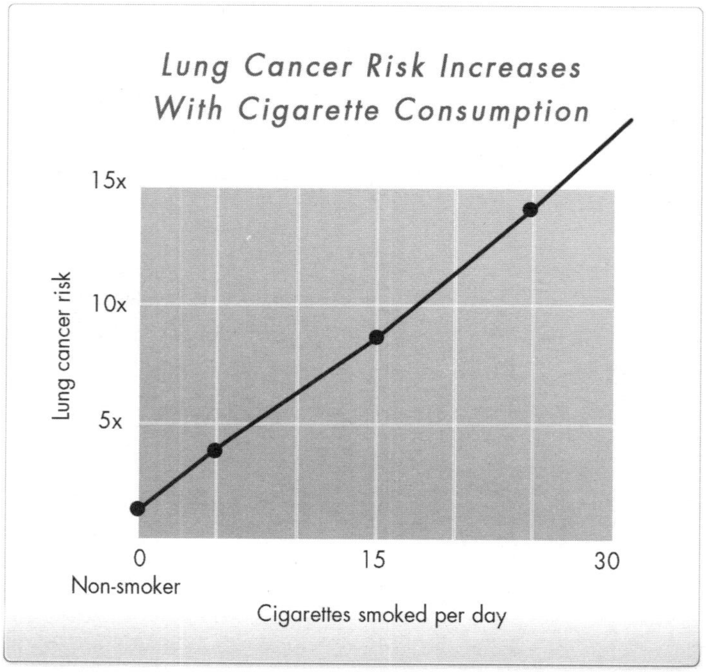

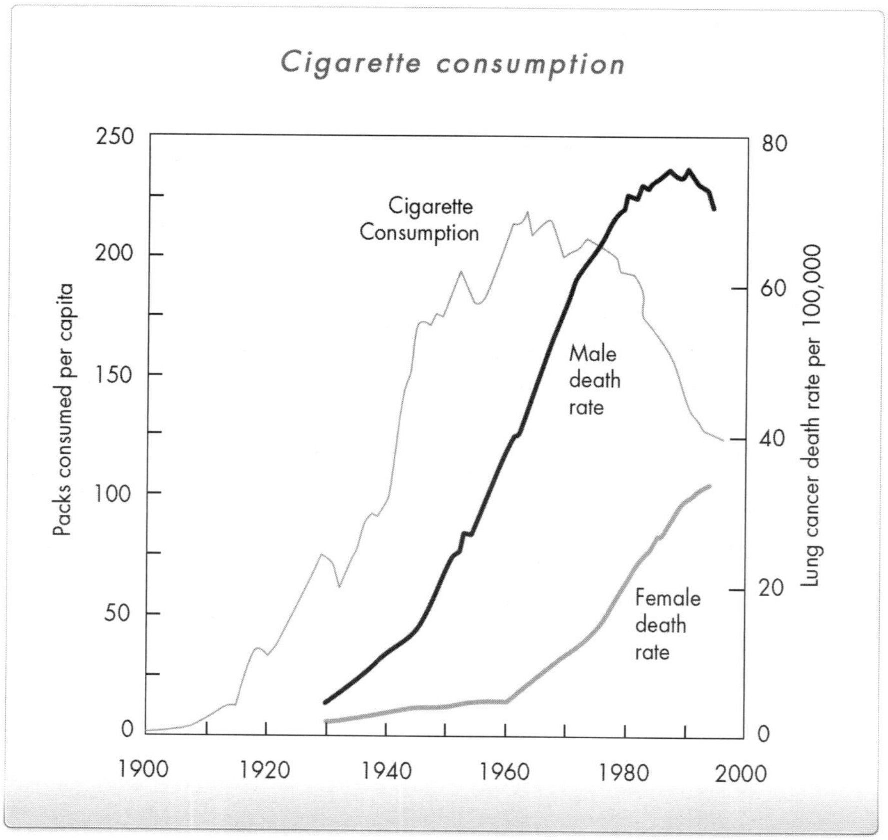

The Stop Smoking Pill

An estimated 32 million smokers would like to quit. A new stop-smoking pill has now been approved by the Food & Drug Administration. The pill (Chantix) is taken twice daily and is reported to have a 20% success rate, slightly better than existing tobacco cessation aids. Surveys show about 8 in 10 smokers have tried to quit at least once. Smoking rates have fallen in the United States to 1951 levels, with a 4.2% decline in 2005 alone. Still, about 22% of high school students smoke tobacco, but the sharp increase in cigarette taxes has driven up the price per pack from $1.74 in 1997 to $3.16 in 2004. However, states are still funding many programs off of these taxes and rely upon young people to continually light up. [Washington Post March 9, 2006]

What smokers and ex-smokers should be doing

Smokers and ex-smokers should habitually take dietary supplements to reduce their risk for lung cancer. A cocktail of dietary supplements might include:

- **Quercetin** + vitamin C 2,000 mg 3 times a day
- **Vitamin E** 400 IU (even better, mixed forms of vitamin E)
- **Beta carotene** 10,000-25,000 IU
- **Selenium**, organically bound to amino acids (selenomethionine, SelenoExcel) 200 mcg
- **Vitamin D** 2,000 IU
- **Folic acid** 800 mcg
- **Lutein** 6-20 mg
- **Lycopene**, from tomato paste or supplements
- **Resveratrol**, 50 mg or more
- **Fish oil or flaxseed oil** 5,000 mg (12,000 mg for active cases of cancer)
- **Melatonin** 10 mg or more for active cases, at bedtime

Outraged yet?

This chapter reveals a great deal of information smokers almost never hear. There are no helpful programs to prevent lung cancer beyond cessation, and cancer risk remains high years after a cigarette habit is abandoned. Doctors offer no advice on how nutrition can help restore health to smoke-damaged tissues after successful smoking cessation. The collusion between government and tobacco companies to give the appearance of an anti-smoking program suggests smokers are considered to be nothing more than pawns who are being fooled out of their money. The prevalent public prejudice, not to tell smokers how to prevent lung cancer via nutritional therapy because it will encourage smokers to continue to puff on cigarettes, is an untenable position. Smokers don't easily put a halt to their habits, there are no truly successful anti-smoking programs, so we continue to lose lives prematurely. Lung cancer is totally preventable in more ways than one.

Vitamin C Cigarette

The most novel idea in tobacco technology is the vitamin C cigarette, introduced in Canada. It is pandered as a way of reducing odor and stains on teeth. Just how much vitamin C is destroyed once the C-vitamin cigarette is lit is unreported. The only safe cigarette is one that's not lit.

Case presentation: Lung cancer disappears

Joan is a 62-year-old woman living in Hawaii, a long-time smoker, who began having fainting spells. She was later diagnosed with kidney cancer in 2001. The kidney was surgically removed but the cancer spread to her lung. She was told she had a year to live, which is what most lung cancer patients are told.

Her son began to manage her care, seeking alternatives from the beginning. Even though Joan had radiation and chemotherapy for her lung cancer, she also flew to the U.S. mainland to undergo Rife Therapy, an electrical frequency treatment that was first developed in the 1930s. She would also undergo cesium treatment, another alternative therapy. Neither of these treatments worked. Her family estimated they spent $20,000 on alternative therapies.

Interleukin therapy was prescribed by her cancer doctors and even though it was very harsh, it served to shrink the primary tumor in the affected lung and cause the small tumors to disappear. Interleukin treatment was buying her time. But she couldn't endure it for long. Surgery was out of the question since the tumor was too close to the heart. Her health plan arranged for Joan to receive a new type of cancer drug, Sutent, which costs $8,000 per course of treatment, but she never opened the bottle.

Instead, thanks to a neighbor who suggested Joan's son investigate nutritional therapy, a regimen of dietary supplements was taken to coincide with radiation treatment. Joan began taking flaxseed oil, IP6 rice bran extract, resveratrol, hyaluronic acid, and Haelan, a fermented source of soy. Initially the radiation treatment was very painful, and it resulted in a collapsed lung and pneumonia. Joan had to be hospitalized. Things were looking very glum. Her son had run out of alternatives to try. He knew conventional cancer treatment is not effective and can only promise short prolongation of life.

Suddenly, after taking the dietary supplement regimen for only a short time, about a month, her health began to improve. The collapsed lung was now 90% healed. She was sent home from the hospital. She was feeling better. Her son hesitatingly took her back to the clinic for x-rays. The tumors had all disappeared! After over four years, the lung cancer had disappeared. Doctors remarked how well she responded to the radiation treatment.

Joan won't know how well this regimen will work on a long-term basis, but conventional treatment alone couldn't produce the improvements in her health that nutritional therapy did. Her son now tries to tell other lung cancer patients of their success with nutritional therapy, but they stand in disbelief. This is another example of the new choices cancer patients have at their disposal today, which are likely more effective and less problematic than conventional cancer therapies.

Cancers you get from smoking

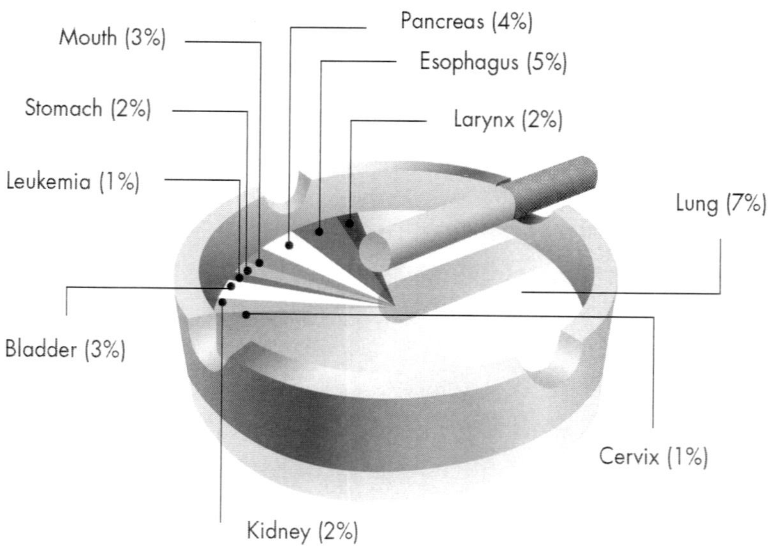

Percentage of total 159,600 individual cases
All numbers are rounded.

CHAPTER 7

Prostate Cancer

p 164 - 218

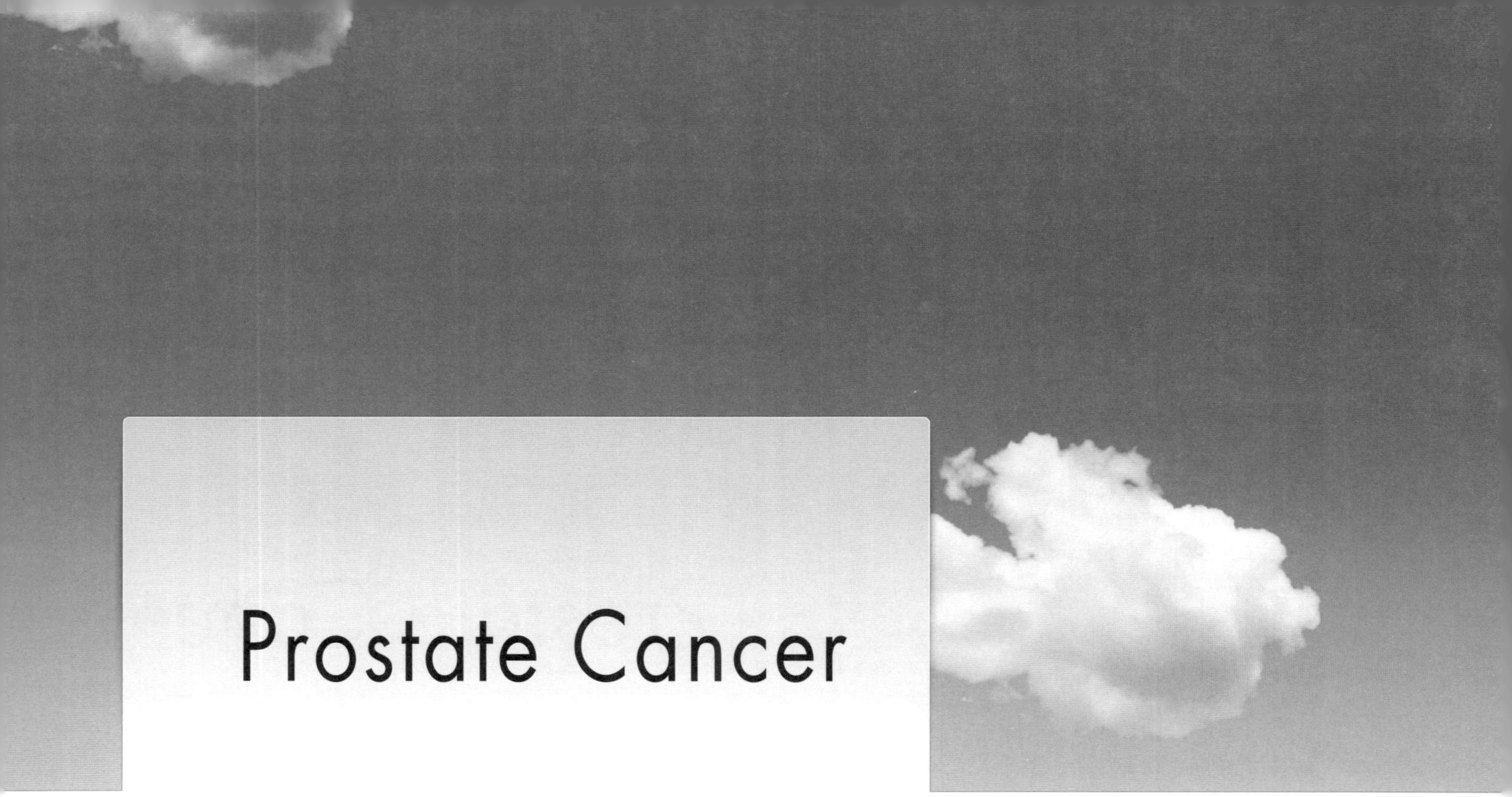

Prostate Cancer

"Prostate cancer choice a coin toss"

Daniel J. DeDoon, WebMD March 28, 2006

Men come daily to a medical center in California have their prostate gland irradiated with proton beams in the hope of a cure. There are only a few of these $100 million proton beam machines available and these men feel they are lucky to live near one of them where they can obtain what is considered the most advanced treatment for prostate cancer in the world.

The medical center that houses the proton beam machines says *"a growing number of patients, clutching internet print-outs and timely new studies...come here seeking proton therapy for their prostate cancer, having done their homework, sorted out the alternatives, and primarily are looking to avoid surgery. Having some peace of mind about their quality of life is a priority."* That may be all these men will obtain from treatment – peace of mind.

With proton beam therapy, positively charged subatomic protons employed at a very low dose increase at the tumor site, where the protons effectively disintegrate the tumor with ions rather than with the photons used in conventional radiation treatment. The radiation dose then rapidly dissipates, leaving surrounding healthy tissue and organs unaffected. It takes these men about six weeks to complete a course of proton beam therapy. The treatment is painless, takes 15 to 90 minutes, and patients leave to resume normal activities. It achieves what most of these men want: treatment without surgery.

> *"It may be the most important decision of their lives, yet most men base their choice of prostate cancer treatments on incomplete information,"* says Daniel J. DeNoon, writing for WebMD.
> *WebMD March 28, 2006*

Because prostate cancer is usually slow growing and remains within the prostate gland, it takes over a decade to ascertain whether treatment like this is effective. So far, no one knows. But that isn't how the medical center describes it.

The medical center where the proton beam treatment is provided says, "*It may now be possible to successfully treat prostate cancer without the risk of life style changes and activity-diminishing side effects commonly associated with conventional radiation or surgery. And, with a track record of significantly less side effects over an extended period, watchful waiting can become a non-issue...Proton treatment for men with prostate cancer has created a proven and highly effective alternative to the traditional options of surgery, radiation or watchful waiting.*"

The medical center goes on to say that "*protons can treat prostate cancer better than traditional radiation and as well as surgery.*" A five-year study is cited where 89% of 643 men with early-to-late prostate cancer experienced overall disease-free survival. The findings also showed that proton therapy resulted in as many or more patients free of disease as those cited in published results of conventional treatments.

Men read this and are impressed. But are these men falling for a sales pitch, or will they really live longer having undergone proton beam therapy?

Let's look at all the factors involved

- The first catch is that men hear "*disease-free survival*" and don't know to inquire about overall survival. Yes, some treatments, particularly surgery and radiation therapy may shrink or remove tumors, but they have toxic side effects that are often mortal. These men may not die of prostate cancer, but they may die from the harsh effects of the treatment. Overall survival may not be quoted in some studies. This is very misleading to prostate cancer patients.

- Another misleading way of presenting data on prostate cancer treatments is to report short-term data. A 14-year government-sponsored study found as many men with prostate cancer who elected to forgo treatment (watchful waiting) survived as those men who elected to undergo surgical removal of their prostate gland. [Agency for Health Care Policy and Research, 1994]

  Nearly all prostate surgery for cancer should have been ruled needless then, but physicians and the medical industry objected and have since sought to eliminate the government agency that produced the report and hide the results of this long-term study. The five-year data on proton beam treatment for prostate cancer is an example of such misleading information.

  These men aren't likely to be fully informed that proton beam radiation, as well as conventional external beam x-ray treatment, carries with it an increased risk for bladder cancer. Bladder or urethral cancer is detected 2.75 years sooner after a proton beam boost to conventional radiation treatment than with standard radiation therapy alone. About 30-45% of men who do not undergo radiation treatment of any kind will develop urinary tract cancer compared to 64% receiving conventional or conventional/proton beam therapy. [The Journal of Urology 175: 2063, 2006]

A biochemical cure

Another problem in understanding prostate cancer treatment is the claim of a "*biochemical cure.*" That is, a decline in the Prostate Specific Antigen (PSA) number. But this number does not equate with survival, particularly overall survival. Men cling to their PSA number. Sometimes it is all they have to cling to.

In one study, a "*biochemical cure*" was reached in 100% of men who underwent surgical prostate gland removal when the PSA number was under 4.0. What this study says is the PSA number never rose if it was under 4.0 immediately following surgery. But this simply means these men probably had slow progressing and less invasive tumors. It has nothing to do with the effectiveness of surgery per se. [International Brazilian Journal Urology 31: 437-44, 2005]

Does any treatment work?

A careful review of research studies published from 1990 to 2004 found that although a lower PSA after treatment with radiation is associated with cancer cure, 5% to 25% of patients ultimately have failure (beyond five years) even with the *"most optimal biochemical response."* The published review says: *"There are only limited data to suggest that early intervention of any type (hormone treatment, radiation or surgery) impacts survival."* [Journal Urology 173: 1456-62, 2005]

And just how are men with diagnosed prostate cancer to compare all the treatments available? In 2004, researchers at the Karolinska Institute, in Stockholm, Sweden, said *"There are no randomized studies that compare the outcome of surgery (radical prostatectomy) with either conventional radiation treatment or implantation of radium seeds (brachytherapy) for patients with low-risk prostate cancer."* And despite some evidence that treatment may lower PSA readings or Gleason scores (severity of tumor as evaluated on a glass slide by a pathologist), *"no overall survival benefit has yet been shown."* There is some evidence that hormone therapy to shrink prostate tumors results in longer overall survival compared with radiation treatment alone, but this is only demonstrated among patients with advanced tumors, which the vast majority of prostate cancer do not have. [Acta Oncology 43:316-81, 2004]

The bottom line is that low-risk patients do well no matter which treatment they receive. [Seminars Urology Urological Oncology 18: 214-25, 2000] This makes every form of treatment look good, since most men with prostate cancer have non-invasive tumors.

Brachytherapy: radium seed implants

Radium seed implants, called brachytherapy, are appealing to men who want to avoid prostate surgery, but a recent analysis found that patients who succumb to cancer within 10 years following brachytherapy *"harbor inherently aggressive cancer."* [International Journal Radiation Oncology Biological Physics 64: 810-16, 2006] In other words, if you have the less aggressive form of prostate cancer, which is usually not mortal, brachytherapy appears to work. By self definition, brachytherapy is far less effective in prolonging life for men who are most in need of life-saving treatment.

Among 1,449 consecutive prostate cancer patients treated with brachytherapy, the 12-year survival was 93% if only considering disease-specific cause of death. But overall, the survival rate was 81%. Brachytherapy is not compared against patients who elected to forgo treatment altogether, so there is no way of knowing the real benefit of brachytherapy. [The Journal of Urology 173:1562-1566, 2005]

The Watchful Wait

A widely cited study that is used to substantiate the effectiveness of surgical removal of the prostate gland versus *"watchful waiting,"* shows an advantage for surgery in real survival. The cumulative incidence of death due to prostate cancer increased from 2.0% at 5 years to 5.3 % at 10 years following diagnosis. This means the relative risk was almost cut in half for men who chose surgery, but in hard numbers, only about three more patients in 100 experienced 10-year survival among those who underwent surgery, and these figures did not include those men who may have died of other causes. Furthermore, this was only a small study of less than 200 men, not sufficient to be used as a conclusive study to share with men considering treatment decisions. [New England Journal of Medicine 352: 1977-84, 2005]

The report of a patient who underwent prostate gland removal and experienced recurrence of cancer 8.5 years later with a nearly non-detectable PSA count (less than 0.02 nanograms per mililiter) shows that cancer can recur despite surgical removal and favorable PSA testing. [Prostate Cancer and Prostatic Diseases 9: 192–194, 2006] Most men concerned about recurrence of prostate cancer are disturbed to find that PSA is not a reliable marker.

An interesting study conducted by Norwegian researchers was published in 1998. The study involved 1,135 specimens of prostate tissue removed during surgical procedures performed between 1974 and 1975. The patients who were operated on were followed for up to 20 years. Then microscopic examination was performed, and only 83 of these 1,135 patients developed new tumors. That is a very small percentage (7%) over a long period of time. Seventy-three (73) of these 83 patients had not undergone additional treatment since their surgery many years prior. A review of Cancer Registry Records found that only 3% of the untreated patients had succumbed to cancer 20 years later compared to 54% of the patients who elected to undergo further treatment following surgery. [Tidsskr Nor Laegeforen 118: 3408-12, 1998] This supports the conclusion that long-term, most prostate tumors are benign and require no treatment.

Age is a factor in treatment decisions

If you are trying to sort out all the treatments and factors involved in prostate cancer in order to make a decision about treatment, join the ranks of the confused. Also add one more factor to your decision making – your age. If you are over age 75, most surgeons won't operate and many doctors will not order other treatments since your remaining life expectancy is shorter than the time it takes for a dormant tumor to begin to become invasive and life threatening. Thus, the statement that most men in their senior years will die with, but not of, prostate cancer, is often quoted. [Journal of the American Medical Association 274: 626-631, 1995]

A study conducted by researchers in Sweden shows that prostate removal surgery produces a small reduction in overall mortality, but that this marginal benefit is greatest, and virtually limited to, men younger than age 65 years. [New England Journal Medicine 352: 1977-84, 2005]

Questions to ask your doctor

The American Cancer Society (ACS) says the death rate from prostate cancer is at an all-time low for both white and black Americans — and a new study suggests that a primary reason may be increased use of the PSA blood test to find prostate cancer early. Prostate cancer incidence rates rose from 1986 – when the PSA test was approved – through 1991, with African-American trends mirroring rates for white men a year or so later. Then after 1991, death rates for white and black men began to drop sharply. The ACS says mortality rates (in 1998-99) were the lowest since 1950 in white men, and the lowest since 1969 (when those rates were first recorded) in black men. [ACS March 31, 2003]

Since there is no effective treatment that prolongs life, just how could the American Cancer Society have come to the conclusion that the PSA test prolongs survival? Experts agree there has been no significant drop in prostate cancer mortality rates for decades. What cancer statisticians are doing is taking the date when prostate cancer is detected, which because of more widespread screening is many years earlier, and adding it to expand survival time. For instance, a man who would, without the PSA test, have his cancer diagnosed at age 70 and pass away at age 75, might now have his cancer diagnosed at age 65 and then succumb to cancer at the same age: 75. Magnify this example by hundreds or thousands and it would appear survival rates have improved, when all that has happened is that cancer is being detected earlier. The irritating part of all this is why the American Cancer Society has to use sleight of hand to mislead the public into thinking more screening saves lives. It doesn't.

Cancer is serious business. If patients can't rely on the major cancer organization to provide accurate information, who can it rely upon?

There is no proven cure for prostate cancer, though there is treatment. Since there are risks involved with surgery and potential long-term side effects, some men choose to forgo the operation since it doesn't prolong life. [Prostate Cancer Prostatic Disease 9:25-9, 2006]

Doctors frequently say when the Gleason score rises (considered the most reliable of all the tests for severity of prostate cancer), when PSA count increases, and when a biopsy is positive, and there may be evidence of metastasis (spreading of tumors to distant locations), then more aggressive treatment may be considered. But then again, aggressive treatment doesn't usually produce a cure in these cases of out-of-control prostate cancer. Treatment only appears to work for men with less aggressive forms of prostate cancer, which may not require treatment at all.

It's difficult to tell men, prostate cancer care is in a state of chaos. That is why this book suggests patients begin to strike out on their own and evaluate valid alternatives, some which appear more promising than the modern armamentarium now used to treat prostate cancer.

QUESTIONS TO ASK YOUR DOCTOR

Getting the answers to the questions below will help clarify which path to take regarding treatment for your prostate condition.

1. Do I have an aggressive (spreading) or localized form of prostate cancer?
2. What is the overall (not disease-specific) survival rate for the type of treatment being considered? (What percentage of men survive 5, 10, 15 years? Survival should mean actual years, not a "*biochemical cure*" by arbitrary evaluation of PSA count)
3. How does the treatment I am considering compare to watchful waiting in terms of overall survival?
4. At my age am I likely to experience a metastasizing (spreading) tumor in my remaining years of life?
5. What percentage of men, electing to undergo the treatment I am considering, experience side effects such as impotence, loss of urinary or bowel control or other symptoms?
6. Does the treatment I am considering in any way increase the risk for secondary tumors? (Radiation damage, etc.)
7. If my tumor is out of control, that is if my Gleason score (severity and invasiveness of the tumor based upon microscopic evaluation of prostate tissue mounted on a glass slide) is elevated, and my PSA count is high and rising, what evidence is there that any treatment will do anything more than shrink the tumor and minimize painful symptoms?
8. Is the planned treatment intended to be a cure or will it just relieve symptoms (palliative treatment)?

Complications from prostate cancer treatment				
Treatment	Reduced sexual function	Urinary Problems	Bowel Problems	Other
Radical Prostatectomy	20% - 70%	15% - 50%		
External Beam Radiation Therapy	20% - 45%	2% - 16%	6% - 25%	
Brachytherapy	36% ?	6% - 12% ?	18%?	
Androgen Deprivation Therapy (LHRH agonists)	40% - 70%			Breast Swelling: 5% - 25%, Hot Flashes: 50% - 60%

Source: Systematic Evidence Review No. 16, Agency for Healthcare Research & Quality, 2006

Prostate cancer care

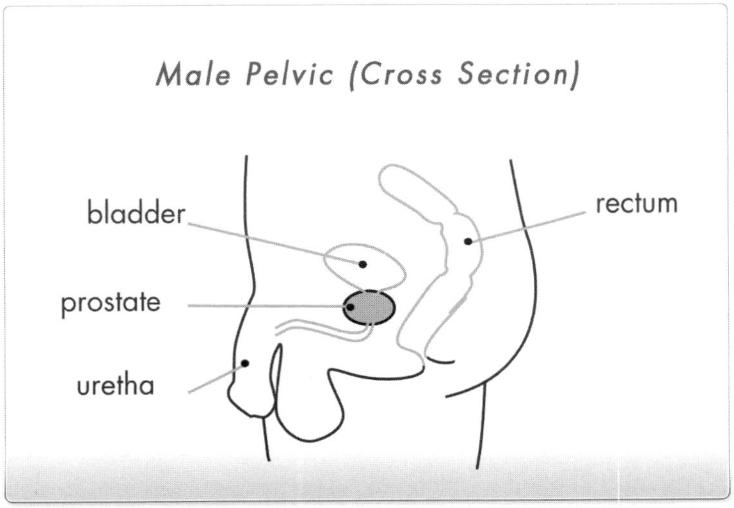

Hormonal therapy

The first line of treatment of advanced prostate cancer involves the reduction, blockage or cessation of testosterone production. Hormonal treatment of advanced stage prostate cancer shrinks the size of the prostate by 25 to 50%. [Minerva Urology Nefrology 57: 71-84, 2005]

Dr. Charles Huggins received a Nobel Prize in 1966 for his discovery that prostate cancer could be successfully treated with hormones. He had proposed the idea in 1941 and it took 25 years for him to be recognized for this discovery. Huggins also recognized that the adrenal hormones played a role in prostate cancer in that they produce testosterone as well as the testes. Huggins advised the double operation of testicular and adrenal gland removal to treat advanced-stage prostate cancer. In 1952, Dr. Huggins reported that four of the first six patients treated in this manner experienced remissions. [Cancer Research 12: 134, 1952] Others reported similar results in 1974. [Urology 3: 223-25, 1974] In a later study involving 50 men who were given a steroid drug and an adrenal inhibitor in addition to hormone therapy, 8 had a partial response and 17 remained stable. The men who underwent both prostatic and adrenal hormone inhibition lived an average of 87.8 weeks, versus 38 weeks for men treated with estrogen alone. [American Journal Clinical Oncology 11: 579-85, 1988] In 1985, doctors wrote that adrenal hormone blockade at the time of initial therapy would prolong survival. [European Journal Cancer Clinical Oncology 21: 1127-31, 1985] Doctors were reporting 30% of men who failed to achieve an improvement via surgical castration or estrogen therapy would experience remission with adrenal blockade. [Seminars Oncology 12: 28-35, 1985]

For about 50 years, blockade of testosterone in prostate cancer has been limited to surgical castration or high doses of estrogens in patients with advanced disease. Then in 1979, the first prostate cancer patient was treated with chemical castration (the cessation of testosterone production with the use of drugs).

Drugs like Lupron and Zoladex inhibit luteinizing hormone-releasing hormone (LHRH) in the hypothalamus of the brain, a hormone that controls the production of testosterone. These drugs are often combined with another anti-testosterone drug, such as flutamide, which slows down aggressive forms of prostate cancer. [Journal Steroid Biochemistry Molecular Biology 92: 327-44, 2004]

One study showed nearly a six-fold increase in response when using flutamide and Lupron together versus surgical castration or the use of an anti-testosterone drug alone. When treatment failure arises, usually at the two-year point following chemical castration, then drugs are used to inhibit testosterone production in the adrenal glands, where up to 50% of testosterone is formed. [Journal Steroid Biochemistry 30: 107-17, 1988]

Steroid anti-inflammatory drugs are widely used as co-treatment in advanced prostate cancer, to improve appetite, weight loss, fatigue, relieve bone pain, diminish urinary obstruction, and to reduce the production of adrenal testosterone. However, steroids induce resistance to several anti-cancer drugs (taxol, gemcitabine, cisplatin, 5-FU and gamma-irradiation). So while steroids are beneficial, they also pose drawbacks. [Cancer Biology Therapy 5: Jan 25, 2006]

The 5 alpha reductase inhibitor finasteride (Propecia) has no detectable effect on the production of testosterone by the adrenal gland, which is why it is of limited value in subduing hormone-sensitive prostate tumors. [Journal Andrology 15:298-301, 1994]

Inhibition of the enzyme 5 alpha reductase interferes with the conversion of testosterone to dihydrotestosterone. The drug finasteride (Propecia) and the herb saw palmetto berry (*Serenoa repens*) are 5 alpha reductase inhibitors. Recent it was discovered that astaxanthin, a red pigment found in crustaceans (krill, crawfish) and made synthetically, also inhibits 5alpha reductase. In a lab dish, astaxanthin inhibited 5 alpha reductase by 98% and worked synergistically with saw palmetto berry to inhibit prostate cancer cell growth. [Journal Herb Pharmacotherapy 5: 17-26, 2005]

A scientific review finds that saw palmetto berry extract is comparable with the drug finasteride in the treatment of prostatitis in regard to symptoms and urinary-flow improvement and has a lower rate of sexual dysfunction. Furthermore, long-term use decreases the progression of pre-cancerous cells in the prostate. [Current Opinion Urology 15: 45-48, 2005]

> The current management of hormone-resistant metastatic prostate cancer is purely palliative.
> *Source: Progressive Urology 15: 398-404, 2005*

Frequently doctors, attempting to cover for the fact that the PSA test is unreliable, will blame the discovery of prostate cancer with long-standing, low PSA numbers on the use of saw palmetto which they say was masking the PSA numbers. But unlike other 5 alpha-reductase inhibitors, saw palmetto induces its effects without interfering with the cellular capacity to secrete PSA. [International Journal Cancer 114: 190-94, 2005] In fact, supplementation with vitamin E, selenium, vitamin C and coenzyme Q10 combined does not affect serum PSA levels or hormone levels of patients with hormonally untreated prostate cancer. [European Urology 47: 433-39, 2005]

Male pattern baldness is also biochemically involved with the conversion of testosterone to dihydrotestosterone, which is facilitated by the 5 alpha reductase enzyme. So drugs that treat baldness, such as Propecia, or herbs like saw palmetto, may be appropriate for treatment of hair loss and prostate problems. [Journal Alternative Complementary Medicine 8: 143-52, 2002]

The use of 160 mg of saw palmetto berry extract twice daily (320 mg total) has been shown to reduce night-time urge to urinate by 33 to 74%, and day-time urinary frequency by 1 to 43%. International Prostate Symptom Score (IPSS) improved by 37% with saw palmetto compared with 39% with Propecia (finasteride). [Drugs Aging 9: 379-95, 1996] (The IPSS is based on answers to seven questions regarding urinary emptying, frequency, intermittency, urgency, strength of urinary stream, straining and number of times awakening to urinate during sleep hours.)

Drawbacks of hormone therapy

The problem with hormone therapy for prostate cancer is that the inhibition of testosterone is too often followed by hormone resistance and the tumor comes roaring back with a seeming vengeance. This is not unlike the use of the anti-estrogen drug tamoxifen for breast cancer, where after five years of use it was found to actually increase the risk for breast cancer in women.

Complete surgical removal of the testes will only eliminate testosterone production from the sex organs, not from the adrenal glands which also produce testosterone. Chemical castration, usually produced with drugs like Zoladex or Lupron, has its drawbacks. Testosterone may drive the growth of prostate tumors, but it is also needed to maintain mood, bone health, and other functions.

Reduction in testosterone may result in hot flashes, breast enlargement, changes in mood, decline in sex drive, fatigue, anemia and bone loss and fractures. [Current Urological Reports 6: 210-16, 2005] Men with prostate cancer may already have low bone mineral density prior to any hormone therapy. [Cancer 91: 2238-45, 2001] Various medications, calcium and vitamin D may be recommended to strengthen bones. However, these measures alone may be ineffective. [Canadian Journal Urology 12: 9-15, 2005S]

As men with prostate cancer live longer, the prevalence of bone loss increases. Many men with prostate cancer who are prescribed hormone therapy are not provided with any preventive measures to help maintain bone health. Exercise, exposure to the sun (vitamin D production), avoidance of excessive alcohol, and cessation of smoking helps to maintain bone integrity. [Cancer 103: 2042-52, 2005]

There has been a long-held belief that osteoporosis is prevented in men by testosterone and in women with estrogen. Recent reports that young men with normal testosterone, but low estrogen levels, developed osteoporosis, reveals that estrogens have a far greater influence on bone healthy than does testosterone. [Joint Bone Spine 72: 202-06, 2005] Even a low-dose estrogen patch or estrogen skin cream has been found to be helpful. [Journal Urology 169: 1735-37, 2003]

Men with prostate cancer placed on hormone deprivation exhibit immediate and delayed memory skills. [Journal Urology 175: 130-35, 2006] One wonders how informed consent for treatment can adequately be obtained from these patients.

Hormone treatment for prostate cancer increases the incidence of diabetes, heart attacks and sudden-death heart attack. One study shows that is 1000 men were treated with hormone therapy for a year, doctors would find 29 new cases of diabetes, 8 more than untreated men, 14 heart attacks, 3 more than untreated men, and 13 sudden-death heart attacks, 4 more than untreated men. [Journal Clinical Oncology 24: 4448-56, 2006]

Why does hormone therapy wear off?

After hormone treatment has successfully calmed PSA levels, the effect wears off. This appears to be due, in part, to the production of testosterone in the adrenal glands rather than the testes. As cited above, surgical removal of the adrenal glands results in long-term survival of prostate cancer patients. [Urology 3: 223-25, 1974] In a more recent study, the use of low-dose diethylstilbestrol plus adrenal suppression with a steroid drug (hydrocortisone, prednisone) reduces PSA levels. Eight of 34 patients experienced greater than a 90% drop in PSA, 13 of 34 a 50-90% drop with clear improvement in symptoms. Blood clotting problems were noted however. [British Journal Urology 85: 1069-73, 2000]

There is an intriguing relationship between hormone cell receptors and folic acid (vitamin B9). Androgen (testosterone) suppression may be prescribed for men with advanced prostate cancer. Estrogen hormones are often employed. For the estrogens to work, they must dock on the surface of prostate cells at what are called receptor sites. Hormone suppression fails when the genes that control the receptor production are silenced. Thereafter, hormone therapy no longer works to suppress testosterone. The genes that control cell receptors are switched off by a process called hypermethylation. [Science Daily March 7, 2002] Folic acid works in an opposite fashion. It's possible that folic acid plus hormone therapy will work better in inhibiting advanced prostate cancer than hormone therapy alone.

Testosterone replacement

Many middle-aged men who want to feel youthful again, vigorously virile, muscular and energetic opt for testosterone replacement therapy (TRT).

TRT is purportedly beneficial for the treatment of erectile dysfunction, decreased sex drive, mental depression, anemia, and age-related bone and muscle loss. Some 1.75 million prescriptions for testosterone products were written in 2002 representing $400 million in sales. [Associated Press, Dec. 11, 2003]

Like estrogen replacement therapy that was prescribed to menopausal women for decades without adequate scientific study, and later found to increase the risk for certain cancers, no randomized controlled studies have been conducted to support the widespread use of testosterone in men for "*andropause*" (the male version of menopause).

There is currently a heated debate about the theoretical association between TRT and the initiation, progression, and aggressiveness of prostate cancer. Although no clear evidence links testosterone therapy to prostate cancer, the possibility of increasing the risk of a clinical manifestation of a latent pre-existing malignancy can influence the decision about testosterone use. Current recommendations are to exclude prostate cancer before initiating TRT in men over age 40 and to closely monitor men in the first year of testosterone replacement, followed by observation in subsequent years. [International Journal Impotence Research, Nov. 10, 2005]

Doctors at St Bartholomew's and The Royal London Hospital School of Medicine, West Smithfield, England, say there has been no conclusive evidence so far, despite numerous studies, that levels of circulating testosterone in individuals with prostate cancer are higher than in controls. In fact, prostate cancers arising in men with low serum testosterone levels are generally more malignant and frequently nonresponsive to hormones. [Drugs Aging 17: 431-39, 2000]

There are a few doctors who have recently begun to suggest testosterone be employed for managing the risk of prostate cancer. This recommendation has drawn strong criticism since it is untested. [New England Journal Medicine 350: 204-06, 2004]

Doctors Ernani L. Rhoden and Abraham Morgentaler at Harvard Medical School write:

> *"One of the greatest concerns among clinicians regarding testosterone replacement therapy is the fear of causing or promoting prostate cancer. We evaluated prostatic changes in castrated men with and without high grade pre-cancerous cells in their prostate. Of 75 men who had taken supplemental testosterone for 12 months, 55 had benign prostate biopsies and 20 had precancerous changes without frank cancer prior to treatment. After 1 year of testosterone treatment, men with precancerous changes did not have a greater increase in PSA or a significantly increased risk of cancer than men without precancerous changes."*
> [Journal Urology 170: 2348-51, 2003]

In an attempt to ascertain whether testosterone replacement therapy ignites prostate cancer, the medical records at six urology practices were reviewed. The records of 20 men undergoing testosterone supplementation for sexual dysfunction or "*rejuvenation*" who were found to have prostate cancer after initiation of exogenous testosterone supplementation were analyzed. Prostate cancer was detected within 2 years of testosterone initiation in 11 men (55%) and from 28 months to 8 years in the remainder. The tumors were of moderate and high grade. Median serum prostate specific antigen (PSA) concentration at diagnosis tended to be low at 5.1 ng/ml (range 1.1 to 329.0). Researchers concluded that prostate cancer may become clinically apparent within months to a few years after the initiation of testosterone treatment. [Journal Urology 174: 534-38, 2005] Was this a mistaken conclusion?

Read the paragraph above again. The percentage of men diagnosed with prostate cancer (55%) in the study above is about the norm for the age range of patients in the study (50-85 years).

A recent review of several prospective studies investigating the incidence of prostate cancer in men receiving testosterone replacement identified only 5 among 461 men (1.1%) observed for 6 to 36 months, a prevalence rate similar to that of the general population. [New England Journal Medicine, 350: 482, 2004]

However, there is grave concern that testosterone therapy may cause a flare-up of an existing low-grade prostate tumor. Autopsy studies reveal that approximately 35% of men have hidden prostate cancer. [International Journal Cancer 29: 611, 1982]

Doctors at the Centre for Advanced Urological Research at Queen's University in Canada indicate testosterone treatment has been used for 70 years and is generally considered safe and effective. While they say *"no evidence exists that appropriate androgen administration with knowledgeable monitoring carries significant or potentially serious adverse effects on the prostate gland, suspicion of prostate cancer is an absolute contraindication for testosterone use."* [Journal Endocrinological Investigation 28: 122-27, 2005]

To the contrary, researchers at Case Western University School of Medicine in Cleveland, Ohio, prescribed testosterone to 10 men who had undergone prior castration and surgical removal of their prostate glands. These men would be considered at high risk for recurrence of tumors. After 19 months, none of the men had a detected rise in PSA and all experienced relief of non-prostatic symptoms associated with low testosterone levels. [Journal Urology 173: 533-36, 2005]

Boston University researchers searched all the known reports involving testosterone published from 1966 to 2004. Of 417 studies, 19 met the criteria they were looking for – testosterone use for at least 90 days among men over age 45 where a testosterone or a placebo tablet was randomly distributed. Among the 651 men who were collectively treated with testosterone, the rate of all undesirable prostate *"events,"* was greater than among the men receiving the inactive placebo tablet. Rates of prostate cancer were higher and the possibility of blood clotting problems was four times higher among the men taking testosterone tablets. [Journal Gerontology 60: 1451-57, 2005]

Something is amiss in the arguments on both sides. Men in youth have high testosterone levels, with some men harboring tumor cells in the prostate gland at an early age, yet prostate cancer usually arises with advancing age when testosterone levels are declining. The knotty question of whether or not TRT contributes to prostate cancer may not be resolved for some time.

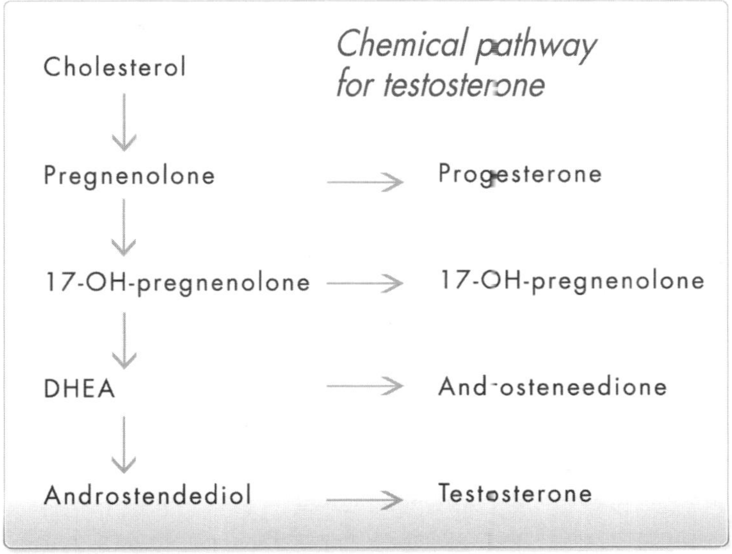

The human prostate gland produces testosterone from a precursor, DHEA (dehydroepiandrosterone), which is often sold in health shops as an anti-aging remedy. [Medical Science 19: 910-19, 2003]

Dehydroepiandrosterone (DHEA) is also produced by the adrenal glands. Serum levels of DHEA peak in men and women in the third decade and decrease progressively and profoundly with age.

DHEA is a precursor for testosterone and estrogen, which are known to accelerate growth of tumors. DHEA produces about 50% of the testosterone in the prostate gland. [Journal Endocrinology 187: 169-96, 2005] But why then don't adults develop breast and prostate cancer earlier in life? [American Journal Physiological Endocrinological Metabolism 288: 573-84E, 2005]

Since DHEA is widely available as an over-the-counter dietary supplement and is widely used as an anti-aging remedy, there is concern that it may stimulate the growth of cancer cells in the prostate and breast.

The age-related decline in DHEA, testosterone, and estrogen is believed to protect against the increasing occurrence of hormone-sensitive cancers.

In aged adults, the use of DHEA as a dietary supplement is of potential concern in that its testosterone or estrogenic actions may stimulate the growth of cancer cells within the prostate or breast. Controversy remains as to whether DHEA enhances or reduces the risk of prostate and breast cancer.

Although DHEA has been reported to increase breast cancer cell proliferation via androgen receptors, studies in small animals suggest that DHEA prevents cancer progression. [Endocrinology 146: 4565-4567, 2005]

Until more is known, DHEA supplements should be continuously used by prostate cancer patients.

Brachytherapy: implantation of radioactive seeds

Brachytherapy is now an often performed procedure when a prostate tumor is discovered. This procedure is usually performed by a urologist and/or a radiation oncologist who insert tiny radioactive seeds into the prostate gland. Brachytherapy is usually recommended when men are reluctant to undergo more invasive treatment or when invasive treatment is known to be of little value. The seeds irradiate and destroy the tumor from the inside.

Long-term data on this treatment is just now becoming available. Men may read about studies that appear very positive. But to be useful, the studies involving brachytherapy need to be compared alongside data from men who elected to forgo care (watchful waiting).

A study of 1561 men who underwent brachytherapy for prostate cancer from 1990 to 2004 is revealing. The 10-year disease-specific survival was 96%, the number that prostate cancer patients are most likely to hear. However, the overall survival rate was 74%. Furthermore, the time from initial treatment to death and PSA failure were so wide ranging (from 1.2 to 10.3 years for mortality and 2 months to 8 years for PSA failure) that it would be very difficult for a man to judge whether he was gaining any significant advantage over his prostate cancer by undergoing brachytherapy. [International Journal Radiation Oncology Biological Physics 64: 810-16, 2006]

The side effects caused by brachytherapy: loss of urinary control, decreased sexual function and erections, appear to subside over time after placement of the seeds. [International Journal Radiation Oncology Biological Physics 62: 956-64, 2005] However, the appeal of seed implants is that they pose the least discomfort and interruption of daily activities as compared to surgery, yet long-term impotency has been reported. [International Journal Radiation Oncology Biological Physics 62: 437-47, 2005]

Brachytherapy may also adversely affect PSA levels. PSA tests are not reliable and should be disregarded, however, when a careful comparison of seed implant and surgical patients was performed over a seven-year period, 98% of surgical patients were found to have PSA levels that were undetectable (less than 0.2) while only 79% of men who underwent seed implants had PSA levels less than 0.5. [Urology 51:884-9, 1998]

Informed consent

Most surgical consent forms deal with the potential risks and benefits of surgery itself. Often numerical data on the probability of side effects is not provided in the consent form. It would be important to know what percentage of men experience sexual dysfunction or urinary control problems following surgery. More important, the option of "*watchful waiting*" is usually not discussed, nor is comparative data presented.

Surgical removal is indicated when there is pain, discomfort, bleeding, blockage of urination and other uncontrollable symptoms caused by the growth of a tumor. For men who are wary of surgery, the radium seed implants appears to be more appealing, but then again, there are significant complications posed by brachytherapy and it is still considered an unproven treatment. Since, for the most part, treatment doesn't appear to be much better than watchful waiting, most patients who elect to undergo treatment usually focus on the potential for side effects.

When men sign a consent form for treatment, the form mentions the risk for side effects, such as impotence and loss of urinary control, but few consent forms say how often these problems occur. Studies indicate the incidence of side ef-

Email from a man with prostate cancer

"My main concern is still that this cancer, even though it is classified as encapsulated, could migrate to other parts of the body. Since there are no foolproof tests, besides bone scans, it then becomes Russian Roulette. All this being conjecture, then it becomes a matter of containment and nutrients that can be used. How does one know when to seek further treatment, when a PSA seems to be the only way to assess the degree of prostate cancer?

Seeing what both my brothers have done now seems to go against the consensus of noted experts. They feel that the mental anguish was reduced greatly after they had their respective treatments. When I informed them that watchful waiting was a viable option, they said that their urologist made it clear that the cancer could spread and they would only know it after it had affected other organs. Such strong dialogue convinced them that they better seek immediate ways to eliminate that possibility. I guess the option of 15 more years of life as opposed to a lesser life span is a strong motivator to accept the current modalities."

Author's note: The urologist in this case misled this man's brothers. Surgical removal does not stop the development or spread of cancer later. There is no surgical, chemical or radiation treatment that can eliminate every cancerous cell, and even if all were eliminated, unless the treatment addresses what caused cancer in the first place, it will return.

Why doctors keep pushing the PSA test: because it leads to more treatment

> *"Men who opt for 'watchful waiting' tend to be older, have lower PSA levels and more favorable characteristics than those men who seek treatment. PSA at diagnosis is the dominant factor for predicting treatment."*
> *Source: Journal Urology 164: 81-88, 2000*

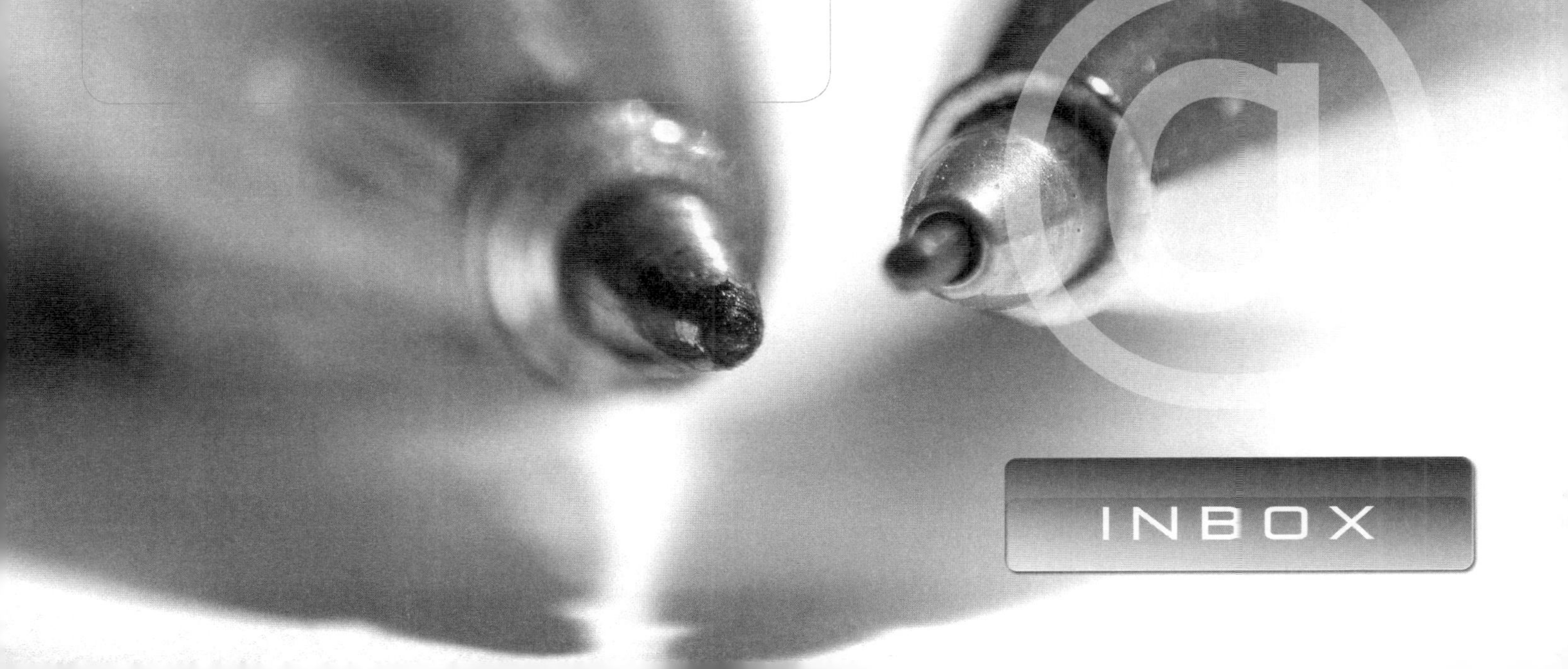

fects can range anywhere from 30 to 70% for impotence, and 1 to 35% for loss of urinary control with all forms of treatment.

Timing of treatment

"A substantial number of men who succumb to prostate cancer have a good prognosis, including low PSA and low Gleason scores. Many had undergone prior screenings."
Source: Journal Urology 174: 553-56, 2005

Patients with diagnosed prostate cancer should be in no hurry to make a treatment decision. Studies show that a delay between biopsy and surgical removal does not influence recurrence of cancer. Experts say: *"Prostate cancer is not a rapidly progressing tumor and therefore it appears inappropriate to rush patients into decision-making and treatment."* [Cancer Dec. 13, 2005]

Patient education, informed consent and decision making

Prostate cancer patients have important treatment decisions to make, and they need their doctor to assist them in making those decisions. Frequently patients hear the word *"cancer"* and elect to undergo treatment out of fear. While males are likely to analyze factual information before making decisions, and most are willing to take an active role in the choice of treatment, they are heavily influenced by the way treatment options are presented.

A survey conducted in Canada found only 5% of men made truly autonomous decisions in regard to their prostate cancer. Most men preferred to share the role with

"Once you've learn you've got cancer, it's very hard to do nothing. You want it out, and you may not want to listen to all the other alternatives."
Claus Roehrborn MD, urologist, University of Texas Southwestern Medical School

their doctors, though fewer desired a totally passive role. [Complementary Therapy Medicine 13: 213-16, 2005]

When physicians encourage more enhanced patient participation, treatment choices change. In a survey of patients who were given standard education and involvement prior to treatment, 90% chose the treatment recommended by the doctor. But, as the surveys described below indicate, this changes significantly when patients are more involved in the decision-making process. Patients may actually trade years of life for maintenance of quality of life (for example- sexual functioning).

Under age 70, otherwise healthy

- Options: surgery, radiation or watchful waiting
- Treatment of choice by doctor: prostate removal surgery

→ Initially, 86% of men chose surgery, but with more participation and education, this dropped to 58%. [BJU International 93: 52-56, 2004]

Over age 70
or with other contraindications for surgery

- Options: radiation, testicle removal, hormonal medicine or watchful waiting
- Treatment of choice by doctor: testicle removal

→ Initially, 50% of men chose testicle removal, but with more participation and education, this dropped to just 8%.

Since no significant differences have been found in survival between surgery and radiation treatment in contained prostate cancer, and no difference is found between various forms of hormone treatment (estrogen, testosterone inhibitors), it is difficult to conclude which treatment is best. [British Journal Urology International 93: 52-56, 2004]

When researchers evaluated patient education materials for patients with early-stage prostate cancer, they found that none of the materials discussed recurrence or success rates. The survey included materials produced by the American Cancer Society, the National Cancer Institute, and other sources. [Annals Internal Medicine 140: 721-29, 2004]

The study concluded by saying: *"Unfortunately, the patient education materials that are currently available... do not contain complete information about prostate cancer treatment and their accompanying side effects, do not provide adequate numeric estimates and are written at reading levels that exceed those of the average U.S. adult. If men are to truly make informed decision about their prostate cancer, better tools for delivering information about the disease and treatment options must be developed."* [Annals Internal Medicine 140: 721-29, 2004]

A survey of urologists appearing in the *Canadian Journal of Urology* found that **information provided to patients should include:**

- Cure rates
- Right to refuse treatment
- Mortality from watchful waiting
- Incontinence rates (loss of urinary control)
- Treatment-related impotence rates

A third of men over age 50 harbor some form of prostate cancer, but only between 6 and 10 percent will acquire the type likely to lead to death or disability. And only about 3% die of it.
Source: Scientific American, September 1996

But there is widespread disparity among urologists as to what information to provide other than the above-listed topics. Doctors frequently indicate they would rather avoid answering patients' questions about selection of a medical center or a doctor's success rate. [Canadian Journal Urology 4: 438-44, 1997]

Comparing doctors

Of course, urologists shudder at the thought of rankings of doctors' performance. Crude data that compares morbidity and mortality among prostate cancer surgeons would be misleading unless adjusted for cancer stage and complicating factors. [Journal Urology 166:968-72, 2001] Probably the best criterion for selecting a physician is experience. However, younger physicians appear to be better trained and more likely to provide patients with more forthright answers regarding the drawbacks of screening and treatment.

From the patient's viewpoint, he often doesn't know what questions to ask his doctor. A survey of patients facing treatment decisions found widespread disagreement as to which questions were the most important to ask doctors. [Medical Decision Making 20: 7-19, 2000]

There are professional guidelines on how to inform patients about treatments for prostate. These differ by health plan, by professional group and by area. However, adherence to these guidelines does not occur in most instances. It is interesting to note that a physician survey found that 73% of female doctors believe it is important for patients to know that PSA screening is controversial and of unproven value, while only 43% of male physicians felt the same way. While physicians have an *"ethical obligation to engage patients in*

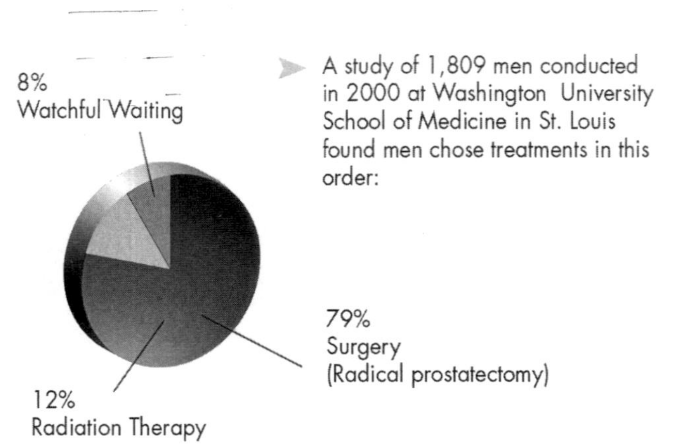

informed decision making for screening tests such as the PSA test, whose net benefit has not yet been proven," the PSA test is taken for granted as being a reliable test and few patients are informed of its drawbacks. [Journal General Internal Medicine 18: 350-56, 2003]

With each additional five years of age, a man was twice as likely to choose watchful waiting over surgery or radiation treatment. [Cancer 88: 1122-30, 2000] A survey published in 2000 found 49% of urologists consider patients are ill prepared to make decisions about prostate cancer care. [CNN May 2, 2000]

A similar survey conducted in 1996, found that the prospect of removing the complete tumor was the strongest factor influencing men to undergo surgery. However, most men are under the misconception that surgery removes all the tumor cells. It doesn't. Men who chose to wait were more influenced by the rate of surgical or treatment- related complications. [Western Journal Medicine 165: 26-30, 1996]

A survey published in 1996, found that prostate cancer patients seem to be uninfluenced by the rather high rate of side effects associated with surgery, even when surgery couldn't offer 10-year survival. [Journal American Geriatrics Association 44: 934-37, 1996]

Between 1984 and 1990 prostate cancer surgery increased by more than 500%, with a complete lack of evidence that it prolonged life or reduced discomfort. [Agency for Health Care Policy Research 1995]

Another survey finds that cancer treatment specialists are more likely to steer patients towards treatment they themselves provide – radiologists recommend radiation treatment, surgeons recommend surgery. Neither surgeons nor radiologists advocated watchful waiting. [Journal American Medical Association 283: 3217-3222, 2000]

While more and more men opt for treatment, men age 65 to 75 years of age with low-grade prostate cancer incur no loss of life expectancy by opting for watching waiting. [Journal American Medical Assn 274: 626-31, 1995] The choice of whether or not to undergo surgery seems to be based on the severity of symptoms experienced. Men with erectile dysfunction, for example, were more willing to go under the knife than men with urinary obstruction. Following is a comparison of men who elected to undergo surgery (radical prostatectomy) versus watching waiting:

Men who elected to undergo surgery (radical prostatectomy) versus watchful waiting:

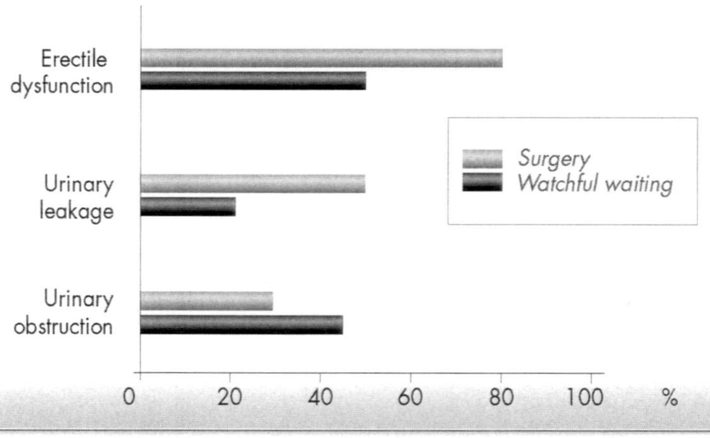

Listen to this straight talk about seed implant treatment from Dr. Nelson N Stone of Mount Sinai School of Medicine in New York:

> *"There is no guidance from well - designed clinical trials, recommendations for one treatment over another are mostly based on the doctor's individual experiences and personal biases. No 'gold standard' exists for localized prostate cancer. As for high-risk prostate cancer, no standard treatment, be it radical prostatectomy (surgery) or brachytherapy (seed implants) yield adequate results."* [British Journal Urology International 93: 5, 2004]

In other words, the slow, progressive form of the disease makes the doctor appear to be providing effective treatment. For the fast-progressing form, there is no proven treatment.

For example, the Scandinavian Prostatic Cancer Group Study drew attention from the worldwide news media when doctors were finally able to say that surgical removal of the prostate gland had been shown to be effective. But the news reports were misleading. While surgery (radical prostatectomy) significantly reduced disease-related mortality at 10 years, the overall survival rate was about the same (5% better for surgically treated patients, which was not considered statistically significant in this small group study). [New England Journal Medicine 352: 1977-84, 2005]

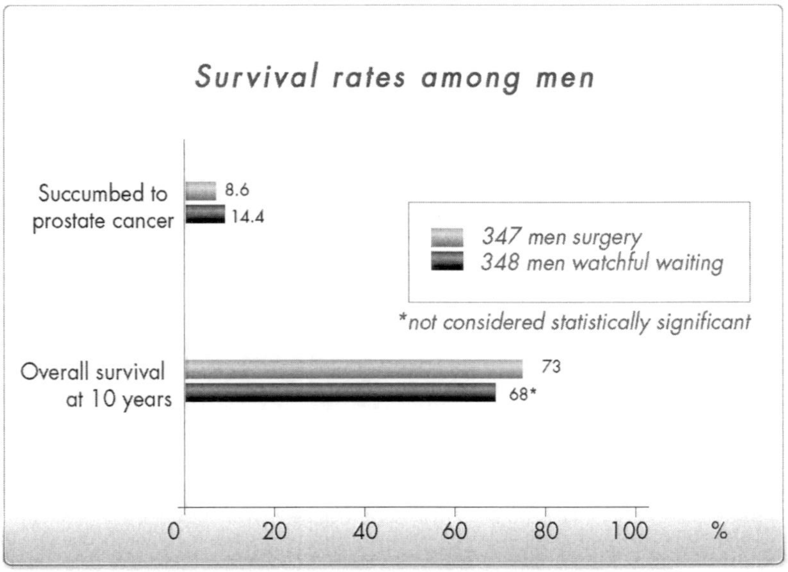

This is the kind of study that is quoted by urologists. It is misleading. First, it did not extend to 14 years. Second, it only considers those who died of prostate cancer. Overall, the death rate was about the same (73% vs 68%), because after 10 years, patients died of treatment-induced problems (heart attacks), not of the prostate cancer itself.

A recent study indicates there should be no rush to undergo prostate removal when cancer is diagnosed. In most cases, the risk for noncurable prostate cancer is the same for men who wait two years before undergoing surgery as for men who undergo immediate surgery. [Journal National Cancer Institute 98:506-7, 2006]

The male hormone testosterone drives the growth of prostate tumors. Studies conducted in the 1970s showed that medical approaches to inhibit testosterone production by sex organs does not prolong survival but does delay progression once it has become advanced disease So hormone drugs like estrogen, Lupron and diethylstilbestrol are used. Again, this is only palliative care used to reduce symptoms among men with the progressive form of prostate cancer.

Chemotherapy, often employed for other types of cancer, should not be considered in most cases of prostate cancer because an analysis of 26 studies done between 1987 and 1999 showed only a small, insignificant response.

Still, prostate cancer patients are subjected to surgery, chemotherapy, and radiation treatment combinations, including the implantation of radium seeds into the prostate sac, in attempts to prolong life. But because prostate cancer is slow to progress, it is not known whether any of these treatments actually prolong survival, and may only result in patients experiencing loss of urinary control, decline in sexual drive or performance, and other complications.

Doctors screen millions of American men and treat thousands, but it appears the various treatments do little to extend life. For the most part, treatment is actually palliative, that is, it only attempts to allay the pain associated with the disease. This misleads many patients into thinking prostate cancer is being cured or at least slowed down. Once cancer has begun to spread, most treatment is aimed at alleviating pain, not effecting a cure.

Since it takes 10-15 years to determine whether a specific treatment is effective, prostate care today has become a giant experiment upon men with prostate cancer. In many instances, treatment that has been disproven is utilized over what is unproven. Since there is often no proven benefit to treatment, and there are significant side effects produced by treatment, modern medicine appears to be violating its rule of *"first do no harm."*

Screening

Surveys reveal that nearly nine in ten Americans believe cancer screening is a good idea. According to a report in the Journal of the American Medical Association, 74% believe that early cancer detection saves lives and many believe that an older adult who refuses to undergo screening tests is irresponsible. Nearly 4 in 10 adults who were surveyed had undergone at least one false positive screening test. Two-thirds said they would want to be tested for cancer even if nothing could be done. This survey reflects public enthusiasm for cancer screening which is not dampened by the lack of effective treatments or false-positive tests. Authors of the survey indicate *"this enthusiasm create an environment ripe for placing the public at risk of overtesting and overtreatment."* [Journal American Medical Assn 291: 71-78, 2004]

Detection and monitoring of prostate cancer is in a state of disarray. This news will likely be dismaying to men with prostate cancer, especially those who have already undergone treatment and are fending off recurrence or are in the midst of making decisions about treatment for the first time.

Even doctors are in a quandary as to what to do now that it has become apparent the PSA test needs to be replaced with a yet-to-be-developed test that will accurately indicate the size of the prostate gland and stage of malignancy.

The current view is that prostate cancer screening is of little value in prolonging life and may prompt many patients to elect for treatment they didn't need. Here is what one report says:

> *Prostate-specific antigen (PSA) screening tests that yield false-positive results (indicate cancer when there is no cancer) can lead to anxiety and repeated biopsies. About 60 % of men who undergo radical prostatectomy (surgical removal of the prostate) cannot have an erection, and 30 % need to wear pads to deal with leaking urine. These relatively common and dramatic personal harms of screening and treatment are readily discounted or explained away. The physician is positively reinforced for recommending screening, regardless of the test result. A negative result makes a patient grateful for reassurance, and a positive result makes a patient grateful for early detection. A patient who is impotent and incontinent after a decision for curative treatment may attribute his survival to surgery and be grateful for having his cancer cured.*

PROSTATE CANCER SCREENING DOESN'T SAVE LIVES
Prostate Cancer Screening Comparison
Seattle/ Connecticut 1987-1997 males age 65-79 years
Source: British Medical Journal 325:740, 2002

	Seattle	Connecticut
PSA testing rate per 100,000	11,803 (5.39 times greater than Conn)	2,199
Biopsy rate per 100,000 per years	1,848 (2.20 times greater than Conn)	840
Cumulative rate of prostate surgery after 10 years	Men in this age group in Seattle underwent 5.9 times more prostate surgery and 2.3 times more radiation treatment than men in Connecticut	
Prostate cancer mortality after 11 years	About the same for both populations	

Whether or not early detection and aggressive treatment of prostate cancer reduces prostate cancer mortality is still not known. There are several ways to curb possible overenthusiasm for aggressive screening and treatment for prostate cancer. One approach is to require that patients complete detailed written informed consent before screening, indicating an understanding that evidence of efficacy is weak or lacking and that adverse effects may occur. By ensuring that patients are informed about the pros and cons of testing and its consequences before they are tested, the chances are much improved that doctors and their patients will make decisions that are not tipped, possibly quite unfairly, toward intervention. [American Journal of Medicine 113: 663-667, 2002]

The researchers examined the rates of screening for prostate cancer, treatment with radical prostatectomy and radiation, and prostate cancer-related deaths from 1987 to 1997 among Medicare beneficiaries aged 65-79 drawn from the Seattle-Puget Sound area and Connecticut.

The PSA testing rate in the Seattle area was 5.39 times that of Connecticut, and the prostate biopsy rate was 2.20 times that of Connecticut during 1987-1990. The 10-year cumulative incidence of radical prostatectomy and external beam radiotherapy up to 1996 were 2.7% and 3.9% for Seattle men compared with 0.5% and 3.1% for Connecticut men. Yet, the adjusted rate of prostate cancer-related deaths up to 1997 was similar for Seattle and Connecticut.

American Cancer Society guidelines (2005) call for doctors to offer PSA testing and digital rectal examinations to men age 50 or older. However, the American Academy of Family Physicians claims there is insufficient evidence to make a recommendation for or against routine screening for prostate cancer using the PSA or the digital rectal exam. The U.S. Preventive Services Task Force advocates PSA testing for early detection of prostate cancer, but concludes there is mixed evidence that early detection leads to improved survival. That's three public health agencies that do not agree on how to address the cancer that kills more men than any other form of cancer. Furthermore, men may be surprised to learn that PSA testing is rarely performed in Great Britain because it is considered unreliable.

Symptoms of cancer or an enlarged prostate?

The harsh reality is that it is difficult, if not impossible, to differentiate prostatic inflammation (prostatitis) from cancer, and benign or idle forms of cancer from aggressive, life-threatening malignancies. Various experts now claim that "*PSA may no longer be an effective marker for early-stage tumors, with PSA elevation failing to discriminate tumor-specific characteristics from benign gland enlargement.*" [Prostate Cancer and Prostatic Diseases 9, 5–13, 2006] Autopsy studies show that by age 30–39, approximately 29% of men have microscopic evidence of pre-cancerous changes in their prostate, which increases to approximately 65% by age 70. [In Vivo 8: 439–443, 1994]

There are four ways to find latent cancer:

1. screening via PSA testing
2. biopsy
3. surgical entry
4. and evidence on the autopsy table

It is said that 80% of men develop prostate cancer by age 80. [Prostate Cancer: Biology, Diagnosis, Pathology, Staging, and Natural History, WebMD, March 10, 2005] Genetic instability leads to abnormal cell growth (neoplasia) and finally to full blown cancer. If so many older men harbor tumor cells in their prostate, what value is there to screening? Most men of advanced age can assume they harbor tumor cells in their prostate almost without confirmation by biopsy. Having non-life threatening tumor cells in the prostate is common and does not demand screening or treatment be performed.

About 17% of American men are diagnosed with prostate cancer during their lifetime and about 16% of those diagnosed will succumb to it, or about 3% of the total male population. [Japanese Journal Clinical Oncology 35: 680-89, 2005] The remaining male population that develops prostate cancer will succumb to other diseases before their prostate cancer becomes life threatening.

Digital rectal exam (DRE)

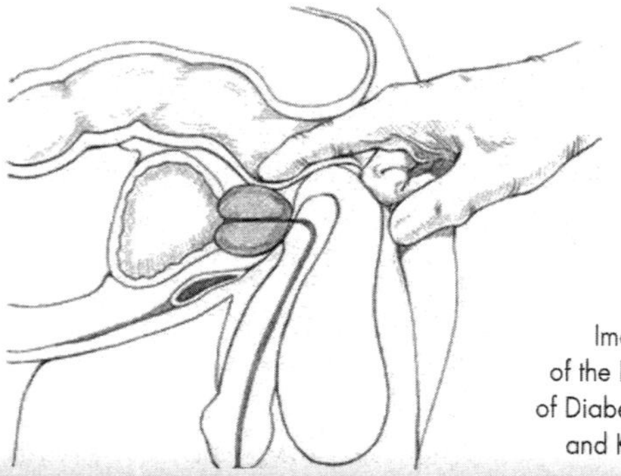

Image courtesy of the National Institute of Diabetes and Digestive and Kidney Diseases

Detection of prostate cancer

"Ideally a doctor should be able to predict the biological behavior of a newly diagnosed cancer and help each patient decide on treatment which avoids over treatment of slow-growing tumors and undertreatment of aggressive ones. At present, making a reliable prediction is not possible."

Gerald W. Chodak, MD, Midwest Urology Research Foundation Chicago, Ill. Prostate Cancer and Prostatic Diseases 9: 25-29, 2006

Prostate cancer diagnosis is a major life altering experience. Among the problems caused by diagnosis alone are:

- Inconvenience
- Uncertainty
- Anxiety
- Discomfort
- Costs
- Embarrassment with incontinence
- Impotence and loss of sexual function

PSA testing

Prostate Specific Antigen (PSA) testing was introduced around 1991.

The normal prostate gland secretes PSA in the seminal fluid, which eventually can be found in trace amounts in the blood circulation. PSA is specific for the prostate gland, but is not specific for cancer since normal, precancerous and inflamed cells all manufacture PSA. However, prostate cancer releases 10 times more PSA into the blood serum than normal or inflamed tissue. By far, the most common reason why PSA is elevated is prostatitis (inflammation of the prostate gland), not prostate cancer. Prostatitis is very common as men age. Monitoring changes in PSA is often performed to watch for the recurrence of prostate cancer after it has been treated or has been in dormancy for a time. But again, PSA numbers are deceiving and unreliable.

With PSA and the digital rectal exam, doctors can only predict with any assurance that a patient has prostate cancer 30-40% of the time. Suspicious exams are followed by a needle biopsy of the prostate. However, prostate cancer detected at any early stage may not produce any symptoms for 10 years or more.

PSA numbers rise with advancing age and there has been debate over when rising numbers indicate it is time to explore further with a biopsy of prostate tissue. In 1994, the FDA settled on a 4.0 nanogram per milliliter (ng/ml) PSA cutoff point where a biopsy is called for. According to the

Cancer Detection Rates In Men Not Previously Biopsied				
Percent of patients with cancer (264 patients studied) Shows PSA varies widely in cases of cancer and non-cancer				
Digital rectal exam	PSA less than 4.0	PSA 4.0-10.0	PSA over 10.0	PSA overall
Normal	27.8%	41.5%	63.2%	42.5%
Abnormal	18.6%	56.6%	75.0%	42.3%
Source: Annual Review of Medicine 53: 355-68, 2002				

FDA standard, a man with a healthy prostate with no prostatitis or prostate cancer should have a PSA count of less than 1.0. But advancing age, recent ejaculation, infection, medications (even finasteride) or inflammation can cause PSA elevation, and mass screening of men with PSA above 1.0 would lead to many needless biopsies and false positive tests. So the FDA set the PSA level considered "*safe*" at 4.0 for healthy men with no additional risk factors. This sounds very arbitrary.

For healthy males 45-50 years of age who have an immediate relative who developed prostate cancer at an early age, or who have black skin pigmentation, doctors now recommend a PSA cutoff of 2.6. [Annual Review Medicine 53: 355-68, 2002]

It has been determined that if men with a PSA of 25.0 did not undergo biopsy, the number of needless biopsies would be reduced by 20% and still 95% of the cancers would have been positively detected biopsying everyone with a PSA of 4-10. [Annual Review Medicine 53: 355-68, 2002]

But all this information is ready to be discarded. Here's why.

PSA invalid

Once a person has consented to PSA testing, he enters a diagnosis mill that can drag him into further testing, biopsies and other invasive treatments, most of which are unnecessary.

It is difficult to imagine that the entire care of prostate cancer is misdirected. But that is exactly what doctors at the Department of Urology at Stanford University School of Medicine report. The Stanford doctors explain how PSA testing deceived the medical profession. In the early days, around 1987, it was reported that PSA levels were proportional to the increasing stages of tumor growth doctors could feel while conducting rectal exams on males. The surgical removal of large nodules of benign, but inflamed, prostate tissues was shown to reduce PSA levels. But since 2001, say Stanford researchers, there has been a turnaround. PSA levels no longer correlate with the size of the prostate gland and the Gleason score, which is an estimate of the stage of cancer based upon microscopic slides of prostate tissue obtained during biopsy. [Journal Urology 172: 1297-1301, 2004]

Men with PSA levels ranging from 2.0 to 4.0 have nearly the same positive biopsy rates as males with PSAs ranging from 2.0 to 20.0. The Stanford doctors say "*the relationship between prostate cancer and PSA is tenuous at best, especially with PSA less than 10.0 and perhaps less than 22.0!*" Careful analysis of data now shows PSA is only related to the size and inflammation of the prostate gland, not to cancer.

When the drive to screen men for prostate cancer began, in the early 1990s, there were many males who had advanced, large palpable (detectable by finger exam) tumors. So the PSA tests were skewed because it appeared the numbers were related to tumor size and stage. As more men were screened, large and advanced stage tumors were found less often, and the correlation with PSA testing faded. The screening programs only appeared successful because the death rate from this cancer is low (about 226 per 100,000), so patients attributed the PSA screening and any subsequent treatment to saving their lives. In fact, relatively few die of prostate cancer.

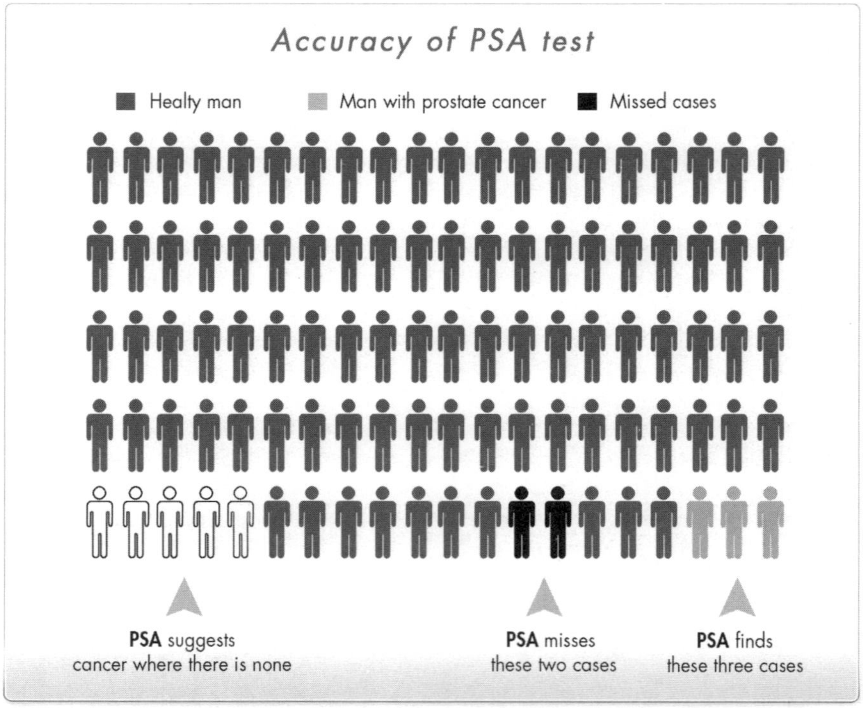

On the autopsy table, it has been found that 14% of males who died of diseases other than prostate cancer had co-existing prostate cancer. In 1996, researchers obtained prostate tissue samples from young males who had been killed in accidents in a major U.S. city. They found 8% of males in their 20s exhibited invasive prostate cancer! With each decade of life there was an increase in prostate cancer until an 80% rate was noted by age 70. This means that any excuse to perform a biopsy is likely to find a tumor among men of advanced age. Biopsy only results in alarming men who have had cancer cells in their prostate gland for decades.

The Stanford doctors say the suggestion to use a lower PSA cutoff point (2.6) to recommend biopsy is misguided because *"this is precisely the range of PSA for most men with benign prostatic hyperplasia (BPH),"* which is common among most males and not life threatening. BPH is inflammation of the prostate gland that causes symptoms such as frequent urination, especially during sleep. Since the PSA numbers for BPH and prostate cancer overlap, and since many older men have BPH, men are likely to get the false impression they have cancer and submit to needless biopsying and treatment. There is no way PSA testing can differentiate between BPH and cancer. [Current Urological Reports 5: 231-40, 2004] Other investigators confirm that PSA testing simply cannot discriminate between the chronic benign condition called benign prostatic hypertrophy (swollen prostate) and cancer. [Current Urological Reports 5: 231-40, 2004]

They ask: "What are we to do in the face of such massive, unwarranted PSA screening?" Lowering the PSA cutoff point only serves to "compound the tragedy by adding millions of men to the biopsy list." They conclude that "we urgently need another marker that correlates with prostate cancer in the current PSA range of 2.0 to 10.0 where most PSA numbers fall." The Stanford doctors say "little is likely to change the current state of overdiagnosis and overtreatment." [Journal Urology 172: 1297-1301, 2004]

What is the accuracy of the PSA test?

For every 100 men over the age of 50 who have the PSA test :

- About 90 will have a normal PSA level, and about 10 will have a higher than normal level.
- And of these 10, as illustrated above, five will be diagnosed with prostate cancer who are free of cancer and two will go undiagnosed .

Another study found that 65%of PSA testing resulted in false positive tests and 20% in false negative tests. [Canadian Journal Urology 4: 6-17, 1997].

Men falsely reassured they don't have prostate cancer

One study shows that 96% of men who underwent PSA testing felt it gave them some level of reassurance they didn't have cancer. [Health Expectations 5: 104-13, 2002]. Another reason for the popularity of PSA testing is that many males are analytical. They like having a number to look at. To many men, even false assurances may appear better than nothing.

The main problem with PSA testing is that even if it does help detect prostate cancer, it doesn't help detect the dangerous life-threatening form of prostate cancer. Most men already have cancerous cells in their prostate gland and are likely to have a positive biopsy test, but few will die of this disease. [Urologe A 42: 1172-87, 2003]

Even men with a PSA test ranging from 4.0 to 10.0 (the level at which a biopsy is usually recommended), have a 70% chance that subsequent biopsies will be negative. Therefore, it is now recommended that men undergo a second PSA test before a biopsy is performed. [Journal American Medical Assn 289: 2695-700, 2003]

While a rise in PSA is considered suspicious, in one study 92% of the increases in PSA were found to be non-cancerous. [Urology 62: 64-69, 2003]

Even more perplexing, an elevated PSA test that normalizes is not necessarily assurance that a man is free of cancer. In one study, 24% of men whose elevated PSA numbers dropped into the normal range were found to have cancer on biopsy. [Prostate Cancer Prostatic Disease 8: 349-52, 2005]

Scientific studies which invalidate PSA testing have not dampened doctors' enthusiasm for the test. One survey found that 88% of doctors still recommend PSA testing even though they, unlike patients, have sufficient training to know that it is not a valid test. [Journal National Cancer Institute 95: 1792-97, 2003]

Finally, if you have acquired PSA phobia from your doctors and cannot take your eye off of this largely meaningless number, consider a study of Japanese men, some who live in Japan and others who live in the United States. For ten years these men were monitored for their PSA level. The Japanese American men had lower PSA levels, but the native Japanese men had half the rate of prostate cancer as the American men. [Journal National Cancer Institute 89: 1716-22, 1997]

To add a final note, a survey shows about 14% of U.S. men who had a PSA test performed are over age 75 and that 27.8% of men in this age group undergo PSA testing. The remaining years of life for men in this age group is generally about 10 years, while the detection of slow-growing prostate cancer would pose a mortal risk for most of these men far beyond the day of their passing. So the value of the screening has been brought into question. [Journal Urology 176: 511-14, 2006] The PSA test only serves to influence men in this age group to elect to undergo needless surgery or further testing.

Yet over 4 million older men undergo PSA testing annually. [Journal National Cancer Institute 95: 1792-97, 2003]

A great many men who are referred by their personal physician to a urologist for further examination of the prostate aren't even aware a PSA test was performed by their doctor and is the sole basis for the referral. [Annals Royal College Surgeons England 88: 284-88, 2006]

Staging

Not only is there disagreement over whether PSA screening is of value, but there is debate over how to determine the stage of cancer progression. There is often disagreement in the Gleason score, which is a judgment made by a pathologist as to the grade of cancer. [Clinical Oncology 17: 655-58, 2005]

PSA, Gleason scores and other data are often used to determine a prognosis, that is, how long does a man have before he will succumb to the disease. Doctors at MD Anderson Cancer Center in Houston report that the prognosis is better determined by whether tumor cells have spread to surrounding lymph nodes or distant organs than by the above measures. In their analysis, males with tumor spread to lymph nodes had a median survival of 134 months and with metastases 42 months. [Cancer, December 20, 2005]

Sleight of hand: Gleason scores

There are a number of doctors who want patients to get accurate information. They began to question just how prostate cancer mortality rates could have improved so abruptly.

It all has to do with the grading score that pathologists give when they examine a biopsy slide of a patient's prostate tissue.

Prostatic Adenocarcinoma (Histologic Grades)

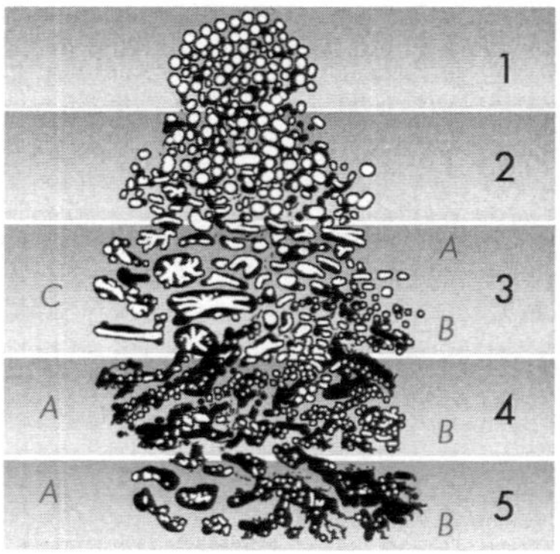

Appearance of cancer cells ranked according to the Gleason grade.

Pathologists rate the severity of prostate cancer by the Gleason score, which measures the severity of the tumor on a scale from 2 to 10, the highest number being the most severe. Twenty years ago pathologists commonly labeled newly diagnosed tumors with relatively low Gleason scores, ranging from 2 to 5, which is a less dangerous cancer. Today, scores this low are rarely given, even though there has been no change in the Gleason scoring system itself. If patients start with higher Gleason scores, this would lead to the false conclusion that improvements in survival have been achieved, when in fact no such improvements occurred.

So some concerned doctors at Stanford University pulled out old pathology slides from years ago (1990-92). They examined 454 old slides with a Gleason score of 6 and compared them with 814 contemporary slides (2002-04) with an actual Gleason score of 6 (that is, what they, not knowing the number given, would have assigned as a 6). When the contemporary slides' scores were revealed it turned out that the pathologists had given them an average score of 6.8. There were 2.08 deaths per 100-person years for the earlier slides, and 1.5 deaths per 100-person years for the contemporary slides. This kind of upgrading led to some reports of declines in mortality rates from prostate cancer by as much as 26%. This results in a false sense of accomplishment. Examiners say *"several factors have conspired to produce a statistically significant upgrading in biopsy Gleason scores, which has, in turn, produced a statistically significant apparent survival improvement."* The examiners recall a statement by Will Rogers, that *"when all the Okies moved from Oklahoma to California, the IQ of both states went up."* Hence, they coined this reclassification scheme for biopsy slides the *"Will Rogers Phenomenon."* [Journal National Cancer Institute 97: 1248-53, 2005]

Biopsy is problematic

Because there may be errors in the tissue samples obtained during needle biopsy, only a series of biopsies are considered to be reliable. For example, one study found 23% of men undergoing initial biopsy had prostate cancer, and a repeat biopsy found that 19% of these men had prostate cancer that was missed on the initial biopsy. [Journal Urology 151: 1571-74, 1994]

As convincing as they are alleged to be, there are some serious drawbacks to biopsies. The chance of finding a *"minimal"* prostate tumor in a man with no other symptoms is substantial. [Canadian Journal Urology 12: 16-20S, 2005] Even after an initial biopsy finds a high-grade, pre-cancer-

What Happens to Prostate Cancer Mortality Rates in the U.K., where PSA Screening Is Rare?

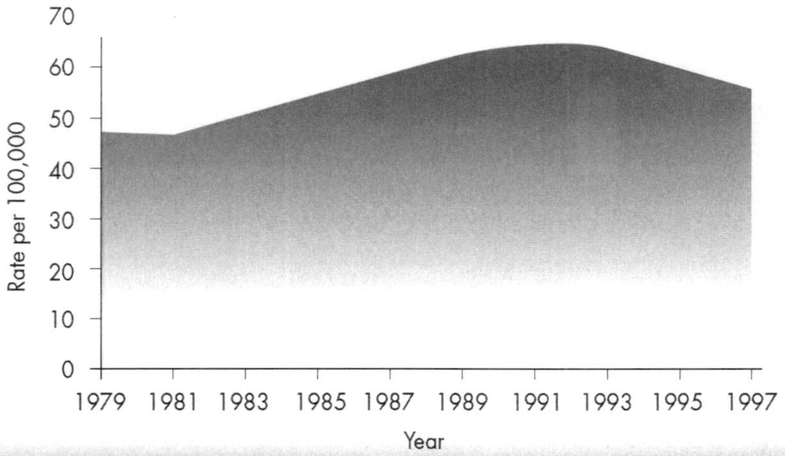

ous condition (intraepithelial neoplasia), repeat biopsy is unlikely to detect cancer and is unnecessary. [Urology 58: 999-1003, 2001]

There is a grey zone when it comes to prostate biopsies. Biopsies are judged to be one of the following: benign, atypical or cancerous. Often if the biopsy finds atypical cells, the doctor will recommend a second biopsy. However, the idea of undergoing another biopsy with an "*atypical*" diagnosis doesn't appear to be worthwhile. In one study only about one-half of one percent of atypical biopsies were found to be cancerous upon second biopsy. [Journal Urology 174: 1390-94, 2005]

Another embarrassment for physicians is that rectal tissue is often seen in needle biopsies of the prostate gland. Distorted rectal tissue can visually mimic prostate cancer, leading to the false diagnosis of cancer. [American Journal Surgical Pathology 30: 866-70, 2006]

The second biopsy

Almost invariably, more tumors are found upon second biopsy of the prostate. Cancer is defined as an abnormal wound healing response. Jabbing needles into the prostate gland sets off inflammation, produces growth factors for wound healing, and releases iron, all of which are factors associated with cancer.

A study of 1,548 men showed there was no difference in the stage at which their cancer was diagnosed regardless of whether they underwent up to 12 biopsies. [Journal Urology 176: 63-69, 2006]

Given the miserable track record of the medical profession regarding accuracy of information on cancer, and the chaotic state of affairs in regards to care of prostate cancer, more men should decline prostate biopsies.

Strategy against prostate cancer

Where do men turn when facing a state of prostate cancer care that is confusing and contradictory?

PSA testing is over-promoted and likely misleading. Biopsies are upgraded by pathologists to encourage more needless treatment and make it appear mortality rates have dropped. More disconcerting, biopsies may spread cancer to other nearby organs or even into the blood circulation by a process of inadvertent "*seeding*" during the procedure.

The hazard of seeding cancer

A common question is why prostate cancer recurs after meticulous surgical removal. It has been found that malignant cells shed during surgery may seed the surgical bed and could actually be responsible for tumor recurrence. [Journal Urology 150: 1169-71, 1993] Prostate cancer surgery including biopsies can "*seed*" cancer elsewhere. [Lancet 346: 1528-30, 1995; Journal Surgical Oncology 35: 184-91, 1987]

The seeding of malignant cells from the prostate to the anal region can occur during prostate biopsy. The tumor may not be apparent for years and never directly related to the performance of a biopsy years earlier. [Urology 51: 158-60, 1998]

Treatments for prostate cancer continue to be performed with little, if any, proven value, and patients are generally kept in the dark about this. The result is that men who have elected to undergo treatment face no better future than those who do not and are more likely to experience complications such as erectile dysfunction, loss of urinary control and other problems. A survey of one-thousand men who have undergone prostate cancer treatment concludes that many doctors minimize treatment side effects. According to Dr. Simon Hall, chairman of the urology department at Mt. Sinai Medical Center in New York, one problem is the ongoing dispute about whether surgery is better than radiation treatment. "*I think certainly — traditionally — there has been a lot of competition between surgeons and radiation oncologists between whose treatment is better,*" says Hall. And when asked if doctors minimize the side effects as part of the sales pitch, Hall says "*yes.*" [NBC News, May 11, 2004]

Furthermore, the prostate cancer care industry parades rich and famous males who have elected to undergo prostate cancer treatment as if it's a mark of bravery to undergo treatment, and characterize it as painless and a "*snap*" with brachytherapy outpatient procedures.

How much longer will men fall for this charade?

Men should develop a mindset that they will inevitably have cancer cells harbored in their prostate gland if they live long enough. For the most part, diagnosis or treatment will not alter the course of the disease. Even when symptoms arise and tumor cells begin to escape from confinement in the prostate gland, treatment is generally only palliative rather than curative.

There must be some better avenues to pursue. This book reveals some of them.

How men make decisions about treatment

The decision to undergo treatment or just wait is wrenching for most males. A real-time survey of 20 men, conducted at the very time they made treatment decisions for diagnosed prostate cancer, reveals that men make decisions based upon fear and a desire for rapid treatment of any kind rather than on rational information provided to them that most prostate tumors are slow growing and pose little danger over the long term.

Doctors will typically advise men to wait a few days before making a decision about treatment, but fearing further spread of cancer, many men impulsively elect to sign up for surgery before they investigate further. Their doctors rarely stand in their way.

The men largely relied upon anecdotal information (experiences of others who have had prostate cancer) and had misconceptions of various treatments. Nineteen of the twenty men elected to undergo treatment, only one was resolved to partner with his doctor and conduct "*watchful waiting.*" Seven of the 20 patients elected to undergo surgical prostate removal, even though most had modest grades of tumors. One patient expressed interest in alternative therapies. [Cancer 107: 620-30, 2006]

Here is how some of the men expressed their feelings after being diagnosed with prostate cancer:

"It's cancer man!.... I try to sleep and get bad dreams.... I don't know how much longer it's going to be for me, you know."

"I think it's a time bomb and you don't know if your time is going to be short or time is going to be long.... my worry is that it will spread into your lungs. Once cancer hits your lungs I think you are fodder, I think it's bye-bye baby."

I'm a little in shock because I had a couple of days of anxiety attacks. I don't know much much cancer I have.... I should just try to retire as soon as I can before I just die off.... But it's a slow-moving cancer so stop freaking yourself out. It's just no serious. All systems go. I'm kind of happy."

"I always had it in my mind that I wanted the surgery before I even went to talk to (the doctor).... You don't wait once you know you got cancer – if you can get rid of it..... They wanted to give me two weeks to think about it, but I didn't want to do that."

"People minimize the danger of having this cancer... that it is slow growing. Yea, a train doesn't look dangerous when it's going 5 miles per hour, but if it runs you over you'll be just as dead."

Participant quotes regarding the advantages and disadvantages of prostatectomy.

"If it's confined to the prostate, and they take (the prostate) out, it's gone. And you're not going to get prostate cancer again, because it's gone."

"With radiation, you are not seeing.... You are going by the PSA score afterwards – basically that would have been tough and I think surgery is just such a positive way to approach it."

"If you have surgery you're in and out. You'll know pretty soon how you are... With radiation you don't know whether or not the cancer cell has jumped the boundary."

Another revealing study was undertaken by investigators at the Erasmus Medical Center in Rotterdam, The Netherlands. Among 1014 prostate cancer detected, 293 men met the criteria for *"watchful waiting."* Yet 136 of these men (46%) elected to undergo surgical removal of their prostate gland, 91 opted for radiation treatment (31%), and just 64 (22%) decided to forgo treatment. Nineteen of these 91 men later opted for treatment of some kind. During a 8-year follow-up period, only three of these 293 men died of prostate cancer, none who were in the watchful waiting group. [European Urology, 50: 475-82, 2006]

Obviously, all the facts aren't going to alter the frightening impact of being told that a man has prostate cancer. However, there is an underlying question of the doctor's role here. Doctors are willing to oblige patients in their decisions, regardless of whether the available data (severity of the cancer, patient's age, ineffectiveness of treatment). Does the doctor perform any treatment the patient desires even though it is inadvisable? The current role of the doctor appears to be to talk patients into treatment which is oftentimes needless or lacking any potential benefit, and the patient's fears, anxieties and desire for rapid treatment are capitalized upon. Yes, doctors tell their patients to wait a couple of weeks before making a decision, but patients often override this recommendation. Should doctor's allow patients to make rush decisions? About 150,000 of the 234,500 men diagnosed with prostate cancer annually move quickly to have surgery, radiation seed implants or a variety of other radiation treatments. [Los Angeles Times, July 3, 2006]

Patients will hear their doctor quote a study which showed a slight survival advantage for patients who elected to undergo surgery versus watchful waiting. But the authors of this study indicate the advantage is not significant and *"at present, making a reliable prediction about the behavior of a newly diagnosed cancer is not possible."* In one study among men who opted for watchful waiting, 74% of these men were able to delay treatment for 2 years, 63% for 3 years and 49% for 5 years, which prolongs the quality of life of these men. [Prostate Cancer and Prostatic Diseases 5: 25-29, 2006]

"Prostate cancer is not a rapidly progressing tumor and therefore it appears inappropriate to rush patients into decision-making and treatment."
Source: Cancer Dec. 13, 2005

Will men, who are gripped with fear following their diagnosis of prostate cancer, hear any of this? Yes, they will hear it, yet this information will be filtered with white knuckles and sweat on the brow. Even with the grim fact more than half of these men will experience an irreversible decline in the quality of their lives (impotence and urinary problems), they will elect to undergo needless treatment. It's so difficult to launch an investigation.

"Prostate cancer is not a rapidly progressing tumor and therefore it appears inappropriate to rush patients into decision-making and treatment." [Cancer Dec. 13, 2005]

Prostatitis

Men may first visit the doctor's office for symptoms of inflamed and enlarged prostate (prostatitis). It is usually at this time that their doctor is likely to suggest PSA testing.

The treatment of prostatitis is as frustrating as the treatment of prostate cancer.

The chestnut-sized prostate gland wraps around the urethra or bladder opening and any swelling can produce uncomfortable symptoms, such as frequent urination, especially during hours of sleep, difficulty urinating, or slow urinary flow.... Many males have urinary symptoms caused by prostatitis. Some 2 million office visits to physicians are generated annually in the United States for prostatic inflammation. Family doctors and urologists report that they are *"frustrated, uncomfortable and lack confidence"* in treating prostatitis. Medical therapy is disappointing. A survey of physicians concluded that that treatment of prostatitis is dismal. [Urology 52: 797-802, 1998]

Prostatis remains a mysterious disease. Some men may initially present with fever and uncomfortable prostatic symptoms, but antibiotics don't remedy the problem. About 9% of men have prostatitis at any given time. About half of all men will experience prostatitis during their lifetime, some beginning as young as age 18. Fortunately, prostatitis often subsides on its own over time. [British Journal Urology 90: 678-81, 2002]

Treatment for prostatitis

Standard treatment for prostatitis is finasteride (Propecia) or alpha blockers. Finasteride shrinks the prostate gland by about 20% and over time helps with symptoms of prostatitis. However, it takes 6-12 months to notice any effects. [Scandinavian Journal Urology Nephrology 203:15-20, 1999] Because these drugs have undesirable side effects, safer alternatives should be sought. [Moleular Cell Biochemistry 250:21-6, 2003]

Saw palmetto berry and prostatitis

Saw palmetto berry extract is the most commonly used dietary supplement for prostatitis. Numerous studies confirm it is effective in shrinking the prostate gland, relieving symptoms of discomfort and nighttime urinary frequency, and is economical. [Public Health Nutrition 3: 459-72, 2000] Symptom relief is generally reported within 4-6 weeks. [American Journal Natural Medicine 1: 8, 1994] Recommended dosage is 160 mg of 85-95% fatty acids and sterol extracts from saw palmetto berry, twice a day. A review of 18 studies confirms saw palmetto berry extract produces similar benefits as Proscar (finasteride) with fewer side effects. [Journal American Medical Assn 280: 1604-09, 1998] The primary reason for failure to relieve prostate symptoms with saw palmetto berry is the use of products that do not provide proper dosage or potency.

	Saw palmetto berry extract	Proscar
Initial urinary flow rate (milliliters per second)	9.53 ml/second	9.6 ml/second
After 3 months	13.15 ml/second	10.4 ml/second

Source: American Journal Natural Medicine 1: 8, 1994

Pygeum and prostatitis

Europeans are more familiar with the use of a tree bark, *Pygeum africanum*, from the evergreen tree, for treatment of enlarged prostate. The usual dosage is 100-200 mg of 71% extract daily. Pygeum has been shown to be effective. [American Journal of Medicine 109: 654-604, 2000]

Stinging nettle and prostatitis

Stinging nettle, *Urtica dioica*, is another commonly used dietary supplement for prostatitis that has been shown to be effective. [MMW Fortschr Med 147: 103-08, 2005]

Vitamin D and prostatitis

An interesting study attempted to find out which life style factors are related to prostatitis. Men who are exposed to more sunlight have fewer prostate symptoms. [Urology 58: 853-58, 2001] This observation suggests vitamin D levels are related to symptoms of prostatitis.

Researchers continue to focus on using synthetic versions of vitamin D to experimentally treat prostates. [J Clinical Endocrinology Metabolism 85:2576-83, 2000]

Higher-dose vitamin D, in the range of 2,000-4,000 IU daily, may be found to be helpful in preventing and treatment prostatitis. Men have been mistakenly directed away from so-called high-dose vitamin D supplements because of studies that incorrectly implicated this nutrient in causing adverse side effects.

Quercetin and prostatitis

The use of quercetin supplements has been shown to mildly improve uncomfortable prostate symptoms compared to an inactive placebo tablet. [Urology 54: 960-63, 1999]

Pollen and prostatitis

Most men are unaware of a considerable number of studies showing that pollen extract is helpful for symptoms of prostatitis. Nearly half of men using pollen extract report good to excellent results in urinary flow and with prolong used, shrinkage of an enlarged prostate. Common dosage is 126mg per day. [Clinical Therapy 17: 82-87, 1995]

A combination of natural products, pollen (cernitin), saw palmetto, B-sistosterol, vitamin E) has been shown to reduce day and nighttime urinary frequency. [International Urology Nephrology 33:217-25, 2001]

Is prostate cancer an infectious disease?

It has recently been shown that men with no symptoms of prostatitis, but with an elevated PSA, will experience a decline in PSA after a 2-4 week course of antibiotics. A significant number (20-30%) of men will avoid subsequent biopsies by undergoing a course of antibiotic therapy prior to biopsy. [Recenti Progress Medicine 96: 365-69, 2005]

This finding suggests underlying infection may be a cause of elevated PSA in many males. Could low-grade infection cause chronic inflammation that leads to prostate cancer? Some experts think so. A study of men in Cuba is instructive. Men studied in Cuba who had more sexual contacts and had a history of venereal disease were more likely to develop prostate cancer. [International Journal Epidemiology 34: 193-97, 2005] An analysis of previous studies confirms there is an association between exposure to any sexually transmitted disease and prostate cancer. [Family Medicine 37: 506-12, 2005]

What to do to prevent prostate cancer

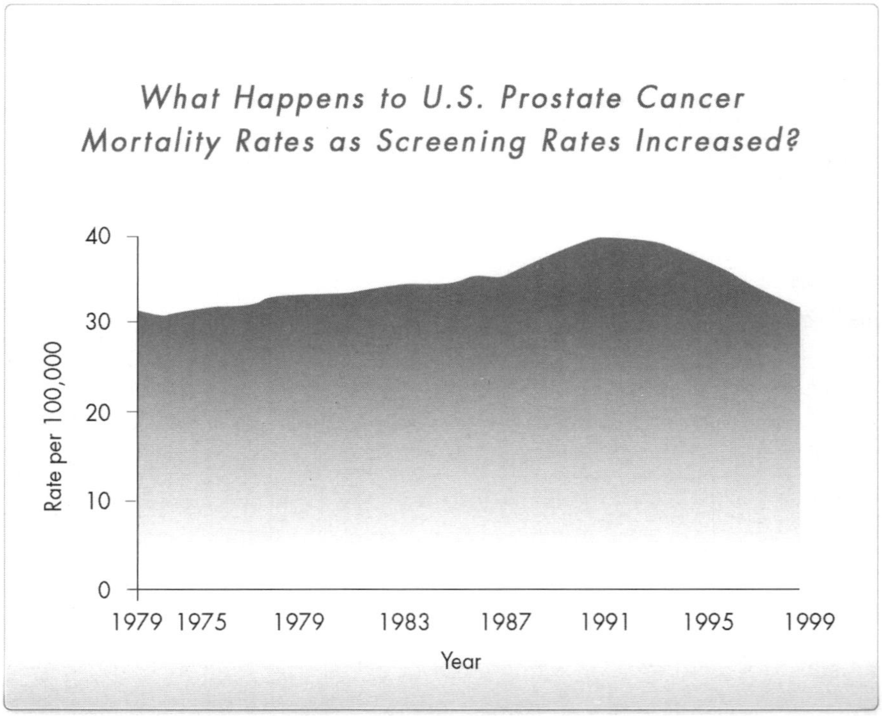

With virtually all men at risk for prostate cancer, and all harboring cancer cells in their prostate gland from early in life, prevention should be emphasized. So far there is no agreement on just what preventive measures should be practiced. While an estimated 57% of men over age 50 in the United States have had a PSA test or have undergone a gloved finger exam prostate exam within the past year, when asked "*What, if anything, are you doing to protect yourself from developing prostate cancer?*" 22% said "*nothing,*" 25% said "*self care,*" 26% said they would rely upon conventional doctoring, and 27% said they would combine doctoring with self care. [Cancer Epidemiology Biomarkers Prevention 13: 78-86, 2004]

Family history

Family history of prostate cancer is a strong predictor of which men are at greatest risk for this form of cancer. [European Urology 47: 761-68, 2005] But this is a very misleading statement.

Frequently men hear they are at greater risk for prostate cancer because their grandfathers died of prostate cancer. But disease that follows along family lines may be due to controllable factors (iron intake, smoking, sun exposure and vitamin D production, infection, etc.). Men can make alterations in their lifestyles and negate the risk for prostate cancer. For example, men who stop smoking experience a decline in their risk for prostate cancer. [Cancer Epidemiology Biomarkers Prevention 12: 604-09, 2003] Doctors frequently ask if a 1st degree relative had prostate cancer, and when the patient nods yes, the doctor indicates the patient had better get a biopsy. This is false reasoning.

Oddly, while it is widely known there is genetic tendency towards prostate cancer, doctors never mention the fact that dark pigmented skin (a genetic trait) reduces the production of vitamin D in the skin upon sun exposure and therefore is a modifiable risk factor. Sunlight in a bottle, vitamin D pills, could reduce the risk. Virtually every black male, if not every male, should be counseled to supplement his diet with vitamin D, to reduce the risk for prostate cancer.

To have a family history for this disease does not condemn men to inevitable prostate cancer.

Baldness and prostate cancer

High testosterone levels are associated with male pattern baldness. In a study of 4,421 males over 21 years, prostate cancer was diagnosed in 214 subjects, more so among balding men (17.5 versus 12.5 per 10,000 person-years of life, or about a 50% increase). [Cancer Epidemiology Biomarkers 9: 523-27, 2000]

Inflammation and prostate cancer

Inflammation is involved in virtually every disease. Studies conducted by Harvard School of Public Health researchers show that two markers of inflammation, C-reactive protein (CRP) and interleukin-6 (IL-6) are raised almost a decade before prostate cancer is diagnosed. [American Association for Cancer Research, Nov. 14, 2006]

The use of anti-inflammatory drugs is associated with reduced risk for many cancers. For example, the Baltimore Longitudinal Study on Aging found any use of aspirin or other non-steroidal anti-inflammatory drugs produced a modest reduction in risk for prostate cancer. [Cancer Epidemiology Biomarkers Prevention 14: 390-96, 2005]

However, other studies do not confirm that aspirin use prevents prostate cancer. [European Journal Cancer Prevention 15: 43-45, 2006]

One of the most positive studies involving anti-inflammatory drugs and prostate cancer was published in 2002. It showed that 23 of 569 men who used anti-inflammatory drugs (4%) compared with 68 of 793 non-users (9%), developed prostate cancer during a six-year period. [Mayo Clinic Proceedings 77: 217-18, 2002]

The increased risk for heart attacks with the use of non-steroidal anti-inflammatory drugs caused an abrupt halt to the idea of life-long use of anti-inflammatory drugs to prevent prostate cancer. [Inflammopharmacology 13: 419-25, 2005]

There appear to be safer and more natural alternatives. For example, vitamin D inhibits COX-2, the inflammatory protein that drugs like Vioxx, Bextra and others attempt to control. [Journal Steroid Biochemistry Molecular Biology 97: 31-36, 2005]

An inflammatory protein called P38 plays a very important role in prostate tumor progression. [Actas Urologia Espana 29: 769-76, 2005] There are many natural molecules, such as quercetin, resveratrol, rosemary, N-acetyl cysteine, that lower P38 levels.

> An article in The New Republic in 1999 called for the National Cancer Institute to show a little fortitude and make it known that PSA screening is not an entirely unmitigated good for all men.
> *Source: The New Republic, March 22, 1999*

5 alpha reductase inhibitors for prostate cancer prevention

In 2003 the Prostate Cancer Prevention Trial, which involved 18,882 men 55 years of age or older, found that administering 5 alpha reductase inhibitors such as finasteride (Propecia, Proscar) delays the appearance of prostate cancer and reduces urinary symptoms, but puzzlingly increased the risk for high-grade prostate cancer (high Gleason score) and produced side effects. [New England Journal Medicine 349: 215-24, 2003]

Finasteride has been shown to reduce risk for prostate cancer by about 25%. But finasteride decreases male sex drive and may induce higher-grade tumors, and it may not save any lives. In fact, with more study, it may actually result in an increase in the mortal form of prostate cancer.

The actual number of years of life saved using a drug like Propecia is minimal (about one month of added life per patient). [Urological Oncology 23: 463, 2005] Studies like this leave doctors scratching their heads. It's not conclusive enough to warrant widespread use of 5 alpha reductase inhibitors as a preventative.

A major finasteride study involved 9,060 men. Among the men taking finasteride, 18.4% developed prostate tumors versus 24% in the placebo group, for a real difference of about 6 in 100 men. This means, over a 7-year period, 94 men taking finasteride would experience no benefit while 6 would. However, while most men develop prostate cancer, few die from it.

In the finasteride study, only 10 men died of prostate cancer, five in each group taking finasteride or placebo. Men taking finasteride who were found to have prostate cancer were more likely to have a fast-growing kind. So finasteride may slightly reduce the risk of prostate cancer, but not dying of prostate cancer. Also, men taking finasteride had more incidences of erectile dysfunction and loss of interest in sex, but fewer urinary problems. [New England Journal of Medicine 349:215-224, 2003]

For a hypothetical group of one thousand 62-year-old men treated with finasteride, an increased survival of 140 life-years is forecasted, or about a month (0.14 years) per individual. [Journal Urology 175:934-8, 2006]

If all at-risk males age 55-80 years were to take Finasteride, it would cost about $3.4 billion per year. [Journal National Cancer Institute 96: 1410-12, 2004]

Some doctors are dubious of the use of finasteride as a preventative and note that weight control, dietary changes, lycopene, soy beans, omega 3 oil, selenium, vitamin E and avoidance of tobacco are without risks, efficient and commendable. [Review Med Suisse 2: 163-65, 2006]

Once prostate cancer has been diagnosed, hormone therapy may be prescribed. Whereas hormone therapy inhibits the production of testosterone, the problem is that cells have a docking or entry port called an androgen receptor (testosterone receptor) that permits entry into cells. (A cell receptor is a structure on the surface of a cell that selectively receives and binds a certain substance, like estrogen or testosterone). Researchers have been stymied to come up with effective therapy that would deal with the hormone receptor sites on prostate gland cells.

Two plant molecules, found in red wine and other botanical sources, quercetin and resveratrol, inhibit the function of androgen receptors. They are potentially useful for prostate cancer prevention. [Cancer Letters 213: 155-63, 2004]

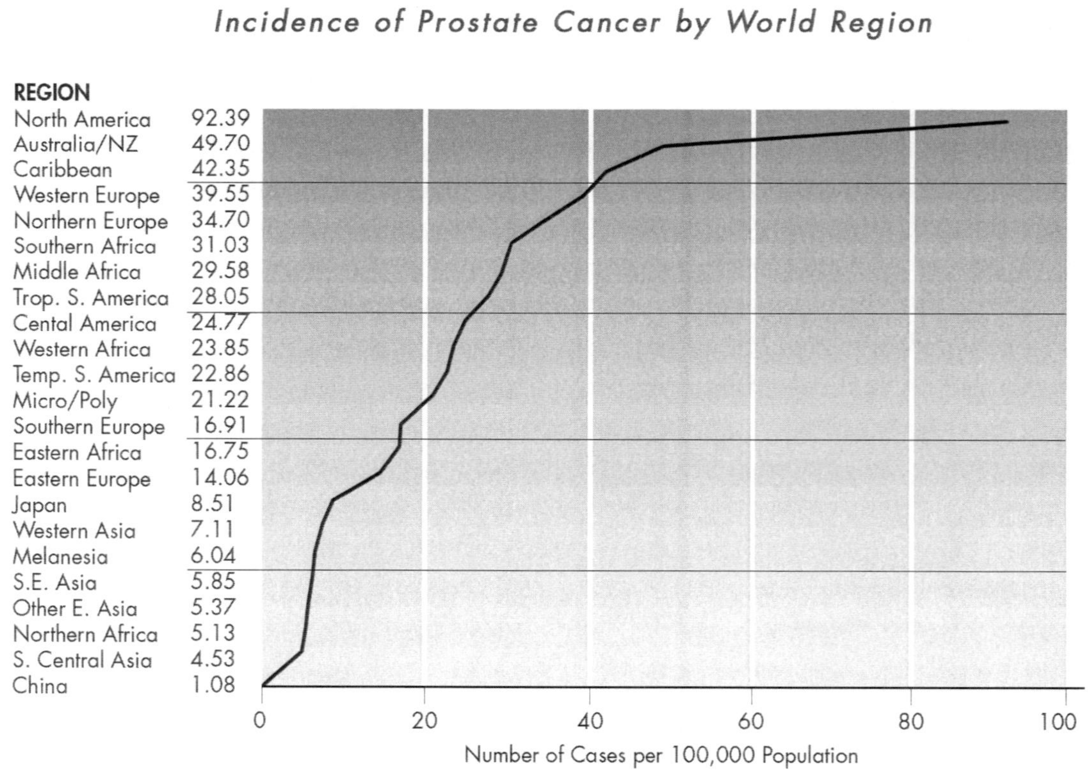

Micro/Poly = Micronesia/Polynesia; NZ = New Zealand; Temp. temperate; Trop. = tropical.

Diet and prostate cancer

It's commonly said that dietary factors are involved in 30-50% of cancers. Certainly the Asian diet which emphasizes soy and fish, comes to mind because prostate cancer rates are so low in Asia.

Soy gains most of the attention in Asian diets, and its weak-plant estrogens (phytoestrogens) are largely given the credit for soy's healthy properties. However, consumption of soy milk, burgers and cereal in Western countries is not likely to produce the same results as in Asian cultures that largely consume fermented sources of soy, such as miso soup and tempeh, in which fermentation concentrates estrogen-like molecules.

Phytoestrogens have a dual nature: being able to lessen the effects of estrogen and testosterone in females and males, and at the same time acting like these hormones when there is a shortage. Overlooked is the fact that soy contains a small amount of omega-3 oil and IP6 that controls iron. These are important cancer fighters as well.

Dieticians often mislead prostate cancer patients into thinking a healthy diet will provide all the beneficial nutrients needed to keep prostate cancer at bay. But there simply is no way to obtain enough vitamin D, vitamin C, vitamin E, folic acid, zinc, or omega-3 oils from the diet to counter prostate cancer growth or prevent the disease altogether.

Men who are most concerned about their diet are those whose cancer has begun to spread and cause symptoms. At this advanced stage, therapeutic levels of nutrients are needed, not just a few more Brussels' sprouts.

A major factor in all cancer is iron. Males have twice the stored iron as females at age 40, and experience twice the rate of cancer. There is no test that tells how much iron is loose (unbound) or how much iron is actually stored in the liver. A great deal of iron is stored in the liver and also carried in red blood cells. If released from transport proteins, free unbound iron is the primary growth factor for tumors. Chelators like IP6 from rice bran, and to a lesser extent green tea, milk thistle, grape seed extract, and other bioflavonoids, help to control loose iron.

Dietary factors are thought to play a role in prostate cancer. Japan has a low rate of prostate cancer, but when Japanese men move to North America their risk for prostate cancer rises by 4 to 9 fold! [British Journal Cancer 63: 963, 1991]

However, the consensus that saturated fat contributes to prostate cancer incidence and mortality simply doesn't hold up in all human populations. Saud Arabian men have very low rates of prostate cancer yet consume high-fat diets. Among 2,270 Saudi men screened, the incidence of prostate cancer was only 3.1/100,000 person-years. A nutritional survey revealed that recent fat consumption was greater than 120 grams per person daily, of which about 40% was from meat and dairy products. Saturated fat comprised about 50% of the total fat intake. There was no difference in the amount of fat in the diet of men with or without prostate cancer. [Journal Urology 164: 1570-72, 2000]

What this confounding information means is that there is more than one way to prevent prostate cancer and that there must be some reversing factors involved in some populations.

Many years ago Dr. John Murray, a cardiologist, went to visit Bedouins in North Africa who ate high-fat diets but had low rates of cardiovascular disease. He brought them iron pills to determine the impact of iron on arterial disease and noticed cholesterol plaques rapidly formed among the men taking iron pills and eating high-fat diets. [Iron Time Bomb, 1999] Maybe something similar to this is happening in Saudi Arabia.

The sale of alcohol is forbidden in Saudi Arabia. Alcohol increases the absorption of iron from foods and iron storage in the liver. [Seminars Liver Disease 24:317-25, 2004]

There is a relationship between iron overload disease (hemochromatosis) and prostate cancer. [Anticancer Research 22:3797-9, 2002]

The mention of a connection between iron and prostate cancer may prompt patients to have blood tests performed.

However, men may be misled by blood tests that measure for bound iron (ferritin levels). The ferritin score is often normal among men with prostate cancer. [J National Medical Assoc. 96:641-9, 2004] The only meaningful iron score would be to know how much iron is being released (free iron) in the prostate gland.

Saudi Arabia is a sunny, desert country located at about 24 degrees North Latitude, so its citizens are likely exposed to more sun. However, Arabic men in Saudi Arabia are often vitamin D deficient due to lack of sun exposure. Their turbans and draping garb are such effective sun blockers that they don't produce enough natural vitamin D from sun exposure. [Tropical Geographical Medicine 36:181-7, 1984]

While there is much quibbling over which specific items in the diet are the most beneficial at preventing prostate cancer, the best overall advice is to eat more plant foods and fewer animal products. [Journal National Cancer Institute 92:61-8, 2000]

Smoking and heavy alcohol use, with the possible exception of moderate red wine drinking, should be abandoned if one treasures a few extra years of life. Remember, most men will live 14 years after their prostate cancer diagnosis and a smaller number will experience the more advanced form of the disease. A change in the diet could keep prostate cancer at bay so it is not life threatening. Most men don't need to be cured of prostate cancer, nor does every tumor cell have to be killed, if they want to leave a fairly long and symptom-free life. The goal should be to keep the prostate cancer cells contained in the prostate gland.

Yet another confounding fact is that prostate cancer patients have lower cholesterol levels than their healthy peers. [Lancet 2:1178-80, Nov. 18, 1989]. Men who participated in the National Health and Nutrition Survey I in the early 1970s, and underwent extended followup through 1987, found males with the lowest cholesterol had a slightly higher risk for prostate cancer. [Cancer Epidemiology Biomarkers Prevention 4:807-11, 1995] Cholesterol accumulates in cancer cells, which may explain why there is less cholesterol in circulation. [Cancer Research 62: 2227-31, 2002] Very low circulating cholesterol (below 160 total cholesterol) increases the risk for cancer. Cholesterol is the carrier to transport fat-soluble antioxidant nutrients, such as vitamin E and lycopene, to cancerous tissues. Low cholesterol levels result in decreased antioxidant defense. [Free Radical Research 25:239-45, 1996]

Dietary Supplements and Prostate Cancer

Whether a man has the slow-growing type of prostate cancer and elects to practice "*watchful waiting*" or undergoes treatment and then is concerned about recurrence, there is an urgent need for prevention. Physicians and researchers are saying that prostate cancer is probably the most promising field for prevention. However, men are often left to fend for themselves when it comes to putting prostate cancer prevention regimens into practice. Dietary supplements are the most frequently used preventive aids, though low-fat diets, smoking cessation and other measures are often relied upon. One study showed that 73% of prostate cancer patients used dietary supplements. The most commonly used were multivitamins, vitamin E, vitamin C and calcium. [Urology 66: 161-66, 2005] Men commonly take saw palmetto berry for prostatitis, but not for prostate cancer.

Cancer doctors are talking about the use of vitamin E, selenium, lycopene, saw palmetto, resveratrol, fish oil and vitamin D, to prevent prostate cancer. [Aging Male 7: 155-69] However, one study found that when prostate cancer patients were given a combination supplement regimen of vitamin E, vitamin C, selenium, and coenzyme Q10, it "*did not affect the serum level of PSA or hormone levels*" in patients who had not received hormone therapy. [European Urology 47: 433-39, 2005] But this is an inappropriate conclusion because these nutrients are designed to prevent, not necessarily treat, prostate cancer, and although they have no reported effects on hormone levels, they still may be beneficial.

Antioxidants may work in a manner that does not affect hormone levels. For example, in a lab dish, it has been found that vitamin C and E combined suppress the formation of survivin, a protein that permits the survival of tumor cells. [Prostate 59: 319-27, 2004]

An interesting study was conducted among 5,141 men who took a low-dose dietary supplement regimen that included 120 mg vitamin C, 30 mg vitamin E, 6 mg beta carotene, 100 mcg selenium and 20 mg zinc daily for 8 years. There were no significant side effects from the supplements reported and no one withdrew from the study due to side effects. In men with a normal PSA, there was nearly a 50% relative reduction in the risk for prostate cancer (estimated by PSA testing) over the eight-year period. (Again, PSA testing is deemed unreliable, but it continues to be used.) For men who had elevated PSA counts and took supplements, there was an increased incidence of prostate cancer of borderline statistical significance. The supplement regimen had no effect upon PSA levels. [International Journal Cancer 116: 182-86, 2005] A conclusion that could be drawn from this study is that low-dose, antioxidant supplements appear to prevent prostate cancer among healthy men, but the dosage is insufficient to prevent development of cancer in men who already exhibited an indicator (elevated PSA) of prostate cancer.

One study found that commonly used dietary supplements vary considerably in actual dosage versus labeled dose, and that some supplements contain virtually no active ingredients. This problem may stall scientific confirmation of the use of supplements for prostate cancer. [Journal Urology 168: 150-54, 2002]

In an animal study, a former associate of Dr. Linus Pauling, Matthias Rath, showed that supplementation with collagen-forming nutrients (lysine, praline, vitamin C) along with arginine (an amino acid) and green tea extract, inhibited the growth of implanted prostate tumors. [In Vivo 19: 179-83, 2005]

1 Citrus pectin and prostate cancer

Modified citrus pectin deserves further investigation into its potential role in inhibiting the growth and spread of prostate cancer. Citrus pectin, added to the diet of small animals, inhibits spread of prostate cancer to other organs, such as the lungs. An animal study found lung metastases was cut in half by adding citrus pectin to the diet. [Journal National Cancer Institute 87: 331-32, 1995] Another animal study showed that modified citrus pectin given to rodents completely blocked the spread of breast cancer cells that had been injected into the animals. [Journal National Cancer Institute 94: 1854-62, 2002] In a lab dish, citrus pectin also inhibits the growth of prostate cancer cells. [Biochemical Molecular Biology International 37: 833-41, 1995] In men with prostate cancer, whose PSA has risen after surgery or radiation, citrus pectin slowed the rate of PSA increase. [Prostate Cancer Prostatic Diseases 6: 301-04, 2003]

2 Vitamin E and prostate cancer

Most people's diets provide about 10-15mg of vitamin E. It is generally believed that doses of vitamin E greater than what the diet provides will help prevent prostate cancer. The first study of the preventive effect for vitamin E was published in 1998 and used 50mg of d-alpha tocopherol, a synthetic form of the vitamin. [Seminar Urology Oncology 17: 85-90, 1999] Smokers appear to derive greater benefit from vitamin E supplement use in preventing prostate cancer. [Cancer Epidemiology Biomarkers Prevention 8: 893-89, 1999]

More recently, various reports have emphasized that both alpha and gamma forms of vitamin E, as well as tocotrienols, the other vitamin E family of molecules, should be utilized and studied in regard to prostate cancer. The gamma form of vitamin E tocopherols is not commonly provided in multivitamins. [Journal National Cancer Institute 92: 2018-23, 2000]

Supplementation with up to 200 IU of d-alpha tocopherol, the natural form of vitamin E from soy, along with ample amounts of gamma tocopherol and mixed tocotrienols appears to be wise for adult males.

3 Vitamin C and prostate cancer

The fact that men, once they develop the hormone-resistant form of advanced prostate cancer, only have a median survival of 9-18 months, and no current treatment produces a significant survival advantage, has led researchers to investigate the use of vitamin C combined with vitamin K. The concept behind this treatment is that these two vitamins are toxic to cancer cells specifically, but not to healthy cells. One study shows the combination of these two vitamins is 5 to 20 times more toxic to cancer cells when administered together. [Cell Biology International 20: 787-97, 1996] Injections of vitamins C and K into tumorous mice increased their remaining life span by 46% compared to untreated animals, and when administered prior to anti-cancer drugs, increased life span by 143%. Some animals who received injected and oral vitamin C showed few, if any, tumors at the completion of one study. [Journal Nutrition 131: 158-60S, 2001] In fact recent studies now show that intravenous vitamin C can achieve concentrations 70 times greater than oral supplementation, and that these concentrations are sufficient to kill cancer cells. This suggests that the day is not far off when all cancer patients will undergo vitamin C treatment. Every prostate cancer patient with advanced metastasizing tumors should undergo intravenous vitamin C treatment.

4 Vitamin D and prostate cancer

A leading researcher said this about prostate cancer:

It is becoming clear that the genesis of prostate cancer involves a variety of pathways. Among the widely accepted risk factors for prostate cancer are age, race, ethnicity, and geographical dependence. This malignancy is uncommon in the Asian population and high in the Scandinavian countries, with the highest incidence and mortality rates occurring in African American males, the latter being two-fold higher than in Caucasian American males. [Biochemical Pharmacology 60: 1051-59, 2000]

It never dawned upon this researcher that all of the above primary factors for prostate cancer revolve around vitamin D.

New understandings of the role of vitamin D in regard to prostate cancer, and compelling data that links low vitamin D levels with early and aggressive forms of prostate cancer, should prompt most adult males to begin supplementing their diet with vitamin D pills.

Review the compelling data below.

- Vitamin D is produced in the skin from sunlight exposure. It is known that cancer develops, on average, about 4 years earlier among those living in less sunny areas. [Lancet 358: 641-42, 2001]

Success story:

Owen Fonorow of The Vitamin C Foundation reports that a man who undergone surgical removal of his prostate gland in 1991, and took medication for 14 years with a PSA of less than 1.0, discovered during a checkup that his PSA was 10 and a mass was discovered. The man elected to undergo intravenous vitamin C therapy along with vitamin K, as he had heard of this regimen advocated by Dr. Steve Hickey of Great Britain. Over a 2-week period he underwent 5 intravenous drip treatments which provided vitamin C, vitamin K and lipoic acid. A subsequent MRI imaging test revealed the mass had disappeared and his PSA had dropped to 8.

Vitamin C Foundation, July 15, 2006

Incidence of Prostate Cancer by Races and Ethnic Groups

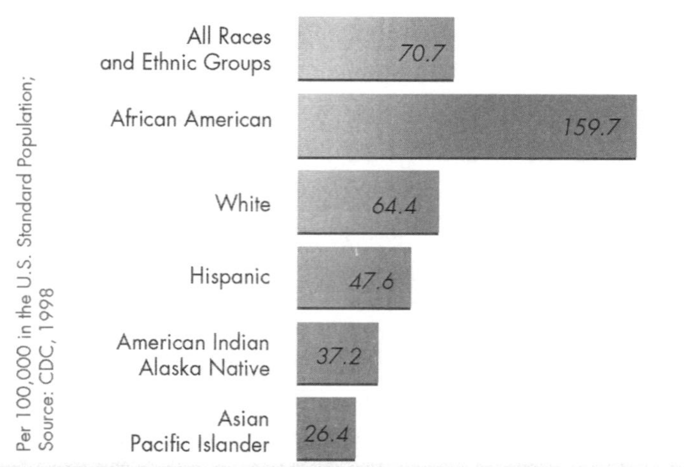

- The prostate cancer belt in the world is in northern climates where vitamin D production from sunlight exposure is low, especially during winter months. [Cancer 70: 2861-69, 1992]

- While it has been said that physical exercise reduces prostate cancer risk, the fact that physical activity often increases hours spent outdoors in the sun may suggest it is vitamin D rather than physical exercise itself that reduces risk for this type of cancer. [Archives Internal Medicine 165: 2538, 2005]

- Blacks experience much higher rates of prostate cancer than do Caucasians and require 5 times as much sunlight exposure to produce the same amount of vitamin D. About 234 Black males per 100,000 develop prostate cancer compared to 144 Caucasian males. Differences in rates of prostate cancer between Blacks and Caucasians are not explained by dietary differences. [Journal National Cancer Institute 92: 2009-17, 2000]

- In a pilot study, of 15 men with prostate cancer who were given 2,000 IU of vitamin D daily, nine experienced a decline in their PSA numbers which remained low for 21 months after completion of the study and cessation of supplementation. Furthermore, PSA doubling time increased from 14 to 25 months. [Nutrition Cancer 51: 32-36, 2005]

- Vitamin D deficiency develops in a significant percent of patients with advanced hormone-resistive prostate cancer. Vitamin D supplementation may improve quality of life and reduce pain in advanced prostate cancer patients. [Journal Urology 163: 187-90, 2000]

- When high-dose vitamin D is used simultaneously with an anti-cancer drug (doxetaxel), men's lives are extended by an additional 8 months. [13th annual meeting of the European Cancer Conference, Nov. 2005]

- It has been hypothesized that high dairy and meat consumption increases the risk for prostate cancer by lowering vitamin D levels. [Cancer Causes Control 9: 567-82, 1998]

- 1,000 IU vitamin D is suggested to reduce prostate cancer risk by 30%. [American Journal of Public Health, February 2006]

Men need to get ahead of the slow-progressing science here. Aggressive forms of prostate cancer appear to be linked with low vitamin D levels. The textbooks on vitamin D are being re-written. Most information is outdated, and most physicians, dieticians and pharmacists are ill informed and likely to warn patients away from so-called high dose vitamin D. This is unnecessary since toxicity of vitamin D doesn't begin till 40,000 IU of vitamin D is consumed daily for many months (the equivalent of about 100 cups of milk). [American Journal Clinical Nutrition 69: 842-56, 1999]

The average diet provides only about 250 IU of vitamin D. Adult males with prostatic enlargement or prostate cancer should supplement with 1,000-4,000 IU of vitamin D daily, and possibly more once cancer has begun to spread.

5 Folic acid and prostate cancer

Folic acid, a B family vitamin, is obtained from green leafy vegetables. A survey has found that the higher the dietary intake of folic acid, the lower the risk for prostate cancer. [Cancer Epidemiology Biomarkers Prevention 14: 944-48, 2005] Another recent study confirms that low folic acid blood levels are associated with increased risk for prostate cancer. Men with the lowest blood levels of folic acid were 4.79 times more likely to develop prostate cancer than were men with higher blood levels. [Annals Epidemiology Dec. 9, 2005]

However, another study measured blood plasma levels of folic acid in relation to prostate cancer risk and came to an opposite conclusion. Higher folic acid and vitamin B12 levels were associated with an increased risk for prostate cancer. [International Journal of Cancer 113: 819-24, 2005] This latter study is a bit puzzling, since no one would suggest that men should avoid a diet rich in plant foods.

6 Zinc and prostate cancer

Many males take zinc supplements to prevent prostate cancer. However, there are three seemingly confusing bits of information in regard to zinc and prostate cancer.

Indeed, prostate cancer patients exhibit lower blood serum levels of zinc. [Asian Journal Andrology 7: 323-28, 2005] However, prostate cancer cells have higher levels of zinc. [Journal Medicinal Chemistry 48: 630-34, 2005]

Men who supplement their diet with 100 mgs or more of zinc increase their risk for prostate cancer by two-fold. [Journal National Cancer Institute 95: 1004-07, 2003]

Actually, prostate cancer cells lose their ability to accumulate zinc. Zinc supplementation may be advantageous, up to a point. Only about 10 mg of zinc is provided in the daily diet and only about 1 mg is actually absorbed.

An investigation into why high-dose zinc supplements may increase the risk for prostate cancer is believed to be due to heavy-metal contaminants in zinc pills. [Cancer Causes Controls 16: 901-15, 2005] Studies show zinc pills may contain relatively high amounts of cadmium, a heavy metal. [International Journal Food Science Nutrition 52: 379-82, 2001] Cadmium accumulates in the human body with advancing age and can produce adverse effects on prostate health. [Cancer Research 61: 455-58, 2001] Zinc gluconate generally contains lower amounts of cadmium than do other forms. [Journal National Cancer Institute 95: 1556, 2003]

7 Selenium

What would happen if there was compelling scientific evidence that an agent could prevent prostate cancer? Would it be met with open arms?

What meticulous scientists want to see is evidence from a *"longitudinal randomized clinical intervention trial."* That means a long-term study where people are randomly assigned to take an alleged anti-cancer agent or an inactive placebo tablet.

Observational studies, that is studies of human populations and what they eat, how much sun they are exposed to, etc, don't always equate with a practice that can be used to prevent cancer because there are so many other variable factors (composition of the diet, intensity of sun exposure, etc.). That's why controlled interventional clinical trials are considered the *"gold standard"* of studies.

So a few years ago, Larry Clark, Ph.D., M.P.H, a cancer researcher at Cornell University and later at the University of Arizona, began such a study. The intent was to measure if the addition of a trace mineral, selenium, would in any way prevent skin cancer. A total of 1,312 patients (mean age, 63 years; range, 18-80 years) with a history of basal cell or squamous cell cancer of the skin randomly received a 200 mcg selenium supplement from 1983 through 1991. The study failed to show that selenium protected against skin cancer. But surprisingly, because Dr. Clark and colleagues monitored for the development of other cancers, it was discovered that selenium supplementation was effective in reducing the risk for a wide variety of non-skin cancers, including prostate cancer. [Journal American Medical Assn 276:1957-63, 1996]

There were 35 cases of prostate cancer in the placebo group and 13 in the selenium-treated group, a two-thirds decline in risk for prostate cancer!

Ironically, a few years after conducting this study, Clark succumbed to prostate cancer at the age of 51.

To this day, Dr. Clark's work is almost forgotten, ignored and diminished by the medical community. Dr. Clark gave the medical community what it demanded and yet his study has been virtually thrown under the bus.

The Center for Science in the Public Interest, in their Nutrition Action Letter, documented the disbelief by the medical community. [Nutrition Action Letter Jan-Feb 1997]

> *"From what we could see, there wasn't anything wrong with the study,"* says Walter Willett, who chairs the nutrition department at the Harvard School of Public Health.
>
> Willett is troubled by how quickly cancer rates dropped in the selenium-takers. *"It's not*

> *impossible, but it's pretty unusual to see cancer rates go down right away."*
>
> Other researchers admit: *"It's unlikely that anything other than selenium explains the differences in their risk."*
>
> *"But it's almost too good to be true,"* adds Dr. Willett. *"If the effect is this large, it would be more important than anything else we know about in cancer prevention."*

The biases and prejudices of the scientific community were further revealed in response to Dr. Clark's study. Researchers were quick to warn of the potential toxic side effects of selenium rather than its proven benefit. This, in spite of the fact the 200-mcg dose used in the study is the *"Estimated Safe and Adequate Daily Intake"* set by the National Academy of Sciences for everyone.

One reviewer said: *"At levels of about 1,000 mcg – or 1 mg – a day people start to lose their hair, they lose their fingernails, and they get gastrointestinal problems. People who ignore those signs can get a lethal overdose. Everybody's scared about the results of this study because you could kill yourself with selenium."* [Nutrition Action Newsletter, Jan-Feb, 1997, Center for Science in the Public Interest]

Of course, none of this is true. There has never been a death from taking selenium supplements. In one clinical trial men awaiting prostate cancer treatment were given up to 3,200 mcgs of supplemental selenium per day and *"no obvious selenium-related serious toxicities"* were observed. [Journal Trace Elements Medicine Biology 18:69-74, 2004] Even occupational selenium poisoning is rare. [Clinical Toxicology 17: 171-230, 1980]

The toxicity of most forms of selenium is low. Also there is a failure to differentiate between elemental selenium, found in soil (sometimes called inorganic), and organically-bound selenium (attached to various amino acids) in plant foods. Forms, such as selenate and selenite, often used in dietary supplements, are not the forms provided in foods. The preferred form in supplements is organically bound to proteins (amino acids), such as selenium attached to methionine (selenomethionine) or to an array of amino acids (SelenoExcel™).

Researchers appear to be intentionally mischaracterizing selenium in order to frighten needy patients away from a proven cancer cure. One has to ask why? Is it because modern medicine can't take its own medicine – a proven preventive agent against prostate cancer in a double-blind, placebo controlled, longitudinal interventional study?

Do oncologists or urologists recommend selenium supplementation to their at-risk patients? Rarely. Patients generally hear about selenium through their own investigation. Then, fearful of potential overdose, they timidly consume 200 mcg of selenium as if somehow they might overdose.

Selenium and DNA damage

A compelling series of studies have been conducted by David J. Waters, DVM, PhD, of the Gerald P. Murphy Cancer Foundation and Purdue University. His first report involving selenium indicates cancer risk in men is more profoundly influenced by selenium than in women. [Mutation Research 55: 91-107, 2004] Subsequently Dr. Waters conducted studies in aged dogs and has shown that DNA damage in the prostate tissues of these dogs is greater when given a standard diet versus a selenium-supplemented diet. Old dogs given a SelenoExcell™ selenium supplement, equivalent to a 200 mcg human dose, had 40% less DNA damage in prostate tissues than unsupplemented animals. [Carcinogenesis 26: 1256-62, 2005; Journal National Cancer Institute 95: 237-41, 2003]

Both Dr. Larry Clark's study and Dr. Waters' study utilized SelenoExcell™, and the researchers said it is the preferred selenium supplement for men.

8 Calcium and prostate cancer

Cancer investigators report that among the many foods that are consumed, milk carries the highest risk for prostate cancer, and tomatoes the lowest. [Alternative Medicine Review 4: 162-69, 1999]

Calcium in foods and supplements is widely promoted for bone health and is generally believed to be healthy. But a series of studies says otherwise in regard to prostate cancer.

In 1998, researchers reported that high calcium intake is related to advanced prostate cancer, nearly tripling the risk. [Cancer Research 58: 442-47, 1998]

In 2001, it was found that men who consume 2.5 servings a day or more of dairy products, in particular skim milk that is richer in calcium than whole milk, are about a third more likely to develop prostate cancer. [American Journal Clinical Nutrition 74: 549-54, 2001]

In 2002, researchers found that men who consume high amounts of dairy calcium have higher rates of prostate cancer. [Urology 60: 1118-23, 2002]

Another study in 2003, found very high intake of calcium, more than 2,000 mg per day, is associated with an increased risk for prostate cancer. [Cancer Epidemiology Biomarkers Prevention 12: 597-603, 2003] For comparison, U.S. men consume about 800 mg of calcium per day, while Japanese men consume about 400 mg per day.

How could calcium, the major mineral component of bone, affect rates of prostate cancer? Researchers believe it is because high calcium intake suppresses the formation of vitamin D. A healthy way to reduce calcium is to eat fructose-containing foods to reduce phosphate levels and stimulate vitamin D production. According to this hypothesis, fruit consumption lowers and milk consumption raises the risk for prostate cancer. [Cancer Research 58: 442-27, 1998]

Men with the highest intake of magnesium appear to have an opposite effect, reducing their risk for prostate cancer. [Journal Toxicology Environmental Health 60: 17-26, 2000]

9 Boron and prostate cancer

Boron is an overlooked mineral that is often used as a dietary supplement to promote bone hardness. Supplemental boron has also been reported to allay symptoms of arthritis. More recently, an animal study reveals that supplemental boron inhibits growth factors and prostate specific antigen (PSA) by 86-88% and reduces the size of tumors in animals by 25-38%. This may be a promising treatment for males with prostate cancer. [Toxicology Pathology 32: 73-78, 2004]

Dietary supplementation may help to reduce the risk for prostate cancer. The consumption of boric acid, the primary form of boron in blood serum, has been proposed as a method to lower PSA levels. Mice given boric acid experience an 88% drop in PSA levels and about a 38% decrease in tumor size with low-dose boric acid (about 140 mg equivalent for a 160 pound human). [Toxicology Pathology 32: 73-78, 2004] There is still much to learn about boron and prostate cancer.

10 Rice bran and prostate cancer

Every cell in the body contains a metal-controlling molecule called inositol hexaphosphate, or IP6. This molecule is derived from grains and seeds, primarily from bran in whole grains. IP6 is required for DNA repair and is the strongest antioxidant known.

When IP6 is added to laboratory dishes where prostate cancer cells are growing, tumor cell growth is inhibited. [Carcinogenesis 21: 2225-35, 2000] IP6 also inhibits the formation of new blood vessels that feed tumors. [Anticancer Research 25: 2891-903, 2005]

When a rye bran diet, rich in IP6, is given to mice bred to develop prostate cancer, it increases normal tumor cell death. [Nutrition Cancer 53: 111-16, 2005]

More encouraging, when IP6 is administered to animals with the hormone-resistant form of prostate cancer, tumor growth was suppressed by 66% and inhibited the spread of the tumors. [Clinical Cancer Research 10: 244-50, 2004]

Why human studies with IP6 have not begun is not explained. It is a non-toxic agent that is a normal component of the human diet. It is extracted from rice bran (~70% IP6, 30% mineral calcium), and is potentially one of the most potent weapons against the worst form of prostate cancer. Men should not wait to incorporate IP6 into their diets, since most men already have tumor cells in their prostate gland.

Since all tumor cells require iron for growth, and IP6 is an iron chelating (removal) agent, it should be utilized with more frequency by men attempting to limit prostate cancer growth. [Nutrition Cancer 4: 223-33, 1983] Daily supplementation with 800 mg of IP6 or use of bran in the diet, would appear to be desirable. Therapeutic use, to treat spreading cancer, can be accomplished with high-dose (2,000-4,000 mg) IP6 taken with water on an empty stomach. Since the body withholds iron from tumors to inhibit their growth, in advanced stages of cancer, the patient may be anemic (cold hands and feet, low hemoglobin levels), and the use of IP6 would cause fatigue.

11 Omega oils and prostate cancer

Fats and oils have been studied in relationship to prostate cancer. The general consensus is that saturated fats increase the risk for prostate cancer. One study shows a three-fold increased risk of dying of prostate cancer among men who consume the most saturated fat. [European Urology 35: 388-91, 1999]

However, some studies misdirect – claiming omega-3 oils (alpha linolenic acid) increase the risk for prostate cancer. [Clinical Biochemistry 32, August 1999] This is highly questionable. While there may have been a statistical relationship between men who had low and high intake of linolenic acid-omega-3 oil, the difference in intake of these oils was only 1 mg. The difference between 1 and 2 mg can be described as a 100% increase, but it is still only a one milligram difference, which is meaningless.

Omega-3 oils have been associated with reduced risk for other forms of cancer, so prostate cancer would be the only exception. When the primary study was examined, it was a dietary study, not a study involving supplements, and it made judgments on the role of linolenic acid in foods, which is only provided in small quantities, primarily in beef along with iron and saturated fats. [International Journal Cancer 71: 5435-51, 1997] So men have been errantly steered away from omega-3 oil, which is quite a tragedy considering its striking ability to inhibit prostate cancer.

The vast majority of studies also implicate omega-6 oils (corn, safflower, sunflower oils) as a contributor to prostate cancer. Omega-6 oils accelerate the growth of prostate cancer cells in a lab. [Proceedings Society Experimental Biology Medicine 216: 224-33, 1997] This is in direct contradiction to a 30-year human study which found that men who ate no fish [which is rich in omega-3 oils) more than doubled their risk for prostate cancer. [Lancet 357: 1764-66, 2001]

Both omega-3 and omega-6 oils are essential for life. The ratio of omega-6s and omega-3s is important in prostate cancer prevention. Sadly, omega-3s have almost been eradicated from Western civilization with the grain-feeding of cattle and the frequent avoidance of fish in the diet. So the ratio of omega-6s to omega-3s is far greater than in previous generations. Omega-3 consumption in the Western diet has become so low that researchers can't find it in lab sample tissues. A study of men found higher concentrations of omega-3s in blood serum samples taken from healthy males, with lower concentrations taken from men with prostatitis. The lowest rates were found in men with prostate cancer. [Clinical Biochemistry 32: 405-09, 1999]

Fish oil has about 30% omega-3 oil while flaxseed oil has about 60% omega-3 oil. So flax is the only oil that can correct the imbalance in omega-3 & 6 oils in the Western diet. Furthermore, flax contains lignans, weak plant estrogen-like molecules (about 1/1000th the potency of estrogen), which further inhibits prostate cancer.

However, men hear the "*bad fats, good fats*" story and think that the more olive oil and fish oil they consume, the healthier they will be. Oils should be used in moderation, cooking oils especially. Monosaturated-oils (omega-9s) such as olive oil, have also been found to reduce prostate cancer risk. [Cancer Causes Control 11: 609-15, 2000] But, again, moderation is advised.

When 25 men awaiting surgical removal of their prostate gland were placed on a low-fat, flaxseed supplemented diet, for 34 days, here is what happened:

	Beginning of study	34 days later
Serum cholesterol - total	201	174
Total testosterone	422	360
Gleason values (tumor spread)	7.1	6.4

[Urology 58: 47-52, 2001]

In regard to prostate cancer and omega-3 oils, these are the best things that can be done to prevent or treat the disease, in this order:

1. Flaxseed meal, 1-2 tablespoons per day, or
2. Flaxseed oil, 1 tablespoon per day (high lignan)
3. Fish oil, omega-3, cod liver source, with vitamins A & D

12 Soy and prostate cancer

Over 150 studies have been published involving soy and its effects on prostate cancer. Asians exhibit far lower rates of prostate cancer and consume 20 times more soy molecules (isoflavones) than men living in Western countries (20 mg versus 1 mg per day).

Many soy studies have looked into the effects that soy has on hormone levels, bone health, reproductiveness, blood sugar, relief of hot flashes, etc. But oddly, many of the studies never looked at the relationship to cancer rates. [Journal National Cancer Institute 97: 1494-95, 2005] A review of eight studies shows that soy foods tend to moderately decrease the risk for prostate cancer. [International Journal Cancer 117: 667-69, 2005] Other reviews have indicated that there is insufficient evidence to show that soy reduces the risk for prostate cancer. [Preventive Medicine 41: 1-6, 2005]

A study of Japanese-American men living in Hawaii found there was little difference in prostate cancer rates among the highest versus the lowest consumers of tofu. [Cancer Epidemiology Biomarkers & Prevention 13: 2277-79, 2004] Yet the annual mortality rate from prostate cancer among Japanese American men is 11.7 versus 24.1 per 100,000 U.S. Caucasian males. Obviously, other dietary factors must be involved. A confounding factor here is that Hawaii is closer to the equator and Hawaiian males are likely to have higher vitamin D levels from sun exposure.

An interesting study was recently conducted among Japanese men, 25 who lived in Japan and 25 U.S.-born Japanese men who lived in California, all of whom were undergoing prostate cancer surgery.

It makes more sense that the Asian diet in its totality, along with other environmental factors such as vitamin D, plays a strong role in prostate cancer prevention. For example, soy and green tea work synergistically to inhibit prostate cancer. [Journal Nutrition 133: 516-21, 2003]

When researchers at the Fred Hutchinson Cancer Research Center in Seattle, Washington gave men a soy beverage containing 83 mg per day of soy isoflavones, no effect was found upon the rate of PSA over a 12-month period. [Cancer Epidemiology Biomarkers Prevention 13: 644-48, 2004]

However, a comparable study in which 52 men were given 60 mg of soy isoflavones over a 12-week period of time,

	Men in Japan	Japanese men in U.S.
Diet	Low fat, high soy	High fat, low soy
Prostate Specific Antigen(PSA)	7.1	8.6
Prostate gland volume cm3	35	38
Gleason score	5.6	6.6
Body fat	19%	24%
Serum triglycerides mg/dL	106	245
Estrogen levels ng/ml	27	31

Source: Urology 64: 765-71, 2004

found that only one experienced more than a 50% reduction in PSA level. [Urology 63: 259-63, 2004] This type of study may indicate PSA is a poor measure of the value of soy rather than the conclusion of researchers that soy appears to be ineffective. Another study also found that soy supplementation did not result in a significant decline in PSA levels and raised levels of insulin-growth factor 1 (IGF-1), which accelerates tumor growth. [Clinical Cancer Research 9: 3282-87, 2003]

In a group of men with a Gleason score of 6 or below, supplementation with a 60 mg soy isoflavone supplement resulted in 61% of men experiencing a reduction or no change in serum-free testosterone versus 33% of the men receiving a placebo. PSA was unchanged or reduced in 69% of men taking the soy supplement versus 55% of the men taking placebo. This study seems to indicate a small beneficial effect for soy isoflavone supplements. [Prostate 59: 141-47, 2004]

13 Soy fractions (genistein) and prostate cancer

Men, in their own study of soy and prostate cancer, may run across studies that show fractions of soy, such as genistein, equol and daidzein, may be potentially troublesome. For example, genistein has been shown to cause genetic damage to human cells in a lab dish, but not in humans. [American Journal Clinical Nutrition 77: 875-82, 2003]

To the contrary, genistein may be very beneficial for prostate cancer patients. An intriguing investigation has begun into the combined role of vitamin D and soy molecules like genistein. Genistein minimizes the breakdown (catabolism) of vitamin D, thus enhancing anti-cancer effects of this vitamin. [Journal Nutrition 134: 1207-12S, 2004] Genistein and vitamin D work synergistically to inhibit prostate cancer cell growth. [Molecular Cell Endocrinology 241:49-61, 2005]

Genistein also helps to reverse the estrogen-receptor resistance (hypermethylation) that occurs over time as men undergo hormone therapy. [Clinical Cancer Research 11: 7033-41, 2005]

Genistein also inhibits an inflammatory protein called P38 that facilitates the invasion of prostate cancer cells through collagen into the blood circulation and other organs. [Cancer Research 65: 3470-78, 2005]

As advantageous as genistein appears to be, fermented soy foods remain superior because they, not only contain concentrated forms of the soy fractions like genistein, but also small amounts of omega-3 oils, and IP6 iron chelator. [Journal Nutrition 125: 733-43S, 1995]

All soy foods and supplements are not the same. [Journal Nutrition 134:1229S-1233S, 2004] There are also many false claims in circulation that soy inhibits thyroid function, something that has been disproven. [Journal Medicinal Food 6:309-16, 2003]

14 Green tea and prostate cancer

Green tea is another component of the Asian diet believed to lower the risk for prostate cancer. Since green tea contains estrogen-like molecules and has iron-controlling factors, it is believed to be one of the reasons for the low rates of prostate cancer in Asia.

However, when a green tea manufacturer applied to the Food & Drug Administration to make a claim that their product reduces the risk of certain types of cancer, the FDA had to turn down the application because of limited human data. The majority of studies involving green tea and cancer have been derived from lab dish or animal studies. In China, one study showed that the more green tea that is consumed, the greater the reduction in risk for prostate cancer. [International Journal Cancer 108: 130-35, 2004]

In a small controlled study, 19 patients with hormone-resistant prostate cancer given green tea extract experienced minimal benefit. Some patients experienced side effects from the caffeine in green tea. [Urological Oncology 23: 108-13, 2005]

15 Saw palmetto berry and prostate cancer

Saw palmetto berry is one of the most frequently used dietary supplements for prostate enlargement.

Only recently have researchers begun to study its effects on prostate cancer. In a lab dish, saw palmetto berry inhibited prostate cancer cell growth. [Cell Biology International 25: 1117-24, 2001] However, saw palmetto berry does not appear to lower PSA levels. [International Journal of Cancer 114: 190-94, 2005]

In a promising study, it was found that astaxanthin, a red carotenoid pigment found in crabs, crawfish and shrimp, and which makes Flamingos pink, is a potent 5alpha reductase enzyme inhibitor similar to saw palmetto berry and inhibits the grown of prostate cancer cells. [Journal Herb Pharmacotherapy 5: 17-26, 2005]

16 Quercetin and prostate cancer

Quercetin is commonly found in red onions and red apple skin. It is a powerful antioxidant in foods and is available as a dietary supplement. It is an estrogen-like molecule that has strong anti-viral, and antihistamine action.

In laboratory dish studies, quercetin was found to inhibit prostate cancer growth. [Nutrition Cancer 38: 116-22, 2000]

When quercetin is combined with the drug finasteride (Propecia), it reduces prostate gland weight in animals. [Journal Endocrinology 181: 493-507, 2004]

Quercetin inhibits genes involved in the growth of prostate cancer cells. [Clinical Diagnostic Lab Immunology 11: 63-69, 2004]

An intriguing approach to inhibit prostate tumor cell growth has been proposed using quercetin combined with the application of heat (hyperthermia). Prostate cancer cells are relatively sensitive to heat stress. [International Journal Urology 8: 623-30, 2001]

The hypothesis is that since cancer cells produce large amounts of lactic acid that is spilled outside of the cell, and since an acid pH enhances the effects of heat, and quercetin inhibits the transport of lactic acid, that it may be an ideal agent to combine with heat treatment. Seventeen years later researchers at Harvard Medical School report that quercetin, when combined with heat treatment, *"drastically inhibited tumor growth in prostate cancer cells."* [International Journal Hyperthermia 17: 347-56, 2001] A concern has been raised that heat may trigger the spread of prostate tumor cells, but experiments disprove this notion. [International Journal Hyperthermia 18: 285-91, 2002]

Researchers propose using moderate heat (40 degrees Centigrade, 104 degrees Fahrenheit) for hyperthermia to treat cancer. [International Journal Hyperthermia 21: 637-47, 2005] One has to wonder about the use of sauna heat, or hot water baths plus oral quercetin to treat prostate cancer at home.

Unfortunately, like many dietary supplements, there is misinformation about quercitin's safety and absorption. Some early erroneous reports claimed quercetin was genotoxic (harmful to genes). Furthermore, claims that quercetin is not absorbed appear to be intentionally misleading. Quercetin metabolites are produced in the gut and it is these molecules that are absorbed. [Annals Nutrition Metabolism 49: 178-82, 2005; Free Radical Research 39: 1139-46, 2005] The International Agency for Research on Cancer has approved quercetin for cancer treatment. [International Journal Molecular Medicine 16: 275-78, 2005]

17 Lycopene and prostate cancer

Lycopene is covered at length in the chapter on herbal remedies for cancer in this book. Readers should refer to that chapter for information about lycopene. Suffice to say, lycopene is one of the most promising dietary and supplemental anti-prostate cancer agents, though shortcomings in the way supplements are made have led to disappointments.

Pomegranate

The consumption of 8 ounces of pomegranate juice daily after prostate surgery or radiation treatment has been shown to prolong the time it takes for PSA number to double (such as from 1 to 2, or from 2 to 4), from a mean of 15 months to 54 months (4.5 years). [Clinical Cancer Research 12: 4018-26, 2006]

18 Resveratrol and prostate cancer

Resveratrol, widely known as a red wine molecule, but also found in mulberries, peanuts and in other botanical sources, is by far the most promising molecule to prevent or treat prostate cancer.

Not only is resveratrol a mild estrogen-like molecule that inhibits hormonal aspects of prostate tumor growth, but as a small molecule it can enter the cell nucleus and "*silence*" genes responsible for tumor growth. There is not one biochemical process involved in the initiation, growth or spread of prostate cancer that resveratrol does not impede. [Cancer Research 59: 5892-95, 1999]

19 Slow aging and block prostate cancer

Slow aging and block prostate cancer – that's what researchers at the Kimmel Cancer Center at Thomas Jefferson University in Philadelphia. Researchers there report that a gene that controls the rate of aging, Sirtuin 1, also influences prostate cancer. Activating the gene "*can almost completely block*" the growth of prostate cancer cells, says Richard Pestell MD, PhD. [Mol. Cell Biol 26: 8122-8135, 2006] Resveratrol is a molecule that activates the Sirtuin 1 gene.

Resveratrol, and genistein, which is a similarly structured molecule from soy, repress the androgen receptor in cells. This is a docking port on the surface of cells that facilitates the entry of hormones for cell growth. Here is what researchers at the MD Anderson Cancer Center in Houston have to say:

"We hypothesize that resveratrol may be especially suitable as a lead agent for prostate cancer prevention given its ability to: 1) inhibit each stage of multistage carcinogenesis, 2) scavenge incipient populations of androgen-dependent prostate cancer cells through androgen receptor antagonism, and 3) scavenge incipient populations of androgen-independent prostate cancer cells by short-circuiting the epidermal growth factor receptor in the cancer cells." [Journal Nutrition 133: 2440-43S, 2003]

"Lab dish and animal studies indicate resveratrol and genistein are promising chemo-preventive agents. Given the clear evidence that androgen receptor pathways are involved in the development and progression of prostate cancer, these data showed that the ability to modulate androgen receptor function would contribute the observed preventive activity of resveratrol and genistein." [Prostate 59: 214-25, 2004]

Resveratrol is superior to genistein and most preferred.

20 Combined herbal ingredients and prostate cancer.

An array of herbal molecules, found in cruciferous vegetables (indole 3-carbinol), turmeric (curcumin), ginseng, pollen, and pygeum, have been shown to have anti-prostate cancer properties. It is likely a combination dietary supplement will be developed to optimally reduce the risk for prostate cancer. European researchers recently provided a dietary supplement containing soy isoflavones, lycopene, milk thistle and other antioxidants to males who had undergone surgery or radiation therapy and found it slowed the progression of the disease. [European Urology 48: 922-30, 2005]

Conclusions and action plan

The major risk factors for prostate cancer have been described in various publications, geographical (northern climates), obesity, skin color (black), calcium (high intake), all which involve the lack of vitamin D. Nary a physician suggests that men, beginning early in life, supplement their diet with ample amounts of vitamin D, despite the obvious evidence of its connection with prostate cancer. Outdated and misleading information about alleged toxicity and hyper-calcemia needs to be dispelled.

Selenium is a proven preventive agent and should be supplemented thoughout adulthood. The particular brand of selenium used in the remarkable cancer study [Journal American Medical Association 276: 1957-63, 1996] was SelenoExcell™, which men should seek out and utilize.

Resveratrol (~25-50 mg trans resveratrol per day, preserved in a sealed capsule) is probably the most significant anti-cancer agent. Its potential preventive and therapeutic value is considered remarkable. Falsehoods regarding resveratrol's lack of bioavailability must be dismissed.

Supplemental vitamin E, 50-200 IU of d-alpha tocopherol (the natural form from soy) along with ample amounts of gamma tocopherol and mixed tocotrienols are suggested.

Supplemental vitamin C is critical to maintain the collagen barrier that keeps tumor cells in place. Quercetin plus vitamin C is a widely available dietary supplement, and repeated use throughout the day (3-5 times) keeps blood levels high. Quercetin + sauna heat therapy may be pursued if the prostate gland is expanding and starting to produce undesirable symptoms.

Omega-3 oils, provided either as pure omega-3 from algae or from flaxseed oil which has the highest natural ratio of omega-3 over omega6 oil (1-2 tablespoons, 3000-6000 mg), will provide omega-3 oils that inhibit prostate cancer cell growth.

Folic acid (vitamin B9) supplements appear to be called for. About 800 mcg per day is a commonly recommended dosage.

Lycopene is a promising anti-cancer agent, both for prevention and treatment. Dietary sources such as tomato paste will have to be relied upon until supplement companies figure out how to preserve the active form of this red pigment molecule (all trans lycopene).

IP6 rice bran extract should be employed in mid-life to reduce iron stores (2,000 mg with water on empty stomach for 30 days) and then periodically in low doses (800-1500 mg) to encourage healthy prostate tissues.

Modified citrus pectin appears to be helpful at the first sign of symptoms. Its use appears to be safe.

Avoidance of tobacco, iron supplements, foods with refined sugar, and excessive alcohol (with the exception of moderate amounts of red wine), should not require any discussion.

Prostatitis and urinary frequency are common. The use of saw palmetto berry extract (160 mg twice a day, 75-85% extract), pollen (cernitin), pygeum, and nettles may be helpful.

Zinc (gluconate, up to 30 mg), boron (3-12 mg), and soy, may be helpful additions to a dietary supplement regimen.

<u>Melatonin and sleep:</u> In advanced stages of prostate cancer, melatonin (~10-20 mg), a pineal gland hormone produced during sleep, should be employed at bedtime as a dietary supplement, as it has been shown to triple the remaining lifespan of cancer patients. Melatonin is secreted at night during sleep, while opening the eyes in the morning to visible light will cause melatonin secretion to cease. Theoretically, blockage of light to the back of the eyes caused by cloudy cataracts would increase melatonin levels and should reduce the risk for prostate cancer. That is exactly what population studies confirm – males with visual impairment have lower rates of prostate cancer. [Cancer Causes Controls 17: 573-76, 2006] Prostate cancer rates are very low inside the Arctic Circle where prolonged periods of winter darkness elevate melatonin levels. [Medical Hypotheses 53: 1-2, 1999] This underscores the importance of sleep for prostate cancer patients. Supplemental melatonin is reported to have stabilized prostate cancer in one patient. [Journal Pineal Research 35: 177-82, 2003] Reduction of

melatonin is most pronounced in patients with advanced prostate cancer. [Advances Experimental Biology Medicine 467: 247-64, 1999]

Once there is an indication that prostate cancer is spreading, it becomes paramount that metastasis (spread) of cancer cells be stopped. Thick blood, which facilitates metastasis, should be thinned naturally with vitamin E, omega-3 oils, resveratrol, magnesium, and garlic. Blood capillaries must be strengthened with high-dose vitamin C (2,000 mg, 3-5 times a day), and the use of enzymes, such as nattokinase, to break up blood clots, should be employed.

Intravenous vitamin C treatment with vitamin K is of value given that it has now been revealed that IV vitamin C can achieve blood concentrations that are toxic to cancer cells but harmless to healthy tissues. If men cannot talk their doctors into administering IV vitamin C, other doctors in the community should be sought. See recommendations under the vitamin C section in this book.

Summary: men have four choices:

1. Submit to PSA testing, repeated biopsies, and treatment, following the doctor's lead.
2. Submit to all that modern medicine has to offer along with the preventive/therapeutic regimen outlined above
3. Practice prevention early in life and employ a regimen that has more promise than existing therapies.
4. Become highly educated about the course of prostate cancer and the advantages and pitfalls of the various treatments available including supplements.

Should any of the measures outlined above begin to work, as occurred when the PC-SPES supplement was available, word will likely spread rapidly. [See addendum to this chapter]. Patient-driven medicine is the only way prostate-cancer care will change for the better.

Suggested readouts

The bottom line is that low-risk patients do well no matter which treatment they receive. [Seminars Urology Urological Oncology 18: 214-25, 2000] This makes every form of treatment look good, since most men with prostate cancer have non-invasive tumors.

Since it takes 10 -15 years to determine whether a specific treatment is effective, prostate care today has become a giant experiment upon men with prostate cancer. In many instances, treatment that has been disproven is utilized over what is unproven.

<u>Special addendum:</u> An herbal remedy prolongs life for end-stage prostate cancer patients, but health authorities remove it from the market.

The most significant event in the recent history of prostate cancer care has been the introduction, for a time, of a combination herbal remedy that caught cancer doctors by surprise. For a time, this herbal dietary supplement captured the attention of prostate cancer patients and doctors alike. The herbal combo began extending the lives of otherwise helpless prostate cancer patients facing the advanced life-threatening form of their disease. How the cancer industry responded to this development, and the events surrounding the decision to withdraw this herbal formula from the marketplace, despite its unprecedented effectiveness, reveals much about the dismal state of cancer care in America. One cannot read this account without becoming outraged at the final outcome.

An herbal remedy captivates

About 230,000 men learn of their prostate cancer each year in the United States. Among them is a group of about 40,000 men who face the aggressive form of the disease where the cancer has begun to spread to bone and other organs, threatening their lives.

In the mid-1990s, men with this progressive form of prostate cancer found a multi-herbal remedy to be quite effective in subduing the pain, inflammation and spread of prostate cancer. Sadly, the product was suddenly recalled for mislabeling problems, never to be re-introduced.

The whole unfortunate tale is indicative of what is going on in the cancer care industry today and worthy of re-analysis here. This is a story that every male with prostate cancer needs to read and understand. If you are familiar with this story, new data places a different ending to the story.

The saga begins

Long about 1996, a research scientist by the name of Sophie Chen, PhD, a graduate of Columbia University and post-doctoral fellow at Cornell University, who spent 14 years working for pharmaceutical companies (Merck Sharp & Dohme and Bayer USA), developed a multi-herbal product for males with advanced prostate cancer. It was named PC-SPES. The PC stood for prostate cancer, and "*spes*" is the Latin word for hope.

In 1988, Dr. Chen began her research into the role that natural herbs can play in healing and curing cancer, and obtained a dozen U.S. patents. In 1993, Dr. Chen co-founded the International Medical Research Corporation with "*Allan*" Xuhui Wang, MD, and John Chen (her brother), which did business under the name BotanicLab, the maker of PC-SPES.

Chen and Wang, who is also an herbalist, collaborated to modify an existing herbal formula used in China to treat urologic problems, which became the PC-SPES product. The first patient to use it was Chen's brother-in-law, a physician in Taiwan with advanced prostate cancer who was alive and well 10 years later. [Journal National Cancer Institute 94: 1266-68, 2002]

Over time Dr. Chen had secured research grants from the National Cancer Institute and prostate cancer survivor/investor Michael Milken's CaP CURE organization. Eventually an $8 million study grant from the National Institutes of Health was obtained, but the study never took place due to product quality problems. [PSA Rising, Dec. 19, 2003]

Many urologists and oncologists believed the herbal mix was prolonging their patients' lives. Over 100 studies were published, validating its beneficial effects.

PC-SPES got spiked

A report published in the Journal of the National Cancer Institute in 2002 said: "*PC-SPES was poised to become the first cancer treatment to emerge from the realm of alternative medicine, pass rigorous clinical testing, and add a powerful natural weapon to the oncologist's arsenal.*"

As positive as the reports were for PC-SPES, there were nagging reports of side effects. Doctors began to suspect that the side effects caused by PC-SPES were similar to those produced by diethylstilbestrol (DES), a testosterone inhibitor that has been used to treat prostate cancer for decades.

The spiking of PC-SPES with drug molecules wasn't apparent at first. A study published in 1998 found estrogen-like effects, but couldn't identify the molecule involved. The study didn't find any DES in PC-SPES at that time. [New England Journal Medicine 339: 785-91, Sept. 17, 1998] Chen denied the presence of any ingredients not on the label. Three times the California FDA tested PC-SPES and found no contamination, but utilized testing methods that could not detect minute amounts.

Then, as reports of side effects began to accumulate in 2001, some men suddenly noticed PC-SPES stopped working for them. PSA levels started to rise. Also a few cases of hemorrhaging were reported. Trace amounts of a blood thinner (warfarin) had been added to subsequent batches of PC-SPES in an apparent effort to counter the reported blood clots.

It was later found that some batches of PC-SPES given to men in a comparative study contained from 0.01 to 3.1 % of DES. [Canadian Journal Urology 9: 1684-88, 2002] However, this wasn't considered to be sufficient to cause the side effects being reported, in particular, the reports of blood clots.

The eight herbs in PC-SPES	The Added Drug Ingredients
Licorice Reishi mushroom Chrysanthemum Dyers woad Rabdosia Saw palmetto Baikal skullcap Ginseng	Diethylstibestrol (DES) (testosterone interruptor) Indomethacin (anti-inflammatory) Warfarin (blood thinner)

Patients take charge

Cancer patients were communicating with each other via the internet, learning of the rising PSA levels among PC-SPES users.

Susan Domizi, wife of a Connecticut man taking PC-SPES, sent samples of the product to a laboratory and found it contained small amounts of DES. A second study also found DES. [International Journal Oncology 20: 583-88, 2002] By October of 2001, doctors had published a case of severe hemorrhaging associated with PC-SPES that was aired in the New England Journal of Medicine. [New England Journal Medicine 345: 1213-14, 2001]

Then the State of California FDA returned to BotanicLab to conduct more sensitive tests and surprisingly found DES in the same lots they had tested before, as well as the presence of another drug, warfarin (coumadin), a blood thinner. Retrospective tests now showed the product had been spiked with DES since 1996, and when side effects were reported, subsequent batches of PC-SPES displayed lower doses of DES, and then eventually the blood thinner, as if someone was attempting to limit the side effects. Sophie Chen responded by saying that none of the drugs was present in therapeutic doses and that *"lots without DES worked equally well."*

Breakthrough in process

Whatever ingredients were in PC-SPES, they were producing a breakthrough in prostate cancer treatment all the while the product was being slammed for adulteration.

Michael Cook is an example. A 49-year-old who was diagnosed with prostate cancer at age 44, his tumors had spread to his ribs and pelvis. PC-SPES dropped his PSA from 80 to 0.2. *"I've been on PC-SPES for three years now, and I seem to be in complete remission,"* said the patient. [LA Times Oct. 21, 2000]

A group of men with prostate cancer, called UsToo, reported that their members maintained a low PSA concentration with PC-SPES in two successive surveys (88% and 93%). *"Even though there were some side effects, a great majority of men are realizing good PSA control while taking the capsules, with some users now into their fourth year of PC-SPES use,"* said their report. [Molecular Urology 4: 289-91, 2000]

Moreover, a study conducted by Eric Small, MD and William Oh, MD at the University of California at San Francisco, showed that PC-SPES produced a 47% response rate compared to just 28% for diethylstiberstrol alone, and reduced PSA levels by more than 80% in all of their prostate cancer patients, with one patient experiencing complete disappearance of a bladder mass. In Dr. Small and Oh's study involving 37 patients, three experienced blood clots. Side effects, however, were deemed to be *"acceptable."* [Journal Clinical Oncology 18: 3595-3603, 2000; Urology 57: 122-26, 2001]

A report in the Journal of Urology stated the side effect profile of PC-SPES was *"comparable to estrogen treatment,"* with 42% experiencing nipple tenderness, 8% breast enlargement and 7% hot flashes. [Journal Urology 164: 1229-34, 2000]

Dr. Charles Myers of the American Institute for Diseases of the Prostate, in Charlottesville, Virginia, reported the case of a man whose PSA was nearly 3,000, an alarming level, but after taking PC-SPES it fell rapidly to below 1. Dr. Myers called PC-SPES "*probably the most active agent*" for treating prostate cancer in patients who no longer get results from conventional, hormone-blocking drugs. [Wall Street Journal May 26, 2002]

Still a mystery

Since no proof existed to show that BotanicLab had purchased any of these drug molecules, the blame for adulteration was cast upon sources of the herbs in China. Chen stated that she was not personally involved in mixing the company's products, saying she was in New York conducting research most of the time, not in their Brea, California headquarters.

But Chen also contradicted herself when she said she had tested the herbal products herself and they were pure prior to encapsulation. She claimed the alcohol extraction of the herbs was conducted by companies in China, not in the United States. One of those suppliers in China also processed pharmaceuticals and could have been to blame. But they would have had to know what was going on in the United States to alter the product as they did.

Strangely, the *Washington Post* report stated that BotanicLab had conducted tests on its own in 2002 and determined bulk herbs coming into the country were free of pharmaceuticals, while packaged products leaving the Brea facility were adulterated. The Washington Post report said:"*Tests conducted after BotanicLab shut down showed changes in pharmaceutical ingredients over time that the people suing BotanicLab regard as evidence of a conscious effort to manage troublesome side effects.*"

Blood clots are common in cancer patients, so this problem may not be attributed to PC-SPES. [Medicine 56:1-37, 1977] But the addition of the anti-clotting drug warfarin, and the cases of hemorrhage, were certainly a concern.

The penalties

It took five years to shut down BotanicLab. PC-SPES was voluntarily recalled in 2002. Under agreements, John Chen, sister Sophie Chen, and Allan Xuhui Wang admitted to single misdemeanors involving the marketing of misbranded and adulterated food. Their defunct company pleaded no contest to the felony count of producing a product that presents a danger to the public. The corporation agreed to pay $350,000, the Chen's agreed to pay $46,500 each, and Wang agreed to pay $56,500. Cancer survivors who had used PC SPES filed a class-action lawsuit against BotanicLab.

Patients sue

Later patients even sued the Milken Prostate Cancer Foundation. "*Giving people prescription drugs without their knowledge is insane. It is total fraud,*" a woman was quoted as saying in a Washington Post article. [Washington Post, Sept. 5, 2004]

What caused the beneficial effects?

In 2000, researchers at Columbia University reported that "*estrogen-like activity is not its [PC-SPES'] sole mechanism of action.*" [Journal Urology 164:1229-34, 2000]

Investigators at New York Medical College obtained samples of single herb extracts used in the PC-SPES product and determined that no single herb could exert the reductions in PSA and testosterone reported in other studies. The authors of that study said "*PC-SPES should be considered a single function unit since the combination of its biological properties appears to be more effective than its individual components.*" [International Journal Oncology 20: 533-88, 2002]

Dr. Oh stated there was something else in PC-SPES causing the beneficial results. Another study found that men taking nine PC-SPES capsules a day could get as much as 0.5

mg of DES per day, compared to the 3.0 mg used in the comparative study of the two drugs. So it appeared a small amount of DES was being added intentionally without being identified on the product label.

The cost

About 10,000 men in advanced stages of prostate cancer were estimated to be taking 6-9 capsules of PC-SPES per day at a retail cost ranging from $400 to $500 per month. An attorney estimated BotanicLab may have taken in $50 million before it was shut down.

For comparison, Canadian pharmacies are selling Lupron kits for $325-486. Lupron stops production of testosterone by the testes. Side effects with Lupron include breast enlargement and decreased libido, similar to those produced by PC-SPES. Over $876 million of Lupron was sold in 2004. Yet one physician, Glenn Bubley, MD, of Harvard Medical School was quoted as saying the manufacturer of PC-SPES *"is making more money than God."* [WebMD August 31, 2000] Another comparison: a 10 milliliter dose of Honvol (diethylstilbestrol) costs about $90 from a Canadian pharmacy.

DES, Lupron and side effects

Jacqueline Strax, whose husband succumbed to prostate cancer in 2001, recalls how PC-SPES had initially helped her husband. In 1984, her 44-year old husband was told he had a month to live. He subsequently underwent orchiectomy (surgical removal of the testes) and the subsequent hormonal suppression was effective for many years. When the tumor later returned with a vengeance, he found PC-SPES on the internet, paid $10,000 to Sophie Chen after speaking with her on the telephone, and soon felt better. In 1998, he died of a hemorrhage. [PSA Rising, December 2003]

Was PC-SPES a killer or a life saver?

On September 5, 2004, the *Washington Post* ran a report with the headline: *"Herbal remedies turn deadly for patients."* How so? PC-SPES by all reports was prolonging life and saving men who were clinging to life. The *Washington Post* asserted the regulatory system of herbal product companies was flawed, claiming BotanicLab spiked its product with rat poison, the blood thinner that was eventually found in PC-SPES. The article called PC-SPES a *"disaster,"* and reported 35 cases where users or their families claimed harm. These were men who were dying without hope.

The *Washington Post* article said: *"Published studies showed that some of the men who took it (PC-SPES) got enlarged breasts, their nipples grew tender, their penises shrank, and they developed other problems."* Yes, but they failed to report that these are the same side effects as are often experienced by those taking Lupron or other estrogen therapy drugs.

The Washington Post article said DES was tested for prostate cancer long ago, *"but produced so many side effects, including blood clots, that most doctors concluded it would do more harm than good. It was largely discarded, but interest in it has cropped up from time to time because of scattered research showing it might work at low doses."* Over 30 years ago doctors used 5 mg of DES. Today, lower doses are used.

PC-SPES was not intended to be used on men with early-stage prostate cancer. When hormone therapy doesn't work any longer and the cancer continues to grow, the herbal treatment (PC-SPES) is *"effective in those patients"* said Dr. Aaron E. Katz. [LA Times, Oct. 21, 2000]

DES reconsidered

One outcome of the PC-SPES debacle is that physicians began to realize they had overlooked DES in favor of more expensive, but maybe not superior drugs, like Lupron. Thirty years ago 5 milligrams of DES was the standard dose prescribed, with considerable side effects noted. Today it is known that low-dose DES, 1 mg, is effective and produces fewer side effects.

Patrick Walsh, MD says that DES may be a more cost-effective agent in reducing PSA than other more aggressive regimens. [Journal Urology 173: 1966-68, 2005].

A more recent study showed that DES plus aspirin can produce a significant drop in PSA (23% experienced a more than 50% drop; 65% experienced a decline overall). [Urology International 75: 217-21, 2005]

DES, which reduces testosterone levels in the body by inhibiting luteinizing hormone in the pituitary gland, is still manufactured under the trade names Honvol (Baxter) and Stibestrol (Wellspring). It is also known to cause blood clots, reduced libido, and cause breast tenderness and related feminization in males. It is listed for primary use for the intensive and selective palliative therapy of inoperable prostate cancer. DES slows growth of tumor cells and may cause shrinkage of prostate tumors.

- Back in the 1970s when diethylstilbestrol was being utilized with regularity among advanced-stage prostate cancer patients, here is what some of the reports said:

- *"High-dose diethylstilbestrol can used effectively in cases of prostate cancer when standard doses of estrogen have failed."* [Canadian Medical Association Journal 109: 697-99, 1973]
- *"Of the conventional chemotherapy drugs available, only diethylstilbestrol has been safe, effective (at least in relieving bone pain) and available for repeat courses of treatment."* [Urology Clinics North America 2: 185-96, 1975]
- In 15 patients with advanced prostate cancer receiving diethylstilbestrol, their disease remained stable without evidence of progression for an average of 25.6 weeks. *"There were no complete remissions, and no significant side effects were seen."* [Urology 8: 231-33, 1976]

- *"Diethylstilbestrol has shown effective symptomatic relief in patients with metastatic carcinoma of the prostate. Diethylstilbestrol is recommended in the treatment of advanced carcinoma of the prostate with soft tissue metastasis. It is safe and effective, and the tumor responses outweigh the side effects of the drug."* [Urology 7: 598-601, 1976]

So why was PC-SPES being recalled for containing trivial doses of DES? Moreover, why weren't oncologists and urologists prescribing low-dose DES more often for their patients with advanced prostate cancer?

Call for greater regulation

Regulatory agencies have been waiting for the opportunity to change public opinion regarding dietary supplements and turn all dietary supplements into high-priced drugs. The calls for greater regulation of the dietary supplement industry during the PC-SPES ordeal were deafening. In one report on PC-SPES, The *Wall Street Journal* said that *"makers of supplements don't have to adhere to as rigorous manufacturing requirements or submit results of clinical trials to the FDA."* [WSJ May 26, 2002] However, current laws require dietary supplements to be pure and contain only the ingredients listed on the label, which PC-SPES failed to do. No new regulations were needed to force BotanicLab to recall PC-SPES.

The journal *CA, A Cancer Journal For Clinicians*, said *"natural products such as PC-SPES should be subject to the same standards and approaches as substances that are classified as pharmaceuticals. And for any anticancer modality to be considered for clinical use, it must compare favorably against a proven therapy in comparable groups of patients."* [CA Cancer Journal Clinicians 51: 199-204, 2001] That's exactly what PC-SPES demonstrated, in both animal and human studies.

The *CA Journal* report tabulated the results from four published studies and found 83% of males who took PC-SPES with advanced prostate cancer experienced greater than a 50% drop in their PSA levels. The report acknowledged that advanced prostate cancer patients have *"limited options,"* noted that most investigators characterized the side effects associated with PC-SPES *"as mild,"* and added that men on estrogen hormone therapy experienced similar side effects. The blood clotting problems that arose later were the most serious side effects. Dr. Aaron E. Katz, of Columbia University College of Physicians & Surgeons said 2 to 4 % of PC-SPES users run the risk of blood clots, which is a potentially fatal problem. [Los Angeles Times, Oct. 21, 2000]

The report in CA Journal stated, that since the herbal formula had not undergone as rigorous studies as would pharmaceuticals, *"physicians and patients must take the place of the agency that provides oversight for the regulated pharmaceuticals."*

The FDA can ban supplements, but do to so it has to show *"a significant or unreasonable risk of illness or injury."* For men who were at the end of their rope, PC-SPES posed no greater risk than many approved drugs, namely DES or Lupron. The herbal products industry was brought to task for poor quality products and cries for greater regulation are still being heard.

Conclusions

What can be concluded from the saga of PC-SPES? Who was responsible for spiking the dietary supplement? Why did drug molecules need to be added when PC-SPES appeared to work well without them? Why was the product recalled, actually taken out of the hands of patients with advanced prostate cancer, when it was by all reports working better than existing drugs and had similar side effect profiles?

The National Center for Complementary and Alternative Medicine, which was ready to sponsor a multi-million dollar study of PC-SPES before the accusations were raised, says it is *"interested in resuming studies of PC-SPES with patients and funding new laboratory studies, but can only do so when a fully characterized and standardized, contaminant-free product using the original formulation becomes available."* [NCCAM Publication No. D149, September 2002]

When BotanicLab conducted studies of its products, certainly any variances in the potency of active ingredients should have been apparent. Herbs can vary in the content of active ingredients, but herbal extracts can be standardized for a certain minimum percentage of the primary active ingredient. Why didn't BotanicLab do this?

The chances of a product like PC-SPES returning to the marketplace with patients and attorneys ready to sue, and regulatory agencies ready to pounce, is nil.

PC-SPES was being asked to demonstrate absolute safety – no side effects, a standard that drugs with all their testing can't achieve.

For comparison, regulated pharmaceutical drugs cause over 100,000 needless deaths annually from side effects caused by their proper use drugs and Public Citizen warns there are 181 unsafe or ineffective prescription drugs on the market. The Vioxx scandal only served to reveal that the FDA approves relatively unsafe drugs that increase mortality rates. The flawed regulatory model should not be used for dietary supplements.

Was there magic inside?

Scientific investigation of PC-SPES continues to this day, with batches of the product still under scrutiny. Researchers at the Keck Science Center in Clarement, California, tested PC-SPES from batches produced in 1998 and 2001. [Cancer Letters 220: 171-75, 2005]

PC-SPES and DES were tested in lab dishes with lung cancer cells. PC-SPES was effective even in cells that had developed resistance against chemotherapy drugs. PC-SPES both killed cancer cells and interrupted their normal immortal state to cause them to naturally die off (apoptosis), whereas none of the contaminants in PC-SPES (warfarin, DES or indomethacin) induced apoptosis (cell death).

Both batches of PC-SPES, even though they varied in the amount of contaminants, were equally effective against this non-sex hormone type of tumor cell. Even adding more DES, indomethacin and warfarin to the less contaminated PC-SPES samples, did not increase its effectiveness.

Researchers conclude that "*natural components in the herbal extract were responsible for the cancer cell destructiveness of PC-SPES.*" PC-SPES also inhibited detoxifying enzymes (cytochrome p450) that are involved in cancer drug resistance. This may have played a part in its unusual effectiveness against drug-resistant strains of tumor cells. [Cancer Letters 220: 171-75, 2005]

Was there some magic synergism in the array of eight botanical herbs in PC-SPES? By examination of the data, this appears to be so.

Dr. Fulton L. Saier, a physician and prostate cancer patient, said the recall of PC-SPES "*will potentially cause the death of thousands of men.*" [Wall Street Journal, May 26, 2002]

Dr. William Oh said "*the worst part (of the PC-SPES saga) was that PC-SPES was a very effective treatment with minimal toxicity for advanced cancer patients. These men don't have many choices for therapy.*"

Dr. Sophie Chen added: "*I feel the patients who had used PC-SPES are the victims of the whole thing.*"

So, in summary, what we have here is multi-herbal dietary supplement......

...whose individual ingredients are commonly sold without noticeable side effects

...that was "contaminated" with small amounts of FDA-approved drugs (DES, ibuprofen, warfarin)

...whose effectiveness was not attributed to minute quantities of drug molecules

...which worked better than the sum of its parts

...which exceeded the effectiveness of existing drug therapies for men with advanced prostate cancer

...and had similar side effect ratios to hormone treatment (Lupron, DES, estrogen)

...whose manufacturer somehow was implicated in covering up the side effects by spiking the product with drugs

... and whose manufacturer and even agencies that funded research studies, were sued by its users and their families

...because its ingredients were "undeclared" on the label and therefore, "could cause serious health effects if not taken under medical supervision"

...however, in most instances, was being prescribed by doctors

...and was therefore recalled by the FDA

Desperate men, for whom hormone therapy had failed, were then asked to return bottles of PC-SPES, thus condemning themselves to an inevitable fate.

Myrna wants to know

Myrna wants to know what to do for her 80-year old father who has prostate cancer that has metastasized to the liver, bones, rectum and elsewhere. She describes her father as healthy up to a few months ago. He had a bout of shingles a few months back. That was a sign his immune system wasn't up to par. One in four 80-year olds develops shingles, which is an eruption of an on-board herpes virus. But in March her father was up on the roof doing some repairs and felt fine. Then it came time for his annual physical. The doctors wanted to do a prostate biopsy. The results were inconclusive. Two months later another biopsy was performed, it was cancer. But two months earlier he felt fine, now the tumor had grown to impair urination. He had to have a urinary catheter. Chemotherapy was ordered. The side effects soon became apparent. Pain pills were ordered. Lupron, a hormonal drug that might shrink the tumor in the prostate, was prescribed. Myrna wanted to know, is there anything that can be done for my dad?

An array of dietary supplements were recommended, even purchased and given to Myrna for her dad, so she wouldn't be confused as to which supplements to obtain. Myrna waited for days, she wasn't sure. Family members were saying only to do what the doctor said. Precious time was passing. Her father's tumor was growing and spreading. Two weeks later she started her dad on the supplements.

It was difficult to explain to Myrna that radiation treatment was not curative, it is palliative care – manage the tumor, keep the patient out of discomfort. The treatment, like all other cancer treatment, never addresses what caused the tumors, or its spread. The metastasis is what threatens life. Nothing was done to stop the spread of the tumor. The initial biopsy is a small surgical procedure. Any biopsy will trigger wound healing and accompanying growth factors. One wonders why biopsies are done on fragile 80-year old men. Most men of this age have precancerous or cancerous cells in their prostate. Why tamper with them and risk igniting the growth and spread of a tumor? The biopsy may have spread the tumor to the rectum and elsewhere. A nephew who is a physician coaxes Myrna's dad to come to his office and reviews his case, and cautions Myrna's dad about the use of herbal supplements. The family doesn't understand. Aren't the doctors trying to cure their dad? No really, they are just attempting to relieve his pain by shrinking the size of the tumor.

"You have already convinced me not to do so with your first email. I instinctively did not want to have the biopsy because it is invasive, no matter what they say. (I refuse to have a colonoscopy for similar reasons). But my wife was bordering on hysterical since my PSA had been fluctuating from 4.6 to 5.3 to 6.2 to 12.6 (probably an aberration) and back to 6.3 over several months. I believe the fluctuations had more to do with sexual activity and diet than cancer. Nevertheless, I succumbed to her emotions. Never again."

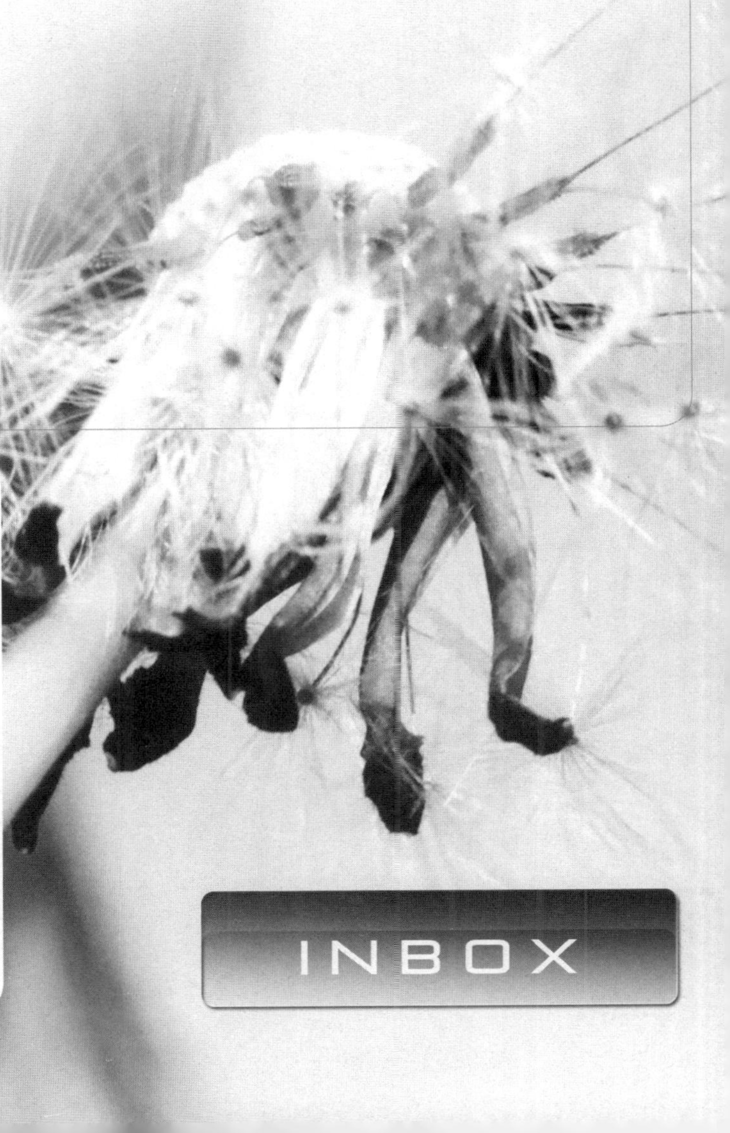

CHAPTER 8

Breast Cancer

p 220 - 292

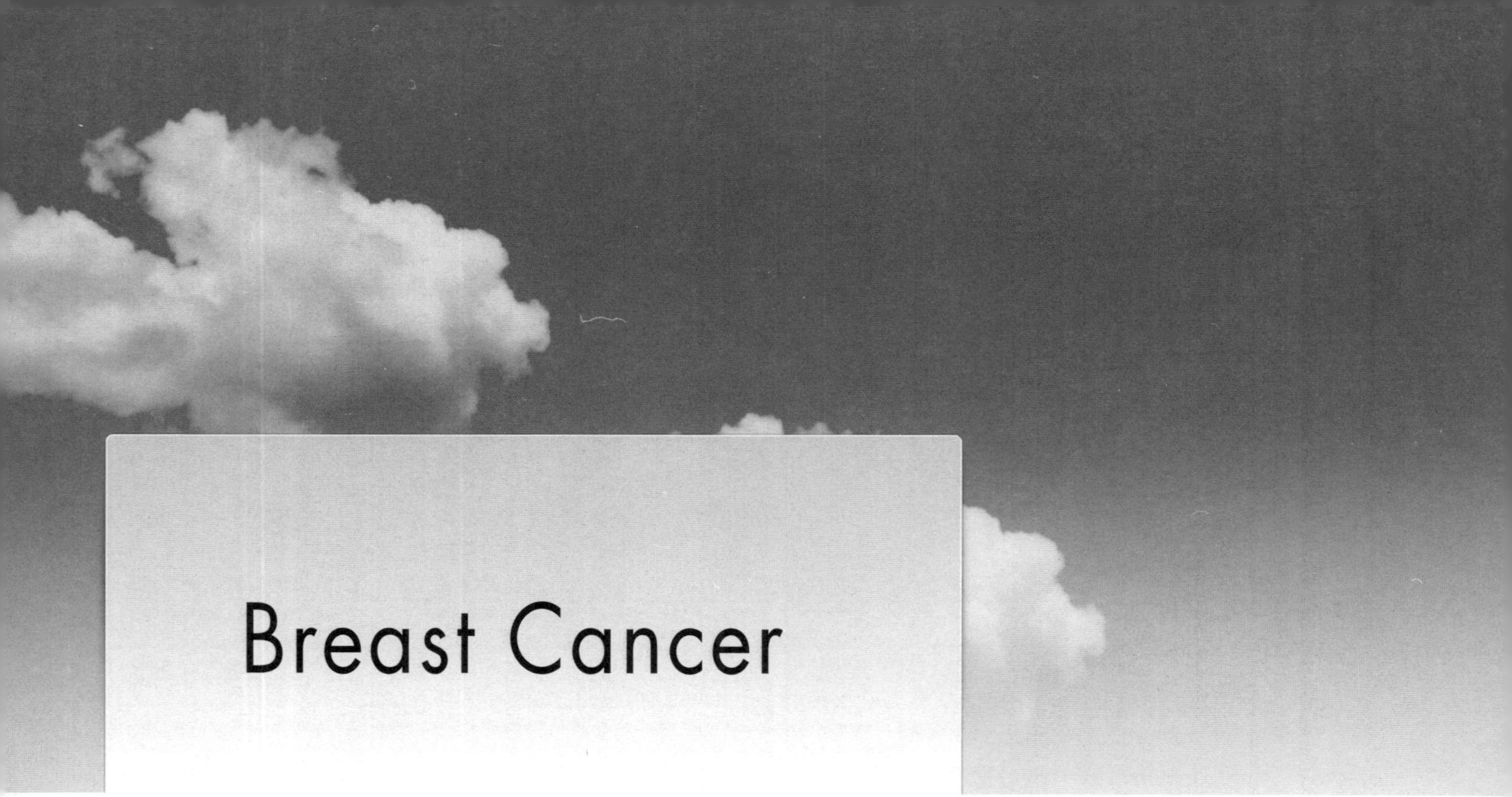

Breast Cancer

THE TRUTH ABOUT BREAST CANCER

The known risk factors for breast cancer account for a small fraction of the population's attributable risk, and new risk factors are required.
Journal Clinical Oncology, April 20, 2006

Introduction

Writing as a journalist, I cannot be so separated from the women who will read this chapter, to not make a plea for them to re-evaluate, if they have the opportunity, their thinking about breast cancer. Research studies show women are more likely to seek solace and emotional support in patient groups, or to lean on the counsel of their doctors, compared to males who are more analytical and may arrive at the doctor's office with a clipboard of notes and questions regarding prostate cancer.

Will information in this chapter on breast cancer change the course of therapy for many women who have the opportunity to read it? I would hope so. The current state of breast cancer care is appalling and shocking. If only women could be told the truth, but the news media are remiss in calling attention to the sorrowful state of breast care provided by the most sophisticated medical centers today. Likewise, alternative medicine is a mixed bag of legitimate cures and fake solutions.

I mulled over how to write this chapter without causing undue alarm among women already dealing with a life-threatening issue centered on an emotionally charged part of their body. Men with prostate cancer don't have to put on their pants and realize their male organ has been permanently removed. It is women who often have to contend with the loss of their breasts and their desirability as females. It's not a situation most men, including this writer, can comprehend emotionally.

There are many well researched but overlooked avenues for women to investigate who have or fear breast cancer. The objective of this chapter is to expose the type of care you may be confronted with once diagnosed with breast cancer, and offer some safe alternatives that provide a better likelihood of survival. This chapter also provides direction for women attempting to prevent the occurrence or reoccurrence of breast cancer.

Some of the issues women with breast cancer must grapple with are:

→ Hormone replacement therapy (HRT), widely prescribed for decades, has fallen into disfavor. Each day, 5,000 women join the ranks of the 40 million American women already in menopause. A smaller percentage of women continue to take HRT, mostly for symptoms of hot flashes and night sweats and *"retaining beauty"* rather than for any health benefits. What now for these women? How will they avoid bone loss, breast cancer, and uterine cancer?

→ With millions of dollars spent on research, there is still no effective preventive measure for breast cancer, only treatment after it has been diagnosed, which consists of estrogen-blocking Tamoxifen after conventional surgical, chemo or radiation therapy. But Tamoxifen itself promotes endometrial cancer and can, with long-term use, promote breast cancer so it cannot be taken for more than five years. For women with a relatively low risk for breast cancer (1.67% over 5 years), Tamoxifen has little effect and the drug actually increases the risk for cancer among women with an intact uterus. [Cancer 107:950-8, 2006] Has the wonder drug Tamoxifen had its day?

→ New aromatase inhibitor drugs, which stop the production of estrogen in fatty tissues, rather than block its entry into cells like Tamoxifen does, are being widely studied because they are said to be more effective at prolonging tumor remissions than Tamoxifen. But in the long run, aromatase inhibitors only delay the inevitable for women with breast cancer. They don't reduce mortality rates and they may accelerate bone loss and mental depression.

→ This pushes American women into the unguided use of phytoestrogens, plant, seeds, beans and herbs that have estrogen-like molecules. But are they any safer or more effective?

→ Why does crushed whole flaxseed exhibit unusual health benefits for the heart, kidneys, bones, prostate and breast tissues? What is it that whole flaxseeds provide that other herbal phytoestrogens do not? By what process does flaxseed produce such incredible health benefits?

Statistical manipulation

There is something odd about the statistics provided about breast cancer. It is widely claimed that the lifetime risk to develop breast cancer is 1 in 8 in the United States. That would amount to 12.5% of women. Most cases of breast cancer occur among women after menopause. There are 40 million women in the U.S. in the postmenopausal age group, but only 2 million are known to be living with breast cancer and another 225,000 or so fresh cases are diagnosed annually. About 40,000 of these women die each year. So, about 5.5 % of postmenopausal American women are suffering with breast cancer at any given time.

Lifetime risk for breast cancer

The American Cancer Society and other women's health groups want to heighten the imagined risk for breast cancer to promote more donations and research grants. So they have unabashedly overstated the lifetime risk for breast cancer, and continue to overstate the risk when it is brought to their attention. Cancer groups claim there is a 1 in 8 lifetime risk of developing breast cancer, but the real risk is more like 1 in 26 for a 40-year old woman.

The lifetime figure of 1 in 8 is a cumulative figure. This figure has been criticized and health authorities concede that this figure is used because it helps to get women to come in for exams on a more regular basis and aids in capturing more funds for research. Over $400 million is spent on breast cancer research annually, or about $200 per active breast cancer patient. How much of those research funds actually go towards true prevention is unknown.

Inventing a pill that would truly prevent breast cancer would stop a whole industry. Too many jobs rely upon the detection of fresh cases of breast cancer to prevent the disease. There are over 14.5 million health care workers in the U.S. representing 10.5% of the workforce. This writer has too often been censored by nurses who guard internet chat rooms for breast cancer patients to *"maintain the status quo"* for the doctors they work for. Getting real answers to women about breast cancer is difficult when health *"authorities"* provide their patients with misinformation.

The real risk factors for breast cancer

What many American women have been taught is that breast cancer may be inevitable, that is, that it's genetically programmed. The fact that women who moved to the United States from countries with low breast cancer rates such as Japan experience the higher risk levels of U.S. women within one generation is unequivocal proof that breast cancer, for the most part, is not genetic. [Network 10: 1-3, 1989] Very little breast cancer is linked to genetic factors. The Council for Responsible Genetics says only 5 to 10 % of breast cancer cases involve inherited mutations. [Breast Cancer Genes, Myths & Facts]

All women have BRCA1 and BRCA2 genes. Mutations in these genes increase the risk for breast cancer. It is misleading to say that there is about an 80% lifetime risk for breast cancer if there are mutations in the BRCA genes. This misstatement is used to sell women on the idea of mastectomy (breast removal). [Journal of the National Cancer Institute, November 7, 93:1585, 2001] Mutations in the BRCA gene do not necessarily result in breast cancer. Colin B. Begg of Memorial Sloan-Kettering Cancer Center in New York said this high risk rate cannot be applied to every woman with mutations of the BRCA genes. The risk is likely much lower than that. [Associated Press, August 20, 2002] But the 80 % lifetime risk figure is frequently quoted, particularly by surgeons.

Here is what one internet resource [www.imaginis.com] advised women about genetic testing and breast cancer:

Regardless of the test results, all women should still take preventive measures to help reduce their risk of breast cancer. These preventive measures include: practicing monthly breast self-examination, having regular clinical breast exams, and having yearly mammograms (at 40 years of age and older). Though testing from BRCA mutations may help identify women who are at a higher risk for breast cancer, 80% of women who develop breast cancer have no known risk factors.

But these measures only detect breast cancer at an earlier stage, they have nothing to do with prevention. Breast care centers are just scouting for more treatment to deliver, not to prevent disease from occurring in the first place.

Age is the master governing factor for risk of breast cancer. The evidence is clear - more tumor cells are found in the breasts of older women than of younger women. Seventy-seven percent of new cases and 84% of breast cancer deaths occur in women over age 50. Over 70% of all breast cancer cases occur among women with no identifiable risk factor. [American Journal Preventive Medicine 20:214-8, 2001]

In developed countries, where women live longer on average, and where there is more doctoring and more sophisticated detection (mammograms), the incidence of breast cancer is greater, about 80 per 100,000, compared to 30 per 100,000 in undeveloped countries. [The Breast Journal 12: S70-80, 2006]

Studies have found that women from China or Japan who move to California, double their risk for breast cancer. [Tidsskr Nor Laegeforen 111: 1745-48, 1991] Women from Poland who migrate to California, increase their rate of breast five-fold! [Tidsskr Nor Laegeforen 111: 1745-48, 1991] What is to blame: the diet or the environment? The answer is neither. The more likely explanation is that all the women in these studies who were found to have breast cancer were harboring the disease for some time but upon moving to the United States they were subjected to exams and screenings that simply detected or even provoked more cases.

- Highest breast cancer risk in the world: San Francisco Bay area, 104 per 100,000
- Lowest breast cancer risk in the world: African women, 5 per 100,000

Source: International Journal Food Sciences Nutrition 46: 373-81, 1995

A report published in the *British Medical Journal* attempted to rank the most important risk factors for breast cancer. Diet, contraceptive use, even alcohol consumption, were not highly ranked risk factors (1.2 to 1.5 times greater risk). The greatest risk factor was advanced age (more than 10 times increased risk) followed by geographical location (5 times greater risk) and exposure to ionizing radiation (3 times greater risk). [British Medical Journal 321: 624-28, 2000]

In this chapter we will examine each of these risk factors and what can be done to overcome them.

Here are factors which are believed to increase the risk for breast cancer

Here are factors which are believed to increase the risk for breast cancer.

- Being overweight (postmenopausal women)
- Alcohol consumption (even moderate consumption is troublesome)
- Red meat consumption
- Lack of whole grains in the diet
- Diets containing corn oil (omega-6 oils) rather than fish oil or flax oil (omega-3 oils)
- Overconsumption of fatty foods
- Smoking tobacco
- Lack of sunshine (vitamin D)
- Environmental carcinogens

Source: J Womens Health 12: 183-92, 2003; Nutrition & Cancer 44: 23-34, 2002; Cancer Causes Control 13: 883-93, 2002

Weight and cancer

Postmenopausal women who carry excess weight (who weigh more than 175 pounds) are at a 2.5 times increase risk of dying from breast cancer compared to thinner women (who weigh less than 133 pounds). [Archives Surgery 139: 954-58, 2004] While there is concern expressed over known carcinogens, such as pesticides, industrial chemicals, etc, excessive weight is a far greater factor in breast cancer incidence and mortality. Women with pear-shaped figures, excessive body hair, or oily skin, are at greater risk for breast cancer. All these factors –weight, body hair and oily skin—are tied in with increased estrogen in breast tissue. [American Journal Clinical Nutrition 45: 283-89, 1987]

However, breast density appears to be more of a factor in determining risk, than is weight. A dense breast has less fat and more glandular and connective tissue. Mammogram films of breasts with higher density are harder to read and interpret than those of less dense breasts. Overweight women tend to have fatty breasts, which decreases density. An overweight woman with dense breasts in connective tissue is nine times more likely to have breast cancer.

One major study of 61,844 women followed for three years, found that the risk of breast cancer associated with extremely dense breasts, compared with entirely fatty breasts, was 4.6 times greater for premenopausal women and 3.9 times greater for postmenopausal women. [Cancer Epidemiology Biomarkers Prevention 13: 715-22, 2004]

A study conducted among postmenopausal women found weight gain (but not necessarily total weight or body mass) is related to breast cancer risk. [Journal Womens Health Gender Based Medicine 8: 1265-72, 1999] However, overall weight has not been found to be a significant factor in breast cancer survival rates (5-year survival only varied by about 5% among leaner versus larger women). [American Journal Epidemiology 163: 101-07, 2006] In younger women, increased body size is commonly associated with a decreased risk for breast cancer. [American Journal Epidemiology 149: 339-46, 1999] This cannot be fully explained as yet by cancer researchers. However, this does say that localized changes within the breast, and less so changes outside the breast, are primarily responsible for breast cancer.

Exercise and breast cancer

Physical exercise can reduce the risk for breast cancer. [Journal National Cancer Institute 97: 1671-79, 2005] After diagnosis of breast cancer, walking 3-5 hours a week reduces death rates by as much as 50%. [Journal American Medical Assn 293: 2479-86, 2005]

Alcohol intake

The preponderance of evidence suggests intake of alcoholic beverages and fatty foods increase the risk for breast cancer. [Annals New York Academy Sciences 963: 247-67, 2002] Women with high estrogen levels were found to consume more alcohol than other women. [Cancer Epidemiology Biomarkers Prevention 7: 189-93, 1998] A total of 53 population studies confirm that the risk for breast cancer increases with the amount of alcohol consumed. However, there is only a 7% increase in risk with each 10 grams of alcohol consumed per day. [Harefuah 145: 39-41, 2006]

According to one large study, consumption of one to two alcoholic drinks per day throughout life was associated with a modest increase in the risk for invasive breast cancer. Risk did not vary with alcohol type (beer, wine, or hard liquor) or by patterns of use, such as recent use, intake prior to age 20 years, or whether use began at an early age.
Alcohol consumption of approximately one drink per day was associated with estrogen receptor positive tumors among lean women, but not among women of larger body size. [Annals Epidemiology 16: 230-40, 2006]

Even less than one drink/day was associated with up to a 30% increase in breast cancer mortality among postmenopausal women compared to non-drinkers. [Cancer Causes Control 12: 895-902, 2001]

In one study conducted in Spain, the consumption of 8 or 20 grams of alcohol per day increase the relative risk for breast cancer by 50% and 70% respectively. [Cancer Causes Control 4: 345-53, 1993]

Environmental carcinogens

The International Agency for Research on Cancer (IARC) in France lists risk factors for breast cancer as: reproductive life, hormonal factors, diet, genetics (BRCA1, BRCA2) and exposure to radiation and selected chemicals. Yet researchers concede that much breast cancer remains unexplained.

The IARC stays *"new etiological links must be sought such as occupational factors and exposure to pesticides and other endocrine disrupters. A recent international summit on breast cancer and the environment outlined the need for more research to be conducted into the effects of exposure in the vicinity of nuclear power plants or chemical landfill sites and, more generally, into contaminants in food, air, water and soil."* [Hormone Research 60 Suppl 3:50, 2003] But none of this makes any sense. As explained earlier in this chapter, the predominant factor in breast cancer is age, not exposure to carcinogens.

In 2002, researchers at the University of North Carolina, School of Public Health, reported that *"there appears to be little or no link between breast cancer and exposure to certain pesticides or air pollutants."* [Cancer Epidemiology Biomarkers Prevention 1: 677-697, 2002]

Industrial xenoestrogens, that is substances that imitate estrogen, comprise 0.0000025% of the daily intake of estrogens in the diet. [Environmental Health Perspectives 103:346-51, 1995] Most of these are weak estrogens that would dull the effect of natural estrogen, thus reducing the risk for hormone-related cancer.

Parabens and breast cancer

There are many estrogen-like molecules in the environment. They are used as preservatives in cosmetics, deodorants and food. Concern has arisen that these estrogen sources may increase the risk for breast cancer. [Journal Applied Toxicology 24: 167-765, 2004] Of course suspicions such as these fuel many research grants for toxicologists, who like to *"blow smoke"* on these issues.

The use of parabens in underarm deodorants has come into question because of proximity to the breast during application and its estrogen-like effects. [Journal Applied Toxicology 24: 5-13, 2004]

Parabens are generally regarded as safe. [Journal Applied Toxicology 23: 285-88, 2003] Animal experiments that have found parabens to be dangerous have employed such unusually high doses of paraben never duplicated in human experience, that one wonders if these experiments have any application to human health. The estrogen-like activity of paraben is many *"orders of magnitude less than estrogen"* and is provided in doses far less than are other estrogen-like molecules in the diet (example: soy). Researchers conclude *"it is biologically implausible that parabens could increase the risk of any estrogen-caused disease."* [Critical Reviews Toxicology 35: 435-58, 2005] Despite this, once women hear of the potential risk of parabens, they may become phobic about their exposure to them while remaining unaware that the production of estrogen itself in the breast during post-menopause poses a far greater risk.

The point here is: women are being distracted by messages that point to estrogen-like molecules in the environment as a primary risk factor for breast cancer, when in fact these molecules are weak estrogens and pale next to the effects of hormone replacement therapy.

Genes and breast cancer

There is the hope that genetic tests will identify those women at highest risk for breast cancer. A woman with a strong family history of breast or ovarian cancer and who carries a mutation of the BRCA1 gene faces roughly an 85% lifetime risk for breast cancer and a 60% risk for ovarian cancer. These are the quoted figures.

The initial assumption was that 1 in 2 high-risk women harbor a BRCA1 mutation, but it has been found that only 7 in 100 do. A report written by Dr. Bernardine Healy, former director of the National Institutes of Health, published in the

New England Journal of Medicine, entitled *"BRCA genes – bookmaking, fortune telling and medical care,"* claims BRCA testing is *"wasteful"* since more than 9 out of 10 times it will be a negative test. [New England Journal Medicine 336:1448-9, 1997]

In addition, the same mutations in the BRCA genes result in different outcomes for women of different ethnic backgrounds. Mutations in BRCA genes, in and of themselves, do not cause cancer. Ashkenazi Jewish women are known to carry mutations in BRCA genes, but mutations for breast cancer are only found in 50% of Jewish women with this gene, not the 85% figure quoted above. Furthermore, dietary or hormonal factors can influence these genes; cancer is not inevitable. Dr. Healy's report says: *"Without facts about these other variables, the fortunetellers are reading a pretty cloudy crystal ball. The problem becomes especially worrisome when statistical prophecies lead to irreversible decisions, like the decision to have both breasts removed based upon genetic testing alone,"* says the report. The five-year survival rates for women who carry a mutation in their BRCA1 gene is essentially identical to the survival rate seen in women who don't carry the gene mutation.

A report written by the Council for Responsible Genetics states: *"Until we have effective prevention strategies, tests for variants of so-called 'cancer genes' benefit mainly the companies that market them, who stand to make huge profits by exploiting women's justifiable fear of cancer."* [Council for Responsible Genetics]

Furthermore, is the test always accurate? The widely used genetic test can miss mutations that provoke breast cancer. The test, which detects mutations in genes called BRCA1 and BRCA2, will fail to detect the mutation in about 12% of women tested. Mutations are not equivalent to breast cancer, but the discovery of these mutations may frighten women into undergoing treatment they don't need. [New York Times, March 22, 2006] Also, only 5-10% of breast cancers in Caucasian women in the U.S. stem from inherited mutations in the BRCA genes. Even in high-risk groups, such as families with four or more cases of breast or ovarian cancer, only 35 mutations could be found in 300 women (11.6%).

A far better indicator of risk of breast cancer is ascertaining women's DNA repair mechanisms. Sub-optimal DNA repair has been found in all women with breast cancer, but only 32% of healthy women. Women at high risk for breast cancer are five times more likely than healthy women to have faulty DNA repair systems. [Journal National Cancer Institute 88: 754-55, 1996] DNA repair is the process of correcting the genetic mistakes that are made each time a cell divides. If the repair process does not go right, it can increase the chances of a person having some forms of cancer.

For unexplained reasons, genetic predisposition for breast cancer has gained more publicity than it deserves. Of the 200,000 American women diagnosed with breast cancer annually, only about 5% or 10,000 women test positive for the BRCA genes. [Canadian Medical Assn Journal 45:104-12, 1999] The treatment and survival is about the same for both women with and without the BRCA mutation unless the genetic mutations are recognized early and preventive measures such as dietary changes are practiced. Instead, the self-serving breast cancer industry has dropped the idea into women's minds they ought to think about total mastectomy. More than half of women who test positive for a genetic predisposition to breast or ovarian cancer opt for total breast removal or surgical removal of their ovaries. [Cancer Genetics Cytogenetics 165:91-7, 2006] Not one medical board declares this practice to be unethical. Out of fear, women elect to undergo surgery, and this does not absolutely remove the risk. Any woman who tests positive on the gene test can elect, on her own, to undergo double mastectomy, and even though she had no disease and may never get the disease, most doctors do not object to performing the operation.

Preventive Mastectomy

The Cochrane Group, which evaluates medical therapies, has determined that most of the women deemed to be high risk by family history, who underwent mastectomy, would not have died from breast cancer, even without prophylactic surgery. [Cochrane Database System Review Oct. 18, 2004] But total breast removal continues to be performed.

Even though there is no measurable improvement in survival, a survey of women who chose preventive mastectomy showed that 86.5% of women said they were satisfied with their decision. [Journal Clinical Oncology 24:1350-6, 2006] One can understand the patient's fear and the desire to remove all the breast tissue in order to reduce mortal risks, but why are doctors allowed to perform these operations with impunity?

Imagine a patient coming to a doctor's office and demanding surgical removal of any expendible organ over a future fear of cancer. Should the doctor comply with the patient's request? The patient would be sent for a psychiatric examination.

Why don't the medical boards prohibit doctors from performing these operations? What about medicine's dictum to *"first do no harm?"* Almost two-thirds of women undergoing bilateral prophylactic mastectomy had at least one complication following surgery. [Journal National Cancer Institute Monograph 35: 61-6, 2005]

MAMMOGRAPHY

Who's telling the truth about mammography?

Millions of women worldwide will undergo mammography to screen for breast cancer annually. Here is what a woman is getting herself into once she submits to the idea of undergoing a mammogram.

Worldwide, an estimated 75 million sets of mammograms are taken each year at 35,000 imaging centers. In the United States, about 37 million mammograms are performed annually, with about 75% of these being screening mammograms for early detection of breast cancer. There are about 200,000 news cases of breast cancer detected annually in the United States.

In a population where the risk of developing breast cancer is 12% and the risk of dying from breast cancer beyond age 50 is 2.5%, screening 250 women may prevent about one death from breast cancer. [British Medical Journal March 3, 2006 online edition] However, another report indicates one tumor is detected for every 1,300 mammograms. [Reuters Health Oct. 16, 2002; Journal National Cancer Institute 94: 1546, 2002] Which source is correct? Is the difference between 1 in 200 and 1 in 1,300 the percentage of needless care being provided?

The American Cancer Society recommends routine screening mammography starting at age 40. As a result, more than 1.2 million women become eligible for mammography screening each year. Imaging centers are only reimbursed about $75 for a screening mammogram and an additional $35 for a diagnostic mammogram. [Radiology 219: 467-73, 2001] The issue of profit is raised because, if clinics cannot make a profit from mammograms, then they must make it off of treatment for disease that is diagnosed.

An assistant professor of surgery at a breast imaging center in New York says:

> *"The reality is that mammography centers simply cannot break even. They must make up for their losses by diagnosing and treating disease. For the time being, breast cancer is not preventable. Mammography is not perfect; in fact, it can miss breast cancer in 17 % of cases."*
>
> *"The cost of malpractice insurance, in addition to poor reimbursement, means that many facilities operate mammography centers at a loss. For some, the resulting business makes up for it. Screening mammography misses about 17% of all breast cancers in women and might mistakenly label an abnormal area as a tumor where none exists. Other studies indicate the error rate could be even higher, closer to 30%. A prominent doctor likens the task of finding breast cancers on a mammogram to 'trying to find a snowstorm in a blizzard'."*
> Source: Medical Imaging Newsletter

One out of three mammograms produce abnormal results that require further testing, but subsequent tests reveal no cancer. About 19% of biopsies are needless and cause 16 million false alarms over 10 years. [New England Journal Medicine, April 16, 1998]

Women should be told about the benefits, limitations, and potential harms associated with regular screening. Mammograms can miss some cancers. However, mammograms, despite their limitations, remain the most effective and valuable tool for decreasing suffering and death from breast cancer.
Source: American Cancer Society

If a group of women begin breast screening at age 40, by age 50 half of them will have at least one false positive test and undergo needless biopsy. [The Ottawa Citizen, Sept. 4, 2002]

Out of 100 positive mammograms, only 20 will actually indicate the presence of cancer. [LA Times Aug. 1, 2002]

The concern is that frightened women, hearing the possibility of breast cancer, and knowing of a family history, will opt for needless breast removal. Out of fear, thousands of women elect to undergo total mastectomy.

Why are so many mammograms misread? One primary reason is that postmenopausal women taking hormone replacement experience a 3.0% incidence of false positive mammograms, which is about 70% higher than women who don't take hormones. [Breast Cancer Research 8:R8, 2006]

The idea that breast screening is effective for women age 50-59 years was shattered when researchers suggested that there are no reliable data to support screening by mammography. When this fact hit the news wires, breast cancer imaging centers and makers of mammography units circled their wagons in defense of their technology. Upon reanalysis, researchers dispelled the idea that mammograms lead to needless care, but still could not produce a meaningful reduction in mortality rates. [Lancet 359: 909-19, 2002] While there has been a reduction in mortality rates for breast cancer in many countries, there is no clear link this is related to screening. A recent report concluded: *"If women choose screening, they should understand their risk of dying may not be reduced."* [Recent Results Cancer Research 163: 115-28, 2003]

By the time a tumor is large enough to be detected on a mammogram it has been growing for 8 to 10 years. [Los Angeles Times, Nov. 13, 2000]

One doctor adamantly maintains mammography offers *"a clear mortality benefit."* What he means to say is that if 1,224 women were screened, one death might be prevented after 14 years. [New York Times Sept. 3, 2002]

By the year 2000, not only have mammograms not been shown in controlled studies to lower mortality rates, but a large Canadian study showed that the death rate from breast cancer was about the same for women who underwent mammograms versus those who underwent physical breast exams by their doctor. [J National Cancer Institute 92: 1490-9 2000]

Data obtained from the National Center for Health Statistics show that 28,230 women died of breast cancer in 1970 (mortality rate 27 per 100,000 women) and 41,737 died of breast cancer in 1997 (mortality rate 30.6 per 100,000 women). Over 30 years, 450 million mammograms in the United States did not reduce breast cancer deaths but pointlessly increased treatments. [Annals Internal Medicine 138: 768-69, 2003]

In terms of dollars, the Swedish mammographic screening program analyzed 605,260 women who had an aggregate of 1,932,353 mammograms between 1987 and 1996. There were 6,713 deaths due to breast cancer, which amounted to 55 deaths (0.8%) fewer than expected without screening. The cost per life saved was $2.36 million. Over 35,000 mammograms had to be performed to save one life. [Lakartidningen 96: 904-908, 1999]

It has been concluded that every-other year breast screening is not frequent enough to detect primary breast cancer for women under 70 years of age. [International Journal Epidemiology 29: 803-06, 2000] For women over age 70, there is only a small gain in life expectancy from annual or bi-annual mammographic screening. While an abnormality will be found in about 8% of women aged 70 years and older who undergo mammography, 85% to 92% of these women do not have cancer, yet all women who have an abnormal mammogram incur additional diagnostic procedures, plus the worry and anxiety of wondering if they have cancer. For every 10,000 women over age 70 screened for breast cancer, 1.4 deaths would be prevented, adding only 7.2 hours of life on average. [Journal American Medical Assn 282: 2156-63, 1999]

John K. Whiteford, MD and John Ryan Whiteford, MD, of Verona, Pennsylvania, share some biting facts about breast cancer.

Based upon autopsy studies, there are projected to be an estimated 16 American million women with undiagnosed breast cancer in the population (2003). While the death toll annually from breast cancer is 40,000, this represents less than 3/10ths of one percent of all women with undiagnosed breast cancer. Among women with detected breast cancer, 88% have not spread and 12% are invasive tumors. There is no justification for treating every breast cancer detected and no sense in detection until the few breast cancers that threaten women can be distinguished from the rest. Most women with breast cancer survive without treatment. [Annals Internal Medicine 138:768-9, 2003]

In the past there were concerns about radiation risks; today if there is a risk, it is very small. Strict guidelines are in place to ensure that mammography equipment is safe and uses the lowest dose of radiation possible. Many people are concerned about the exposure to x-rays, but the level of radiation in modern mammography does not significantly increase the risk for breast cancer.

Source: American Cancer Society

The Cochrane Collaboration, an international not-for-profit and independent organization, dedicated to making up-to-date, accurate information about the effects of healthcare readily available worldwide, issues systematic reviews of healthcare interventions. The Cochrane Collaboration reviewed published studies involving mammography and determined that the absolute risk reduction for breast cancer achieved by mammography is 0.05% (1/20th of 1%), and that 0.05% of women undergoing mammography are mistakenly diagnosed. Over a 10-year period, for every 2000 women undergoing mammography only 1 woman would have her life prolonged while 10 healthy women would be errantly diagnosed as having breast cancer and undergo unnecessary treatment. Cochrane reviewers state that *"it is not clear whether screening does more good than harm."* [Cochrane Database System Review Oct, 18, 2006 CD 001877]

The idea is, if breast tumors are growing for 8-10 years before detection, that mammograms in younger age groups should produce earlier detection and reduce mortality rates. One problem is that radiation from mammography increases the risk for death from breast cancer so that the advantages of screening in younger women are offset by the increased risk of radiation-induced cancer. [Journal Medical Screening 5: 81-87, 1998]

The promotion of mammography screening began in 1972. For most of the years following, high-dose radiation was used, posing a greater theoretical net increase in breast cancer mortality than the benefit of early detection. [British Journal Cancer 82: 220-28, 2000] In the 1970s, industrial type x-ray film was used and required doses of radiation 20 times greater than what is used today with more sensitive film. [Rofo 173: 79-91, 2001] Women were made into guinea pigs and subjected to potentially harmful radiation. Then, when it was realized the radiation dose was too high and it was reduced, and there still was no benefit in regard to reduction in mortality rates, these facts were hidden from women. Most women who dutifully showed up for their annual mammograms were simply *"cooking their breasts."*

Women should be told about the benefits, limitations, and potential harms associated with regular screening. Mammograms can miss some cancers. However, mammograms, despite their limitations, remain the most effective and valuable tool for decreasing suffering and death from breast cancer.

Source: American Cancer Society

Many women remain unaware of the extent to which efforts to achieve breast cancer control through mammography screening may be doing harm as well as good. An unacknowledged harm is that for up to 11 years after the initiation of breast cancer screening in women aged 40–49 years, screened women face a higher death rate from breast cancer than unscreened control women. ...We live in an era in which lip service is paid to the concept of the informed patient sharing in decision making. If we practice what we preach, physicians must let frightened women know that, even without screening, most women who get breast cancer will not die of it and that, despite screening, some women will still die of breast cancer.

Cornelia J. Baines
Department of Public Health
Sciences, University of Toronto

Source: Journal National Cancer Institute 95:1508-11, 2006

Up to 92% of women report that mammogram examination is painful. [Pain 108: 170-79, 2004]

Breast cancer prevention is a contradiction. On the one hand, women, fearful they will develop breast cancer as their family members have, take precautions not to be exposed to xenoestrogens (man-made chemicals that mimic estrogen), avoid hormone replacement drugs, pesticides, smoking, underarm deodorants, and alcohol, and then walk right into a clinic on an annual basis and expose their breasts to the physical trauma and ionizing x-ray radiation that is called a mammogram, unwittingly increasing their risk for breast cancer.

Breast trauma from mammography

Scientists have known for over a decade that a link exists between wound healing and cancer. [Proceedings National Academy Science 102: 3738-3743, 2005] For instance, in a 1994 experiment at the Lawrence Berkeley National Laboratory, chickens infected with a cancer virus developed tumors in areas of their body that had undergone wounding or scarring, while no tumors developed in infected areas that had not suffered wounds.

Women with breast cancer are 3.3 times more likely to report physical trauma to the breast in the previous five years than healthy women. [European Journal Cancer Prevention 11:307-11, 2002] Women submit their breasts to be clamped during mammography, which is painful for most when undergoing filming. [Pain 108:170-9, 2004; Journal Pain Symptom Management 25:53-63, 2003] Furthermore, many women are in a mammogram-induced state of anxiety while they await results of their test. [Archives Internal Medicine 163: 833-6, 2003]

Radiation exposure during mammography

From the 1920s through the 1950s, radiation therapy was used in Sweden as treatment for benign breast disease and was found to increase the risk for subsequent breast cancer. [Journal National Cancer Institute 85: 1679-85, 1993] Exposure to x-ray radiation is known to increase the risk for breast cancer. [Lancet 363: 345-51, 2004]

> The three unequivocal contributors to cancer – ionizing radiation (example- x-rays), estrogen replacement and alcohol consumption–, still do not explain the vast majority of breast cancers that occur in the absence of these factors. [International Journal Cancer, Dec. 15, 2005]

In 1976, Drs. Irwin Bross and Leslie Blumenson of Buffalo's Roswell Park Memorial Laboratory estimated that, based on radiation dosage exposure, twice as many deaths as cures could result from mammographic screenings of mostly healthy women. [Journal Surgical Oncology 8: 437-45, 1976]

Dr. Bross became an outspoken critic of mammography, calling it a *"disastrous mistake"* that would *"produce the worst . . . epidemic of cancer in medical history."* At a meeting sponsored by the National Cancer Institute, Bross accused the American Cancer Society and the American College of Radiology of subjecting a quarter million American women to X-ray dosages equivalent *"to death warrants with a 15-year delay in the execution."* Cumulatively, mass mammography screening could have produced 12 times more cases of cancer than it detected. [I. D. Bross, Written Statement Submitted for the NIH/NCI Consensus Development Meeting on Breast Cancer Screening, Sept. 14-16, 1977]

Some patients are more genetically predisposed to breast cancer. Should these patients be exposed to repeated radiation mammography? [Clinical Oncology Royal College Radiology 18: 257-67, 2006] Even exposure to chest x-rays, particularly before the age of 20, heightens the risk for breast cancer with BRCA mutations. [Journal Clinical Oncology 24:3361-6, 2006]

Quietly, the radiation emitted during mammography was reduced as digital films were introduced. How many women have now developed breast cancer from these early screenings is unknown. Virtually every woman exposed to high-dose radiation mammography should have been placed on antioxidant therapy. None were.

Certification of mammogram readers and imaging centers

In a woman's lifetime, if she begins breast screening at the age of 50, she could experience as many as three false-positive mammograms. [Journal National Cancer Institute 92: 1657-66, 2000] The false-positive rates (percent of the time cancer is diagnosed when in fact it doesn't exist) among radiologists varies by 1.5 to 24.1%. [Breast Cancer Research Treatment, July 4, 2006 online]

Doctors who interpret mammograms only need to read 480 films a year to maintain their standing whereas studies indicate doctors need to read 2,500 films a year to stay sharp. Canada and Britain requires that many readings a year to maintain certification. Doctors who read more than 3,600 mammograms per year are about 76% accurate while doctors who read 1,200 or fewer films have only a 65% accuracy rate. Of the 20,000 doctors who read over 30 million mammograms per year, the average miss 1 in 10 breast tumors, the stated error rate, but skills vary and some doctors may miss up to 4 in 10. An audit of breast clinics in North Carolina found the best centers found 347 cancers and missed 70 while the worst found 178 and missed 94. [New York Times, June 27, 2002]

Breast self examination

Teaching women to perform breast self-exams does not lower their risk of death from cancer and may only lead to unnecessary biopsies. [Journal National Cancer Institute 94: 1445-57, 2002] Breast self examination should be abandoned.

Another obstacle in detecting breast cancer at its earliest stages is that breast self examination has not been shown to be useful as a screening tool. [Lancet 357: 9274, 2001] A nursing journal article asks: *"Why are we still promoting breast self-examination?"* [International Journal Nursing Studies, Jan. 19, 2006]

Reliability of estrogen receptor tests

Even testing for estrogen receptor status is not foolproof. This is a laboratory test that measures the percentage of tumor cells that are sensitive to estrogen. Somewhere around 10 to 20% of the tumor cells must be sensitive to estrogen before the test is judged to be positive. About 200,000 breast cancer patients have this test done annually, and some labs use a 10% cutoff point, while others use higher numbers. [Washington Post Dec. 4, 2000] It appears arbitrary cut-off points are used, which can obviously lead to unnecessary treatment. The test obviously does not catch estrogen-negative tumors.

With all of the screening, breast exams, mammograms, and biopsies for breast cancer being performed today, it seems that the end result has paradoxically been to produce more disease.

The U.S. Food and Drug Administration (FDA) must certify each mammography facility. In order to be certified, the equipment, personnel, and practice of the facility must be reviewed by an FDA-approved accreditation body. Each mammogram machine has to be accredited. Certain staff members must meet strict standards including radiologists (the doctors who interpret the mammograms)

Source: The American Cancer Society

A woman participating in breast screening from age 50 to 64 increases her chances of surviving to age 75 by 0.6%.

Source: Journal Medical Screening 10: 22-26, 2003

PREVENTION

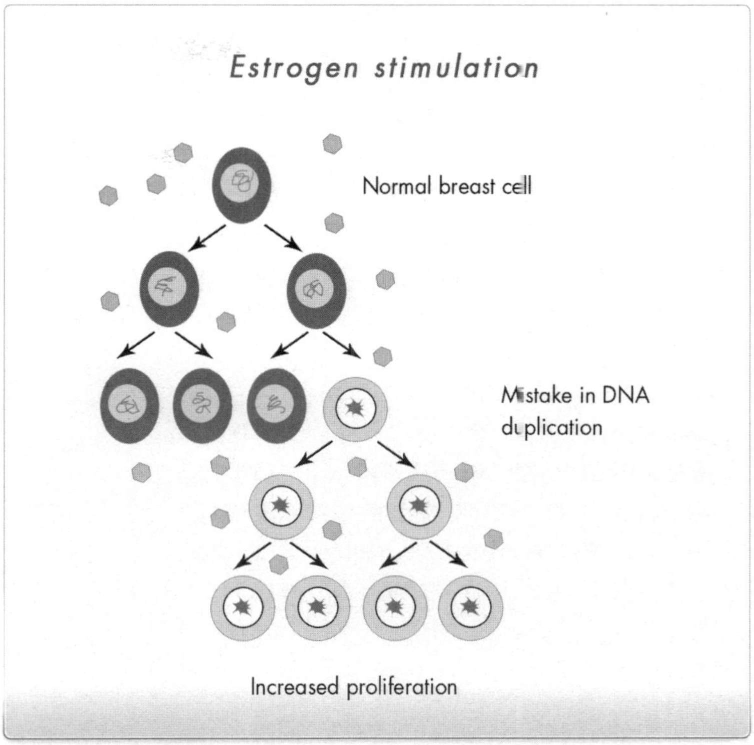

Does prevention exist?

Little is done to promote healthy breast tissue, and everything is done to invade, disturb, destroy and remove breast tissue. The National Cancer Institute defines prevention as *"reduction in the incidence of invasive breast cancer, which should lead in turn to a decrease in breast cancer mortality."* In the minds of doctors and clinics, more breasts to treat equals prevention. There is no economic incentive for true prevention. When clinics spend as much as $1 million to purchase mammography equipment, they expect a return on their investment. They have to churn a given number of women through the turnstiles to pay off loans to purchase equipment. There are 15,000 mammography units in the United States, about 30,000 worldwide.
The grey area where clinics can pad the number of patients undergoing mammography and subsequent treatment is among women with *ductal carcinoma in situ*. Somehow the word *"carcinoma"* was attached to these breast abnormalities, and with the proliferation of mammography equipment, business boomed. (More about ductal carcinoma below.)

In a report published in *Postgraduate Medicine* entitled *"Who's liable for breast cancer prevention? Your patient can sue–and win–if preventive options aren't made clear,"* the emphasis is on doctors diagnosing breast cancer early and treating it, not addressing what caused it in the first place. [Postgraduate Medicine 111: 83, 2002]

Mastectomy is still characterized as prevention. Chemoprevention is solely comprised of drugs like Tamoxifen and aromatase inhibitors, all prescribed after diagnosis (called secondary prevention.) [CA Cancer Journal Clinicians 50: 156-70, 2000]

Phytoestrogen

The rate of breast cancer varies widely worldwide. Japanese and other Asian women experience a risk of breast cancer that is about a third to half that of American Caucasian women. [European J Cancer Prevention 11: 519-22, 2002] The reduced risk for breast cancer is often attributed to the consumption of phytoestrogens, primarily soy in Asian diets. However, the effect is not consistent. In a telephone survey of women who were diagnosed with breast cancer, the consumption of plant estrogens was found to have little or no effect upon cancer risk with the average intake of less than one serving of tofu per week. [Am J Epidemiology 154: 434-41, 2001] Possibly much higher consumption is required to exhibit a protective effect.

The assumption has been, since vegetarian women have lower circulating estrogen levels, that this is the primary reason why they exhibit lower rates of breast cancer and that the inclusion of phytoestrogens in plant-food diets is the primary dietary factor involved. This is only partly correct. Estrogen is dumped into the digestive tract at the end of the monthly cycle and women who consume more meat will reabsorb more of their dumped estrogen and thus exhibit higher circulating levels of estrogen and longer menstrual periods. To the contrary, women who consume fiber-rich plant foods excrete 2 to 3 times more estrogen in their feces and thus have lower circulating estrogen levels and shorter monthly cycles. [Cancer Research 41: 3771-73, 1981] But while estrogen is a major player in the onset of breast cancer, it's not the only factor. There are other overlooked factors, explained later in this chapter.

Estrogen is dumped into the digestive tract at the end of the monthly cycle and women who consume more meat will reabsorb more of their dumped estrogen and thus exhibit higher circulating levels of estrogen and longer periods.

A review of scientific data reveals that advancing age, not necessarily a change in sex hormone levels, is the major factor involved in the onset of breast cancer. More than 80% of cases of breast cancer occur after age 50 and only 1.5 % occur under age 35. [Clinical Obstetrics Gynecology 25: 387-92, 1982] But age itself may be just a marker. The cessation of menstruation and the loss of control over iron, may be a major factor in the rising risk for breast cancer after menopause. Up until menopause, women increase the level of iron in their bloodstream due to menstrual flow each month and therefore avoid the iron overload that males commonly experience. A middle-aged male will harbor twice the iron as a middle-aged female (who is still menstruating) and incur twice the risk of developing cancer in any part of the body.

Tamoxifen

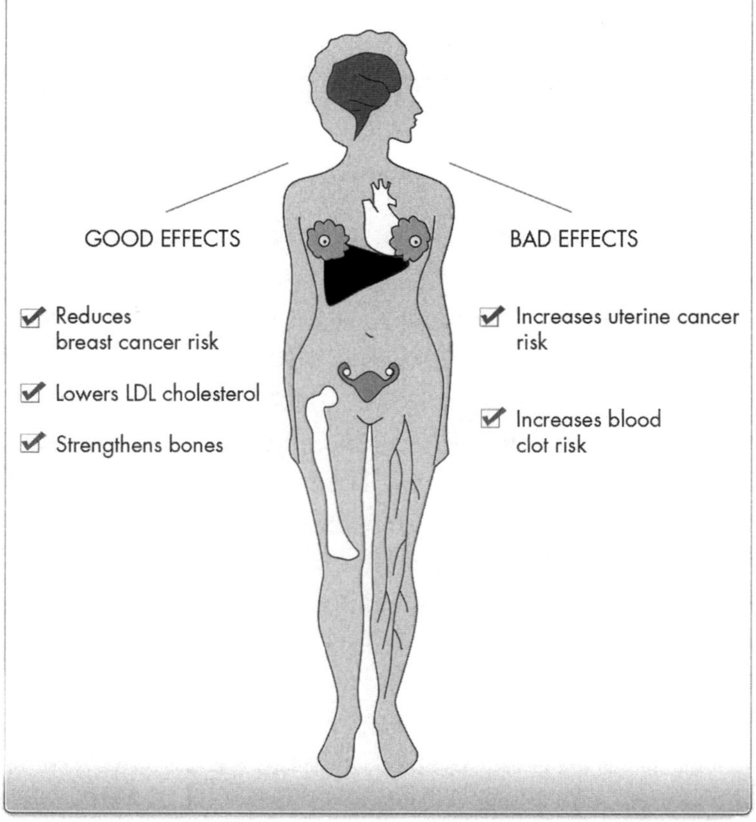

Estrogen effects associated with hormone replacement therapy during menopause

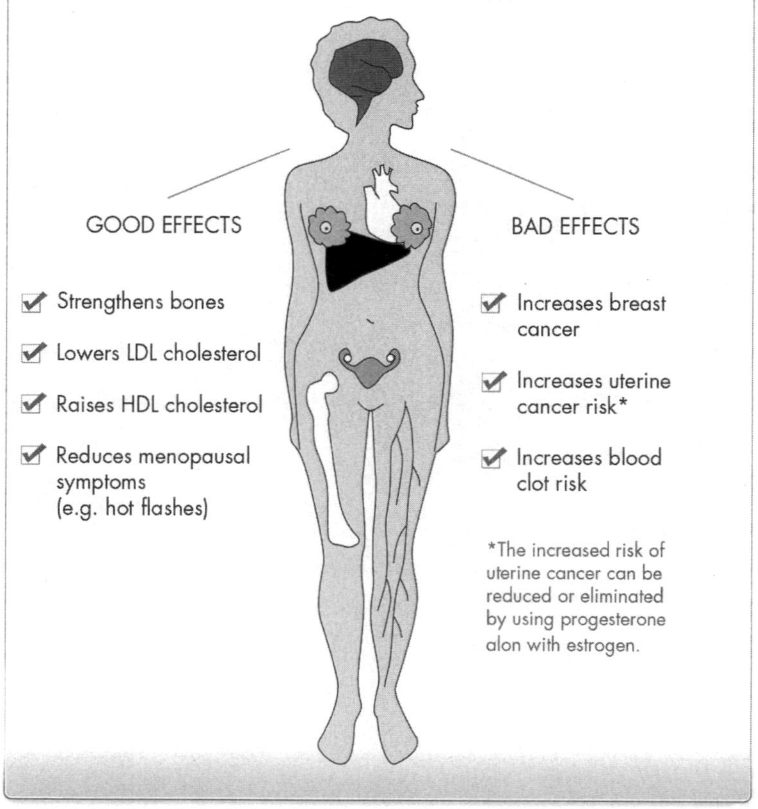

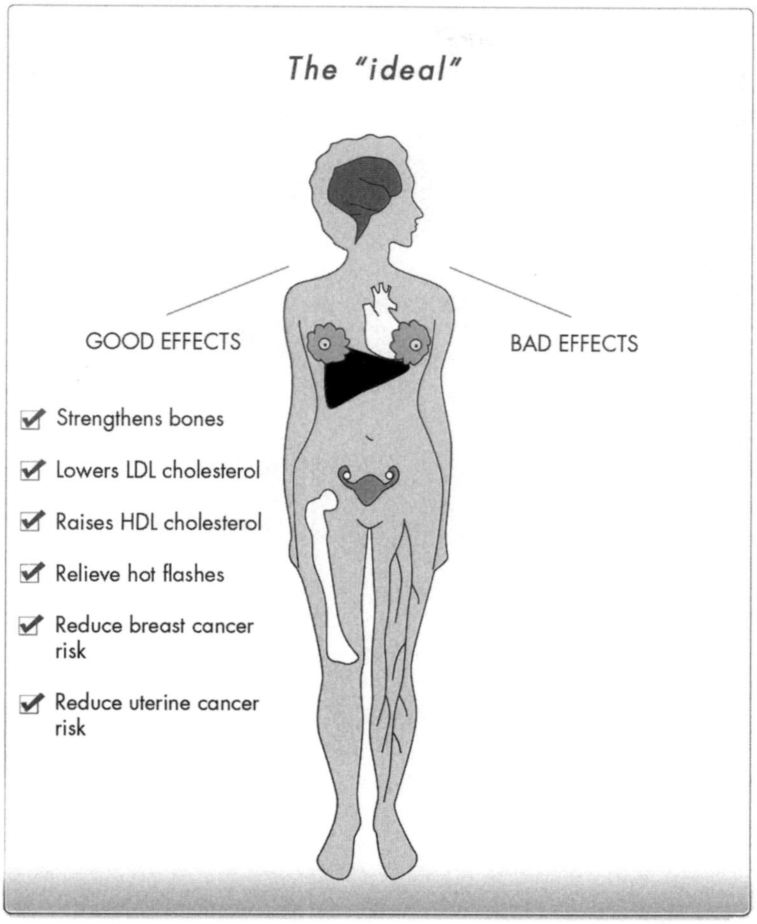

horse mare urine), prescribed for the change of life, first to calm the hot flashes and mood issues associated with the change of life, and second to allegedly improve bone health, reduce cardiovascular risk and inhibit the onset of breast cancer.

In 1976, *Consumer Reports* said the use of hormone replacement had almost tripled from 1965 to 1976 and during that same time period the incidence of cancer increased in women over age 50 who were in high-socioeconomic groups– the same group most likely to use estrogen therapy.

"Earlier reports suggested estrogen might protect against breast cancer; most recent studies suggest the opposite." [Consumer Reports 41: 642-45, 1976] Estrogen therapy was supposed to be restricted solely to women with vaginal shrinkage and a few other narrow indications. Consumer Reports said: Doctors weren't there to step into the breech and protect American women. Doctors acquiesced to the pharmaceutical companies and the greatest yet-to-be-proven medical experiment was underway.

Hormone replacement therapy

There simply is no way to begin a discussion about breast cancer without addressing the issue of hormone replacement. Despite concerns over health risks, many millions of women still take hormone replacement drugs.

So much has been said about hormone replacement therapy and the state of breast cancer treatment, yet so many questions still remain. This limited report will never be able to answer all the remaining questions American women have about supplemental hormones, but it may provide a clearer picture of what is really going on. And it may, for the first time, give interested readers a valid scenario for the prevention of breast cancer altogether.

For almost three decades American women have had estrogen and progesterone, (pharmaceutically extracted from

Phytoestrogens dismissed

In the meantime, non-prescription, plant-based estrogens (called phytoestrogens) were cast aside and mis-characterized. A 1978 report said phytoestrogens *"can markedly enhance tumor cell proliferation."* [Endocrinology 103: 1860-67, 1978] Of course, this conclusion was drawn from test-tube studies where cells were flooded with plant estrogens rather than being given in doses commonly found in raw plant-food diets. One of the biases revealed in animal and test-tube studies is that they may utilize very high, if not unobtainable, levels of plant estrogens which would then induce the same side effects as estrogen. For example, one study using black cohosh (a source of phytoestrogens) gave rodents 300 mg of black cohosh per kilogram (2.2 pounds) of body weight. That is equivalent to nearly 22,000 mg of black cohosh in an adult human, or 1,100 black cohosh pills. [J Medicinal Food 4: 171-78, 2001]. Not surprisingly the study found that black cohosh had damaging effects.

So doctors proceeded to prescribe to millions of American women pharmaceutical-grade estrogen, and while they conceded that estrogen replacement increased the risk of endometrial cancer, this risk was addressed by prescribing progesterone and advising women on hormone replacement to come in for frequent checkups. [Postgraduate Medicine 62: 73-79, 1977] All the while, doctors were saying food supplements like flaxseed, black cohosh and red clover were unproven, even "*snake oil.*"

With the news that hormone replacement therapy posed health risks, doctors were so overwhelmed by phone calls from millions of women that they simply shut off their office phones.

The bomb drops on hormone replacement therapy

For decades doctors continued to prescribe hormones to postmenopausal women under the assumption they improved health for postmenopausal women. But after years of customary use it was time for a scientific review. Did hormone replacement therapy really improve health?

The bomb dropped in July of 2002 with reports that hormone replacement slightly increased the risk of breast cancer and cardiovascular events like strokes. At the time the news report hit, 6 million women were taking these prescribed hormones. [National Institutes of Health Press release July 9, 2002] Some physicians were so overwhelmed by phone calls to their offices over this startling news that they simply shut off their office phones.

Specific study findings for the estrogen plus progestin study compared to placebo include:

- A 41 % increase in strokes
- A 29 % increase in heart attacks
- A doubling of rates of venous thromboembolism (blood clots)
- A 22 % increase in total cardiovascular disease
- A 26 % increase in breast cancer
- A 37 % reduction in cases of colorectal cancer
- A one-third reduction in hip fracture rates
- A 24 % reduction in total fractures
- No difference in total mortality (of all causes)
- It could no longer be said hormone replacement therapy saved lives.

Then just 11 months later, a news article reported that hormone replacement therapy could increase the risk of being mentally demented in later years of life. Among 2,229 postmenopausal women who took estrogen plus progesterone replacement pills beginning in 1996 through 2002, 40 were diagnosed with probable dementia compared with just 21 in a group of 2,303 women who did not use hormone pills. The relative risk doubled among the hormone users. The absolute risk was low, 1.8% among hormone users, just 0.9% among non-users. Among the 6 million American women now taking hormone replacement therapy, this could increase the number of cases of Alzheimer's disease by about 13,800 annually. [J Am Med Assoc 289: 2651-62, 2003] The increased risk was still small, but the point had been made. A small increased risk weighed against no potential benefits meant the widespread use of hormone pills had to be re-evaluated. In March of 2003, the FDA approved a lower dose of Prempro, the most popular hormone replacement pill, due to concerns over side effects. By May of 2003 postmenopausal women were being told still more bad news.

"Some women said they could never give up the pills, not because they needed them for severe menopause symptoms but because they were convinced that estrogen prevented wrinkles or because it staved off mental fogginess."
[New York Times July 5, 2003]

Here is what Judy Siegel-Itzkovich of the *Jerusalem Post* had to say about hormone replacement therapy. It couldn't be said any better than this: *"Middle-aged women should think twice before taking combined progestin-estrogen pills to alleviate their hot flashes, night sweats, and other disturbing menopausal symptoms, according to an analysis of data from last year's U.S. Woman's Health Institute study on the effects of hormone replacement therapy. What pharmaceutical companies have pushed for decades as a 'preventive fountain of youth' for menopausal women, now seems to increase the risk of breast cancer even when taken for only one year."* [Jerusalem Post June 25, 2003; J Am Med Assoc 289: 3243-53, 3254-63, 2003]

Due to the negative scientific studies, the use of estrogen therapy in Canada dropped an astonishing 32% from 2001 to 2002. [J Am Med Assoc 289: 3241-42, 2003] In the United States, hormone replacement therapy declined by about 30%. [Journal General Internal Medicine 20:1026-31, 2005] In Britain, the decline was about 16%. [Am J Public Health 96:1219-25. 2006]

But, a few million women kept taking the pills. Some women continued to take HRT because they simply didn't want to face a return to all those hot flashes and mood problems and the increased risk for breast cancer was considered statistically small. Other women continued to take the hormone pills for more frivolous reasons. As a report in New York Times said, *"Some women said they could never give up the pills, not because they needed them for severe menopause symptoms but because they were convinced that estrogen prevented wrinkles or because it staved off mental fogginess."* [New York Times, July 5, 2003]

Annual increased risk from use of estrogen/progesterone		
Risk/benefit	Change per year Source: National Institute on Aging	Annual increase/decrease among estimated 4 million users of hormone replacement
Heart attacks	7 more cases in 10,000 women	+2,800 new cases
Breast cancer	8 more cases in 10,000 women	+3,200 new cases
Strokes	8 more cases in 10,000 women	+3,200 new cases
Blood clots	18 more cases in 10,000 women	+7,200 new cases
Dementia	23 more cases in 10,000 women*	+9,200 new cases
Hip fractures	5 fewer cases in 10,000 women	-2,000 fewer cases
Colon cancer	6 fewer cases in 10,000 women	-2,400 fewer cases
	* Over age 65	

Increased risk for uterine cancer with use of estrogen	
Using no hormones after 10-19 years	+4.4 cases in 10,000 women
Using estrogen alone for 20 years or more	+14 cases in 10,000 women

Women have been conditioned to accept menopause as a period of life when life-long medication with hormones is a normal process. Although there have been many warnings against the use of hormone replacement, *"they have either been ignored or trivialized."* [Int J Health Services 31: 769-92, 2001] Not counting the cost of doctor's office visits, hormone replacement pills sales were nearly $2.7 billion in the United States annually. A year after the fateful announcement of health risks associated with hormone replacement, sales declined to $1.9 billion [Business Week November 5, 2004]

Anatomy of the female breast

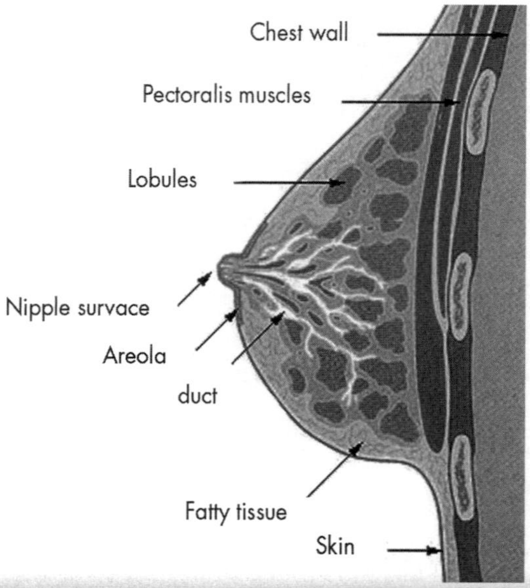

What will American women do now as menopause approaches and they experience all those related symptoms: night sweats, hot flashes and mood changes? It's quite a dilemma since there are about 5,000 more American women who reach menopause, the permanent end of menstruation, each day, added to the 40 million who are already in their menopausal years.

Reactions to menopause appear to be culturally conditioned in females. Mayan women from Guatemala look forward to menopause and their newfound freedom and consider the symptoms of menopause as evidence of their improved status. [Maturitas 44: 293-97, 2003] In contrast, many women in America have been conditioned to run to the doctor for a pill for their hot flashes and night sweats.

TREATMENT

Breast cancer treatment

A lot of the success of treatment depends upon just how extensive breast cancer is on the day of its discovery. If it hasn't spread to the lymph nodes and other sites, treatment success is about 70%. In the other 30% of patients the cancer will come roaring back after treatment. That is the figure that is quoted for the success rate of cancer care. [National Cancer Institute Benchmarks Volume 6, Issue 3, 2006] The fact is, many breast tumors have already spread to lymph nodes and beyond on the day of diagnosis.

Breast cancer surgery, when performed among younger premenopausal women, can provoke the growth and spread of remaining tumor cells. Researchers have noted that 20 percent of pre-menopausal breast cancer patients undergoing surgery, whose cancer had spread to lymph nodes, experienced relapse within 10 months of surgery to remove the primary tumor. [Breast Cancer Research 6:R689-96, 2004]

Breast cancer researchers from Britain say that:

> *"A new crisis is upon us now in that trials of early detection have resulted in unexpected disadvantages to certain subgroups...there is a previously unreported early hazard of relapse. Clinical data suggests the act of surgery might accelerate the appearance of distant metastases. There is the very real possibility of doing more harm than good by operating upon women with breast cancer. Surgical resection should be avoided for disease much more advanced than very early stage tumors."*
> [European Journal Cancer 41:508-15, 2005]

The three treatments for breast cancer: surgery (mastectomy or lumpectomy, with or without removal of lymph glands), radiation and chemotherapy, need to be scrutinized.

Radiation therapy

The general consensus is that women who undergo conservative treatment (lumpectomy) without removal of underarm lymph nodes and forgo radiation therapy will experience shorter survival. [Breast Cancer Research Treatment 72: 23-31, 2002] This is the prevalent thinking of oncologists today.

Women who are quick to accept the advice of their oncologists need to take a step back and ponder what they are told about treatment options.

For example, according to the latest studies, widely publicized in the news media, radiation treatment for millions of women with early-stage breast cancer will significantly reduce their chances of dying.

> *"We've shown very clearly, for the first time, there is a benefit," said one expert. "The message for women is that if their doctors are offering them radiotherapy, they should consider it very seriously. It does save lives."*
> [Washington Post Dec. 16, 2005]

Should you follow the latest advice? Probably not. Here's why.

After two and a half decades of attempts, studies do show that radiation therapy applied after breast cancer surgery, chemotherapy and anti-estrogen drugs (Tamoxifen), *slightly* increases survival of women with early-stage breast cancer. The new data shows breast cancer mortality rates were reduced by only 5%. [Lancet 366: 2087-2106, 2005]

For women who underwent a mastectomy, but whose cancer had spread to the lymph nodes under their arms, the 15-year breast cancer mortality risk was 54.7% with radiation vs. 60.1%t without – a reduction of 5.4 percentage points. There was a similar reduction in overall death risk. Radiation was previously shown to reduce the breast cancer mortality rate, but the new study is the first to show a decrease in overall mortality. [Lancet 366: 2087-2106, 2005]

The reduction in mortality is modest. Just four years earlier, a similar study showed that for women whose risk of relapse is low (no spread to lymph nodes), the benefits of radiation are small, if any. [Lancet 355: 1739-40, 2000]

Is this new data justification enough to warrant all women getting radiation treatment? Patients need to ask their doctors, how many patients have to be treated with radiation for one patient to experience any benefit? It appears to be 20. Cancer doctors need to stop recommending marginally beneficial treatments for all just because the statistical pendulum slightly swings in favor of treatment.

Since 1978, radiation treatment has been routinely applied following breast cancer surgery without evidence of any benefit, yet with certain evidence of long-term harm.

High doses of radiation used in the 1970s and 1980s produced long-term increased risk for heart problems. Radiation dosage has been reduced after doctors recognized that the radiation itself resulted in an increased risk for heart disease and cancer in the opposing breast.

Frankly, the latest data does show that reduced-dose radiation doesn't appear to increase the risk for heart disease. [Lancet Oncology 6: 557-65, 2005] Most of the data on radiation exposure and risk for breast cancer is collected from younger women, not 75- year- olds who are much more vulnerable to tissue damage and cancer recurrence from radiation exposure. Women over 65 years of age comprise most of the breast cancer cases.

Furthermore, what oncologists are reporting is a slight increased survival rate, without consideration of morbidity. Patients undergoing radiation treatment have to endure more than the long-term risk for heart problems.

- For example, about 25% of radiation-treated, breast cancer patients experience immediate lung damage. [Acta Oncologica 45:16-22, 2006]

- Recent reports demonstrate a dramatically increased rate of secondary leukemia for breast cancer patients receiving high-dose chemotherapy (anthracycline) with radiation treatment, with radiation being an independent factor for the development of leukemia. [International Journal Radiation Oncology Biology Physics Jan 31, 2006]

- Radiation treatment after breast cancer surgery increases the incidence of local artery disease and hemorrhagic arterial plaque. [American Journal Pathology 168:649-58, 2006] Cancer doctors will blame the death

Estrogen receptors: Positive/Negative Cancer

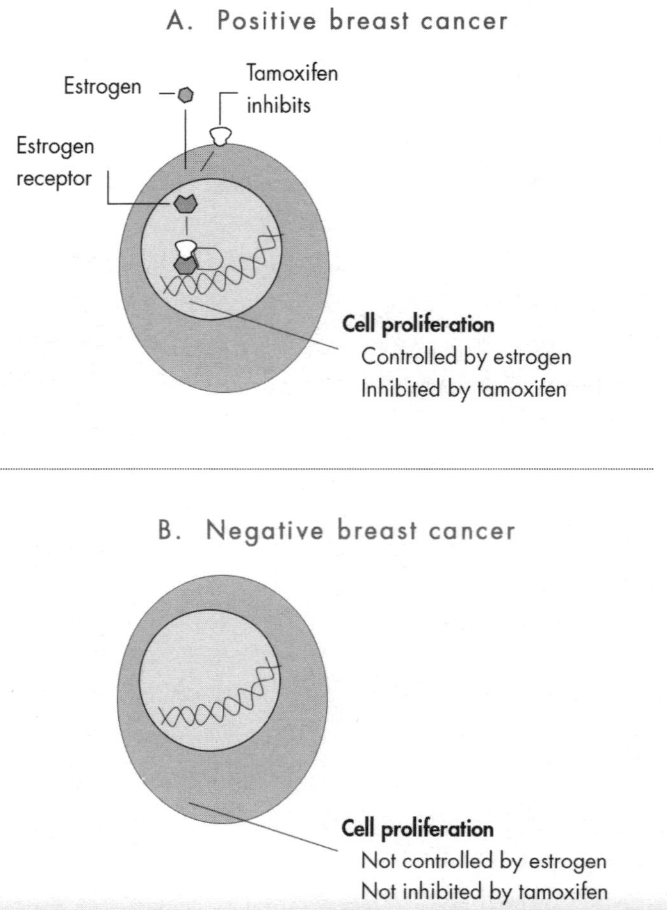

Tamoxifen Insert

WARNING - For Women with Ductal Carcinoma in Situ (DCIS) and Women at High Risk for Breast Cancer: Serious and life-threatening events associated with **NOLVADEX (tamoxifen citrate)** in the risk reduction setting (women at high risk for cancer and women with DCIS) include uterine malignancies, stroke, and pulmonary embolism.

Incidence rates for these events were estimated from the NSABP P-1 trial. Uterine malignancies consist of both endometrial adenocarcinoma (incidence rate per 1,000 women-years of 2.20 for NOLVADEX vs. 0.71 for placebo) and uterine sarcoma (incidence rate per 1,000 women-years of 0.17 for NOLVADEX vs. 0.0 for placebo*). For stroke, the incidence rate per 1,000 women-years was 1.43 for NOLVADEX vs. 1.00 for placebo**. For pulmonary embolism, the incidence rate per 1,000 women-years was 0.75 for NOLVADEX vs. 0.25 for placebo. Some of the strokes, pulmonary emboli, and uterine malignancies were fatal.

Health care providers should discuss the potential benefits versus the potential risks of these serious events with women at high risk of breast cancer and women with DCIS considering NOLVADEX to reduce their risk of developing breast cancer.The benefits of NOLVADEX outweigh its risks in women already diagnosed with breast cancer.

of a loved one on heart problems without informing the family that the treatment may have induced cardiac death.

→ Among women who smoked tobacco at the time of their breast cancer diagnosis, treatment with radiation increases their risk for lung cancer. [Journal Clinical Oncology 23:7467-74, 2005]

→ If radiation therapy is so desirable, why hasn't the FDA approved implantable radiation seeds after breast cancer surgery? The answer is because many women don't want to endure 6-7 weeks of radiation treatment with external burns to their breast tissue. [Expert Review Medical Devices 2: 387-94, 2005]

→ Women who survive breast cancer and are treated with radiation therapy are at a higher risk for leukemia, esophageal cancer and second breast cancer in the years following initial care. [British Journal Cancer 91: 868-72, 2004]

So, if you are a typical patient with newly detected breast cancer, and it has spread to the lymph nodes, radiation treatment does improve survival slightly, with significant pain and discomfort, and does not address the cause of the cancer. In fact, it is a *cause* of cancer. Roaming tumor cells that have spread to other locations will not be killed off by application of radiation to the breast or lymph nodes. It is the tumor cells that have escaped beyond capture in the lymph nodes that result in metastasis and mortality.

Tamoxifen

Tamoxifen is the "*gold standard*" of breast cancer treatment, heralded as the "*most important drug in the history of the management of breast cancer.*"

In 1896, Dr. George Beatson discovered that surgical removal of a woman's ovaries shrinks breast tumors. [Lancet 2: 104-07, 1896] Thereafter efforts have focused on controlling estrogen to limit the growth of breast cancer. Tamoxifen doesn't inhibit the production of estrogen, but it blocks its entry into cells.

Tamoxifen has been credited with decreasing mortality from breast cancer by 20-30%. It is said that more than 400,000 women are alive today thanks to Tamoxifen therapy.

The data used to back the claims that Tamoxifen is a wonder drug are specious. On April 7, 1998 a news story proclaimed that a research study on Tamoxifen was so convincing that researchers halted the study a year early so more women could benefit from the drug. Researchers called their study a "*historic milestone*" and said the drug cut the risk of breast cancer in half. [Associated Press, April 7, 1998] But these studies are supposed to be done in a "*blind*" fashion, without knowing which patients received Tamoxifen and who received a placebo. Tamoxifen was found to reduce the percentage of women who developed

> If Tamoxifen is such a godsend, why has only the U.S. approved Tamoxifen for use among healthy women?

breast cancer from 2.4 to 1.3%, but this was recorded as the difference between these two numbers, which is an 84% relative difference. However, if using solid numbers, the results would break down as follows: if 1,000 women took Tamoxifen, two would develop breast cancer versus 3.5 among 1,000 women who did not take the drug. It would require that 998.5 women take Tamoxifen, with risks for significant side effects, for 1.5 women to delay or prevent breast cancer. How could this be a major breakthrough? [Journal Orthomolecular Medicine 13 67, 1998]

Was the American study intentionally halted to produce a positive result? Longer-term studies in Italy and Britain (4 and 8 years) did not confirm the earlier study which was abruptly halted. [Orv Hetil 144: 597-603, 2003] The U.S. Food & Drug Administration widened the use of Tamoxifen to high-risk but otherwise healthy American women. If Tamoxifen is such a godsend, why has only the United States approved Tamoxifen for use among healthy women? [Gynecology Obstetrics Fertility 31: 327-36, 2003]

It is frequently said that the benefits of Tamoxifen outweigh the risk for serious side effects. But the potential benefits only apply to the 1.5 out of 1000 women who take Tamoxifen for 10 years and avert or delay the diagnosis of breast cancer. The other 998.5 women are only at risk for drug side effects since they would not develop cancer anyway.

Tamoxifen fraud?

Surprisingly, the American Cancer Society also hailed Tamoxifen as an anti-cancer drug. While data shows it may prevent breast cancer, it also may cause uterine cancer and blood clots. Not only did subsequent studies fail to confirm the effectiveness of Tamoxifen, but a Duke University Medical Center study revealed that Tamoxifen eventually loses its effectiveness and "*actually may help cancer grow.*" [Associated Press, July 30, 1999, from Science 285 (5428):744-6, 1999] This is another example which shows that reports of scientific breakthroughs in the news media may not be trustworthy and are likely to be swayed by economic interests.

Here is how the National Cancer Institute (NCI) helps to promote drugs like Tamoxifen to the public, essentially acting as public relations shill for the drug companies.

> Concerning potential side effects caused by Tamoxifen, the National Women's Health Network asked: *"Does this represent disease prevention, or disease substitution?"*

The NCI reports that 10 million American women are at high risk for breast cancer and maybe ought to see their doctors about taking Tamoxifen. The NCI concedes only 2.4 million of these women are likely to benefit from taking the drug, and out of this group of 2.4 million the number of cases of breast cancer is likely to be reduced from 58,148 to 28,492. The number of cases of breast cancer appears to be cut in half (49%) when viewed as a relative percentage. But in reality, only 2.4% of the 2.4 million women would be expected to develop breast cancer if they didn't take Tamoxifen and 1.2% if they did. So the difference in hard numbers is only 1.2%, hardly a way to sell Tamoxifen to American women. [J National Cancer Institute 95: 526-32, 2003; University of Iowa Press Release, April 4, 2003] So the relative numbers are used instead.

It's very misleading. Yes, admittedly when looking at hard numbers about 20,000 additional women would be spared from breast cancer. The problem is you have to get over 2 million women to take the drug to realize this benefit. Most women taking Tamoxifen are at greater risk for drug side effects than they are of experiencing any health benefit.

Another one of the hidden facts about Tamoxifen is that half of the women with advanced estrogen-positive tumors fail to respond to this drug and are removed from drug therapy. The studies don't always include these failures. [Drugs 61: 1721-33, 2001]

Current efforts to expand Tamoxifen therapy as a preventive agent for breast cancer have begun. High-risk but otherwise healthy women derive some risk reduction if given Tamoxifen. In one important study, of the 6,600 women who took Tamoxifen, there were 69 fewer tumors compared to 6,000 women who took a dummy pill. In other words, Tamoxifen benefited only about 1 in 100 high-risk women as a preventive measure. Yet it was widely hailed as a breakthrough! [Associated Press Oct. 30, 1998] There has been resistance to the idea of giving healthy women a drug that runs the risk of serious side effects. The National Women's Health Network asked: "*Does this trial represent disease prevention, or disease substitution?* [Breast Cancer Action, Feb. 26, 1996]

Side effects of Tamoxifen

How did Tamoxifen ever get approved as a cancer treatment drug? For one thing, it was initially confined to be used on those with advanced cases of cancer following surgery, chemotherapy and radiation (if that isn't an admission those other conventional treatments don't work, I don't know what is.) Most likely, the Food & Drug Administration was coaxed into approving this drug for this group of patients because of the risks of mortality facing post-treatment breast cancer patients. In other words, the side effects could be overlooked given the potentially mortal consequences from an otherwise unimpeded tumor.

Because Tamoxifen permits estrogen to continue being produced from androgens (adrenal hormones, mostly testosterone), women may also experience some menopausal symptom relief. Women's estrogen production is not blocked, rather its entry into cells is prevented. The existing estrogen helps to minimize age-related bone loss. Since about two-thirds of breast tumors are estrogen-positive, Tamoxifen may be helpful in prolonging regression and delaying a relapse, as well as preventing or delaying onset in the opposing breast.

But the list of potential benefits of Tamoxifen stops there. The realization that this drug can turn into a carcinogen can cause shivers. Here are the major drawbacks of Tamoxifen.

Tamoxifen is listed as a carcinogen (cancer-causing substance) in the 9th edition of the RAC list (reasonably anticipated to cause cancer) prepared by the National Toxicology Program of the Department of Health and Human Services.

1 Tamoxifen is listed as a carcinogen (cancer-causing substance) in the 9th edition of the RAC list (reasonably anticipated to cause cancer) prepared by the National Toxicology Program of the Department of Health and Human Services. [National Toxicology Program, Factsheet, May 2000] Canadian health authorities issued a health warning in 2002 regarding Tamoxifen and its side effects. [Health Canada, Nov. 26, 2002]

2 That is because Tamoxifen is only an organ-specific anti-cancer agent. It blocks breast tumors but encourages endometrial cancer. It has been known since 1975 that the use of Tamoxifen increases the risk of endometrial cancer by 450%. [New England Journal Med 293: 1164-67, 1975; International J Gynecology 12: 496-500, 2002] Some physicians suggest women undergo a complete hysterectomy before they start on the drug to eliminate the risk of endometrial cancer.

3 Estrogen blockers like Tamoxifen eventually lead to a dead-end street. Due to what is called *"Tamoxifen resistance,"* the drug inevitably turns on every woman within five years. Tamoxifen must be stopped after five years when cellular resistance materializes and turns this drug into a cancer-promoter. [J Steroid Biochemistry Molecular Biology79: 143-49, 2001; Drugs 61: 1721-33, 2001]

4 While it is said the risk of second breast cancer is reduced with Tamoxifen, in fact there is a five-times increased risk of estrogen-negative breast tumors in the breast opposite the first diagnosed tumor. [Fred Hutchinson Cancer Research Center, July 3, 2001] Despite its acclaim, Tamoxifen has not been found to increase life expectancy after five years of use. [British Journal Cancer 85: 1280-88, 2001]

Other side effects of Tamoxifen

Tamoxifen may induce irreversible blindness. It is possible for Tamoxifen to cause retinal blindness. [Am J Ophthalmology 131: 386-87, 2001; Cancer Treatment Reports 62: 315-20, 1978; Bulletin Society Belge Ophtalmol 238: 161-63, 1990] Tamoxifen also increases the risk of blinding cataracts, as much as 400%. [Breast Cancer Research Treatment 60: 167-72, 2000]

Tamoxifen may cause premature menopause, weight gain and mental depression. It may also induce hot flashes, night sweats and vaginal discharge in addition to blood clots, and stroke. [J National Cancer Institute Monograph 30: 130-34, 2001]

Scientists are currently mulling over data to determine if Tamoxifen is actually toxic to DNA. [Mutagenesis 18: 395-99, 2003]

Because of the long list of potential side effects, "*Women should be given all of the information about the benefits and risks of Tamoxifen use so that they can make an informed decision based on the best data available.*" [Annals Pharmacotherapy 37: 268-73, 2003] But are they?

After all the side effects generated by more than 20 years of prescribing Tamoxifen, and threatened with a new competitor (aromatase inhibitors), researchers finally decided to reduce the standard prescribed dosage of Tamoxifen from 20 mg to just 5 mg. This, researchers have recently concluded, may be enough to prevent relapse of breast cancer after conventional treatment (surgery, chemotherapy, radiation). [American Assoc Cancer Research, April 8, 2003; J National Cancer Institute 95: 779-90, 2003]

Chemoprevention of breast cancer

Cancer doctors have hopes that, some day, breast cancer can be prevented before it occurs. In 1998, Tamoxifen became the first drug employed to prevent breast cancer.

Women aren't buying into the idea of taking Tamoxifen to prevent breast cancer. They are wary of side effects. [Journal National Cancer Institute 96: 1410-12, 2004]

In a study where women at risk for breast cancer were offered Tamoxifen, only 43% elected to take it, mostly out of fear of side effects. [Annals Surgical Oncology 2004]

In another study, out of 51 women eligible for Tamoxifen breast cancer prevention, only 12% chose the drug and another 12% said they were uncertain. [Breast Cancer Research Treatment 94:153-9, 2005]

In yet another study, only 1 of 89 (1.2%) at-risk women elected to take Tamoxifen for prevention of breast cancer and 42% of the women made their decision to pass up Tamoxifen based upon advice from their family doctors. [Annals Family Medicine 3:242-7, 2005]

In a survey of 250 women deemed to be at higher risk for breast cancer, only about 18% of these women chose to take Tamoxifen even though 32% of them felt a high self-perceived risk of developing breast cancer. [Cancer 103:1996-2005, 2005]

While Tamoxifen increases the risk for blood clots in the legs from $5/10^{th}$ to $8/10^{ths}$ of one percent, that is still a 63% increase. [British Journal Clinical Pharmacology 45:608-12, 1998]

Despite its acclaimed achievements, health authorities are now asking: "*Has Tamoxifen had its day?*" [Breast Cancer Research 4: 213-17, 2002; Nat Review Drug Discovery 2: 205-13, 2003] That's because of a new class of drugs called aromatase inhibitors.

Aromatase inhibitors

Breast and prostate cells can produce enough sex hormones via activation by the aromatase enzyme to stimulate growth of tumors. [Clinical Cancer Research 9: 455-59S, 2003] Whereas Tamoxifen permits production of estrogen and then blocks its entry into cells, the aromatase inhibitors dampen the production of an enzyme responsible for production of estrogen itself.

Oral aromatase inhibitors are now being employed with results superior to that of Tamoxifen. [Breast Cancer Research 4: 213-17, 2002; Nature Review Drug Discovery 2: 205-13, 2003]

The superiority of aromatase inhibitors over Tamoxifen was demonstrated in a recent study. After 4 months of treatment, about 6 out of 10 women taking Femara (letrozole, an aromatase inhibitor) showed tumor shrinkage versus only 4 out of 10 women taking Tamoxifen. [24th Annual San Antonio Breast Cancer Symposium]

Letrozole compared to Tamoxifen

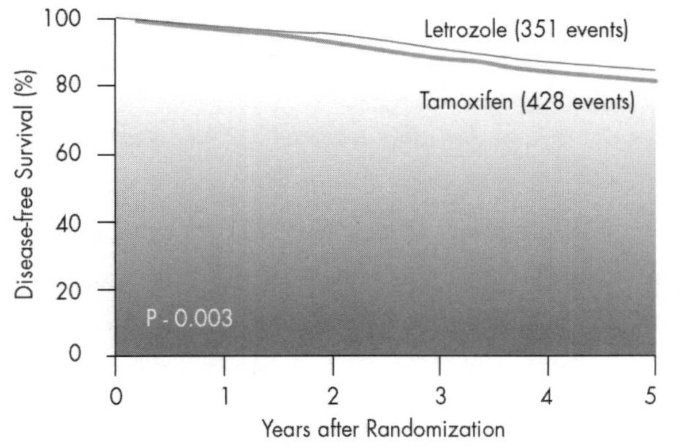

Letrozole						
No. at risk	4003	3892	2964	1261	892	567
Disease-free survival (%)		97.7	95.1	90.5	86.8	84.0
Tamoxifen						
No. at risk	4007	37.96	2926	1238	866	544
Disease-free survival (%)		97.6	93.4	89.0	84.6	81.4

Now that aromatase inhibitors are under widespread study and about to be prescribed to millions more American women, *The New England Journal of Medicine* has just published an extensive report on aromatase inhibitors. [New Eng J Med 348: 2431-42, 2003] The report says "*these drugs are effectively challenging Tamoxifen for use in postmenopausal patients with estrogen-receptor-positive cancer,*" the majority of breast cancer cases. Aromatase inhibitors don't induce tumor resistance as does Tamoxifen. [Endrocrin Relat Cancer 6: 75-92, 1999]

Aromatase inhibitors are also being considered as primary prevention. What this means is that the pharmaceutical companies want to put every woman on these drugs throughout life. Whereas Tamoxifen increases the risk of endometrial cancer and blood clots and becomes a cancer promoter over time, the aromatase inhibitors have no such side effects. But they have their own set of problems.

The aromatase enzyme is found in high concentrations in the ovaries, and in low levels in fat, liver, muscle, brain, normal and abnormal breast tissues. The production of residual estrogen production after menopause is solely from these non-glandular sources, particularly from subcutaneous fat. (This is the probable reason why obesity increases the risk for breast cancer in postmenopausal women.) Whereas menopause causes a 16-fold drop in the blood plasma levels of estrogen, menopausal breast tissue will exhibit concentrations of estrogen 10 times that found in blood plasma. This makes the breast the most likely tissue for estrogen-related tumors to emanate.

The first generation aromatase inhibitor, aminoglutethimide, previously used as an anticonvulsant, induced adrenal insufficiency, drowsiness and skin rashes. The newer versions were supposed to be milder, but the third-generation aromatase inhibitors were found to be three times more potent than aminoglutethimide! [Clinical Breast Cancer 1: 9-14S, 2000] Pharmaceutical aromatase inhibitors are "*remarkably potent*" at inhibiting aromatase activity. [Expert Opinion Investigative Drugs 12: 337-51, 2003] Letrozole (a

HEALTH EFFECTS OF LOW ESTROGEN	HEALTH EFFECTS OF HIGH ESTROGEN
→ Causes bone thinning (osteoporosis)	→ Maintains bone mineralization
→ Causes depressed mood	→ Maintains elevated mood
→ Promotes loss of moisture-holding hyaluronic acid (skin, eyes, joints, hair)	→ Sends "grow" signal to cells
→ May promote calcifications from calcium being released from bone (breast, arteries, heart valves, kidney stones, bone spurs)	→ Releases iron from carrier molecule; increases ability for iron to enter cells

Tamoxifen Currently about 1 million American women receiving Tamoxifen	Aromatase Inhibitors Under clinical investigation Femara (letrozole, Novartis) Aromasin (exemestane, Pharmacia) Arimidex (anastrozole, AstraZeneca)
Primary use: *"gold standard"* for treatment and recurrence of advanced breast cancer following surgery, chemo or radiation therapy.	Primary use: after 5-year Tamoxifen therapy or in place of Tamoxifen; combined or alternate use with Tamoxifen of no extra benefit; potential use as 1st preventive breast cancer drug; possible use for uterine fibroids, endometriosis, prostate cancer; not indicated for premenopausal women with breast cancer who have normal ovarian function nor for women with estrogen or progesterone-receptor-negative tumors.
Action: blocks entry of estrogen into cells; does not impair estrogen production. Increases fertility; evidence this drug acts as a pro-estrogen over time.	Action: inhibits aromatase enzyme required to produce estrogen; 3rd generation drugs more potent
Proposed benefits: heralded 49% reduction in invasive breast cancer is a relative number; in hard numbers, improvement in survival compared to no treatment, in hard numbers: 3.5% (The Lancet 339: 71-85, 1992) About 1 in 10 women will benefit from taking Tamoxifen; only 1% benefit among high-risk women when taken for prevention	Proposed benefits: prevents estrogen from being formed in the first place; prolongs remission after conventional breast cancer treatment, but no significant decrease in mortality rates
Active against estrogen-positive and negative breast tumors (different mechanisms)	Active against estrogen-positive tumors
Bone: Retains bone integrity because it does not impair estrogen synthesis	Bone: weakens bone due to loss of estrogen production
Side effects: • Claim is that *"benefits far outweigh the risks"* • Can only be taken for 5 years; then Tamoxifen resistance begins • Increases risk of uterine cancer; 400% increased-risk among women over 50; increase of 2 cases of uterine cancer per 1,000 women; increased risk of uterine sarcoma of 2 per 10,000 users; doctors often recommend surgical removal of uterus to eliminate this risk • Cataracts, retinal blindness • Migraines • Blood clotting, strokes • Hot flushes	Side effects: • Decreased mood • Headache, nausea, peripheral edema, fatigue, vomiting, indigestion, hot flushes and vaginal dryness. [Endocrine Related Cancer 6: 325-32, 1999] • Possible calcifications throughout the body including breast tissue

third- generation aromatase inhibitor) is such a strong estrogen inhibitor that only 1 mg is needed to produce an effect. [Annals Oncology 14: 62-70, 2003]

Strong inhibition of estrogen is likely to result in depressed mood. [Cell Molecular Neurobiology. 16:325-44, 1996; J Clinical Psychopharmacology 11: 121-26, 1991] The long-term effect of aromatase inhibitors on mood is unknown. Doctors are likely to dismiss this biological origin of depression and attribute it to psychogenic factors surrounding diagnosis and treatment. Therefore, many women undergoing cancer treatment with these drugs may be inappropriately placed on antidepressant drugs.

There is no question that aromatase inhibitors are going to replace Tamoxifen since they result in prolonged tumor regression. But the use of aromatase inhibiting drugs is not indicated for premenopausal women with breast cancer who have normal ovarian function, nor for women with estrogen or progesterone-receptor-negative tumors. [J Clinical Oncology 19: 2596-2606, 2001]

Many studies are now underway with aromatase inhibitor drugs. One study has been ongoing for the past seven years. Even though tumor regression is prolonged, absolute freedom from relapse *"appears to be very small so far, and no survival benefit has emerged."* [New England J Medicine 348: 2431-42, 2003] A more recent report, even when viewed in the most encouraging way, still only shows a mild benefit for aromatase inhibitors (8.0% recurrence of cancer on Tamoxifen, 4.6% for aromatase drugs, a 3.4% difference. [Journal National Cancer Institute 98: 86-87, 2006]

Below is data from a five-year study comparing survival with Tamoxifen compared to letrozole, an aromatase inhibitor. A slight edge goes to letrozole, but not enough to herald this as a breakthrough. What is missing from the chart below is whether overall survival (not just from breast cancer) was any better with this new class of drugs. Mortal side effects can alter the final analysis. The aromatase inhibitors may reduce recurrence of breast cancer but not have any effect upon death rates. [New England Journal Medicine 353:2747-57, 2005] The jury is still out on this new class of drugs, and women are participating in a giant experiment similar to hormone replacement therapy.

Aromatase inhibitors: side effects

Side effects, reported as mild in most studies, include headache, vaginal dryness, hot flashes and musculoskeletal pain, similar to those experienced with Tamoxifen. [New England J Medicine 348: 2431-42, 2003] There is a clear reduced risk of blood clots and uterine cancer with the aromatase inhibitors. However, one aromatase inhibitor, anastrozole (Arimidex), produces a higher incidence of musculoskeletal symptoms and fractures than reported with Tamoxifen. [Lancet 359: 2131-39, 2002] Arthritis is another prominent problem with aromatase inhibitors, caused by the lack of estrogen and the resultant decline in the production of hyaluronic acid, a joint-cushioning molecule. [Arthritis Rheumatism 52:2594-8, 2005]

Since aromatase inhibitors lower circulating estrogen levels to almost unrecordable levels in postmenopausal women, women taking them may experience rapid withering of their bones, and more fractures and face being bedridden. [British Journal of Cancer 93 Suppl 1:S16-22, 2005] The risk of fracture in the postmenopausal woman given aromatase inhibitors may be increased by up to 60%. [Journal Steroid Biochemistry Molecular Biology 95:151-4, 2005]

The importance of maintaining some estrogen production in the body is underscored by the report of a man who could not produce aromatase, had no detectable levels of estrogen and experienced rapid bone loss. In other words, widespread use of aromatase inhibitors could make osteoporosis a bigger epidemic among postmenopausal women than it is today. [Calcified Tissue International 59: 179-83, 1996]

Aromatase inhibitors in postmenopausal women also increase total serum cholesterol. [European J Cancer 37: 1510-13, 2001] Since sex hormones are made from cholesterol, the reduced estrogen synthesis facilitated by the aromatase inhibitors probably sends a signal to the liver to produce more cholesterol in an attempt to maintain youthful levels of hormones. [Med Hypotheses 59:751-6, 2002]

Aromatase inhibitors are being promoted not only for breast cancer treatment, but for uterine fibroids and endometriosis as well as male prostate cancer. [Cancer Investigations 19: 649-59, 2001]

Combinations of Tamoxifen and aromatase inhibitors have not been shown to be advantageous. [Forum 12: 45-59, 2002]

Since aromatase inhibitors strongly reduce production of estrogen, they may induce calcifications throughout the body. Low levels of estrogen apparently induce loss of calcium from bones which results in calcifications throughout the body, including the arteries and breast. [J Medical Screening 9: 38-39, 2002; Acta Pathology Microbiology Immunology Scandinavia 93: 13-16, 1985; Arteriosclerosis Thrombosis Vascular Biology 20: 1926-31, 2000; Atherosclerosis 34: 469-74, 1979] Of interest is a study where researchers noted that the rapid disappearance of calcifications in breast mammograms was indicative of the onset of breast malignancies. [British J Radiology 72: 3-8, 1999] This spontaneous resolution of calcifications in breast tissue could indicate a rise or resumption in estrogen production and thus a signal for tumors to grow. Hormone replacement therapy is associated with a lower incidence of calcifications in postmenopausal women. [British J Radiology 60: 457-58, 1987]

Should Women Switch From Tamoxifen to Raloxifene (Evista)?

Pharmaceutical companies hire some big publicity agencies, but there is no bigger publicity agent than the National Institutes of Health (NIH), which decided to preempt the planned summer release date for its study of two breast cancer drugs with a press release that extols the virtues of Raloxifene. [National Cancer Institute press release, April 17, 2006] The NIH study said that Tamoxifen reduces the risk for invasive breast cancer by about 50% (in hard numbers, it's a reduction of only about 1.2%) and that Raloxifene results in about the same reduction, with fewer side effects. According to the NIH press release, Raloxifene reduces the risk for blood clots in the legs (deep vein thrombosis) by about 29%, and the risk for uterine cancer by 36%. Forgotten is the evidence that high-dose vitamin D can reduce the overall risk for breast cancer by about 50%.

Now before women go running to their doctors to ask about Raloxifene, this data needs translation. If you were taking Tamoxifen and you switched to Raloxifene, an additional 13 out of 4,700 women would avoid uterine cancer, or 2/10th of one percent. In other words about 500 women would have to take Raloxifene for one additional woman to avoid uterine cancer. An additional 22 women out of 9,700 would avoid blood clots, or about 1 in 442 women taking the drug. Is this a breakthrough worthy of worldwide headlines? Hardly.

But the NIH had to drum up business for the drug companies. The National Cancer Institute's Dr. Worta McCaskill Stevens says, *"Not as many women have been participating in Tamoxifen therapy because of the side effects of the drug. So now women have a choice."*

"With Tamoxifen, it put women in a very difficult situation of balancing really scary problems," said Dr. Hope Rugo, director of breast oncology clinical trials at UC San Francisco. [Journal Immunology 175: 2666-75, 2005] *"Now you can take raloxifene. It may be that your risk of blood clots and uterine cancer is a little higher than if you didn't take anything at all, but it's markedly less than if you took Tamoxifen. You want to get a drug that is good and has less serious side effects, and we've definitely got that now."*

Wait, did Dr. Rugo say the risk for side effects was still higher, just not as high as Tamoxifen? Yep, that's what she said. The risk is elevated, but not as elevated as taking Tamoxifen. The risk reduction is miniscule. By sleight of hand with numbers, it makes it sound like Raloxifene is far safer. In fact, it's a very slight drop in side effects.

Since 1998 it has been known that Raloxifene (Evista) reduces the incidence of breast cancer by a reported 76%. But even that figure is specious. The Canada Drug Guide

Project explains Raloxifene this way:

> Raloxifene (Evista) reduces incidence of breast cancer by 76% with only a 1% risk of side effects. What it doesn't make clear is the fact that the patients who took the drug in the study went from having a 1% absolute risk of having breast cancer down to a 0.24% absolute risk of having breast cancer over three years (hence, the *"76%"* reduction). If measured in relative terms, many of the side effects increased much more than 76%–in fact some risks, such as those for blood clots, increased, relatively speaking, by 300%.

Both Tamoxifen and Raloxifene interfere with the human immune system, lowering the ability of healthy adults to ward off or treat existing breast cancer. [Journal Immunology 175: 2666-75, 2005]

Herceptin

The gene-targeted drug

Herceptin has been called the new hope for many women with breast cancer. An editorial published in the British journal Lancet in 2005, described the results of a study on Herceptin as *"simply stunning"* and *"revolutionary."* [Lancet 366:1673, 2005]

The author even went so far as to say that Herceptin *"may even be a cure"* for breast cancer. Naturally this comment was picked up and repeated across the world, fueling demand for rapid access to Herceptin. The excitement is premature. Comparisons (with other drugs) have been hampered by the omission of crucial overall and disease-free survival data, as well as information on cardio toxicity. It has been shown that Herceptin can precipitate severe heart failure in some patients.

Nevertheless, Herceptin has been approved for use in late-stage breast cancer in Britain. But pharmaceutical companies weren't able to make much money from the drug because patients who are considered to have late-stage breast cancer don't have long to live. Since 1998, it has been used to treat more than 230,000 breast cancer patients worldwide, all with late-stage disease. *The London Times* reports Herceptin will not cure the disease, *"but it may extend life by a couple of months, at best".* [*The London Times*, April 29, 2006] A debate then ensued over whether Herceptin can be used for earlier-stage disease.

In 2006, a terminal breast cancer patient lobbied health authorities for the right to use Herceptin. The High Court in Britain ruled that health authorities must pay for her care, including Herceptin. Advocates for the drug (mostly its maker) point to a study showing a 46% reduction in risk for recurrence of breast cancer after standard chemotherapy. The drug costs around $45,000 for a course of treatment. The woman who served to make a public example out of her plight said she believed refusal to provide Herceptin was a *"death sentence."* [British Medical Journal 332: 443, 2006] She is being hailed as a heroine today.

Here are the hard facts surrounding Herceptin:

- For every 100 patients with early breast cancer treated with Herceptin, only 3 will actually benefit (improvement in disease-free survival). [British Medical Journal 332: 727: 2006]
- In May of 2000, the manufacturer of Herceptin mailed a letter to doctors warning of 15 deaths and other adverse reactions associated with the use of the drug. [New York Times May 5, 2000]
- In a recent drug trial, 143 of 1,694 women (8.4 %) could not continue taking Herceptin due to side effects. [New England Journal Medicine 353: 1659-72, 2005]
- In one study, after 4 years the survival rate with chemotherapy plus Herceptin was 91.4% versus 86.6% (4.8% difference) with chemotherapy alone. While Herceptin was said to reduce the occurrence of metastases in distant organs, there was an increased incidence (up to 300%) of tumors that had spread to the brain. [New England Journal Medicine 353: 1673-84, 2005]

In 2001, a report showed that Herceptin (trastuzumab) improved survival over chemotherapy alone from 20.3 to 25.1 months. The most common side effect is heart failure which occurred in 27% of patients given chemotherapy plus Herceptin, which is more than double the rate for chemotherapy alone. [New England Journal Medicine 344: 783-92, 2001]

For the small percentage of women with HER-2 positive (genetically predisposed) breast cancer, (15-30% of cases), Herceptin appears to offer a slight improvement in survival – three to four months of added life, with the increased risk of heart failure, and thousands of dollars in costs. For the up to 30% of breast cancer patients who produce the HER2 protein, there is no explaining to them that such a drug could be withheld from use, even if it does increase the risk for mortal heart problems. [Globe and Mail, November 24, 2005]

The enthusiasm over Herceptin caused a woman in India sold her house to pay for Herceptin, not knowing she was buying a few more months of life at best.

Doctors continue to express misplaced enthusiasm for Herceptin. One doctor at Memorial Sloan Kettering Cancer Center said Herceptin was *"the biggest difference I've ever seen in stage IV disease."* Editorials in medical journals and news reports claim Herceptin is *"astounding," "jaw dropping,"* and *"revolutionary."*

"In 1991, I didn't know we would cure breast cancer, and in 2005, I'm convinced we have," said a doctor at the National Cancer Institute. In one study, 227 women developed recurrence of breast cancer after a year of chemotherapy whereas only 127 did when Herceptin was added to the regimen. These figures do not include those women who died of heart failure caused by the drug. Recurrence is one thing, survival is another.

After three years of follow-up, about 0.8% of women on chemotherapy experience heart failure compared to 4.1% with chemotherapy plus Herceptin.

It's difficult to imagine where the enthusiasm for Herceptin emanates from. Criticism has been raised over the use of Herceptin among women with less invasive forms of breast cancer. A British newspaper wanted to know why one top medical journal called Herceptin a cure, another said it was inadequate, while a third said, because of its cost, there should be a process for women to access such a highly effective drug. [Globe and Mail, Nov. 24, 2005]

The question arises, should a drug that reduces recurrence, but not necessarily mortality of breast cancer be approved for use even if it would bankrupt the public health system? This is the dilemma surrounding Herceptin, which costs from $35,000 to $50,000 for a year of treatment and reduces recurrence of breast cancer by 8% or 17% (hard numbers) according to two published studies.

An alternative to Herceptin appears to be oleic acid, a component of olive oil, which decreases the proteins produced by the breast cancer gene HER-2 by 36-46%, which is almost as strong as Herceptin, which reduces HER-2 proteins by 48%. [Annals Oncology 16: 358-71, 2005] Why isn't oleic acid called *"jaw dropping," "stupendous,"* and *"revolutionary?"*

One combined study showed that oleic acid plus Herceptin had a dramatic synergistic effect, reducing the HER-2 gene/protein by 70%. [Annals Oncology 16:359-71, 2005] Since resveratrol, a component of red wine, has been found to inhibit HER-2 in a manner similar to Herceptin [International Journal Cancer 115: 36-45, 2005], it would be interesting to measure the effect of resveratrol plus oleic acid/olive oil.

Breast Cancer Surgery - Mastectomy

The scenario is a familiar one: the surgeon exits the surgery suite, locates the patient's family, and promptly declares, *"I got it all."* It is difficult to understand the reasoning why surgeons carefully excise breast tumors with wide surgical margins. The spread of most breast tumors is via the blood circulation, not by direct extension of the tumor itself. Abnormal blood vessels grow out towards the tumor, they do not extend from the tumor. Most breast tumors aren't detectable until they can be felt by physical exam and thus have been developing for 7-9 years. By then, a small number of tumor cells have likely escaped into the blood circulation. [Treatment of Breast Cancer, Clinical Symposia, 49: 4-32, 1997]

In 2002, it was reported that women with small breast tumors (2 centimeters, or about 1 inch in size), who elected to undergo subsequent chemotherapy due to spread of the tumor to lymph nodes, experienced about the same survival rate whether they had a total mastectomy (breast removal) or a lumpectomy. [New England Journal Medicine 347: 1227-32, 2002]

Another report shows that women with tumors up to 2 inches (~4 centimeters) in size that had spread to the lymph nodes, experienced the same 20-year survival rate regardless of whether they had undergone mastectomy or lumpectomy. Additional radiation treatment reduced the occurrence of cancer occurring in the same breast from 40% to 14%. [New England Journal Medicine 347: 1233-41, 2002] But then again, recall the long-term side effects of radiation treatment cited above. Less cancer in the breast is traded for mortal side effects elsewhere.

Dr. Shahla Masood, editor-in-chief of *The Breast Journal*, recounts his experience with a 30-year-old mother who had undergone right-sided breast removal and who had come to his office for counsel. She was devastated by her appearance. Dr. Masood reviewed her medical records and found her breast tumor was less than 1 centimeter (half an inch) in size with no spread to lymph nodes. He questioned whether total mastectomy was the right decision for her. The patient responded by saying *"No one ever discussed any other treatment option with me following my cancer diagnosis."* [The Breast Journal 9: 69: 2003]

Even though 75-80% of newly diagnosed breast cancer patients have early-stage breast cancer and are eligible for lumpectomy, most women still undergo mastectomy.

Understand, oncologists were performing bone marrow transplants on women with breast cancer for years without knowing if they worked. When data became available that they may not be worthwhile, doctors continued performing bone marrow transplants. In 2000, insurers finally stopped paying for ineffective bone marrow transplants for women with breast cancer. The treatment was costing $100,000 per patient. [New York Times, Feb. 16, 2000]

Survival and chemotherapy

It is difficult to comprehend the disarray breast cancer care is in today. A report in the New York Times states: *"After years of adding more and more to the regimen – more drugs, shorter intervals between chemotherapy sessions, higher doses, longer periods of harsh therapy – doctors are now wondering whether many women could skip chemotherapy altogether."* Dr. Eric P. Winer, of the Dana-Farber Cancer Institute in Boston, says *"It's an uncomfortable time."* For women facing breast cancer, the uncertainty is agonizing. *"If the medical profession is not even close to being of one mind, how is the woman to know?"* asks Donald A. Berry, statistician at the University of Texas MD Anderson Cancer Center.

Doctors are likely to respond to this new study by saying to patients: *"Well, but just to be on the safe side, why don't we at least try one course of chemotherapy."* They leave treatment decisions in the patient's hands, and these uncertain patients generally elect to undergo more aggressive treatment.

Here is how oncologists justify chemotherapy for breast cancer. Young women who receive chemotherapy gain on average about 5.4 months of life, compared to those who do not elect chemotherapy. For older women, the benefit is smaller: just 2.9 months. [Lancet 358: 9278, 2001] It has been established, that for women in whom breast cancer has not spread to lymph nodes, the benefit of undergoing chemotherapy is less than 1%. [Breast Disease 21: 33-40, 2004]

There is long-term morbidity associated with chemotherapy. Women who receive chemotherapy for breast cancer may experience long-term memory impairment. [Cancer 85: 640-50, 1999]

It appears that for women with small estrogen-sensitive (estrogen positive) tumors and who are taking estrogen-blockers like Tamoxifen, chemotherapy may not show any added benefit because the estrogen-blocker is working effectively, at least for a period of time. Women with estrogen-negative tumors may theoretically benefit from chemotherapy. [Journal American Medical Assn 295:1658-1667, 2006] It is estimated that as many as 50% of women with breast cancer receive unnecessary chemotherapy treatments.

Dr. R.E. MacCormick of the Cape Breton Cancer Clinic at Dalhousie University in Nova Scotia, Canada, writes that chemotherapy is only a secondary treatment for breast cancer and while it claims a 30% improvement in long-term overall survival, it "*demonstrates significantly less absolute improvement.*" What Dr. MacCormick is saying is that chemotherapy is very harmful in itself. Long-term side effects include a decline in mental function, muscle and bone complications such as early onset of osteoporosis, premature aging of the skin and eyes as well as profound fatigue.

In one survey only 22% of cancer patients were satisfied with the information they had received about treatment benefits and side effects.
Source: Behavioral Medicine 23: 36-45, 1997

Dr. MacCormick concludes that chemotherapy accelerates the aging process. He says: "*Whereas short-term toxicity of chemotherapy can usually be considered acceptable even for a small improvement in survival, long-term toxicity and early onset of frailty can have an impact that lasts for years.*" [Medical Hypotheses March 16, 2006, online] Statistically, chemotherapy sounds goods. In practice, it lowers the quality of life and women struggle with its side effects for years. These side effects will then be attributed to heart disease or some other form of cancer rather than to the chemotherapy.

Treatment decision making

Surprisingly, as patients exert more control over the types of treatment they receive, studies show women more often elect to have more aggressive surgery that removes the entire breast even though survival rates are about the same for breast-conserving surgery. It is patients themselves who are a driving force behind aggressive treatment. The fear- factor predominates.

According to a survey published in the *Journal of Clinical Oncology,* 27% of women who said they made their own treatment decision, elected to undergo mastectomy compared to only 5.3% of women who said their surgeon made the decision. [J Clinical Oncology 23: 754-67, 2005]

Selection of surgeon

Patients treated by lower-volume surgeons tend to have a greater likelihood of undergoing mastectomy. [Health Services Research 36: 166-79, 2001]

Most patients who undergo breast cancer surgery are operated on by surgeons who perform fewer than 30 operations per year. The five-year survival rate of breast cancer patients is lower, by as much as 16%, when their surgery was done by a surgeon who performed only 15-30 operations annually. [Cancer 101: 1323-29, 2004] More experienced surgeons produce better survival outcomes. About

9 in 10 breast cancer operations are done by surgeons who perform fewer than 30 operations annually.

The milk duct caper

"Well, have I got cancer, or haven't I?"

Don't expect a clear answer to that question when it comes to Ductal Carcinoma In Situ (DCIS).

With the great amount of confusion that surrounds ductal carcinoma in situ, another problem has recently been revealed that doctors don't talk about. Tumor cells within the milk ducts of the breast that do not spread (noninvasive) are not likely to pose a threat to life. Doctors only become suspicious of cancer because of calcification and irregular appearance of mammograms. So they perform biopsies.

DCIS, by definition, cannot spread to the underarm lymph glands. The cells are trapped in the duct. So lymph gland removal is not indicated. But there is a prevalent idea that there are micrometastases (miniscule tumor cells, observed only under a microscope,) that have spread to the lymph glands.

Researchers conducted a study of 508 consecutive patients with pure DCIS of the breast who underwent lymph node biopsy, to determine if any tumor cells had spread or leaked from the milk duct. Most of the patients underwent conservative surgery (removal of the sentinel lymph nodes) and biopsy specimens were sent for conclusive analysis. Metastases were detected in only 9 of 508 (1.8%) patients. Eight patients underwent complete surgical lymph gland removal. In none of these patients did researchers find additional cancerous underarm lymph nodes. So the widespread practice of biopsy and surgical removal of lymph glands in DCIS patients is unsubstantiated. [Breast 14: 520-2, 2005]

When a more sophisticated tissue-staining method is used to detect invasive cancer in lymph node biopsies, the incidence of micro-metastases rises, but does not influence survival. [European Journal Surgical Oncology, March 25, 2006, online]

When the lymph nodes of women with DCIS are biopsied, surgeons often find noninvasive tumor cells or benign epithelial cells. These cells are displaced outside the milk ducts in the breast where they can then travel to the lymph nodes, to spread real cancer or give the false impression that invasion is occurring. This has given rise to the false notion that ductal carcinoma in situ "*may be a precursor rather than just an ambiguous risk factor for invasive breast cancer,*" and once that is established in the minds of oncologists, women will forever be over-treated and unduly frightened. [Cancer, April 10 2006 online]

Many women are inappropriately alarmed that they have invasive cancer and are subsequently prescribed radiation and other toxic therapies, when they have noninvasive, non-life threatening growths within their milk ducts, nothing more. [Journal Clinical Oncology 24: April 11, 2006 online] Doctors are manufacturing the appearance of disease where none exists. [Journal Clinical Oncology, April 10, 2006] How often this occurs, no one knows. One thing is for sure: more and more surgeons are carefully searching to find cancer cells that have spread from the breast to the lymph nodes.

Until 1980, DCIS represented only 1% of all newly diagnosed cases of breast cancer in the United States. There are now about 40,000 cases reported annually (or about 18% of all breast tumors) which are not counted as part of the 180,000 cases of invasive breast cancer diagnosed each year. Ductal carcinoma in situ represents only 7% of the breast tumors diagnosed in Japan. [Biomedical Pharmacotherapy 56 Suppl 1:182s-186s, 2002]

The hallmark sign of ductal cancer of the breast is calcifications shown in a mammogram. [Cancer Treatment Reviews 26: 103-25, 2000] About 1 in 1,300 mammograms reveal a ductal cancer, more often in younger women. [Journal National Cancer Institute 94: 1546-54, 2002] Most women who undergo lymph node biopsies are post-menopausal. However, younger women with ductal carcinoma in situ, are far more are likely to experience recurrence (26.1%) than are older women (8.6%). [New York Times Jan. 15, 2000]

Here is how one Mayo Clinic doctor explains microcalcifications in the breast:

"Calcifications are tiny deposits of calcium within the breast tissue that show up as white spots on a mammogram. Breast calcifications are common. Many women have at least one calcification that can be seen on a mammogram. Most breast calcifications aren't associated with cancer. But certain patterns of calcifications, such as tight clusters with irregular shapes, can be associated with cancer."

Noncancerous (benign) causes of breast calcifications include:

- Calcium within the fluid of a noncancerous cyst (milk of calcium)
- Calcifications associated with a dilated milk duct
- Previous injury to the breast (post-traumatic fat necrosis calcification)
- Inflammation due to infection (mastitis)
- Skin (dermal) calcifications such as caused by dermatitis or residue from metallic particles in powders, ointments and deodorants
- Radiation therapy for breast cancer
- Calcification of the arteries (vascular calcifications)
- Calcifications in a fibroadenoma, a noncancerous growth

If the microcalcifications appear suspect, your doctor will recommend a biopsy.

An online health encyclopedia provided by a health center says:

Macrocalcifications usually are degenerative changes in the breast resulting from old injuries, inflammations, or aging of the breast arteries and are usually not related to cancer. Most often they do not require a biopsy. Macrocalcifications occur in about half the women in the U.S. who are over 50, and in about 10% of women under the age of 50.
Microcalcifications are specks of calcium that may be found in an area of rapidly dividing cells. The residue left by rapidly dividing cells can appear as microcalcifications. When many are seen in a cluster, they may indicate a small cancer. About half the cancers detected appear as these clusters.

The question is, are microcalcifications cancer? Answer: no. Here are some typical responses from women who have been diagnosed with microcalcifications:

"My surgeon said I was riddled with cancer."

"Yes, it's definitely cancer."

"Well, I feel like I'm on some see-saw of medical incompetence."

"Why did my doctor recommend surgery for a pre-cancerous condition?"
Source: Health Expectations 5: 310-18, 2002

Investigators reviewed the treatment of 172 women with ductal carcinoma in situ, all of whom underwent biopsy, with 65% undergoing repeat biopsy. Surgery (lumpectomy) was performed in 18% of these women, radiation in 82%. Of the 172 patients, 15 (8.7 %) experienced a recurrence, and only one death was recorded over a 10-year period. [Annals Surgery 231: 235-45, 2000] The question is, was treatment responsible for the high cure rate? We don't know. Treatment may have had no effect. These women may not

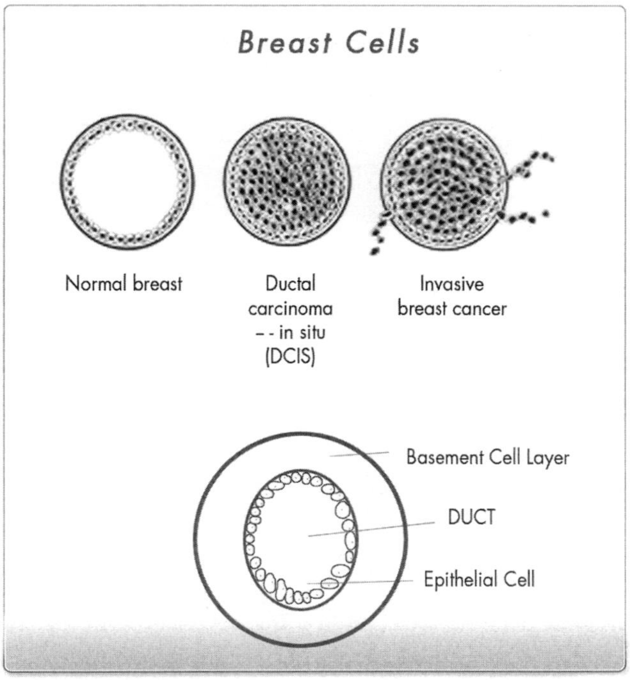

have had invasive breast cancer to begin with.

Studies show that only 16-20% of patients with ductal carcinoma in situ, as diagnosed by biopsy, will subsequently be diagnosed with invasive disease. [Radiology 202: 843-47, 1997] But does the biopsy itself provoke the invasiveness of the pre-tumorous condition?

Melvin J. Silverstein, MD, a Los Angeles physician, describes ductal carcinoma in situ of the breast as a *"surgeon's disease."* While DCIS represented only 1% of newly diagnosed breast disease decades ago, since the introduction of mammography it may represent 30-40% of the new cases that are treated. [Annals Surgical Oncology 6: 802-10, 1999]
Dr. Silverstein goes on to say that *"many patients with DCIS are in a state of terror after having been told that they have breast cancer."* But is DCIS really breast cancer? Yes, up to 40% of cases may develop into invasive breast cancer, but only after 25-30 years. Maybe 1 in 5 patients with DCIS will die of breast cancer. In Dr. Silverstein's experience with 803 patients with DCIS, the absolute mortality rate was less than 1% (5 died). Among, the DCIS patients who underwent mastectomy, none died and among those who underwent lumpectomy, 1.9% died.

Dr. Silverstein also says that the treatment of DCIS is based upon the size and appearance of breast tissue rather than its origins. *"With sufficient time, most noninvasive lesions will learn how to invade and metastasize. We must learn how to prevent this."* [Annals Surgical Oncology 6: 802-10, 1999]

Where does the calcium come from?

Where do calcium deposits originate from in women's breasts? Women with breast cancer are five times more likely to experience vertebral fractures. [British Journal Cancer 79: 1179-81, 1999] Calcifications of the mitral heart valves increase among women with osteoporosis. [American Heart Journal 147: 1113-16, 2004] The calcium being lost from the bones with the onset of menopause is being deposited in the breast.

The loss of estrogen production from the ovaries results in bone loss and deposition of calcium in distant organs. Breast calcification is normal in post-menopause. Bone mineral density is predictive of breast cancer in postmenopausal women. [Journal American Medical Association 276: 1404-08, 1996] Significantly increased levels of breast arterial calcification are observed among women who never have used hormone replacement. [Journal Medical Screening 9: 38-39, 2002] Postmenopausal women taking estrogen replacement experience a 14.6% increase in arterial calcium deposits annually compared to 22.3% among non-estrogen users. [Journal Women's Health 14: 410-17, 2005] Arterial and breast calcification often accompany each other. [Journal Medical Screening 9: 38-39, 2002]

Calcium-blocking drugs inhibit the entry of calcium into breast cancer cells. [Cell Calcium 22: 75-82, 1997] Vitamin D helps to regulate calcium inside cells and may represent *"a novel approach to the treatment and prevention of breast cancer."* [Endocrine 9: 321-27 1998]

Do breast microcalcifications ever disappear on their own? Yes, though this is rarely seen. Only 33 cases were found among 108,000 mammograms, one study reported. [British Journal Radiology 72: 3-8, 1999] But women who appropriately control their hormonal issues, such as Japanese women who obtain phytoestrogens from their diet, would likely be at less risk for DCIS.

Confused?
So's your doctor

Treatment decisions are difficult to make in a timely fashion when faced with breast cancer. Most patients rely on their doctors to help them make decisions. But do the doctors really know the best course of action? There is considerable disagreement among breast cancer specialists as to how to treat breast cancer. The *"easy"* way out is a mastectomy. Usually patients demand this surgical approach in the mistaken belief that this is the best way to ensure complete removal of cancer, but doctors comply with their requests too quickly.

A report in the New York Times reveals the state of confusion within the ranks of oncologists. [New York Times, May 12, 2006]

Facing little progress in survival times, doctors have been adding more drugs, increasing doses of chemotherapy, and shortening intervals between treatment sessions. Now they are wondering if more women should skip chemotherapy altogether.

Doctors now think chemotherapy is more appropriate for patients with non-hormone related (estrogen-negative) breast cancer, which is only about 30% of breast cancer patients. *"It's a slightly uncomfortable time,"* says a doctor who directs the breast oncology center at the Dana-Farber Cancer Institute in Boston
Gina Kolata, the New York Times health writer, says: *"For women with breast cancer, of course, the uncertainty is excruciating. Faced with a disease that already causes indecision and anxiety, they are now confronted with incomplete data, differing opinions from different doctors and a choice that can seem almost impossible: Should they give up a taxing treatment when all the answers are not in and they have what may be a fatal disease?"* [New York Times, May 12, 2006]

One university-based statistician asks: *"If the medical profession is not even close to being of one mind, how is the woman to know?"* Higher doses of chemotherapy have failed to prolong survival times. [Journal Clinical Oncology 22:2061-8, 2004]

Barbara Brenner, who has had breast cancer and is executive director of the advocacy group Breast Cancer Action, said, *"We finally tell people at the end of the day: 'You're going to get a lot of information. Trust your gut. Nobody has the answers."* But this kind of advice usually results in the decision to have a mastectomy.

Says one doctor who was interviewed for the New York Times article: *"Part of it is that this area of medicine we're practicing in is kind of a high wire act. It is more comfortable to adopt things that are aggressive."*

The frank truth is that most treatments for breast cancer were developed prior to the introduction of tests which can distinguish which patients have estrogen-positive (also called estrogen-sensitive) or estrogen-negative tumors.

Patients are being asked: *"Do you want to take something that is potentially toxic when you have a 90% chance of remission without it?"* One doctor responded to this question by saying: *"In my experience, more want to get chemo than not."*

But where are the ethics of the medical profession? Will doctors ever admit that there is ever any inappropriate or needless treatment? Or is all treatment OK as long as the patient elects to have it? Only when doctors begin refunding insurance payments for inappropriate or ineffective treatment will real reform within the ranks of physicians take place.

Imagine an automobile mechanic telling his customers: *"worn engine valves need to be removed and replaced, but to be on the safe side, maybe we should replace the whole engine."* That's what is going on daily in breast cancer clinics across the globe.

NUTRIENTS AND BREAST CANCER

Breast cancer and diet

Many women with breast cancer, or at risk for breast cancer, or recurrence of breast cancer, receive little if any counseling regarding their diet.

A survey of breast cancer patients in Finland found that about 9% of women believed diet contributes to the onset of breast cancer and 32% changed their dietary habits after diagnosis of breast cancer. The main reason for the dietary change was to be cured while others altered their diet to reduce painful symptoms of disease. The primary changes were a shift away from red meat, fat and sugar to consumption of fruit and vegetables. [European Journal Clinical Nutrition 54: 844-48, 2000]

An authoritative review published in 1997 concluded that low intake of vegetables increases the risk for breast cancer, but only in a very modest way. Researchers concluded then that the nutrients responsible for reduction of breast cancer risk *"remain elusive."* [Cancer Causes Control 7: 56-68, 1996]

Researchers appear puzzled, asking *"why only among postmenopausal women is increased breast cancer risk associated with either general obesity or abdominal obesity, and why is per capita fat intake related more to breast cancer incidence in postmenopausal than premenopausal women?"* [Breast Cancer Research Treatment 38: 239-46, 1996] Restriction of dietary fat for 10-22 weeks in healthy postmenopausal women is reported to reduce circulating estrogen levels by 17% on average. [Journal National Cancer Institute 82: 129-34, 1990]

In one study, lifelong vegetarians only showed a slight reduction in risk for breast cancer relative to lifelong meat-eaters. [International Journal Cancer 99: 238-44, 2002] It is true that vegetarian women excrete two to three times more estrogen in their feces than meat eaters and meat-eating women have about 50% higher plasma levels of estrogen compared to vegetarians. [Cancer Research 41: 3771-73, 1981]

Japanese women who move to the United States and consume western diets experience an increased risk for breast cancer within one generation. [Network 10: 1-2, 1989]

Breast Cancer Mortality And Sugar Consumption
Source: Medical Hypotheses 11: 319-27, 1983

	Mortality per 100,000 by age groups				
Country	35-44	45-54	55-64	65-74	Average grams sugar intake per day
Britain	23.0	64.7	96.9	122.2	131.8
Holland	20.7	56.5	94.2	117.6	125.1
Ireland	19.3	69.0	72.2	112.5	126.8
United States	16.9	51.0	83.0	98.9	133.7
Sweden	13.4	33.9	66.2	94.0	117.4
France	13.4	39.5	64.1	85.6	92.2
Italy	17.2	42.6	64.6	77.5	71.4
Greece	14.2	36.2	46.2	50.2	51.9
Japan	6.8	14.6	18.2	17.0	57.4

Researchers in Italy attempted to sort out which dietary or lifestyle factors can be attributed to breast cancer risk. The results of their study were as follows:

Lifestyle factors	breast cancer risk
High alcohol intake	10.7%
Low beta carotene intake	15.0%
Low vitamin E intake	8.6%
Low physical activity	11.6%

This still only explains about 40% of cases. [Journal National Cancer Institute 90: 389-94, 1998]

Other studies estimate dietary and lifestyle factors may be responsible for 33-55% of breast cancer cases. [Asia Pacific Journal Clinical Nutrition 11: S618-31, 2002]

What about survival? Once diagnosed with breast cancer, do women live longer if they consume more fruits and vegetables? The latest studies don't confirm the correlation between a plant-based diet and reduced risk of breast cancer. [Breast Cancer Research Treatment, March 15, 2006; Annals Epidemiology 15: 789-95, 2005]

Among women in Italy, high glycemic foods such as bread, cereal and sugar, along with iron/fat-rich foods such as pork, were associated with increased risk for breast cancer while vegetable oils (olive oil), raw vegetables, fish, beta carotene and vitamin E were associated with reduced risk. [Biomed & Pharmacotherapy 52: 109-115, 1998]

Sugar and breast cancer

There is a strong correlation between the incidence of breast cancer and diabetes and a strong link between breast cancer mortality and sugar intake. [Medical Hypotheses 11: 319-27, 1983]

The link between sugar and breast cancer has been known for a long time and has gone beyond being just a hypothesis. The question is, why don't most women attending breast cancer clinics ever hear, or have emphasized, the importance of sugar reduction in their diet?

One wonders if women, after diagnosis of breast cancer, don't alter their diet, reduce refined sugar intake, and experience prolonged remission from disease, which is mistakenly attributed to their treatment (surgery, radiation, Tamoxifen)?

In Italy, the diets of more than 2,500 women were analyzed and it was found that sugary foods were associated with a small increased risk for breast cancer. [Annals Oncology 17: 341-45, 2006] A study of 49,000 Canadian women produced similar findings. [International Journal Cancer 114: 653-58, 2005]

The provision of Metformin, an anti-diabetic drug, has been shown to be moderately helpful in prolonging the life (by 8%) of animals with breast cancer. [Experimental Gerontology 40: 685-93, 2005]

Milk

There are concerns that milk or dairy products may increase the risk for breast cancer. One concern is that milk is produced from pregnant and lactating cows. Their milk is markedly high in estrogen and progesterone. [Medical Hypotheses 65: 1028-37, 2005]

A review of 52 published studies does not confirm the notion that cow's milk raises the risk for breast cancer. [Journal American College Nutrition 24: 556-68S, 2005] A 25-year study of women in Finland found milk drinking was associated with a reduced risk for breast cancer. [British

Journal Cancer 73: 687-91, 1996] The fortification of milk with vitamin D may actually counter any cancer-promoting effects of cow's milk.

Second, cow's milk has growth factors, in particular, insulin-like growth factor-I (IGF-I). Serum IGF-I levels rise by about 10% among milk drinkers. IGF-1 may not be related to breast cancer risk, but rather to breast cancer growth. [Journal Womens Health Gender Based medicine 8: 1265-72, 1999] With consumption of high glycemic foods, IGF levels are raised, which may spur the growth of breast cancer cells. [Cancer Epidemiology Biomarkers Prevention 12: 573-77, 2003]

A hidden cancer-causing factor in cow's milk may be Mycobacterium Paratuberculosis, which is found in 2.5% of milk cartons in stores. [Journal Food Protection 68: 966-72, 2005] Pasteurization doesn't kill this germ. *Mycobacterium paratuberculosis* is associated with the formation of cysts in the body. Younger women who have breast cysts are six times more likely to develop breast cancer. [Lancet 353: 1742-45, 1999] Para-TB is also found in cheese curds. [Molecular Cells Probes March 15, 2006]

Fats

A number of studies do not show a link between high dietary fat consumption and breast cancer. [Cancer 61: 181-85, 1988] High intake of dietary fat is associated with higher blood levels of estrogen in postmenopausal women. [Journal Nutrition 135: 2862-65, 2005] A 5% increase in dietary fat has been shown to raise estrogen levels by about 12%. [Journal Nutrition 135: 2862-65, 2005]

Intake of animal fat, particularly from red meat and high-fat dairy foods, is modestly related to breast cancer risk in premenopause. [J National Cancer Institute 95: 1079-85, 2003] However, the Nurses Health Study, comprised of 44,000 women, could find no increase in the rate of breast cancer with greater intake of dietary fat of any type, among postmenopausal women. [Cancer Epidemiology Biomarkers Prevention 11:261-5, 2002; Journal American Medical Assn 281:914-20, 1999]

Weight of breast tumors in rodents given various oils in their diet
Source: British Journal Surgery 76: 1069-73, 1989

Type of oil	Weight of tumor
No oils added to diet	270 mg
Olive oil	212 mg
Evening primrose oil (omega-6)	133 mg
Fish oil	70 mg

Breast cancer growth rate in animals given omega-3 and omega-6 oils
(66% reduction in growth with omega-3 oil)

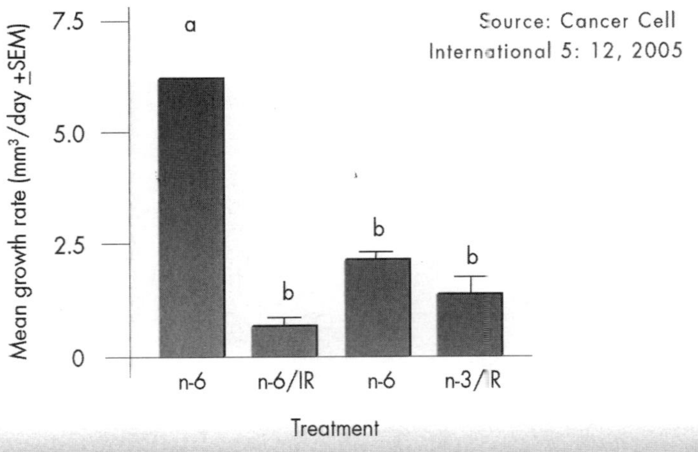

Initially, it was thought that reduction of dietary fat from 38 to 22% of total calories would increase disease-free intervals or 5-year survival rates for postmenopausal breast cancer patients. But researchers later recalculated and suggested fat intake be reduced to 15% of total calories. [Nutrition Cancer 19: 1-10, 1993] This is such a low-fat diet it would leave most women yearning for fatty foods and push them into such low circulating hormone levels that they would experience mental depression.

The most recent study did not find that dietary fat was related to the invasiveness of breast cancer. [Journal American Medical Assn 295: 629-42, 2006]

A survey comparing breast cancer patients with healthy family members found vegetable oils and fat were associated with reduced risk for breast cancer among premenopausal women and consumption of carbohydrates and sweetened beverages increased risk. [Breast Cancer Research Treatment 42: 243-51, 1997]

A diet rich in the trace mineral selenium, indole-3 carbinol from cruciferous vegetables, and lycopene from red vegetables like tomatoes and watermelon, have been recommended to enhance DNA repair in susceptible individuals with BRCA gene mutations.
However, this would require the consumption of two glasses of tomato juice and two pounds of cruciferous vegetables per day. [Cancer Causes Control 16:125-38, 2005] Similarly, omega-3 oils from flaxseed or fish beneficially control genes and prevent breast cancer. [Advances Experimental Medicine Biology 375: 85-95, 1995] Dietary supplements would be a more practical way of reaching these protective intake levels.

Oils

Consumption of unsaturated vegetable oils is associated with lower risk for breast cancer. [Lancet 347: 1351-56, 1996]

Time after time, laboratory experiments have been conducted to show that omega-6 oils (corn oil is the predominant omega-6 oil in the American diet) promote growth of breast cancer cells while omega-3 oils inhibit their growth. Olive oil also inhibits tumor cell growth. [Breast Cancer Research Treatment 86: 225-35, 2004]

Breast cancer growth rate in animals given omega-3 and omega-6 oils (66% reduction in growth with omega-3 oil). Source: Cancer Cell International 5: 12, 2005

An intriguing study of breast cancer was performed in animals at Michigan State University Department of Food Science and Nutrition. Rodents had breast cancer cells implanted in their breast tissue and then were given either corn oil (omega-6 is predominant), fish oil (rich in omega-3 with some omega-6), or either oil plus antioxidants (vitamin E). There was greater suppression of breast tumor growth in animals given fish oil versus corn oil, but the effect was erased when antioxidants were co-administered. [Lipids 28: 827-32, 1993] Fish oil plus chemotherapy may further inhibit tumor growth. [Nutrition & Cancer 51: 178-83, 2005]

The lesson here might be that oxidation kills cancer cells, fish oil induces oxidation, but vitamin E as an antioxidant counters this cancer-cell killing activity. High doses of antioxidants like vitamin E may prevent breast cancer, but once cancer growth has started, and omega-3 oils are employed, their benefit is negated by vitamin E, which is not selective in which cells it spares from oxidative damage. Human studies appear to confirm that high-dose supplemental vitamin E may raise the risk for breast cancer compared to dietary doses. [Breast 12:128-35, 2003]

Dietary Factors Among Japanese Women's Low Incidence of Breast Cancer

- Seaweed consumption (source of iodine, selenium)
- Fermented sources of soy (miso, tofu for phytoestrogens)
- Fish (omega-3 oils, selenium, iodine)
- Low-calorie diets
- Low sugar intake

Vitamin E should not be mischaracterized as a cancer-promoting nutrient. It strongly inhibits breast cancer. [Journal Nutrition 134(12 Suppl): 3458S-3462S, 2005] Both forms of vitamin E, tocopherols and tocotrienols, inhibit breast cancer. [Frontiers Bioscience 10: 699-709, 2005] Vitamin E may inhibit estrogen-positive cell growth by altering the cellular response to estrogen. [Annals Internal Medicine 138: 168-75, 2003]

Vitamin E is not entirely contraindicated during courses of chemotherapy. Vitamin E counters some of the side effects of chemotherapy. [Cancer 101: 1058-64, 2004] For example, vitamin E supplements may prevent nerve damage caused by chemotherapy. [Neurology 64: 26-31, 2005]

Vitamin E supplement use only modestly improves survival or limits recurrence of breast cancer, but this is in the face of toxic treatment. [Nutrition & Cancer 46:15-22, 2003] The point here is that supplemental vitamin E doesn't appear to raise mortality risk among patients being treated for breast cancer.

In breast cancer prevention, the ratio of omega-3 to omega-6 may be more important than the total omega-3 oils provided. [Preventive Medicine 16: 493-502, 1987] Low-dose omega-3 oil is believed by some researchers to be more useful in cancer prevention than treatment. [Oncology 53: 398-405, 1996] High-dose omega-3 oil is appropriate for treatment of breast cancer.

Fiber

In regard to fiber intake, there are both reports showing that it reduces the risk of breast cancer and reports stating that it is ineffective in regard to breast cancer risk.

One rationale for fiber is that it may reduce insulin resistance and levels of estrogen. [European Journal Clinical Nutrition 61: 573-77, 1997] A high-fiber diet might reduce circulating estrogen levels by reducing the liver recirculation of estrogen. [British Journal Cancer 73: 557-9, 1996]

Alcohol and breast cancer

The elevated risk for breast cancer among alcohol drinkers is modest at best and actually declines with about 3 glasses of wine(per day), but rises with excessive consumption (6 or more drinks per day). The very high consumption of alcohol combined with low intake of folic acid produces the greatest risk for breast cancer among drinkers compared to abstainers. [British Medical Journal 331: 807, 2005; Preventive Medicine 17: 683-85, 1988] The lower risk of breast cancer among moderate wine drinkers could be explained by the resveratrol in wine. [Pathophysiology 10:83-92, 2004; American Journal Surgery 180:357-61, 2000]

Estrogen replacement and alcohol

It appears that estrogen replacement and alcohol may be a deadly combination. Researchers in Sweden found a 5.6 times increased risk for lobular breast cancer and 6.5 times increased risk for tubular cancer, and 2.3 times increases risk for ductal cancer, with 5 or more years of use of estrogen-progestone therapy. [Breast Cancer Research 8: R11, 2006] This study means that millions of female alcohol drinkers are literally creating a recipe for breast cancer when they are on estrogen replacement therapy.

Alcohol appears to increase the percentage of women who develop estrogen-sensitive (estrogen-positive) breast tumors. [Journal National Cancer Institute 97: 1601-08, 2005]

Alcohol works by another pathway to promote breast cancer. Both the Iowa Women's Health Study (1992) and the Nurses' Health Study (1995) found that only women who consume alcohol exhibit an increase risk for breast cancer when taking estrogen replacement. The blood levels of estrogen rises by as much as 300% in a postmenopausal woman who takes estrogen replacement and consumes alcohol. [Journal Clinical Endocrinology Metabolism 82:2378, 1997]

Barnett Zumoff, MD, of Beth Israel Medical Center in New York, writes that estrogen is inherently capable of promoting the growth of breast cancer, and therefore of increasing the incidence of clinical breast cancer but large doses are needed to produce this effect. Estrogen replacement therapy provides only about the same amount of estrogen as produced naturally by the ovaries in premenopause. Alcohol plus estrogen replacement results in the elevation of circulating estrogen levels. Eliminating or minimizing alcohol intake and diminishing changes in estrogen by consumption of cruciferous vegetables (indole-3-carbinol) can theoretically reduce the risk for breast cancer. [Proceedings Society Experimental Biology Medicine 217:30-7, 1998]

Alcohol, folic acid and breast cancer

Higher folic acid intake reduces the risk of developing estrogen receptor negative breast cancer. Ensuring adequate folate (folic acid) intake seems particularly important for women at higher risk of breast cancer because of alcohol consumption. [Cancer Epidemiology Biomarkers Prevention 14: 2004-8, 2005]

The risk of breast cancer is slightly elevated among alcohol drinkers who consume less than 300 mcg of folic acid per day. The elevated risk disappears among women who consume more than 400 mcg of folic acid per day. [European Journal Clinical Nutrition 60: 280-06, 2006] Dark-green, leafy vegetables, oranges, orange juice, asparagus, beans, eggs and fortified foods (cereal) are good dietary sources of folic acid, though most adults will benefit from taking a supplement since this vitamin is destroyed by heat during cooking. [American Journal Clinical Nutrition 28:459-64, 1975]

There is a relative 59% increased risk for breast cancer among women who consume alcohol and have low intake of folic acid. Use of a multivitamin that contains folic acid along with other B vitamins has been shown to decrease the risk for breast cancer. [Journal American Medical Assn 281: 1632-37, 1999]

Alcohol also may induce a shortage of vitamin B12 which can increase the risk for breast cancer. [European Journal Clinical Nutrition 58: 1518-24, 2004] A vitamin B12 deficiency is now considered a risk factor for breast cancer. [Nutrition Reviews 57: 250-60, 1999]

Studies show that folic acid deficiencies are related to estrogen-negative breast cancer, but not estrogen-positive breast cancer. The primary group found to develop estrogen-negative breast cancer is women who drink alcohol and have low intake of folic acid. [Cancer Epidemiology Biomarkers Prevention 14: 2004-08, 2005] What seems very odd here is that women treated for estrogen-negative breast cancer in one breast, usually with surgery, chemotherapy and/or radiation, may never be advised by their doctors to limit alcohol intake and take folic acid supplements. This is all part of the strange disconnect between scientific findings involving cancer prevention, and the lack of interest shown by those who deliver treatment.

Alcohol and DNA

Researchers have unraveled the mechanisms and steps involved in the development of breast cancer. DNA strands in breast cells are broken by free radicals (species of oxygen that are destructive). For example, mutations in the DNA genetic material can be produced by alcohol and alcohol also increases the absorption of iron from foods. The combination of iron plus free radicals damage DNA, and promote mutations that result in cells becoming abnormal. [Free Radical Biology Medicine 26: 348-54, 1999]

Wine and breast cancer

While wine does contain antioxidants known as polyphenols, including resveratrol which is a potent anti-cancer agent, the consumption of wine does not reduce the risk for breast cancer over and above the consumption of any other alcoholic beverage. However, the consumption of grapes, which also provides resveratrol, significantly reduces the risk for breast cancer. [European Journal Cancer Prevention 14: 139-42, 2005]

Plant estrogens (phytoestrogens) and breast cancer

Effect of Digitalis on Breast Cancer Recurrence, Spread and Death Rate		
	Digitalis Users	Non-digitalis users
1982 study: recurrence or spread of breast cancer	1 in 40 (2.5%)	21 of 88 (24%)
1999 study: death rate from breast cancer	2 of 32 (6%)	46 of 143 (32%)

Most women are warned away from plant estrogens as soon as they are diagnosed with breast cancer. This is because plant estrogens (called phytoestrogens) may interfere with Tamoxifen, the most often-used drug for breast cancer. [Cancer Research 65: 879-86, 2005] This is understandable, since Tamoxifen is an anti-estrogen and phytoestrogens are mild estrogens.

However, studies show there is no evidence that plant estrogens increase the risk for breast cancer. [International J Fertility Womens Medicine 50:250-8, 2005] The only study that had to be halted because of the discovery of a risk to promote breast cancer was for hormone replacement therapy, not for any plant estrogen supplement.

Women who consume soy and flax have less dense breast tissue. [European J Medical Research 10: 389-94, 2005]

One of the puzzling problems posed by analysis of the myriad studies involving phytoestrogens like soy in relation to breast cancer is the obvious contradiction in terms. On the one hand, pooled analysis of studies shows soy intake may be associated with only a small reduction in breast cancer risk. [Journal National Cancer Institute 98: 459-71, 2006] However, many studies show that consumption of soy and other plant estrogens in the diet is very low in Western populations. [Journal Nutrition 131: 1826-32, 2001] Low intake should equal minimal prevention.

Asian populations that consume large amounts of soy obtain a 17-73% reduction in risk for breast cancer. [European Journal Cancer Prevention 11: 519-22, 2002]

Concern has arisen over the potential detrimental effect of soy in breast cancer patients because of estrogen-like effects. [Journal Nutrition 131: 3095-3108, 2001] However, women in Asia do not consume soy burgers, cereal and milk as do Western populations. They consume fermented sources of soy, like tempeh and miso, which concentrate the estrogen-like molecules. An important study conducted in Japan shows that increasing consumption of miso soup but not other soy foods confers a decreased risk for breast cancer. [Journal National Cancer Institute 95: 906-13, 2002] Fermented sources of soy have more anti-cancer properties. [Journal Agriculture Food Chemistry 41: 1961-67, 1993]

One study showed women in Japan who ate tofu were more likely to develop breast cancer, but this type of study must be discounted since women at high risk are known to consume more tofu. [Journal National Cancer Institute 95: 1881, 2003] There may be no cause and effect relationship here.

Dual role of plant estrogens

A common mistake made by cancer doctors and nurses is their communicated fear that plant estrogens promote cancer growth. But plant estrogens act both as estrogen and anti-estrogens. [Oncology Reports 6: 1383-87, 1999] Phytoestrogens are very weak, about [illegible],000th the activity of natural estrogen, with resveratrol exhibiting 1/7,000th the activity of estrogen. Furthermore, while plant estrogens may promote tumor cell growth in lab dishes, they may not in the body. Resveratrol has been shown to exhibit no breast cancer promotional effects. [Journal Steroid Biochemistry Molecular Biology 94: 431-43, 2005] A recent study shows that flaxseed inhibits any potential growth-stimulating effect of soy protein, and therefore may be a superior source of phytoestrogens. In animals that had their ovaries removed, soy initially inhibited and then stimulated breast cancer cell growth, in a manner similar to Tamoxifen. However, the combination of flaxseed and soy did not stimulate breast cancer growth. [International Journal Cancer March 23, 2006 online]

Digitalis and breast cancer

An interesting group of studies come to light. Digitalis is a drug often prescribed for heart failure. Digitalis is a molecule of similar structure to estrogen. A study performed in 1979 showed that women with breast cancer taking digitalis experienced nearly a 10 times decreased risk for recurrence or spread of their cancer compared to women not taking digitalis. Only 1 woman among 40 taking digitalis experienced recurrence or metastasis versus 21 out of 88 among non-digitalis users. [The Lancet, June 2, 8127, 1196-97, 1979; New England Journal Medicine, Feb. 25, 1982] A more recent long-term study of 175 patients over a period of 22 years found only a 6% death rate among 32 women with breast cancer versus a 34% death rate among the remaining patients. This is almost a 600% difference! [Oncology Reports 6: 493-96, 1999] If interpreted correctly, it means that modern medicine is overlooking one of the most potent weapons against breast cancer in favor of Tamoxifen, a drug that turns against women over time, increasing their risk for death.

Alternative to hormone replacement: phytoestrogens

Hormone replacement therapy during menopause is only utilized by 8-10% of eligible women, mostly due to concern over health risks. Furthermore, there is no proven drug that women in their fertile years can take to ward off future breast cancer. So the door is wide open for plant estrogens, called phytoestrogens, to be self employed by American women. No question, many American women are increasing their consumption of soy, flax and other plant foods, primarily for health reasons. In addition to the widely advertised herbal phytoestrogens, the diet has some natural ones. Green beans, alfalfa sprout, mung bean sprout and kudzu root also exhibit estrogenic properties. [J Agriculture Food Chemistry 51: 2193-99, 2003]

Women are trying extracts of black cohosh, red clover, vitex, dong quai and a host of other plant estrogens in an attempt to beat the sometimes difficult symptoms of menopause.

Generally speaking, phytoestrogen extracts in pill form all deliver about 50-100 mg of active ingredient. Doses below 2 mg per kilogram of body weight are considered safe. Thus, a 100-pound female could safely consume up to 90 mg, a 160-pound female up to 145 mg and a 200-pound female up to 180 mg of plant estrogen extract. [British Journal Nutrition 89: 898-906, 2003]

Plant estrogens reduce the number and intensity of hot flashes by a modest 10-20 %. [J Nutrition 133: 1983-86S, 2003] That's not enough to be considered reliable. However, one recent study found that flaxseed (40 grams a day) reduced symptoms of menopause equivalent to hormone replacement therapy. However, another study found flaxseed reduces menopausal symptoms by 60-70 %. [Obstetrics Gynecology 100:495-504, 2002]

Researchers point out the lack of studies to indicate proper dosage, and to identify the active ingredients in herbal products for hormone replacement or cancer prevention, is a major drawback of these natural remedies. [International Journal Fertility Womens Medicine 48: 64-68, 2003]

In a landmark study published in 1997, researchers obtained urine and blood samples from women who were newly diagnosed with breast cancer and compared them with healthy women in regard to plant estrogen levels. Among the soy plant estrogens (genistein, daidzen and equol) and the lignans from fiber-rich foods like rye and flax (enterodiol, enterolactone and matairesinol), only equol from soy and enterolactone from flax were associated with substantial risk reduction for breast cancer. [Lancet 350: 990-94, 1997]

BLACK COHOSH

Black cohosh is an herb widely used in Europe and marketed in the United Staes under the brand name Remifemin.

Standardized extracts of black cohosh (Remifemin) have demonstrated an ability to reduce postmenopausal complaints and are also useful for women who have undergone hysterectomy. [Alternative Therapy Health Med 7: 93-100, 2001] Black cohosh appears to improve complaints surrounding the monthly cycle. [J Steroid Biochemical Molecular Biology 83: 133-47, 2002]

However, a study published in 2001, did not find that women who had completed breast cancer treatment experienced a reduction of hot flashes when taking black cohosh. [J Clinical Oncology 19: 2739-45, 2001]

Approximately 30% of women experience menstrually-related migraine attacks. The provision of soy, black cohosh or dong quai extracts has been shown to relieve symptoms and reduce frequency of these attacks. [Biomed Pharmacotherapy 56: 283-88, 2002]

The current recommended dose of black cohosh is 40-80 mg per day. A popular commercial extract of black cohosh, Remifemin, provides 20 mg per pill. Weight gain, nausea, vomiting, headaches and dizziness have been reported as side effects. [Nutrition Clinical Care 5: 283-89, 2002] Gastrointestinal upset and rashes are the most common among the few reported side effects from black cohosh. [Menopause 10: 58-64, 2003]

Surprisingly, even though this herb is classified among the phytoestrogens, recent studies have not confirmed it has estrogen-like properties. Since 1985 it has been believed that an isoflavonone called formononetin in black cohosh is responsible for its mechanism of action. But a recent laboratory analysis has been unable to detect formononetin in samples of this herb. [Phytomedicine 9: 461-67, 2002] A study conducted in Austria confirmed the estrogen-like activity of soy and red clover, but not black cohosh. [J Steroid Biochemistry Molecular Biology 84: 259-68, 2003] One report says that while biological action of black cohosh may involve estrogen effects, *"new data dispute the estrogen theory and indicate that extracts of black cohosh do not bind to the estrogen receptor, up-regulate estrogen-dependent genes, or stimulate the growth of estrogen-dependent tumors in animal models."* [Nutrition Reviews 61: 183-86, 2003] Non-estrogenic components of black cohosh are believed to relieve symptoms of menopause and lower doses (~40 mg) appear to work as well as higher doses (~125 mg). [J Womens Health Gender Based Medicine 11: 163-74, 2002]

When black cohosh is combined with Tamoxifen, it appears to enhance the anti-estrogen effects of the drug. [Breast Cancer Research Treatment 76: 1-10, 2002]

A recent review declared black cohosh to be relatively safe. [Menopause 10: 58-64, 2003] Black cohosh also appears to be safe for women to use during menopause. [Breast Cancer Research Treatment 76: 1-10, 2002]

Despite its widespread use in Europe, a review of four studies involving black cohosh extract did not yield *"compelling evidence"* for this herb as a hormone-replacement agent in menopause. [European J Clinical Pharmacology 58: 235-41, 2002]

While available evidence on the effects of plant estrogens in regards to breast cancer is contradictory, extracts from black cohosh have been shown inhibit the growth of breast cancer cells. [J Steroid Biochemical Molecular Biology 80: 125-30, 2002] Components of black cohosh also serve as antioxidants and may help protect DNA from damage. [J Agriculture Food Chem 50: 7022-28, 2002] However, one researcher recently gave mice bred to develop breast cancer the human equivalent dose of black cohosh. These mice were more than twice as likely to develop breast tumors and for the tumors to spread to the lung. American Association Cancer Research, Vicki Davis, Mylan School of Pharmacy, Duquesne University, Reuters July 12 2003] But this is an unpublished study and various methods (MTT tetrazolium assay) of testing for growth in breast cancer cells may produce false positive results. Thus, until the method of testing can be scrutinized, this recent report must be withheld from evidence used to judge black cohosh. [Planta Medica 68: 445-48, 2002]

Bottom line: black cohosh is probably safe to use for symptoms of PMS and menopause. The reported skin rashes appear to be similar to side effects reported with the first-generation aromatase inhibitors. The contrary results surrounding black cohosh in regard to growth of breast cancer cells raise questions as to the validity of the testing.

A recent report states that "*evidence from in vitro, animal and clinical studies all suggest that black cohosh is a safe, herbal therapy for menopausal women if taken for a limited period.*" [Expert Opinion Drug Safety 3:615-23, 2004]

CHASTEBERRY (Vitex)

This fruit extract from a shrub native to west Asia and southwestern Europe has been traditionally used for thousands of years to quell symptoms involving menstrual difficulties. In a study of 1,634 patients, a remarkable 93% reported a decrease in the number of premenstrual symptoms, with no serious side effects. [J Womens Health Gender Based Med 9: 315-20, 2000]

DONG QUAI

Dong quai is an herbal phytoestrogen from China. It is not as popular as red clover, soy or black cohosh.

Dong quai may thin the blood, induce skin light sensitivity, and induce abnormal heart rhythm. It should not be used with blood thinners. [Pharmacotherapy 19: 870-76, 1999] Like red clover, because of its potential to over-thin the blood or interfere with drugs, its widespread use may be unwise.

In one study, dong quai and ginseng induced the growth of human breast cancer cells in a laboratory dish, while black cohosh and licorice root did not. [Menopause 9: 145-50, 2002]

RED CLOVER

Red clover extract, widely marketed in the United States as Promensil or Rimostil, has been shown to reduce hot flushes among menopausal women. [Maturitas 42: 187-93, 2002] However, a recent study of Rimostil (57 mg plant estrogens) and Promensil (82 mg plant estrogens) did not provide evidence that it relieved hot flushes among postmenopausal women experiencing 35 or more hot flushes per week. [J American Medical Assn 290: 207-14, 2003]

Red clover does not seem to have a protective effect upon uterine tissue. [Menopause 8: 338-46, 2001]

Red clover has a higher affinity to block androgens and progesterone receptors than do soy products. For comparison, black cohosh exhibits very little if any ability to block androgens and progesterone. [J Steroid Biochemical Molecular Biology 84: 259-68, 2003; Reproductive Fertility Development 13: 325-29, 2001]

A test conducted in Australia shows that red clover extract taken in doses ranging from 28 to 85 mg per day significantly raised HDL cholesterol and improved bone mineral density by 4.1%. [Menopause 8: 259-65, 2001]

However, in another study, an 86-mg extract of red clover was not found to exhibit cholesterol-lowering properties. [British Journal Nutrition 89: 467-74, 2003] But while red clover may or may not alter cholesterol profiles, it appears to improve the elasticity of large arteries and prevent high blood pressure. [J Clinical Endocrinology Metabolism 84: 895-98, 1999]

Molecules called coumarins in red clover raise concerns over blood clotting effects. [Atherosclerosis 152: 143-37, 2000; Menopause 8: 333-37, 2001] For this reason, widespread use of red clover extract may not be wise. When millions of women are likely to be involved, the potential for side effects, particularly serious ones like blood clotting problems, must be almost nonexistent.

SOY PHYTOESTROGENS

Phytoestrogens from soy (genistein, equol, daidzein) are widely promoted as cancer fighters. Much more can be said about soy than in this short report. Suffice to say that there is a royal battle going on in scientific circles over the use of soy to combat symptoms of menopause and prevent breast cancer.

There is also cause for concern. Soy phytoestrogens may stimulate growth of breast cancer cells under certain circumstances. [Journal Nutrition 133: 1983-86S, 2003] But is this concern pose a real threat?

A world authority on soy, Mark Messina, says *"the available data justify the recommendation that patients with frequent hot flushes consider trying soy foods or isoflavone supplements for the alleviation of their symptoms."* [J Med Food 6: 1-11, 2003] However, another researcher (MS Kurzer) from the University of Minnesota writes that *"until safety with respect to breast cancer is established, phytoestrogen supplements (like soy) should not be recommended."* [J Nutrition 133: 1983-86S, 2003] Other researchers in Finland say *"no negative effects of soy on breast cancer have been observed"* and that soy may be *"slightly protective"* against breast cancer. [J Steroid Biochemical Molecular Biology 83: 113-18, 2002]

Soy provides a unique combination of estrogen-like molecules, iron binders (IP6 phytic acid), and a small amount of omega-3 oils, only exceeded in quantity by flaxseed oil in nature, all three of which are anti-breast cancer agents. [J Nutr. 130: 820-6, 2000; Am J Clin Nutr 51:809-14, 1990] The importance of this triad in the prevention of breast cancer will be described more fully below.

A remarkable study has recently been published which sheds light on why there may be variability in the rates of breast and prostate cancer among populations that consume significant amounts of phytoestrogens. Japanese researchers found no protective effects from soyfoods among 21,852 Japanese females age 40-59 years. However, researchers did discover a marked reduction in breast cancer risk with increasing consumption of miso soup, which is made from soybean paste. The incidence of breast cancer dropped from 109.7 to 57.2 per 100,000 Japanese women when they increased their miso soup consumption from one to three cups a day. [Journal National Cancer Institute 95: 906-13, 2003] It is obvious that the hot water in soup making produced a hot-water extract of the soy isoflavones which produced the health benefits.

1 cup miso soup (soybean paste)	109.7 per 100,000 risk for breast cancer
3 cups miso soup (soybean paste)	57.2 per 100,000 risk for breast cancer

GENISTEIN

Genistein is a principal plant estrogen molecule found in red clover and soy and deserves special attention.

Genistein inhibits breast cancer growth at low concentrations and promotes growth of breast cancer at high concentrations. When soy is consumed as a whole food, it doesn't appear to significantly increase or decrease the risk for breast cancer. [J Nutrition 3095-3108S, 2001; Oncology Reports 6: 1383-87, 1999]

In one study, only genistein from soy, and not lignans, were found to be protective for prostate cancer. [Yonsei Med J 43: 236-41, 2002]

FLAX LIGNANS

Lignans started out as unidentified estrogen-like compounds in urine extracts of females which were called Compound X. Their dietary source was only confirmed later. [Nature 287: 738-40, 1980] They are the most promising of all the plant estrogen modifiers and probably the safest.

Lignans are estrogen-like molecules found in whole grains, like rye and flaxseed. Very small amounts of lignans are provided in coffee and tea. [Brit J Nut 79: 37-45, 1998]

Flaxseed provides an unusually high amount of lignans, from 80 to 700 times more than found in other grains. It does not seem possible to experience estrogen-related adverse effects from consuming a diet rich in lignans because they exhibit only 1/10,000th the effect of estrogen. Flaxseed lignans do more than just block the hormone receptor sites on living cells like Tamoxifen does. As early as 1993, it

Phytoestrogen source	Botanical or latin name and trade names	Potential drawbacks
Red clover (genistein)	Trifolium pratense L; Promensil, Rimostil	Blood thinning; may promote tumor growth
Chasteberry	Vitex agnus castus	May promote tumor growth
Kudzu	Pueraria lobata L	May promote tumor growth
Hops	Humulus lupulus L	May promote tumor growth
Dong quai	Angelica sinensis	Blood thinning; may promote tumor growth
Licorice root	Glycyrrhiza glabra	May promote tumor growth
Black cohosh	Cimicifuga racemosa L; Remifemin	Relatively safe (rashes?); may not be a true phytoestrogen
Soy isoflavones (genistein, daidzen, equol); provides phytoestrogens with small amounts of iron-binding phytic acid and omega-3 oil.	Glycine max; many trade names - Soylife	Soy phytoestrogens alone, under certain circumstances, may promote growth of tumors.

was determined that lignans are mild inhibitors of estrogen production by virtue of their ability to inhibit aromatase, the enzyme responsible for estrogen production. [J Steroid Biochemical Molecular Biology 44: 147-53, 1993]

Widespread health benefits of flaxseed and lignans

While the focus of this report centers on breast cancer, the health benefits of lignans are not confined to breast or prostate tissue.

Flax lignans and heart disease

In a recently published study conducted in Finland, high circulating levels of lignans were associated with reduced coronary heart disease and mortality from heart disease in middle aged men. [Archives Internal Medicine 163: 1099-1104, 2003]

Lignans may partly accomplish a reduction in coronary heart disease in males by moderating cholesterol levels. Flaxseed consumption lowers cholesterol. [J Clinical Endodrinol Metabol 87: 1527-32, 2002] While concentrated lignan extracts have not been evaluated for cholesterol profiles, it is known that healthy men with the highest circulating levels of enterolactone, the primary lignan component in flaxseed, exhibit much lower rates of acute heart attacks than men with low levels of enterolactone. [Lancet 354: 2112-15, 1999]

Almost two decades ago studies were conducted showing that lignans also had some properties similar to digitalis (Lanoxin, Digoxin), a drug used to strengthen heart pump action. [J Hypertension 4: 161-64S, 1986; Biochemical Biophysical Research Communications 134: 1064-70, 1986]

Flax lignans and kidney disease

The provision of flaxseed lignans to the diet of animals and humans has been shown to spare the kidneys from assault in autoimmune diseases like lupus. [Lupus. 9:429-36, 2000; Am J Kidney Dis. 22:326-32, 1993; Kidney Int. 48:475-80, 1995]

Flaxseed lignans and breast cancer

In Finland, Sweden and Australia, low dietary intake levels of lignans are associated with an increased of risk of breast, prostate and colon cancer. [Baillieres Clinical Endocrinology Metabolism 12: 605-23, 1998] Excretion of lignans is low among women with breast cancer, a fact that has been known for nearly two decades. [Clin Chim Acta 158: 147-54, 1986] This means the consumption of lignan-rich foods is also low in women with breast tumors.

Lignans in the diet work in the fat cells of the body to inhibit estrogen production by calming down estrogen production. [J Steroid Biochemical Molecular Biology 50: 205-12, 1994] Essentially, flaxseed lignans are aromatase inhibitors.

The addition of ground flaxseed and flaxseed oil to the daily diet increases the circulating levels of enterolactone, the primary phytoestrogen in flaxseed. [European J Clinical Nutrition 56: 157-65, 2002] Generally, very low circulation levels of enterolactone are associated with breast cancer, though sporadic cases can be found among females who have high enterolactone levels. [European J Nutrition 41: 168-76, 200] Apparently it's important to find the right amount for daily consumption.

Flaxseed, about three tablespoons a day, appears to slow the growth of breast and prostate tumors once diagnosed. [US Berkeley Wellness Letter, May 2002] Chemically induced breast tumors in rats became 67% smaller when the rats were fed flaxseed powder. But the effect was not consistent. [Nutrition Cancer 17: 153-59, 1992] This is likely attributed to the variable amount of lignans in the flax or other factors discussed below.

Flax lignans and bone strength

Another compelling potential health benefit from flaxseed is its ability to help maintain bone strength. Women with osteoporosis excrete less enterolactone, the primary estrogen molecule in flaxseed, meaning their dietary consumption of lignans is low. [Clin Endocrinol 56: 321-28, 2002] Flaxseed and flaxseed oil, along with fish oils, inhibit the production of chemicals that lead to loss of bone density. [Alternative Medicine Review 6: 61-77, 2001]

In Korea, higher consumption of lignans as evidenced by concentrated urinary excretion, in particular enterolactone, was found to be related to strong bone mineral density. [Clinical Endocrinology 56: 321-28, 2002]

Whereas pharmaceutical aromatase inhibitors inhibit the production of estrogen to the point where they compromise bone health, flaxseed supplementation appears to mildly reduce estrogen levels, LDL cholesterol and triglycerides, but does not prevent age-related bone loss. [J Clinical Endocrinology Metabolism 87: 1527-32, 2002]

In rodents, flaxseed lignans appear to enhance bone mineral content, but in later life this protective quality does not persist. [British J Nut 86: 499-505, 2001] But at least flaxseed lignans do not promote degradation of bone as do pharmaceutical aromatase inhibitors.

Lignans and antibiotics

Another confounding factor that increases the risk of breast cancer in developed countries is the overuse of antibiotics. Lignans in the diet convert into protective enterolactone by intestinal bacteria. One study reveals that recent users of antibiotics exhibit lower concentrations of enterolactone in their blood circulation. [Am J Epidemiology 155: 472-77, 2002]

Other benefits of flaxseed lignans

It has been known for some time that consumption of flaxseed powder, by virtue of its ability to reduce estrogen production, slightly raises relative concentrations of testosterone in women at a certain time during the month. [J Clinical Endocrinology Metabolism 77: 1215-19, 1993] Since testosterone drives sexual interest in females (as it does in males), this means that flaxseed lignans may increase women's desire for sexual activity.

While virtually all the studies concerning flaxseed and health involved the provision of whole flaxseed, the emphasis has been solely upon its phytoestrogen lignan content. Yet it is apparent that flaxseed exhibits unusual health benefits not observed in other herbal phytoestrogens such as red clover or black cohosh. A possible explanation for the reasons for the widespread health benefits attributed to whole ground flaxseeds is described below.

The recent introduction of the world's first lignan extract (Brevail, Lignan Research) is noteworthy. Brevail assuredly provides 50 mg of lignans extracted from flaxseed whereas the lignan content of flaxseeds themselves can vary considerably. The omega-3 and IP6 phytate content of this product is currently unknown and the product may be more appropriate for women dealing with symptoms of PMS or the onset of menopause than for breast cancer itself. Many women have reported improved well-being, stronger nails, more interest in midlife bedroom activity, and fewer menopausal symptoms using Brevail.

Whole grains

The issue of whether fiber reduces the risk for breast cancer continues to be debated. Some researchers suggest differences in fiber sources may explain whether fiber reduces risk or is ineffective. [European Journal Cancer Prevention Supp. 2: S25-28, 1998]

Only some fiber sources, such as bran and seeds, contain phytate (IP6) that binds to iron and has been shown to reduce cancer risk. [Cancer 56: 717-8, 1985] Fiber from apples, pears, and processed grains do not provide iron-binding components. This explains why various studies involving fiber are inconclusive.

It is known that whole grains contain many other compounds that may protect against chronic disease including cancer. These include the mineral chelator phytate (IP6) as well as lignans, phytoestrogens and vitamins and minerals. [Proceedings Nutrition Society 62: 129-34, 2003]

Iron, estrogen and breast cancer

While the etiology of breast cancer is linked to high life-time exposure to estrogen, there are disparities in studies that attempt to establish this association. [J Steroid Biochemical Molecular Biology 80: 163-74, 2002] Estrogen alone is not the sole governing factor in breast cancer.

If estrogens alone were the primary factor in breast cancer, then why don't more women get this form of cancer during their fertile years when hormone levels are very high?

One answer to this question is that these high hormone levels occur when iron levels are low and metallic minerals like iron are either being lost in the monthly menstrual flow or being donated to a developing baby.

It should not be a surprise that precisely when women lose their ability to control iron, when monthly blood loss with accompanying iron depletion ceases, is exactly when the risk of breast cancer rises dramatically. For example, the liver stores iron and iron stores in the liver are higher among women in whom menstruation has stopped before the age of 50. [Ann Internal Med 127: 105-10, 1997]

When women are still having monthly cycles in their fertile years the likelihood of developing breast cancer is only 1 in 231 up to age 39. But there is an abrupt elevation in risk from age 40 to 59 years to 1 in 25 women, and from 60-79 years of age to 1 in 15 women, [Breast Cancer Family Foundation] which coincides with the buildup of iron.

It is well established that the iron content of cells increases the risk of cancer. [Environmental Health Perspectives 87: 291-300, 1990; Pathobiology 60: 2-9, 1992] *"Iron has not received much attention in discussions of estrogen-induced carcinogenesis and human hormone-associated cancer."* An elevated dietary intake of iron enhances the incidence of breast tumors in animals. The buildup of iron in the body has been specifically linked to higher mortality rates due to cancer among postmenopausal women. [International J Epidemiology 24: 665-70, 1995]

Why do a woman's hormones turn against her when she is mature, rather than when she is young and has higher hormone levels? The answer is simple. Menstruation has ceased and with it, the loss of control of iron.

Factors that involve iron in breast cancer

→ Alcohol consumption (increases iron absorption, elevates estrogen levels that release iron)

→ Whole grain intake (provides molecules that control iron)

→ Menopause/ cessation of menstruation (loss of iron control with the change of life)

→ Red meat: One study shows that red meat consumption raises the risk for breast cancer by 85%.

[Nutrition Cancer 44: 23-34, 2002]

An interesting study to prove the importance of local production of estrogen in breast cancer was conducted. The study found no difference in circulating hormone levels (estrogen, testosterone) between postmenopausal women with and without breast cancer. [J National Cancer Institute 98:110 – 15, 2006]

How could this be? Estrogen levels inside breast tumors can be 10-to 20-fold higher than blood serum levels due to local production of estrogen. [J Steroid Biochemistry Molecular Biology 86: 245-53, 2003] Some, but not all studies, indicate breast cancer is not related to blood serum hormone levels. [Disease Markers 16: 151-57, 2000] The reduced risk of invasive breast cancer in Tamoxifen-treated women is not associated with circulating sex hormone levels. [Journal National Cancer Institute 98: 110-15, 2006]

Estrogen releases iron in breast tissues which then causes gene mutations that can lead to cancer. Consumption of whole grains (like bran or flaxseed meal) can help to control iron and minimize the potentially harmful effects of supplemental estrogen.

Some herbal products that bind to iron may be effective in the treatment of breast cancer. For example, artemisia, an herbal extract from the wormwood herb, is toxic to cancer

	Growth Years	Years of Fertility	Change of Life
Males	High iron needs	Markedly lower iron needs	Lower iron needs
Females	High iron needs	High iron needs (unless hysterectomy)	Markedly lower iron needs

RISKS FOR BREAST CANCER	REGULATION OF IRON
Menopause; advanced age	Loss of menstruation and blood loss of iron
Alcohol	Increases dietary absorption of iron
Plant food diets	Iron more difficult to absorb from plants
Red meat consumption	Contains highly absorbable form of iron

cells in the presence of iron and "*may be a simple, effective, and economical treatment for breast cancer.*" [Life Sciences 70: 49-56, 2001]

Estrogen administration increases iron accumulation. [Current Medical Chemistry 8: 839-49, 2001] Metabolites of estrogen (4-hydroxyestrogens) can induce release of iron from its carrier molecule (ferritin) to generate the dreaded hydroxyl radical, the rusting agent that contributes to the initiation of breast tumors via DNA mutation. [Archives Biochemistry Biophysics 346: 180-86, 1997; Mutation Research 475: 153-59, 2001; Zentralbl Gynakol 124: 559-65, 2002]

The accumulation of iron is also attributed to other common health problems among postmenopausal women such as high cholesterol and coronary heart disease. [Arteriosclerosis Thrombosis 14: 857-61, 1994]

While iron is necessary for life and the production of hemoglobin in red blood cells, when it is unbound from its carrier proteins (what is called "*free iron*"), then it becomes a rusting agent that can induce the hydroxyl radical which is the primary "*culprit in cancer.*" [Stem Cells 12: 289-303, 1994] Metastatic (spreading) breast tumors exhibit a 2-fold increase in hydroxyl radical damage compared to non-spreading tumor cells. [Proceedings Natl Acad Sci 93: 2557-63, 1996]

> The removal of iron via chelation is believed to be a viable method of preventing and treating cancer.

The role of iron in breast cancer is demonstrated by experiments where animals are given estrogen supplements along with an iron-fortified diet. The incidence of kidney tumors is two to four times higher with an estrogen + iron regimen than when estrogen is given with an iron-poor diet. No tumors were observed in animals treated with low or high-iron diets. Circulating levels of iron are much higher in animals given a high-iron diet plus estrogen. [Carcinogenesis 19: 1285-90, 1998] Of particular interest is the fact that breast cancer cells exhibit 5 to 15 times more receptors for iron deposition (transferrin receptors) than normal cells. Iron-carrying proteins like transferrin are growth factors for breast tumors. [Med Oncology Tumor Pharmacotherapy 8: 229-33, 1991]

The removal of iron via chelation is believed to be a viable method of preventing and treating cancer. [European J Cancer Prevention 5: 19-36, 1996] Bran obtained from whole grains, which contain the iron-binding molecule called IP6 phytate, have been shown to inhibit the growth of breast tumors in laboratory dish experiments and in animals. [Archives Latinoamerica Nutrition 49: 309-17, 1999] IP6 phytate, found in relatively high amounts in flaxseed, sesame seed and rice bran, reproducibly inhibits experimental breast tumors in laboratory animals. [Carcinogenesis 16: 1055-58, 1995]

Conventional medicine is not unaware of or ignores the important role iron plays in breast cancer. It's just that researchers are attempting to develop patentable molecules for use as drugs to treat existing cases of breast cancer rather than study flaxseed which could potentially be used for prevention on a widespread basis. For example, researchers are studying an iron-binding drug to treat mammary tumors. [Anticancer Research 22: 2685-92, 2002]

It is interesting to note that alcohol consumption is associated with increased risk for breast cancer. Alcohol increases the absorption of iron from the diet and "*accumulation of iron coupled with diminished antioxidant defenses in breast tissue with advancing age*" explains the associated between breast cancer and alcohol. [Free Radical Biology Medicine 26: 348-54, 1999]

Widely overlooked is that fact that the risk for breast cancer dramatically increases as females cease menstruation and thus lose their ability to control iron build up via blood loss.

Another widely known risk for breast cancer is the increased consumption of animal meat combined with a decrease in the consumption of plant foods. Animal meat provides iron in a form (heme iron) that is more readily absorbed than the form in plant foods (non-heme iron). [Oncology Reports 6: 865-70, 1999]

The body attempts to withhold iron when tumors, infection or chronic inflammation arise. This appears to be a survival mechanism. [Blood Rev 9: 33-45, 1995] So the withholding of iron via dietary binding or chelating factors like IP6 phytate would also inhibit the growth of tumors.

Transferrin is the transport molecule or delivery truck for iron in the blood circulation. Transferrin carries iron back to the liver for storage and transferrin receptors permit transferrin to carry iron into cells. Malignant cells have more transferrin receptors. It would make sense that estrogen increases transferrin receptors in female tissues so as to facilitate the delivery of iron as a growth factor for a developing baby. [Proceedings Annual Meet American Society Clinical Oncology 11:A75, 1992]

Widely overlooked is that fact that the risk for breast cancer dramatically increases as females cease menstruation and thus lose their ability to control iron build up via blood loss. About 80 % of the iron in the body is found in red blood cells. The increased stores of iron in postmenopausal females are linked to an increased mortality from cancer. [International J Epidemiology. 24:665-70, 1995] The parallel rise in heart disease in postmenopausal females can also be attributed to an increase in iron stores due to cessation of menstrual blood loss. [Arterioscler Thromb. 14:857-61, 1994] Menstruating females exhibit half the stores of iron compared to middle-aged men and have half the rates of heart disease, diabetes and cancer. [Lancet 1: 1293-4; 1981; Iron Time Bomb, B Sardi, 2001]

Flax lignans and iron control

It has been known for some time that breast tumors thrive in an environment rich in omega-6 fatty acids, as provided in corn, safflower and sunflower oil for example, compared to a diet rich in omega-3 fatty acids provided in flaxseed. The risk to develop breast cancer is significantly diminished by the consumption of omega-3 fatty acids as provided in flaxseed. [J Nutrition 133:1409-14, 2003]

In an animal study, flaxseed inhibited growth in established human breast tumors and inhibited metastasis (spreading), and this effect is partly due to its inhibition of growth factors (insulin-like growth factor I and epidermal growth factor receptor expression). [Nutrition Cancer. 43:187-92, 2002]

The consumption of omega-3 oils in a favorable balance over omega-6 oils is attributed to the prevention of a variety of diseases seen commonly in populations consuming western diets. [Biomed Pharmacotherapy 56:365-79]

Miracle triad of flaxseed

Too much has been made of the phytoestrogen content of flaxseed, and for that matter all herbal estrogen modifiers, while its other components have been overlooked. Whole ground flaxseed exhibits unique properties for health promotion over and above those provided by other plant estrogens such as red clover, black cohosh or vitex. Flaxseed has unique components that (1) inhibit the synthesis of estrogen; (2) control iron (IP6 phytate); (3) and favorably balance omega-3s over omega-6 fatty acids. While soy also provides phytoestrogens with omega-3 oil and phytate, these are minor components of soy. Crushed flaxseeds are far richer in omega-3 and phytate.

Two tablespoons (15 grams) of ground flaxseed (Forti-Flax from Barleans), an organically-grown, herbicide-free source of cold-milled flaxseeds, which is low in calories (70), provides more than 50 mg of flax lignans, 320 mg of iron-binding IP6 phytate and 3,000 mg of omega-3 fatty acids in a 3-to-1 ratio over omega-6 fatty acids. This is an unusual array of the right nutrients to prevent, treat and block the recurrence of breast and prostate cancers. Crushed flaxseed must be utilized to obtain the lignans and omega-3 oils. Capsules containing standardized amounts of flax lignans, phytic acid and omega-3 fatty acids provide a more assured source of these nutritional factors.

Summary

It is obvious that commercial interests reign supreme over women's health concerns. Profiteering off of women's monthly hormonal swings and the cessation of their menstrual cycle in mid-life is widespread. It is a chilling fact that, after decades of research, that there still is no effective preventive measure for breast cancer.

The expansion of Tamoxifen for use among healthy women is not justified by the scientific data and pronouncements by health agencies for at-risk women to take this drug are irresponsible. The use of a drug that can turn on its users and become a cancer promoter is certainly playing with fire.

Newer aromatase inhibitors eliminate some of the side effects posed by Tamoxifen for breast cancer patients following conventional cancer treatment, but cannot be safely used as a preventive measure among healthy women who are still having a monthly cycle. The widespread use of aromatase inhibitor drugs would likely cause rates of osteoporosis and mental depression to skyrocket.

As for Herceptin, a new drug which had been heralded as a cure, the best that can be said about its efficacy and safety for the treatment of early breast cancer is that the available evidence is insufficient to make reliable judgments. It is profoundly misleading to suggest, even rhetorically, that the published data may be indicative of a cure for breast cancer. [Lancet 366:1673, 2005]

Phytoestrogens are being used by women who do not want to rely on modern medicine for hormonal regulation, but their use is generally unguided. Some phytoestrogens (red clover, dong quai) may over-thin the blood and thus not be safe for use by large numbers of women. The use of phytoestrogens may quell some of the symptoms of PMS and menopause, but they, too, are likely be found to increase the risk and spread of breast tumors because they mimic the "*grow*" signal in cells. The use of concentrated phytoestrogen extracts as dietary supplements, over and above levels provided by typical plant-food diets, may actually increase the risk of breast cancer over time.

Herbal phytoestrogens (red clover, dong quai, vitex) should be distinguished from phytoestrogens provided in beans and seeds, such as soybeans and flaxseed. Soy and flaxseed phytoestrogens are provided in a natural matrix of iron controllers (IP6 phytate) and omega-3 oils, with flaxseed providing the only significant source of all three of these nutrients.

It is evident, when estrogen levels are the highest, during pregnancy and the fertile years, that breast cancer rates are very low, which discounts the idea that estrogen is the sole governing factor in breast health. It is also obvious that women's risk for breast cancer rises upon the loss of their control of iron, either by surgical or age-induced menopause. Iron plays the preeminent governing role in breast cancer and estrogen plays an important role as a release agent for iron. Iron bound to proteins is harmless, proven by iron bound to the red hemoglobin pigment which does not induce oxidation, tissue damage or DNA mutation. On the other hand, unbound iron is a *"rusting agent"* that can induce the feared hydroxyl radical, believed to be the primary agent that initiates breast cancer. [Archives Biochemistry Biophysics 346: 180-6, 1997; Proc National Academy Science USA. 93:2557-63, 1996]
Efforts to prevent breast tumors prior to menopause are not likely to be fruitful and may not even be necessary. Fertile women control iron effectively via menstruation.

The idea of lifetime exposure to estrogen as a risk factor for breast cancer is a flawed concept. Except for vitamin D, nearly every major risk factor or preventive measure for breast cancer (alcohol consumption, red meat, exercise, age, vegetable consumption), involves the control of iron.

Prevention of breast cancer should ensue immediately following cessation of menstruation and continue throughout the remainder of life and consist of iron chelation, provision of omega-3 oils and the calming of estrogen production via safe and natural plant molecules such as low-dose lignans.

Flaxseed meal provides a unique concentrated source of omega-3 oils, iron binders (IP6 phytate) and lignan as an estrogen-controlling agent. Flaxseed does not have any of the drawbacks of Tamoxifen or pharmaceutical aromatase inhibitors and is inexpensive. The superiority of lignan compounds was recently demonstrated in a laboratory test which revealed their ability to inhibit DNA mutation and to chelate iron. [Free Radical Research 31: 149-60, 1999]

While whole grains and flaxseed are rich in IP6 phytate, this natural grain and seed component may only serve to help prevent rather than treat existing tumors. In laboratory experiments where breast tumors were chemically induced, IP6 phytic acid in bran cereal was not nearly as effective at inhibition of tumor growth or the quantity of tumors as was purified IP6 extracted from rice bran. [Nutrition Cancer 28: 7-13, 1997; Anticancer Research 19: 3671-74, 1999] Purified IP6 phytic as a dietary supplement, of which about 70 % is unbound to minerals and ready to attach and remove unbound iron, has both a preventive and therapeutic effect.

Flaxseed meal provides a unique concentrated source of omega-3 oils, iron binders (IP6 phytate) and lignan as an estrogen-controlling agent. Flaxseed does not have any of the drawbacks of Tamoxifen or pharmaceutical aromatase inhibitors and is inexpensive.

In two other laboratory experiments where mammary tumors were induced in rats by feeding them corn or sesame oil, the provision of purified IP6 phytic acid extracted from rice bran reduced the number and size of breast tumors. [Carcinogenesis 16: 1055-58, 1995; Cancer Letters 75: 95-102, 1993] In a telling experiment, the provision of supplemental iron or calcium to mice increased markers for breast tumor growth, while the provision of IP6 phytic acid as a mineral-binder brought about reductions in tumor markers. More remarkable, the provision of IP6 phytic acid simultaneously with supplemental iron and calcium still brought about a reduction in tumor markers! [Carcinogenesis 12: 2041-45, 1991]

The complete blockage of estrogen production or estrogen entry into cells during the post-menopausal years is counterproductive because it trades the risk of breast and uterine cancer for the onset of osteoporosis and mental depression. Hormonal harmony must be pursued by more reliable means than what is currently practiced today.

Melatonin and breast cancer

Melatonin is a hormone, produced in the pineal gland at the base of the brain, during sleep. Close your eyes and a signal is sent to produce melatonin. Melatonin is known as the sleep hormone and is often used as a sleep aid for travelers crossing time zones. Its peak production occurs around 2 to 3: a.m. Melatonin is a strong antioxidant and influences the immune system. It is also known as a cancer-fighting hormone. [Pathological Biology 53: 265-68, 2005]

Even low intensity light for short periods can reduce melatonin production at night. [Neuro Endocrinology Letters 23: 17-22, 2002] Scientific discussion is centered on the possibility that night-shift work may increase the risk for cancer by its inhibition of melatonin production. A modest increase in breast cancer risk is found among female night-shift workers. [Epidemiology 17: 108-11, 2006]

Physical exercise, particularly of longer duration in the later hours of the day, helps to boost melatonin production at night. The mechanism is not fully understood. [American Journal Epidemiology 162: 1114-22, 2005]

Cancer researchers already are aware that cancer patients frequently exhibit sleep problems [Clinical Cornerstone 6: S6-14, 2004], that breast cancer patients have urinary melatonin levels that are lower than in healthy women [Journal Neural Transmission 52: 281-94, 1981], and that long-sleepers (9 hours or more per night) exhibit a modest decrease in the risk for breast cancer. [Cancer Research 65: 9595-6000, 2005]

Melatonin interacts with estrogen, behaving much like an anti-estrogen. [International Journal Cancer 118: 274-78, 2006] Melatonin inhibits production of the aromatase enzyme required for estrogen synthesis. [Breast Cancer Research 64: 287-96, 2000] Therefore, it works much like Tamoxifen or aromatase inhibitors.

If rodents are given melatonin supplements, growth of tumors will be suppressed. [Endocrine 27: 179-88, 2005] When blood samples are taken from premenopausal women who are exposed to light at night, and infused into animals with tumors, the tumors grow more profusely than when melatonin-rich blood is given to the animals. [Cancer Research 65: 11174-84, 2005]

In an intriguing experiment, mice with breast tumors were given omega-3 flaxseed oil, melatonin or a combination of both. Melatonin alone delayed the growth of breast tumors, but the combination of flaxseed oil and melatonin inhibited tumor growth more so than melatonin alone. [Breast Cancer Research Treatment 64: 287-96, 2000]

Supplemental melatonin should become a mainstay among women undergoing chemotherapy for breast cancer as it reduces many of the side effects and reduces mortality rates in animals subjected to chemotherapy. [Journal Cardiovascular Pharmacology 46: 200-10, 2005]

Put your cancer literally *"to sleep"* by getting enough sleep. Melatonin is a beneficial supplement for women with active forms of breast cancer. Melatonin's use as a supplement for breast cancer prevention is yet to be tested.

Coenzyme Q10 and breast cancer

Coenzyme Q10 (CoQ10) is a naturally produced antioxidant within living tissues. Studies indicate CoQ10 concentrations are much lower in breast tissues of cancer patients as compared to surrounding healthy tissues. [Clinical Biochemistry 33: 279-84, 2000]

Some animal and three human studies have been published involving coenzyme Q10 and breast cancer. Cancer cells are known to lack energy, as measured by ATP levels (adenotriphosphate). The provision of coenzyme Q10 to cells elevates ATP.

In one study, energy-elevating nutrients, such as riboflavin, niacin and coenzyme Q10, were given to rodents with chemically-induced breast tumors. The cellular energy levels were improved. [British Journal Nutrition 93: 901-09, 2005]

Dietary supplementation with oral CoQ10 has been proposed as breast cancer therapy. [International Journal Clinical Pharmacological Therapy 36: 506-09, 1998]

Tamoxifen is a drug frequently used in the treatment of breast cancer. Extremely high-dose coenzyme Q10 along with Tamoxifen given to rodents with chemically induced breast cancer was found to restore energy levels to tumor cells. [Molecular Cell Biochemistry 273: 151-60, 2005]

The most recent human study involved 90 breast cancer patients, 36 of whom took CoQ10 along with varying amounts of beta carotene, niacin, vitamin C, selenium and zinc. Breast cancer-specific survival and disease-free survival times were not improved for the vitamin/mineral treated group over those of patients who did not take supplements. [Breast Cancer Research Treatment 76: 137-43, 2002] But this study failed to note the dosage of coenzyme Q10 and whether it was encapsulated with oil to enhance absorption.

The other human studies are compelling. A review by Dr. Karl Folkers of previous studies involving coenzyme Q10 among breast cancer patients was published in 1994.

Thirty-two patients with breast cancer were given CoQ10, 90 mg per day, along with 3,500 mg of omega-3 fatty acids, 385 mcg of selenium, 58 mg of beta carotene, and 2,500 IU of vitamin E. During the 18-month trial, none of the patients died and when monitoring was extended to 24 months, no patients died. All expressed a feeling of well being. Remission was reported in 6 of 32 patients. In one of the 32 patients the dosage of coenzyme Q10 was increased to 390 mg per day with disappearance of the tumor by touch in one month and absence of the tumor by mammography in two months.

Another breast cancer patient, age 59 years, with a palpable tumor (could be felt by touch) in her left breast, taking 390 mg of coenzyme Q10 daily over a two-year period, experienced an apparent complete remission (disappearance of the palpable tumor), confirmed by mammography.

Encouraged by the above experience, doctors then prescribed 390 mg of coenzyme Q10 to a 74-year-old female who had undergone breast tumor removal and refused further surgery. Coenzyme Q10 therapy was begun in October of 1993 and within one month it could no longer be felt by physical examination and within two months it was no longer detectable by mammography. [Biochem Biophysical Research Communications 199: 1504-08, 1994]

Vitamin A and breast cancer

Tumors from some breast cancer patients lose their ability to produce a protein called cellular retinol-binding protein (vitamin A-binding protein), which is believed to be involved in the conversion of vitamin A. This gives a growth advantage to tumor cells. [Journal National Cancer Institute 92: 438-39, 2000]

Vitamin A is derived directly from foods (such as butter, eggs, cheese, liver) or indirectly from beta carotene that is converted to vitamin A in the liver when consumed with a small amount of fat. Disease detectives have determined by study of human populations that women who consume fewer colored vegetables that contain carotenoids (lutein, beta carotene, lycopene) incur more than twice the risk for breast cancer compared to women who consume large amounts of these foods. Researchers conclude that "*low intake of carotenoids, through poor diet and/or lack of vitamin supplementation, may be associated with increased risk of breast cancer.*" [American Journal Epidemiology 153: 1142-47, 2001]

Other studies confirm that the risk of developing breast cancer is cut in half among women who consume plenty of foods that contain vitamin A, beta carotene and vitamin E, as compared to women who do not eat sufficient amounts of these foods. [Cancer Epidemiology Biomarkers Prevention 11: 451-57, 2002]

Carotenoids are target antioxidants. They accumulate in certain tissues only. For example, lycopene accumulates in the prostate and skin, lutein in the eyes and breast, and beta carotene in the skin. So certain carotenoids may be protective against certain cancers and not others. [American Journal Epidemiology 135: 115-21, 1992] Oddly, most cancer studies involving carotenoids test for their concentration in the blood circulation, but not in tissues.

When breast cancer cells are placed in a laboratory dish and vitamins A and C are added, together these vitamins inhibit the growth of tumor cells by altering the genetic commands to produce more of these abnormal cells. [Journal Nutritional Biochemistry Nov. 15, 2006 online]

Oddly, while doctors shun vitamin supplements for breast cancer, they are avidly studying a synthetic form of vitamin A to treat breast cancer. The synthetic form, called Fenretinide, has been described in the medical literature since 1980. [Prostaglandins Medicine 4:285-96, 1980] Somehow what nature provides is characterized as toxic and what is re-engineered is approved for use. Fenretinide, a derivative of vitamin A, has been shown to inhibit the recurrence of breast cancer among younger premenopausal women. [Journal of the National Cancer Institute 91: 1847-1856, 1999]

Vitamin A has been found to work in a synergistic manner with Tamoxifen, but not Fenretinide. [Journal Endocrinology 183: 395-404, 2004; Journal Clinical Oncology 24: 129-35, 2006]

Breast tumor cells can become resistant to vitamin A. But agents that control genes, known as histone deacetylase inhibitors, such as resveratrol, can overcome this resistance. [Anticancer Research 24: 4019-24, 2004]

A study conducted in 1984 in the *Journal of Preventive Medicine* is interesting. Twelve women with benign breast disease who had breast masses were treated with 150,000 units (IU) of oral vitamin A daily for three months. Complete or partial response was noted in five patients and marked pain reduction was noted in nine patients. Side effects were mild, consisting of skin and mucus changes and reversed with discontinuance of vitamin A. There were no cases of liver toxicity. [Preventive Medicine 13: 549-54, 1984]

In 1998, researchers attempted to determine whether women with breast cancer have low circulating levels of vitamin A in their blood serum. Blood serum vitamin A levels were not low in early breast cancer patients, but they declined in metastatic (spreading) breast cancer patients. Researchers concluded that vitamin A supplementation may *"have potential benefit for metastatic breast cancer patients."* [Kaohsiung Journal Medical Science 14: 673-78, 1998] Do oncologists recommend vitamin A for these types of patients? Rarely.

Vitamin D

The geographical breast cancer belt in the world is in areas where there is less sunshine. Northern latitudes have the highest breast cancer rates. For over a decade it has been known that the worldwide incidence of breast cancer is higher in geographical areas of less sunlight. [International Journal Epidemiology 19:820-4, 1990] Women living in sunnier areas of the United States experience a relative 35-75% drop in their risk for breast cancer. [Cancer Epidemiology Biomarkers Prevention 8: 399-406, 1999] Annual age-adjusted mortality rates for breast cancer varied over a 1.8-fold range, from 17-19 per 100,000 in the South and Southwest United States to 33 per 100,000 in the Northeast. [Preventive Medicine 19:614-22, 1990]

Women who have breast cancer generally have lower blood circulating levels of vitamin D. [Public Health Nutrition 2: 283-91, 1999] Women with low blood circulating levels of vitamin D (below 50 nanomolar) exhibit a 354% increased risk for breast cancer compared to women with high levels of vitamin D. [Anticancer Research 26:2573-80, 2006]

There has been concern that farmers exposed to pesticides would incur more breast cancer. However, outdoor work, like farming, has been found to be protective against breast cancer. [Epidemiology 11:523-31, 2000] Obviously, vitamin D offers protection here, and the worry about pesticides may be overblown.

Vitamin D can be successfully combined with cancer treatment:

Researchers have concluded that vitamin D, by itself or in conjunction with chemotherapy, *"may be beneficial for the treatment of estrogen independent (negative) breast cancer."* [Journal Steroid Biochemistry Molecular Biology 84: 181-92, 2003]

In a lab dish study, when breast cancer cells were doused with vitamins A and/or D and then a chemotherapy drug like Adriamycin was employed, the vitamins were found to lower the threshold needed to induce tumor cell death. [Cancer Research 60: 2040-48, 2000]

Vitamin D inhibits breast cancer in various ways:

Vitamin D inhibits the growth and invasion of breast tumors by its ability to inhibit a protein called Tenascin-C which breaks down collagen so that tumors can spread. [FEBS Letters 426: 225-28, 1998]

Insulin-like growth factor (IGF-1) is implicated in breast cancer. IGF-1 cells receptors are over-produced in breast cancer. Vitamin D inhibits IGF-1 and promotes normal cell death and renewal. [European Journal Cancer 35: 1717-23, 1999]

Vitamin D helps reduce breast density among premenopausal women. [Cancer Research 66:588-97, 2006]

There is a report of the successful use of a form of topical vitamin D on breast tissue that reduced the diameter of tumors by 50% among 3 of 14 patients. [Lancet 337: 701-02, 1991]

If undergoing cancer treatment, cumulative sunlight exposure in the months preceding treatment is a predictor of subsequent survival. [International Journal Cancer, May 2, 2006 online] Place sunshine or vitamin D pills on your list of preventive or therapeutic measures.

A daily intake of 2,600 units of vitamin D (65 mcg) is recommended to attain blood concentrations that will optimally protect against disease. [Journal Nutrition 136: 1123-5, 2006] There is no way the diet can provide this much vitamin D. Sun-starved females are at great risk for breast cancer, particularly women living in northern latitudes where wintertime sun exposure produces little vitamin D because of a decline in UV radiation in solar light. Dietary supplements are strongly recommended. Warnings that adults can overdose on vitamin D with daily oral doses exceeding 2,000 units are ill founded.

Vitamin D's ability to inhibit breast cancer cell growth is enhanced by resveratrol, a red wine molecule. Resveratrol increases the vitamin D receptor sites on cells which sensitize the cells to vitamin D. Co-treatment of resveratrol and vitamin D would be synergistic. [Journal Steroid Biochemistry Molecular Biology 84: 149-57, 2003]

Folic acid

Folic acid, an essential B vitamin, is needed for DNA repair and to inhibit the production of homocysteine, an undesirable blood protein. Folic acid may be protective against certain cancers, particularly breast cancer among postmenopausal women who drink alcohol.

In an animal experiment, a folic acid deficiency was found to increase the *"rate of appearance, incidence, weight and volume of tumors compared with animals given sufficient amounts of folic acid."* [Carcinogenesis 26: 1603-12, 2005] This makes sense. A shortage of folic acid will make it difficult for tumor cells to grow and repair breaks in their DNA.

Mortality, breast cancer, by country, latitude		
Country	Rate per 100,000	Latitude
Gambia	3.4	13 North
India	19.9	13 North (Madras)
China	21.2	31 North (Shanghai)
Japan	21.9	34 North (Osaka)
Singapore	23.2	14 North (Singapore)
Portugal	35.7	38 North (Lisbon)
Spain	47.5	41 North (Barcelona)
Ireland	53.7	54 North (Belfast)
England / Wales	56.1	51 North (London)
Germany	56.3	52 North (Berlin)
Switzerland	61.6	47 North (Zurich)
Sweden	62.5	59 North (Stockholm)
Italy	65.4	43 North (Florence)
Denmark	68.6	55 North (Copenhagen)
Canada	71.1	43 North (Toronto)
The Netherlands	72.7	52 North (Amsterdam)
United States	89.2	40 North (New York)

Higher levels of folic acid, vitamin B6 and vitamin B12 confer a reduction in the risk for breast cancer. [Journal National Cancer Institute 95: 373-80, 2003] Folic acid and vitamin B12 appear to have a more marked protective effect against breast cancer among postmenopausal women. [Cancer Epidemiology Biomarkers Prevention 15: 443-48, 2006]

Among the first anti-cancer drugs were those that interfere with folic acid. The problem is, in the long term, healthy cells that are deprived of folic acid cannot repair their DNA. The whole idea of using folic acid-depleting drugs, called anti-folates, to treat cancer, should be called into question.

A common claim by clinicians is that vitamins interfere with toxic treatments. There is some truth to this, though it is mischaracterized. Chemotherapy is toxic and vitamins help to prevent side effects from the drugs themselves. A 14-year study of women who developed breast cancer found that high folic acid intake does not worsen survival. In fact, women who consume more folic acid have a moderately reduced mortality rate. Mayo Clinic researchers conclude that "*folic acid supplementation is unlikely to have a significant adverse effect on survival after chemotherapy for breast cancer.*" [Nutrition & Cancer 44: 139-44, 2002]

Folic acid is compatible with certain types of chemotherapy, reducing drug toxicity and increasing anti-tumor activity. [Cancer Chemotherapy Pharmacology Dec. 15, 2005]

Vitamin E and breast cancer

Breasts are largely filled with adipose tissue, in other words: fat. Vitamin E is the primary antioxidant that protects fats. Average dietary consumption of vitamin E is less than 10 mg per day, so most children and adults run short of the recommended 15 mg dietary intake.

In discussions about vitamin E and its role in breast cancer, readers need to pay careful attention to specifics, namely differences between breast cancer prevention, treatment and use with chemotherapy.

There is evidence that vitamin E plays a key role in protecting breast tissues and may be a strong preventive agent. [Advances Experimental Medicine Biology 364: 119-27, 1994]

Women taking a 600 IU daily regimen of supplemental vitamin E did not report any significant reduction in breast pain for benign breast disease. [Surgery 97: 490-94, 1985]

Nor did a daily intake of 600 IU of vitamin E appear to reduce evidence of benign breast disease as viewed on a mammogram. [Surgery 107: 549-51, 1990] However, among women with confirmed breast cancer, lower tissue levels of vitamin E and lower dietary intake of vitamin E have been found. [Cancer Causes Control 7:591-95, 1996]

In lab dish experiments, vitamin E succinate was found to inhibit breast tumor cell growth. [Journal Surgical Research 93: 163-70, 2000] This form of vitamin E appears to be especially appropriate for women with estrogen-negative breast tumors. [Cancer Research 57: 881-90, 1997]

More than 20 reports confirm that vitamin E-fed animals exhibit fewer and later appearing tumors after exposure to carcinogens than animals not fed vitamin E. [Nutrition and Cancer 27: 109-17, 1997] A few studies show that vitamin E was ineffective, but none show that vitamin E increased the growth of breast tumors.

Many studies involving vitamin E and breast cancer rely upon patients recalling their intake of foods that provide vitamin E. This can be unreliable. So researchers in France conducted a study where they actually measured the amount of vitamin E in breast tissues. Women with invasive breast cancer had more than 7 times less vitamin E in their breast tissues compared to women with non-malignant breast tumors. It's quite a striking study. [International Journal Cancer 67: 170-75, 1996]

When populations of women are analyzed, the consumption of vitamin E from food sources, but not supplements, appears to lower the risk for breast cancer. [Cancer Causes Control 3: 503-12, 1992] This has puzzled investigators and the public.

M. J. Friedrich addressed questions about vitamin E and cancer in his article "*To 'E' or Not to 'E,' Vitamin E's Role in Health and Disease Is the Question,*" published in the Journal of the American Medical Association. [Journal American Medical Assn 292: 671–673, 2004]

Friedrich writes that most clinical trials designed to examine the ability of vitamin E to prevent disease have included the form of vitamin E called alpha-tocopherol, the most abundant form of the vitamin and the primary compound used in dietary supplements. But recent molecular and epidemiological studies have prompted researchers to look beyond alpha-tocopherol to the other forms of vitamin E such as gamma-tocopherol.

Naturally occurring vitamin E is actually available in eight molecular forms, as alpha, beta, delta and gamma, in two families, the tocopherols and tocotrienols. While gamma-tocopherol (found in corn, soybean, and sesame oils and walnuts, peanuts and pecans) is the most common form of vitamin E in the U.S. diet, gamma-tocopherol levels are generally 10 times lower than levels of alpha-tocopherol in blood plasma. Also, alpha tocopherol sticks around in tissues longer than other forms of vitamin E. For these reasons, scientists have placed a greater focus on alpha-tocopherol.

But Friedrich writes that cancer researchers have begun to pay closer attention to gamma-tocopherol, in particular, mainly because studies with alpha tocopherol have been inconsistent. This may be due to the problems of dietary intake reporting by patients, but studies where supplements have been used in humans have also been inconsistent.

Friedrich asks the question: could alpha-tocopherol be more effective when paired with the gamma compound? Some studies with other forms of cancer appear to confirm this theory. Researchers have also found that protective effects of high concentrations of selenium and alpha-tocopherol were only observed when gamma-tocopherol concentrations were high. This study and others are raising questions about gamma-tocopherol's effects on other types of cancer.

While gamma tocopherol is a very similar molecule to alpha tocopherol, it appears to inhibit cancer cell growth by a mechanism apart from its antioxidant properties. [FASEB Journal 16: 1952-54, 2002]

Then there is the other family of vitamin E, the tocotrienols, primarily derived from palm and rice bran oil in dietary supplements. The body naturally concentrates these compounds in adipose tissue, the main type of tissue that constitutes the breast.

It has been demonstrated in lab dish and animal studies that tocotrienols—primarily the gamma and delta versions—inhibit breast cancer cell growth in both estrogen-dependent (positive) and estrogen-independent (negative) cells. [Lipids 33:461–469, 1998] Much larger amounts of tocopherols than tocotrienols are needed to show beast cancer inhibition.

In breast cancer cell-dish studies, tocotrienols have been found to inhibit growth of both estrogen-negative and estrogen-positive tumor cells and work well with Tamoxifen. [Journal Nutrition 127: 544-48S, 1997]

Studies suggest dietary supplements that provide the whole array of vitamin E molecules, both tocopherols and tocotrienols, may be the best option for breast cancer prevention and treatment. [Nutrition Cancer 33: 26-32, 1999]

The dynamics of cancer growth or abolition are being uncovered. When omega-3 oils are combined with iron-chelating drugs (anthracyclines), this combination enhances tumor cell destruction. In rodents, the combination of the above two agents decreased breast tumor size by 50%, but the addition of vitamin E increased tumor size by 188%. [Nutrition & Cancer 51: 178-83, 2005] This is predictable. Vitamin E indiscriminately protects living cells, including cancer cells, from toxic agents like anti-cancer drugs. The lesson here is that high-dose vitamin E taken during chemotherapy may be counter-productive. But chemo and radiation treatment are very toxic and studies show vitamin E protects patients from treatment-induced side effects. [Urology International 75:340-4, 2005; J Clinical Oncology 23:8570-9, 2005; Neurology 64:26-31, 2005]

Dr. Kedar N. Prasad, at the Center for Vitamin and Cancer Research, Department of Radiology, University of Colorado Health Sciences Center, Denver, says most oncologists do not recommend antioxidants to their patients during standard therapy, but some may recommend them at low doses after completion of therapy. However, about 60% of patients take antioxidants during standard therapy without the knowledge of their oncologists. According to Prasad, laboratory experiments show that antioxidants undesirably protect cancer cells when administered only one time, at low doses, shortly before administering chemo or radiation treatment. [Journal Nutrition 134:3182-3S, 2004]

However, laboratory experiments also show that growth-inhibiting doses of vitamin E (alpha tocopherol succinate), vitamin C and vitamin A administered before and after irradiation enhance the effect of x-ray radiation on cancer cells and protect normal cells against some radiation damage. Vitamin A and beta-carotene at high doses, administered daily before x-ray-irradiation produces more than a 90% cure rate in mice with implanted breast cancer cells, whereas treatment with radiation alone or antioxidants alone are ineffective.

Prasad cites a study where breast cancer patients with stage 0-III cancer undergoing radiation treatment were given antioxidants (8,000 mg of vitamin C as calcium ascorbate, 800 IU of vitamin E [alpha tocopherol succinate], and 60 mg of natural ß-carotene—administered orally, divided into two doses, half in the morning and half in the evening). Among 25 patients who were not given antioxidants, two new breast cancers arose over a 22-month observation period. Among 22 patients given antioxidants, no new tumors developed. [Journal Nutrition 134:3182S-3S, 2004]

Iodine and breast cancer

Iodine is another intriguing nutrient to study in regard to breast cancer because it is consumed widely in Japan where breast cancer rates are very low. [Nutrition & Cancer 4:217-22, 1983]

Women in Japan commonly consume seaweed, known for its iodine content. Seaweed is reported to reduce the risk for breast cancer. [Japanese Journal Cancer Research 92: 483-87, 2001]

In one study, thyroid disease incidence was higher in breast cancer patients than in healthy women (58% versus 18%). But other studies do not confirm that abnormal thyroid hormone levels are associated with breast cancer. [Nutrition Cancer 27: 48-52, 1997] It may be that an increased ratio of thyroid hormone over estrogen sets up a growth-promoting effect on breast tumors. [Brazilian Journal Medical Biology Research 38: 761-5, 2005]

Low thyroid is also associated with a reduced risk for breast cancer. [Cancer 103:1122-8, 2005]

A study of 4,575 women with breast cancer in the United States did not reveal a higher rate of thyroid disorders compared to healthy women. [Cancer Epidemiology Biomarkers Prevention 12: 1574-78, 2003]

But to get back to the topic of seaweed and breast cancer, there is more in seaweed than just iodine. Seaweed as a popular dietary component in Japan is a rich source of both iodine and selenium. Selenium acts synergistically with iodine. Selenium status may affect both thyroid hormone regulation and iodine availability. [Cancer Causes Control 11: 121-27, 2000]

The high consumption of iodine-rich seaweed (25 times more than in Western countries) has been associated with the low incidence of benign and cancer breast disease in Japanese women. In animal and human studies, molecular iodine supplementation exerts a suppressive effect on the development and size of both benign and cancerous growths. [Journal Mammary Gland Biology Neoplasia 10: 189-96, 2005]

Researchers hypothesize that the dietary preference for seaweed in Japan may be associated with the low incidence of benign and malignant breast disease. In animal and human studies, iodine supplementation induces regression of both iodine-deficient goiter and benign pathological breast tissue. [Cancer Causes Control 11: 121-27, 2000]

Does seaweed prevent breast cancer? Because of the iodine content of seaweed, some experts think so. The seaweed's wakame and mekabu suppress chemically induced breast cancer in rodents. Researchers in Japan believe mekabu is a potential preventive agent of human breast cancer. [Japanese Journal Cancer Research 92: 483-87, 2001]

D-limonene and breast cancer

Limonene, a natural solvent and degreasing agent found in a variety of plants, is available as a dietary supplement, usually from orange peel oil. Limonene contains molecules called monoterpenes that have detoxification and anticancer properties. [Journal Cell Biochemistry 22: 139-44, 1995]

Limonene has multiple actions against breast tumors. [Breast Cancer Research Treatment 46: 191-97, 1997] One study shows that adults who often consume citrus peel exhibit a lower risk for cancer. [Nutrition Cancer 37: 161-68, 2000]

Limonene increases the production of a protein called TGF-beta (transforming growth factor) that programs breast cancer cells to self destruct. Orange peel oil (limonene), added to the diet of rats with advanced mammary tumors, causes complete regression of the cancers. [Cancer Research 53: 3849-52, 1993]

Researchers report that cancer regressions are not observed with dietary consumption levels of limonene, but supplemental limonene (greater than dietary intake levels) causes "*a majority of tumors to completely regress. Removal (of limonene) from the diet results in a significant number of tumor recurrences.*" [Cancer Research 52: 4021-26, 1992] In animal studies, limonene not only prevents but shrinks existing breast tumors. [Carcinogenesis 5: 661-64, 1984] It has minimal if any toxicity. [Cancer Chemotherapy Pharmacology 42: 111-17, 1998]

A less promising human study was conducted in 1998, employing D-limonene on just 10 breast cancer patients for whom other treatments were ineffective. Limonene in doses of 500-12,000 mg per day was given for fifteen 21-day courses. One breast cancer patient experienced a partial response for 11 months. [Cancer Chemotherapy Pharmacology 42: 111-17, 1998] This study refutes the effectiveness of limonene.

Limonene represents a novel class of anticancer drugs with the potential to cause tumor regressions with limited toxicity. [Cancer Research 52: 4021-6, 1992] The demonstrated ability of limonene to cause breast tumors to regress has been documented since 1986. [Journal National Cancer Institute 76: 323-5, 1986] For unexplained reasons, large human trials have never been conducted. Rather, researchers have suggested that altered forms of limonene, that would be patentable as a drug, should be utilized. [Journal Cell Biochemistry Supplement 22:139-44, 1995]

Despite limonene's promising activity against breast cancer, it has disappeared from view in research studies. The last studies were reported in the late 1990s.

Resveratrol and breast cancer

Resveratrol, known as a red wine molecule, is the most profound anti-breast cancer molecule found in nature.

Grapes and mushrooms contain chemicals that mildly inhibit aromatase, the enzyme that generates estrogen. [Annals NY Academy Science 963: 229-38, 2002] Red wine has anti-aromatase molecules. [Annals New York Academy Sciences 963:239-46, 2002] Resveratrol, a red wine molecule, is the most advantageous of all estrogen-like plant molecules. [Journal Steroid Biochemistry Molecular Biology 94:431-43, 2005] Resveratrol acts as an estrogen receptor antagonist (blocks entry of estrogen into cells) in the presence of estrogen which leads to growth inhibition of human breast cancer cells. [Journal Cell Physiology 179:297-304, 1999] Resveratrol also inhibits production of estrogen from the adrenal glands. [Hormone Research 64:280-6, 2005]

Resveratrol blocks all three major steps in breast cancer, initiation, growth and spread (metastasis). It works in many ways to thwart breast cancer: it repairs DNA, chelates copper that tumors rely upon for growth, blocks estrogen and aromatase in a safer manner than drugs, switches off genes that control tumor cell growth, reduces inflammation, and inhibits new blood vessel formation that supplies nutrients to tumors. [International Journal Cancer 115: 36-45, 2005] Resveratrol has not been shown to be toxic in any animal studies. It is a more promising anti-breast cancer agent than the currently used gene-targeted drugs like Gleevec or Erbitux. [Current Drug Targets 7: 423-42, 2006] See the section in this book on resveratrol.

Ginseng and breast cancer

Researchers in China were surprised to find, in a recently conducted survey of over 1,000 women diagnosed with breast cancer, that ginseng may have some beneficial properties for women. Compared with patients who never used ginseng, regular users had a significantly reduced risk of death (~29% relative risk reduction) and had better psychological and social well-being. [American Journal Epidemiology 163:645-53, 2006] Another study conducted in China found ginseng plus another herbal ingredient was more effective than most drugs used to treat breast cancer. [Life Science 76:191-200, 2004]

Ginseng not only has mild phytoestrogen molecules that calm natural estrogen [Archives Pharmacological Research 26:58-63, 2003], but it also appears to control blood sugar, which is a risk factor for breast cancer. [Journal American College Nutrition 25:100-7, 2006]

Oddly, ginseng is one of the herbs doctors attempt to steer cancer patients away from.

Dietary supplements

Surveys show about 80% of women at risk for breast cancer recurrence take vitamin pills. [Journal American Dietetic Assn 98: 285-92, 1998]

A study was conducted by researchers at the University of Victoria in British Columbia, Canada, to ascertain whether a dietary supplement regimen would improve survival times for women with non-spreading breast cancer in one breast. The women took what was identified as a mega dose formula of beta carotene, vitamin C, niacin, selenium and CoQ10. However, this was not a controlled study, but rather one in which women took varying amounts of these nutrients which were recorded by investigators. Survival for the vitamin-taking patients and the non-vitamin supplement users was about the same. This study is often used to assert that vitamin supplement use does not cure breast cancer. The problem here is that the dosage of nutrients employed by these patients may have been sufficient for cancer prevention, but insufficient to treat existing tumors. There is a big difference between the two. Also, we have no data on whether these women smoked tobacco, changed their diet, or other factors. [Breast Cancer Research Treatment 76: 137-43, 2002] This type of study was designed to fail before it started.

Stress and breast cancer

Many women claim that their breast cancer diagnosis occurred after a period of emotional turmoil in their lives. Emotional stress may work in a way not anticipated. It may actually *prevent* rather than *promote* breast cancer. Researchers believe stress raises levels of adrenal hormones and lowers levels of ovarian hormones, resulting in a decreased risk for breast cancer. [British Medical Journal 331: 548, 2005] The preventive effect is modest, but it certainly dispels the idea that stress increases the risk for breast cancer.

SUMMARY

What should women do?

When buxom actress Suzanne Somers, then in her mid-50s, shunned conventional breast cancer treatment, opting not to have surgery and to undergo radiation treatment only, and also to take an herbal remedy (mistletoe), the cancer industry treated her with disdain, saying she was setting a poor example. Compare this to when First Lady Nancy Reagan chose to undergo a mastectomy over the simple lumpectomy that her doctors advised. There was no outcry against her choice, even though her decision influenced many women to have their breasts surgically removed when there has been no evidence that this is advantageous. Somers is alive and thriving years after her diagnosis.

Dr. Lorraine Day, a prominent orthopedist, underwent surgery in 1992 but rejected further conventional breast cancer treatment substituting instead a regimen that included sunlight, clean water, and a good diet, and has experienced a prolonged remission since 1992. For her success she was branded as a *health quack* by Quackwatch. If any woman finds a way to remedy her cancer outside of conventional regimens, they are likely be ridiculed. Such is the current state of breast cancer care.

Health practices to prevent breast cancer:

- If alcohol is consumed, consume red wine in moderation, supplement with folic acid
- Avoid tobacco; if smoking, supplement with vitamin C, vitamin E, beta carotene, lutein, chondroitin sulfate.
- Obtain sunlight for vitamin D
- Exercise to calm estrogen production

Foods to eat

- Brussels' sprouts (steamed, not boiled)
- Orange peel, lemon peel, whole kumquats
- Garlic
- Flaxseed meal (1-2 tablespoons)
- Bran
- Seaweed
- Tofu or miso
- Olive oil, virgin, should be dark color
  Drink bottled, unchlorinated water

Foods and beverages to avoid

- refined sugar
- milk

Supplements for prevention

- Selenium (organically bound to amino acids, such as selenomethionine or SelenoExcel rather than selenite or selenate) 200 mcg
- Iodine, 150 mcg
- Vitamin D, 2,000 IU or more
- Vitamin E (tocopherols and tocotrienols) 200+ IU
- Folic acid, 800 mcg

- Quercetin + vitamin C
- Resveratrol
- Lignan capsule for menopausal symptoms or in place of Tamoxifen or Arimidex (www.brevail.com)

Supplements to avoid

- iron supplements

Supplements for treatment of active cancer

- IP6 rice bran extract (if not anemic- cold hands and feet) with water on empty stomach 2,000-4,000 mg
- Flaxseed oil, 12,000 mg
- Vitamin A, 5,000+ IU
- D-limonene orange p
- Chondroitin sulfate (to rebuild tissues) 1,000-1,500 mg
- Nattokinase enzymes to prevent cancer spread
- Fresh crushed garlic clove, or in food blender, for allicin, active ingredient in garlic; or Garli-eze® garlic powder in various brands of garlic pills
- Resveratrol, 200 mg
- Melatonin, 10 mg or more at bedtime
- Coenzyme Q10, 100 mg or more
- Intravenous vitamin C

This book is written for information purposes only. It cannot diagnose nor prescribe. The nutritional regimens and doses published in this book are general in nature and not specifically prescribed for any individual. The author is not a doctor and does not accept consultations or examine patients. Regardless of the shortcomings of cancer doctoring today, this book is not a substitute for professional care. While readers are urged to seek other sources of information before adopting any health regimen, this book recognizes there are few health authorities available who can provide you with an up-to-date unbiased opinion. The cancer patient faces difficult choices with few sources of reliable information.

Hello,

My 65-year old sister (she seems and looks 20 years younger and never sick) was just diagnosed with breast cancer much to our shock and amazement breast cancer she has led a healthy lifestyle all of her life. No history of hormone therapy and she has eaten healthfully, never smoked nor does she drink alcohol and there is no family history. We both try to read all we can when it comes to taking care of our bodies and do take some supplements. Do you have any recommendations for me to pass along to her. -BG

Follow-up: will heed your advice on both IP6 and progressive cancer. I am frantically trying to find out all I can about breast cancer....the first cancer of any kind in our large family and we are in shock b/c of my sister's healthy life style..she did all the right things. She did start chemo last week and has a fighting spirit but it has spread to bones and liver, not a good sign at all, and we are devastated.

If you don't mind I really need your advice concerning my mother. She is to go in for radiation on the 30th and this is really bothering me. After her biopsy she went in for the surgery and they removed the tumor and one of her lymph nodes. After examining the lymph node they said that it was fine and there was no indication in it that the cancer was spreading, yet they still want her to do radiation.

I have suggested to her that maybe she should check out all her options, including natural medicine, before making a treatment decision. I have told her about the IP6 rice bran and showed her your advice in your response to my email. I have downloaded several guides and pamphlets detailing all the various options and organizations at her disposal. I read a report which claims needle biopsies increased risk of cancer of the lymphatic nodes located under the armpit by 50%. I also read that mammography brings in the big $$$ for the cancer society so they continue to encourage its use, despite being aware of its dangers and ineffectiveness. I also read a report from the professor emeritus of molecular and cellular biology at UC Berkeley concerning all the destruction caused by radiation.

I am very upset that they have now turned my mother into one of their "manageable patients" and are possibly exploiting her and deceiving her. They put her on these pills, arimidex, that cost $200 (she only has to pay $20) for one bottle of 30 tablets - she has to take them, one a day, for the next 5 years. They told her that this drug has the ability to, and will, heal her. (She is also on diclofenac for her rheumatoid arthritis she was recently diagnosed with.) I told her drugs have no power to heal but, of course, she believes them over me.

They have her believing that she has to do this. I even had to offer to give her a ride, which I am very conflicted about, for I feel that to give her a ride to this is to condone it. What do I tell her to make her think twice? Or am I looking at it all wrong? I don't know what to do. -BG

Mary has breast cancer

For Mary, the discovery of breast cancer was a shock. There was no family history and she had no friends who could share with her their experiences with breast cancer. When a sore breast lump presented itself, she ignored it, thinking at her age, 62, that it was like the soreness she experienced when she was younger. She had developed tough fibrocystic breasts over the years. When the discomfort became so severe that it deprived her of sleep, she visited her family doctor, who referred her to a breast cancer specialist. She immediately took to her doctor. He was very qualified and the nurses bragged about him. He was handsome, too. She had to develop complete confidence in him as she felt lost dealing with her medical problem.

What seemed like endless tests were ordered including mammograms, blood tests, and the like. The doctor asked what she wanted to do. There was the option of lumpectomy or mastectomy (breast removal). Her husband had no idea of how to help. Too frightened to even make a decision, she asked her doctor to decide what was best. He recommended surgical removal of the entire breast plus surrounding lymph nodes.

Family and friends were now chiming in, offering natural remedies, even suggesting cancer clinics in Mexico. She would have nothing to do with this advice. Her insurance covered most of the costs of care the doctor ordered and she simply didn't have money for all the other therapies suggested to her. Her doctors told her herbal and vitamin therapies were not safe and often conflicted with treatment. So she stayed away from them.

The loss of the breast was disfiguring, but she endured. She was encouraged by the option of reconstructive surgery in the future, and utilized bras that hid the visibility of breast removal surgery.

After surgery she was prescribed Tamoxifen, an estrogen-blocking drug. This caused her hair began to fall out, and she began to slowly develop cataracts. She became so depressed that her doctor prescribed an anti-depressant. Her facial skin aged rapidly. She was tired most of the time.

She remembers, after surgery, her husband told her that her surgeon had said "*They got it all.*" So, eight months later when the cancer had spread beyond the lymph nodes and an unremitting headache was evidence it had grown in the brain, she didn't know what to think. Radiation therapy was ordered to shrink the brain tu-

Incidence of Breast Cancer in Females by World Region

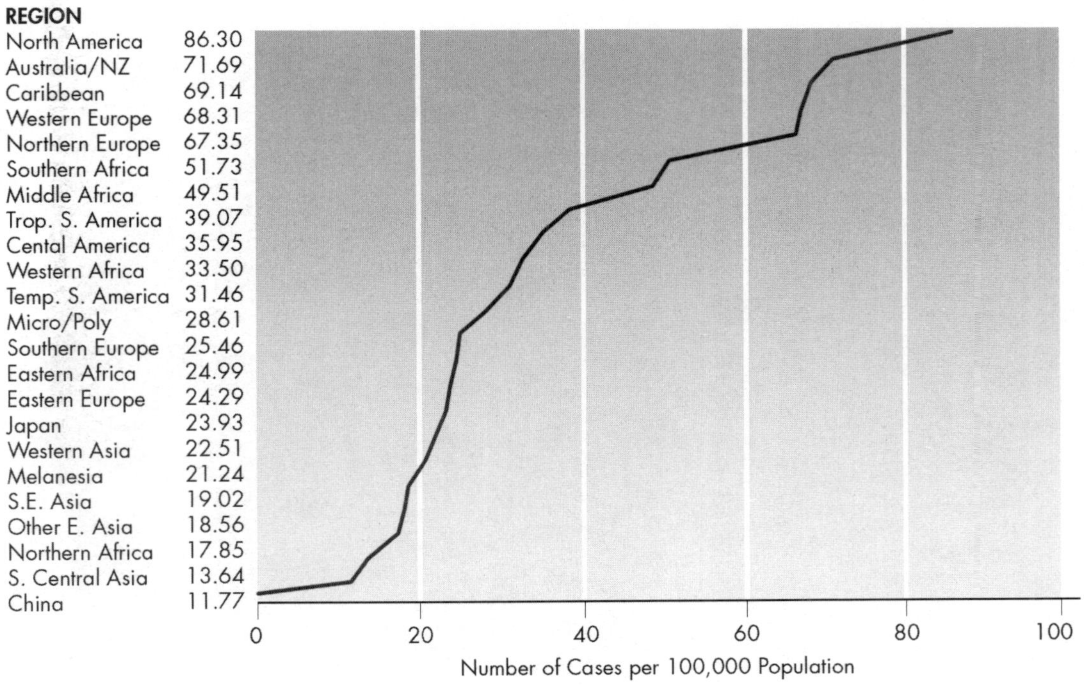

Micro/Poly = Micronesia/Polynesia; NZ = New Zealand; Temp. temperate; Trop. = tropical.

mor that was inaccessible to other treatment. She did everything the doctor had told her, but she was losing the battle.

Maybe now it was the time to consider some alternative therapy. A friend had said something about Essiac tea, so her husband got some.

Fourteen months after her initial diagnosis, she experienced a stroke and has been paralyzed and bedridden since.

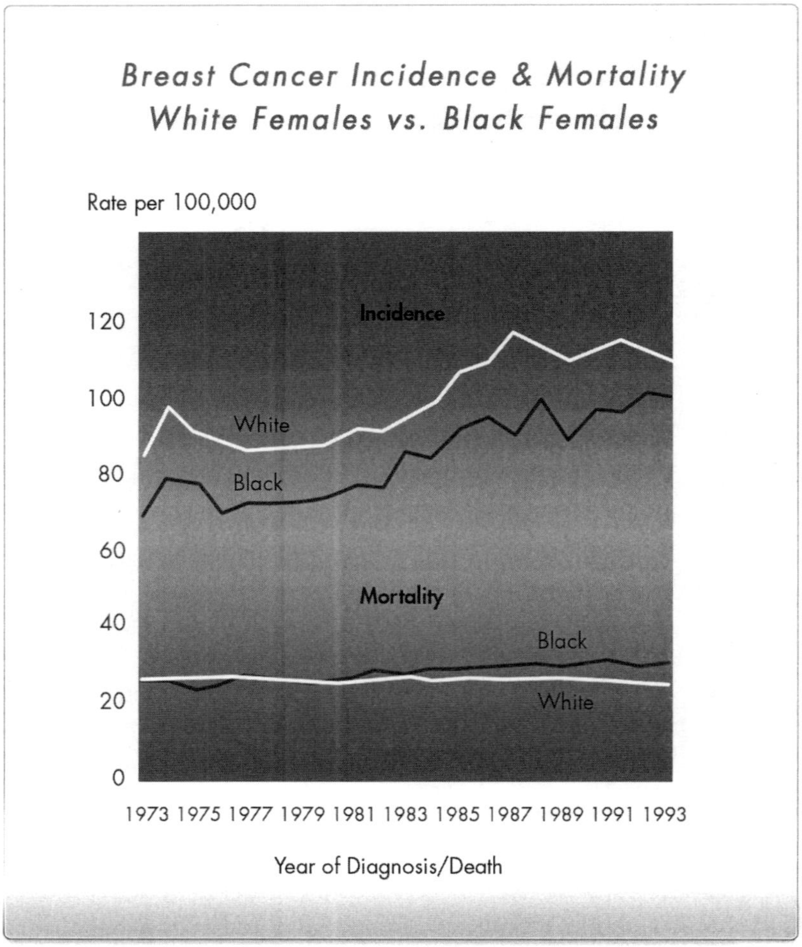

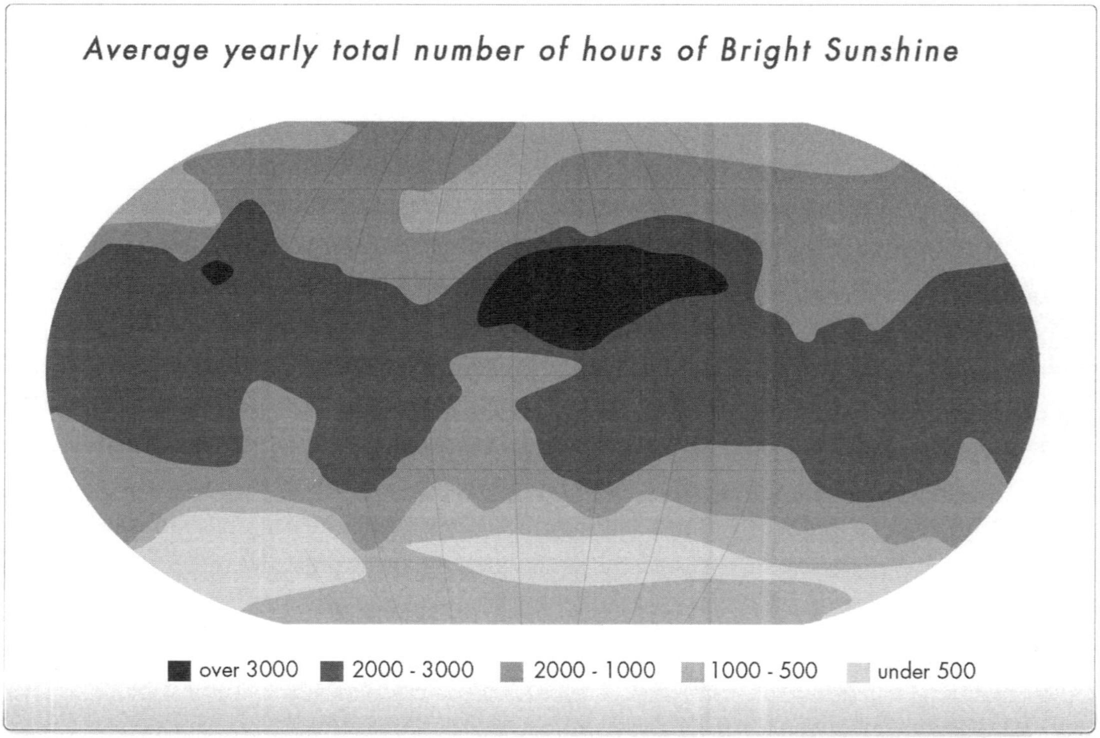

About 80% of our lifetime exposure to UV radiation occurs before the age of 20.

A report published in the British Medical Journal attempted to rank the most important risk factors for breast cancer. Diet, contraceptive use, even alcohol consumption, were not highly ranked risk factors (1.2 to 1.5 times greater risk). The greatest risk factor was advanced age (more than 10 times increased risk) followed by geographical location (5 times greater risk) and exposure to ionizing radiation (3 times greater risk). [British Medical Journal 321: 624-28, 2000]

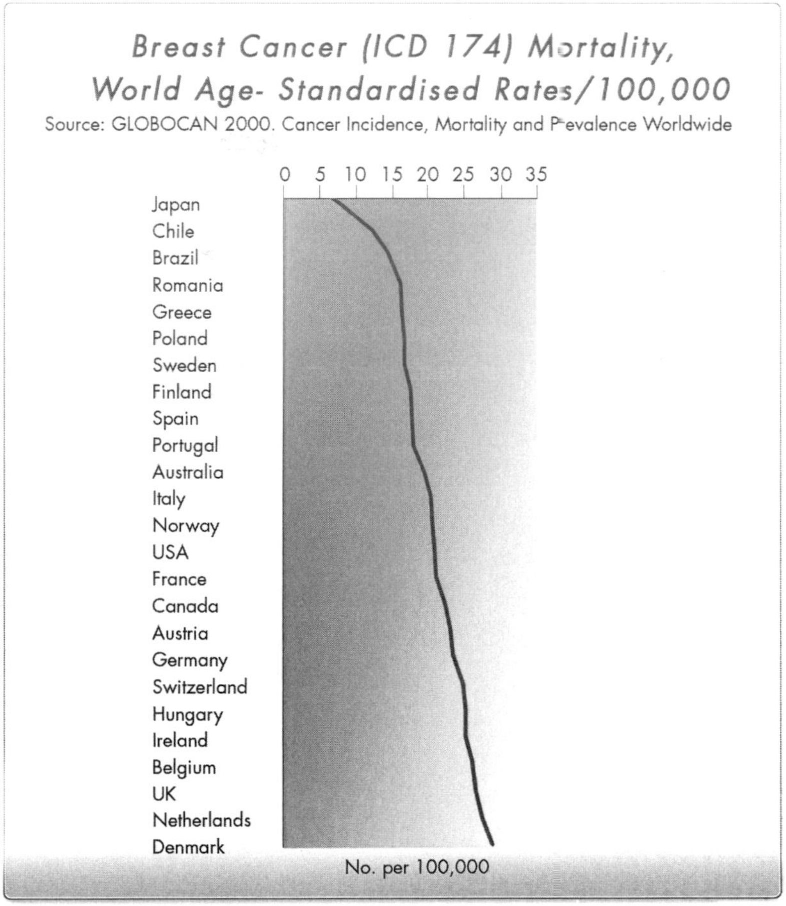

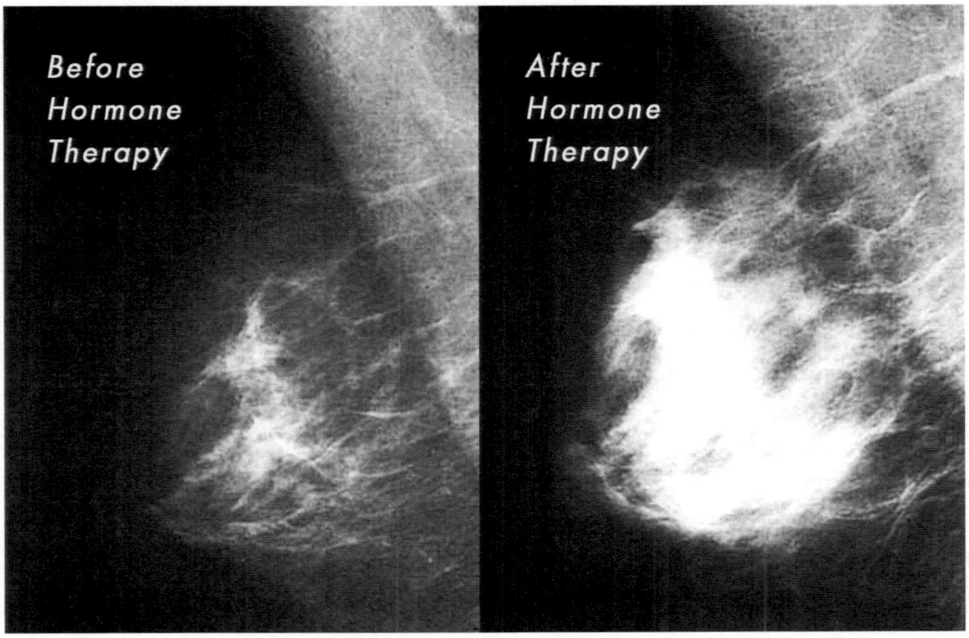

Age-standardised incidence of and mortality from female breast cancer, England, 1971-2003

CHAPTER 9

Colon Cancer

p 294 - 326

Colon Cancer

There are so many appalling facts and unanswered questions regarding colon cancer.

- It's said that colon cancer is preventable, mostly through dietary measures. But there are currently no conclusive preventive measures in practice, only screening to find more disease to treat.

- It's said that colon cancer stems from abnormal growths in the colon called adenomas or polyps. Colon polyps occur on the inside lining of the large intestine. But while the vast majority of colon cancers involve polyps, not all cases of colon cancer can be traced to polyps. [American Family Physician 61: 1759-70, 2000] Some colon cancer emanates from flat or depressed growths. [American Journal Gastroenterology 101:172-80, 2006] This goes unexplained.

- It's said that colonoscopy, the insertion of a scope into the digestive tract, is the best prevention for adults, beginning around age 50. But for the highest risk group, adults over age 80, it offers little in the way of added days of life.

- It's said that removal of adenamatous (cancerous) polyps saves lives, but polyp removal does not address the cause of polyp formation and polyps often reappear after removal.

- While colonoscopy is widely promoted, most family physicians rely on an occult (hidden) blood/stool test, which is highly inaccurate.

- Many health professionals including gastroenterologists themselves never undergo colonoscopy. Many say they haven't the time to undergo this examination.

- Colonoscopy can detect large cancerous polyps, but doctors often cannot detect smaller polyps, which is the whole purpose of the examination, to detect cancer at its earliest stage.

- Promotion of colonoscopy in detecting colon cancer at earlier stages, gives the false impression of improved survival. In fact, most colon/rectal cancer patients succumb to their disease on the same calendar day despite colonoscopy and subsequent treatment. Improvements in survival times are only statistical.

- The discovery of colon cancer usually results in surgical removal of a part of the colon and resection of remaining tissue. However, this treatment does not address the cause of colon cancer.

- A course of chemotherapy usually follows surgery, but only about 20% of the tumors in the colon and rectum are sensitive to these drugs which produce harsh side effects that many patients cannot endure.

- Benefits of treatment for colon cancer are often presented in terms of percent increase in survival, but in calendar numbers, treatment often only adds a few weeks to life.

- Rates of colon cancer vary by as much as a 20-fold difference between those countries with the highest rates versus those with the lowest rates. North American and European Countries have the highest rates, India the lowest. The factors responsible for this wide difference (vitamin D, iron intake) are mostly disregarded by modern medicine.

- Inherited predisposition for colon cancer accounts for only 5% of all cases. But this less frequent form of colon cancer receives great attention.

- Almost half of all patients thought *"cured"* of colon cancer develop recurrence within five years — usually due to undetected metastases.

- Secondary prevention, recommended after detection of polyps or cancer itself, has largely consisted of non-steroidal anti-inflammatory drugs. A 1999 issue of the Harvard Health Letter suggested COX-2 inhibitor drugs such as Vioxx and Celebrex are preferred over aspirin to avoid gastric bleeding. But now it has come to light that the COX-2 inhibitors don't really reduce the risk for bleeding gastric ulcers and may have induced cardiac death among thousands of Americans who were prescribed these drugs for prevention or treatment of colon cancer.

A typical colon cancer patient

Manny Ramirez is thankful for United States doctors who he believes deliver the best care in the world. His immigrant parents came to America a couple of decades ago from South America, where health care was substandard. And he is thankful his employer pays for his physical exams. Preventive exams are encouraged by his employer.

So when the doctor performed a gloved examination of his rectum and feels a growth there, it was time for urgent action. Manny, age 55, followed the doctor's instructions completely. He was immediately scheduled for deeper examination, and visual observation of his colon and rectum with insertable scopes. A test for blood in his stool is also performed. Tissue was removed from the rectum (called a biopsy) and sent to analysis by a pathologist, who searched for cancerous cells. An abnormal mass in the rectum prompts the doctor to schedule immediate surgery. Polyps in the colon are removed.

His family is thankful the doctors are doing all they can to cure the cancer. The surgeon announces they *"got it all"* and the family is relieved. His family believes the doctors may have cured Manny.

To prevent recurrence of Manny's malignancy, secondary follow-up (adjuvant) care is provided. The oncologist prescribes two drugs, 5-FU, a chemotherapy drug that interferes with folic acid (a B vitamin), and levamisole, a drug that boosts the immune system. Manny is informed this is necessary to keep tumor cells from returning. The drugs are administered into a vein in his arm. He also receives an anti-inflammatory drug, a COX-2 inhibitor, thought to be a colon cancer preventive agent. He is unaware that only 20% of cancer patients have colon/rectal tumors that are sensitive to 5-FU. For the remaining 80% of patients, 5-FU will be ineffective and the patients will endure suffering from side effects needlessly.

Furthermore, colon cancer is a solid tumor, and all forms of chemotherapy cannot penetrate solid tumors and over time drug resistance will occur, rendering the treatment useless.

Manny soon loses his appetite, and he is bothered when he goes outside in the sunlight. There is tingling in his hands and feet. His hair falls out. The doctor provides a medicine to treat his blistering lips. Then the diarrhea begins. His legs begin to swell. He starts to cough at night. He has lost energy. His joints ache. After three months of this he cannot go on. He misses a scheduled chemotherapy appointment. His family doesn't know what to do. He is too sick to go to the clinic.

Manny has always had a strong heart, his doctors told him in the past. But suddenly he has a heart attack. His family wonders how such a strong man could now have a heart attack in addition to cancer. After a night in the intensive care unit, more medicines are prescribed although the cardiologist says the event was mild. His family asks the doctor if something can be done for his pain. Morphine is prescribed.

Only now does Manny's family think of alternatives. A neighbor suggests an herbal tea. An acquaintance of the family who went to Mexico to undergo treatment at a border cancer clinic recommends that he try it. They make phone calls to ask what it would cost for Manny to receive care there. But Manny doesn't go to Mexico because the oncologist gives them new hope. He says there is a new drug, Avastin (a drug that inhibits growth of new blood vessels that feeds tumors), and many patients on it are surviving much longer. The doctor orders the expensive drug after having gained approval from Manny's health plan.

The reason why the approval is required is that the drug costs $10,000 per month. The health plan says they will pay for the drug, but Manny has to come up with $1,000 per month as a co-payment. To come up with the money, the family sells Manny's car since he is not using it any more to go to work. They will rely on a medical bus service to transport him to the doctor's office. The family is encouraged to think the new drug may cure Manny.

Then suddenly they hear on television that the drug is being recalled by the manufacturer. Manny's family is devastated. What will they do now?

Manny's battle with colon-rectal cancer is typical. His life is threatened more by his treatment than by his tumors. But Manny's family has no idea that none of his treatment was ever intended for cure. In fact, some of it was totally inappropriate or already proven ineffective. It was prescribed as palliative care, a term in modern medicine which means treatment to relieve symptoms rather than cure the disease.

It would be too harsh to tell Manny and his family there is no cure for colon cancer. Patients and families demand something be done. So treatment is provided. If doctors didn't provide treatment the family would go elsewhere, or complain to the health plan that the doctors aren't doing anything to save Manny's life.

Massive efforts are made to screen for colon cancer. The public is told that colon cancer is curable if caught in time. But the smallest of tumors often go undetected even with colonoscopy and larger tumors have likely spread to the liver which means there is far less chance of extended survival.

Earlier detection simply means tumors like Manny's will be smaller on the day of their discovery and it will give the statistical appearance that treatment is helping patients live longer. But Manny will still succumb to his cancer on the same calendar day. Doctors know the statistics they quote are misleading, but they continue using them.

Age and colon/rectal cancer

Age is the overriding factor in colon cancer. Incidence rates rise from 10 per 100,000 at age 40 - 45 to 300 per 100,000 at age 75 - 80, a 30-fold increase. [Centers for Disease Control statistics]

Polyps also increase with age. One study showed that abnormal growths were found among 14% of people in their early 50s, almost 27% of adults in their late 70s, and about 29% of people 80 years of age or older. Screening for colon cancer at age 80 has diminishing returns. Colonoscopy after age 80 results in only 15% increase in life expectancy, which amounts to about 10 months of extra life. [Journal American Medical Assn 295: 2357-65, 2006] Colonoscopy requires anesthesia, which itself is a risk for

Colon cancer is assigned stages I through IV (also called Dukes stage A,B,C,D) based on the following general criteria:			
Stage	Definition	Percent of cases	5-year survival
Stage I (Dukes A)	Confined to surface cells (epithelium) and has not penetrated bowel wall	15%	85-90%
Stage II (Dukes B)	Invaded through bowel wall	20-30%	50-65%
Stage III (Dukes C)	Spread to lymph nodes	30-40%	25-40%
Stage IV (Dukes D)	Spread to distant organs	20-25%	5%

older patients. The population that is most likely to develop colon cancer is the least likely to benefit from screening colonoscopies.

Colorectal Cancer Survival Rates

The most encouraging statistics for survival are the most often published – that 90% of colon cancer is curable with early detection. The doctors' definition of a cure is survival for five years. However, cure rates are almost totally dependent upon the stage of development on the day of discovery, rather than treatment. Treatment appears to only offer a slight increase in survival, usually a few months.

A startling report by Swiss researchers was recently released. Colonoscopy was performed on 1,514 patients age 50-80 during the period 1991 to 2000 and analyzed retrospectively. Most of the screened patients reported symptoms that prompted colonoscopy. Only 0.3% of the cancers were detected among patients without symptoms versus 12.3% of the patients with suspicious symptoms. The stage of colon cancer was advanced in 82% of screened patients. Treatment of advanced-stage colon cancer has not yet been proven to prolong survival. If the results of this study are universally experienced by other populations, colonoscopy is worthless in regard to lowering mortality rates. Additionally, too many colonoscopies (at least 300) would have to be done to detect just one case of early-stage colon cancer. [Swiss Medical Weekly 135: 679-83, 2005]

While it is said that 90% of colon cancer can be cured with early detection, only about 15% of cases are detected in this early stage. This is because colon cancer doesn't produce symptoms until it has reached a more advanced stage. *"By the time this disease becomes symptomatic, it's often in the late stage,"* says Robert Kurtz, M.D., chief of gastroenterology and nutrition at Memorial Sloan-Kettering Cancer Center in New York. [FDA Consumer Nov-Dec 2000] About 65% of colon/rectal cancer patients have advanced disease on the day of detection.

Even the most encouraging statistics do not include the patients who succumbed to other maladies during their treatment, many of these (heart attack, hemorrhage) being caused by the treatment itself.

By the time the primary tumor is detected, it is usually larger than 0.4in (1 cm) in size and has over a million cells. This amount of growth itself is estimated to take about three to seven years.

A more accurate picture of survival rates is provided by a European report. In a review of 1,073 patients who had undergone surgery for colon-rectal cancer, only 31 had more than a five-year survival rate and seven lived more than 10 years. Rectal cancer had a five-year survival rate of about

5% compared to 1% for colon cancer. Half of these long-term survivors had no additional treatment. [Langenbecks Archives Chir 113: 133-35, 1996]

A few months of extra life over and above the normal course of the disease is often all that modern cancer care has to offer. None of the current treatments, except one, addresses metastasis (the spread of colon cancer), which is the life-threatening factor of the disease. Polyps are detected and removed during colonoscopies, but recur in the same location. Patients are prescribed aspirin or COX-2 inhibitor anti-inflammatory drugs after polyp removal, but the COX-2 inhibitors raise the risk for fatal heart attacks and aspirin may cause bleeding ulcers. Survival rates do not include figures for patients who succumbed to other causes, even if they were induced by treatment.

As ineffective as treatment is for colon cancer, the practice of modern medicine is driven by insurance billing codes. The treatment of colon cancer is an example of how oncologists attempt to get every billable examination and treatment performed before the patient meets her demise. Regardless of how ineffective or harsh the treatment, it is all justified because of the mortal threat to life. No treatment can be deemed unnecessary. Only when doctors have to return insurance checks for needless care will there be reform in cancer treatment. Most patients are totally in the dark over these facts.

The polyp chasers: colonoscopy

As patients begin to experience symptoms of colon cancer, often rectal bleeding or anemia, they make appointments to see the doctor. In one study the mean time from first symptom to first medical exam was about 83 days. [Age Ageing 22: 260-64, 1993]

However, many patients undergo screening exams by colonoscopy or sigmoidoscopy (introduction of tubes into the colon or rectum to visualize the presence of abnormal growths, called adenomas or polyps) before they experience symptoms. Most polyps are benign. Among average-risk patients who report no symptoms, adenoma (polyp) prevalence averages approximately 10% when sigmoidoscopy (rectal exam) is performed and more than 25% when colonoscopy is performed. However, the prevalence of colorectal cancer among these patients is less than 1%. [Technology Coloproctology 8: 243-47s, 2004]

Somewhere between 1 in 10 and 1 in 100 polyps are cancerous. In one study, 1,235 colonoscopies were examined and yielded a total of 1,933 small or diminutive cancerous polyps. Cancer was found on the biopsy tissue slides by the pathologists in 10.1% of the small adenomas (5-10 mm in size) and 1.7% of diminutive adenomas (less than 4 mm). [Clinical Gastroenterology Hepatology 4:343-8, 2006]

Just what percentage of the polyps/adenomas that are surgically removed annually are non-cancerous is unreported. It appears to be 99%.

Findings from the National Polyp Study, however, suggest that periodic colonoscopy could prevent 76% to 90% of colon cancers. These figures are based upon a study of 1,418 patients who were found to have at least one polyp on their first colonoscopy, 80% (1,134) of whom returned for follow-up colonoscopies every 1-3 years. So, among at least 3,000 colonoscopies performed on 1,134 patients, five (5) non-symptomatic, early-stage colorectal cancers (malignant polyps) were detected by colonoscopy (three at three years, one at six years, and one at seven years).

This means even among patients who are believed to be at higher risk (already had a polyp removed), only 4/10th of one-percent, or in less than 1 in 200, was a subsequent malignant polyp found.

Based upon rates in three other reference studies where patients underwent colonoscopy with discovery of polyps but who did not elect to undergo polyp removal, researchers anticipated they would find between 20 and 48 polyps, among the 3,000 colonoscopies performed, compared to the five actually detected.

Researchers estimate the reduction in colon cancer risk from repeat follow-up colonoscopy ranges from 76 to 90%. [New England Journal Medicine 329: 1977-81, 1993] However, these figures only apply to the smaller percentage of patients who have a malignant polyp upon initial colonoscopy, not to the population at large.

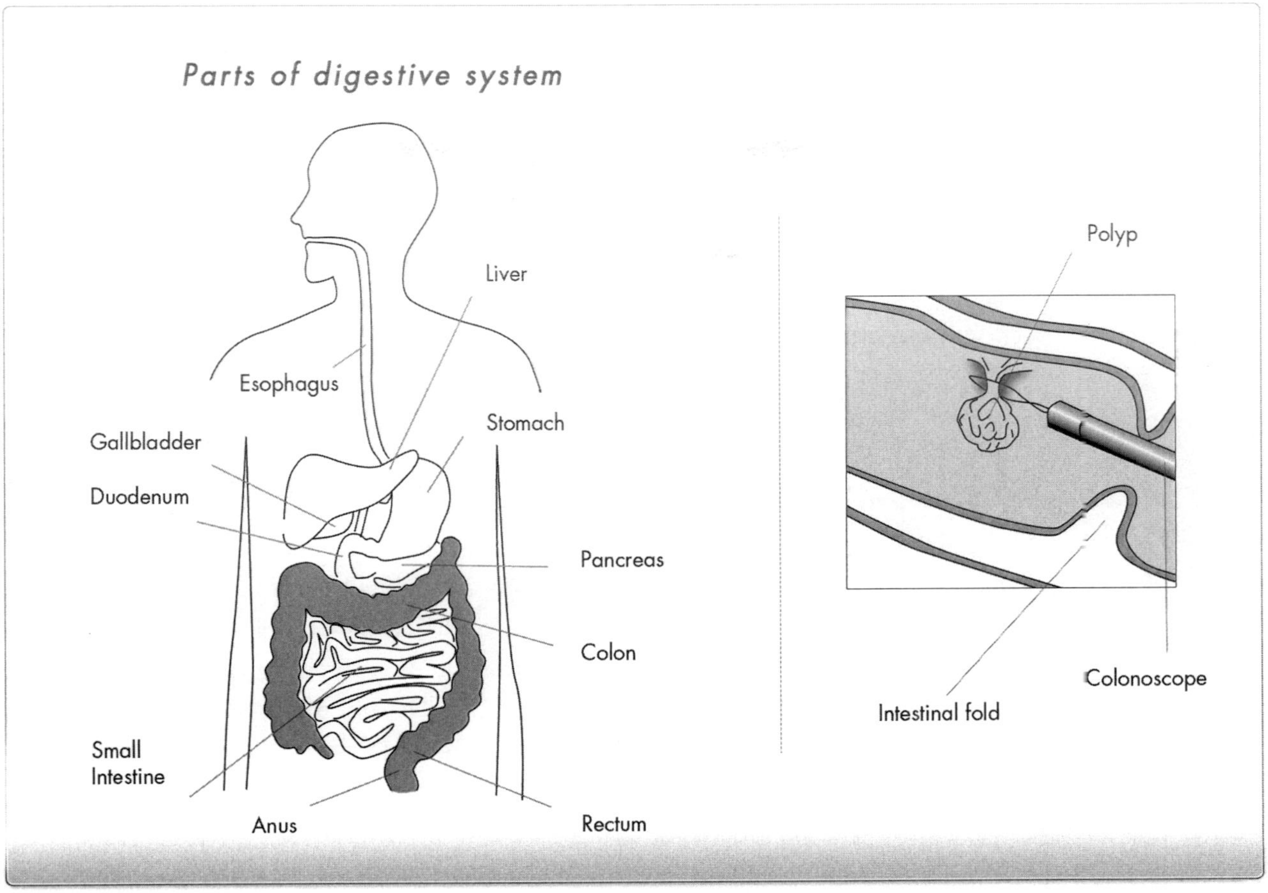

Since about 25% of patients undergoing colonoscopy have polyps, it would take about 4,500 patients to be screened to find these recurrent colon tumors if all polyps found were malignant. [New England Journal of Medicine 329: 1977-81, 1993]

However, only about 1-2% are malignant, so it would require over 110,000 patients to be screened to find 1,134 malignant polyps and at least 3,000 subsequent colonoscopies to find another five tumorous polyps over a seven-year follow-up period. The 110,000 colonoscopies would cost between $880-1200 each, or $88-132 million. The follow-up colonoscopies would cost an additional $2.4-3.6 million. Ongoing colonoscopies would have to be performed to continue to prevent the appearance of colon tumors, adding up to more cost. So, for about $90 million, five lives can be saved, assuming the five detected tumors were not reversible through other methods (diet, smoking cessation, avoidance of alcohol, folic acid and vitamin D supplements).

It is easy to see that doctors prefer treatment over prevention. There is no economic incentive for true prevention, which would reduce the occurrence or recurrence of tumors altogether and eliminate the need for treatment and colonoscopy.

There are approximately 80 million Americans over age 50 who are candidates for colonoscopy. Three-year interval colonoscopies performed on 80 million Americans at an estimated cost of $1,000 each would run up an incredible tab in the nation's healthcare budget. Fortunately, those patients with a negative first colonoscopy wouldn't need to return for another exam for another 10 years. These figures are weighed against the 155,000 new cases annually and 65,000 deaths from colon/rectal cancer. However, most people who undergo colon/rectal cancer screening will not receive much assurance that they will never get colon cancer and if adenomas are discovered, will subject themselves to lifelong colonoscopies thereafter.

It is estimated 50% of people over age 60 will develop at least one polyp, and discovery and removal of polyps may give patients the false impression their life has been saved. But most polyps are noncancerous, so colonoscopy only saves about 1 in 100 of these patients.

The miss rate

Even then, the best physician can miss small tumors in the colon. [Gastroenterology 112: 24-28, 1997] The miss rate for the smallest growths (less than 5 mm in size) is around 25%. Furthermore, the discovery of a tumor and its surgical removal does not address the cause of the malignancy. It only buys some time.

The American Cancer Society (ACS) set a nationwide goal to increase the proportion of people aged 50 and older who have colorectal cancer (CRC) screening via colonoscopy from 25% to 75% by 2015, but a survey of physicians in Wisconsin found only 38.2% of doctors would be willing to screen a moderate-risk patient. [Wisconsin Medical Journal 101:39-43, 2002]

An estimated 31% of Medicare consumers have never been tested for colon cancer and 28% report they have not received a recommendation to be screened from their physician. [American Journal Preventive Medicine 30:313-9, 2006]

Do doctors take their own medicine?

One has to wonder if doctors really believe colonoscopy saves lives. If so, you would think they would line up for their own medicine. Surveys show only about half of doctors over age 50 undergo colon cancer screening, many citing lack of time (47% of doctors) or insufficient data (14% of doctors) to warrant such testing. [Canadian Journal Gastroenterology 20:281-4, 2006] Only 25% (13 of 52) of physicians over age 50 belonging to the Colorectal Surgical Society of Australia report participating in colon cancer screening. [Australia New Zealand Journal Surgery 73: 1028-31, 2003]

Surgical removal of the polyps appears to reduce the incidence of subsequent cancer. [New England Journal Medicine 343:1603–7, 2000] But with the discovery of polyps, patients may actually alter dietary habits, smoking and alcohol intake after a cancer scare. It is difficult to know whether polyp removal is curative.

Doctors' enthusiasm for annual colonoscopies must be tempered since a three-year interval (the generally recommended interval if a polyp is found) is usually as effective as 1-year exams. American Cancer Society suggests patients only need colonoscopies every 10 years once they have undergone an initial colonoscopy where no polyps are found. [Journal American Medical Assn 295: 2366-73, 2006]

Hidden blood test

Most doctors rely upon the fecal occult (hidden) blood test to detect colon cancer. This is a test where a stool sample is placed on a chemically treated card or wipe and a chemical developer is poured on top. If the card or wipe turns to a blue color, this is an indication there is blood in the stool. Colon tumors usually bleed and small, otherwise undetectable, blood in the stool can be a sign of colon of cancer. Dark stools are another overt sign. Fresh blood in the anus usually is from hemorrhoids.

Published studies indicate the fecal occult-blood test *"significantly reduces the incidence of colorectal cancer,"* but in reality it only detects, it does not reduce incidence. [New England Journal Medicine 343:1603–7, 2000]

The occult blood test has a false negative rate of 20-31%. [CA Cancer Journal Clinicians 44: 22-42, 1994] This means you could have colon cancer and this test wouldn't detect it.

Recent studies have found that 24% to 64% of primary care providers use only the fecal occult blood test (FOBT) as their primary screening test. [Annals Internal Medicine 142: 81-5, 2005] But this test is only accurate about 5% of the time. One doctor who studied the problem with the test calls it *"worthless."* Yet it is performed by doctors every day and patients leave their doctor's offices with a false sense of assurance they don't have colon cancer. A 95% failure rate is enough for insurance companies to stop paying for the test. Home testing has been shown to be more accurate. [Annals Internal Medicine 142: 81-5, 2005]

It is easy to see that the current scheme of colon/rectal cancer screening is designed to find more disease to treat rather than true prevention.

Surgery

Surgery is the standard treatment for colon cancer. A section of the large intestine is surgically removed and the remaining segments are reattached.

In a study of 290 patients who underwent surgery for colon cancer, 53% experienced polyp recurrences within two years. [American Journal Gastroenterology 91: 2096-2102, 1996]

As a report in the journal of *Hospital Practice* states, *"colon-rectal cancer is responsible for 200,000 deaths each year, despite continuing improvements in surgical technique and postoperative care. Among the 300,000 new cases, some 80% exhibit no microscopic evidence of residual tumor cells after surgery, yet more than half of these patients experience a local recurrence or spread of their disease and succumb to it."* [Hospital Practice 35: 55-62, 2000] This speaks for the futility of treatment.

For patients undergoing surgery, minimally invasive surgery, performed through a scope, produces about the same results as open incision colon/rectal surgery. [Annals Surgery 223: 790-96, 1996]

The bigger problem in colon cancer is when tumors have spread to the liver. Surgical removal of liver tissue may prolong survival time. [World Journal Surgery 19:59–71, 1995]

Chemotherapy

Metastatic colon/rectal cancer is *"generally incurable."* But many patients have advanced-stage colon/rectal cancer on the day of their diagnosis. Doctors already know treatment is likely to be useless. However, patients and their families are not likely to forego treatment. Following surgery the patient will likely be subjected to chemotherapy.

Prior to 1990, there was considerable doubt regarding the role of chemotherapy after surgery (called adjuvant therapy) for the treatment of colon cancer. Analysis of 25 trial studies conducted in 1988 failed to show significantly improved survival. [Journal American Medical Association 259: 3571-78, 1988] Treatment regimens haven't changed much and continue to be prescribed.

5-Fluorouracil (5-FU) is the most commonly used chemotherapy drug, however it only works in about 20-25% of patients. [Cancer 76: 1709-14, 1995; Nature Medicine 3: 1233-41, 1997] But virtually every colon cancer patient receives this drug.

While most colon cancer patients are able to complete courses of chemotherapy, not all can. About 2 in 10 patients cannot finish their chemotherapy, which speaks for the harshness of the treatment. [Journal National Cancer Institute 98: 610-19, 2006] For those who must stop chemotherapy due to side effects, short-course chemotherapy is no better than no therapy at all. While the patients who do complete chemotherapy experience a statistical increase in survival, the gain is only slight in terms of months of life added. [Journal Clinical Oncology, April 17, 2006, online]

Patients with advanced (stage III or IV) colon cancer have a median survival of only 6-9 months from the diagnosis of their disease. The adverse effects of treatment must be weighed against the symptoms of their disease. [European Journal Cancer 35: 1640-49, 1999] When compared against studies where no chemotherapy was employed, drug therapy improved survival by about 3-6 months. Doctors are making decisions to treat these patients on a paucity of data. Infusion of 5-FU into a vein following colon cancer surgery improves 5-year survival by a small percentage (6%). [Journal National Cancer Institute 89: 497-505, 1997]

5-FU interferes with folic acid, a B vitamin needed for DNA repair. 5-FU is indiscriminate and also interferes with DNA repair in healthy cells, leading to serious side effects that many patients cannot tolerate.

Levamisole, an immune-boosting drug, often accompanies 5-FU. But it doesn't appear to help treatment very much.

If interferon is added to the combination of 5-FU and levamisole, studies show it is so toxic that most patients can't handle it. Interferon as a drug is a mimic of natural interferon which is a protein produced by the body's cells in response to viral infections. More severe toxic reactions (Grades III and IV) were recorded in 9.9% of patients receiving 5-FU or levamisole alone, but in 31% of patients receiving the two drugs plus interferon. [Annals Surgery 242: 178-87, 2005] In another study, at least one Grade IV toxic reaction occurred among 39% of patients receiving two chemotherapy drugs. [Journal Clinical Oncology 23: 1819-25, 2005]

When studies using 5-FU-based regimens were analyzed, after adjustment for deaths caused by the treatment itself, 5-FU resulted in only a 2.3–5.7% absolute improvement in 5-year overall survival (a month or two more of life). [Diseases Colon Rectum 40: 35–41, 1997].

A more recent survey of 39 clinical trials shows that 5-FU and other drugs only modestly improve survival. Five-year survival increases by about 5% for colon cancer and 9% for rectal cancer. [Diseases Colon Rectum 40: 35-41, 1997]

Chemotherapy and antioxidant supplements

While it is frequently said that supplemental vitamins are not compatible with chemotherapy, the combination of 5-FU and folic acid allows for a doubling of survival time, with median survival improved by about 10 months. [Rev Med Brux 18: 209-12, 1997]

A study published in 1997 by researchers at Vanderbilt University found vitamin E increases the effectiveness of the most commonly used chemotherapy drug (5-FU) for colon cancer. [Nature Medicine 3: 1233-41, 1997]

An interesting case draws attention. Methotrexate is a drug that is frequently used to treat rheumatoid (autoimmune) arthritis. Methotrexate interferes with folic acid. A case was described in a medical journal where a 79-year-old patient who had been taking Methotrexate for rheumatoid arthritis since 1990 and was therefore immune compromised, was diagnosed in 2002 with a colon tumor which had spread cancer to the liver. This is the most deadly form of cancer. Methotrexate therapy was discontinued to avoid liver toxicity and the patient began to experience tumor remission. At last report the patient was alive and without symptoms in the spring of 2005. This case would indicate that discontinuation of long-term Methotrexate therapy should be considered in patients with colon cancer. [American Journal Medicine 119: 366-68, 2006]

One has to wonder why drugs that interfere with folic acid such as methotrexate are used to treat colon cancer at all. It appears that patients will never get well using these drugs. Over 30 years of failure has not caused modern medicine to back away from toxic chemotherapy for colon cancer.

Avastin and colon cancer

In Israel, colon cancer patients participated in a hunger strike, pleading for government agencies to pay for newest colon cancer drug, Avastin. A woman in Great Britain gained public attention in the news media for her fight to get health authorities to pay for Avastin to treat her otherwise hopeless case of colon cancer. A woman in India sold her home to pay for Avastin.

With other treatments for colon cancer so ineffective, the newest promoted drug is all that many colon cancer patients can hang their hopes upon. Avastin is that drug.

The New York Times reports that Avastin costs $100,000 a year, yet even with health plans kicking in most of the costs for the drug, co-payments by patients are $1,000 and upwards per month. Many patients simply haven't the money, but they use up their life savings in the hope that the drug will cure them. However, Avastin is more likely to just financially impoverish them and their family in the last months of life. *The New York Times* article said: *"families are selling their houses, mortgaging their homes for a few months of extra life for their loved ones."* [New York Times, Feb. 15, 2006]

The actual cost of producing Avastin is a fraction of what the drug company charges for it, but the manufacturer is attempting to recover research and development costs in a short time.

The Food & Drug Administration approved Avastin in 2004. Avastin inhibits the formation of new blood vessels (called angiogenesis) that feeds tumors so they can grow. This is the most promising of the chemotherapy agents in use for colon cancer. However, Avastin offers, at best, only a few months more of life.

Ethics problems have riddled the FDA, and the National Institutes of Health, and it's obvious that cancer patients are just pawns while researchers and drug companies make billions of dollars for trivial improvements in survival rates. Cancer patients and their families have no time to investigate all this. They can only accept what their doctors tell them. They have no idea they are being shepherded to a dead end street. [APMIS 112: 496-507, 2004]

The advancements in colon cancer survival are small but the headlines and costs of the treatments are large. For example, news sources heralded the combination of Avastin and Eloxatin. Stock prices of the drug companies involved rose and analysts predicted billions of dollars in sales. But the patients were short changed. The overall improvement in survival went from 10.7 to 12.5 months using the combination of Avastin and Eloxatin rather than just Avastin. News reports claimed a 26% reduction in risk of death from colon cancer, but the translation into actual months of added life was often left out of the news reports or buried in lower paragraphs of the reports. All this over-hyping of the drug-combo was done under the auspices of the National Institutes of Health.

The National Cancer Institute lauded itself, saying *"by working with biotechnology and pharmaceutical companies, NCI was able to coordinate the drug development of these two agents."* The NCI said *"These results are simply more good news for people with colorectal cancer."* [ASCO Gastrointestinal Cancers Symposium, Hollywood, Fla., Jan. 27-29, 2005]

In the pivotal Phase III study, the addition of Avastin to chemotherapy (irinotecan/5-fluorouracil/leucovorin) significantly extended survival by, on average, 4.7 months (20.3 months versus 15.6 months) for people with previously untreated metastatic colorectal cancer. [New England Journal of Medicine 350: 2335–2342, 2004] But this was at a cost of tens of thousands of dollars. Shall we bankrupt government and private health insurance plans to provide colon cancer patients with a few more months of life?

The provision of three months of Avastin treatment for the 65,000 patients who succumb to colon cancer each year in the United States would cost $1.5 billion (or $23,000 per patient).

In February of 2006 the maker of Avastin issued a bulletin halting the study of the drug for early stage colon cancer due to a 5% increase in mortal blood-clotting events. [Nature Biotechnology 22: 1198, 2004] In May of 2006 the manufacturer of Avastin issued a press release stating it intends to resume patient enrollment in this study. Worldwide sales of Avastin reached $1.3 billion in 2005 and the halt in the clinical study hardly made an impact upon sales, which surpassed $500 million in the first three months of 2006. [Pharmaceutical Business Review Online, May 23, 2006]

Radiation treatment

In North America there is an emphasis on postoperative radiation treatment and there is evidence that this is more effective when combined with 5-FU-based chemotherapy. The combination treatment has demonstrated a reduction in local recurrence from 8% to 2%. However, most treated patients experience no benefit. In order to benefit six patients it is necessary to treat 100 patients. [Diseases Colon Rectum 41:543–9, 1998]

In a review of 22 published studies, overall survival was the same for patients who were allocated to radiation therapy alone as for those allocated to surgery alone (62% versus 63%). Attempts have been made to improve survival and treatment success by utilizing radiation treatment prior to surgery. However, rates of cure for surgical resection of the colon were not improved by preoperative radiation treatment (85% radiotherapy vs 86% control). About the same percentage of patients who had preoperative radiation treatment died from cancer than did those who had surgery alone (45% vs 50%) and deaths from other causes increased (8% vs 4%). [Lancet 358:1291-304, 2001] Despite this, most oncologists try to coax patients into a short-course of radiation treatment.

Non-steroidal anti-inflammatory drugs

After cancerous (adenomatous) polyps are discovered and surgically removed, medicines are usually prescribed to prevent recurrence.

Studies show that anti-inflammatory drugs are very strong preventive agents. Various population and laboratory studies indicate non-steroidal anti-inflammatory drugs reduce the risk for colon cancer, the primary preventive action being realized by inhibiting COX-2 enzymes. Animal studies have found that COX-2 inhibitors reduce the risk for colon cancer by up to 97%! [Cancer Research 58: 409-12, 1998] However, animal studies do not reveal the mortal side effects that humans who take this type of drug experience. These studies were performed prior to knowledge that COX-2 inhibitors can cause mortal heart attacks or strokes.

An example of the potential dangers posed by COX-2 inhibitors is seen in a study of patients with familial adenomatous polyposis, a genetic predisposition to develop polyps and colon cancer. Some gastroenterologists have begun using non-steroidal anti-inflammatory COX-2 inhibitors (Vioxx, Celebrex) to prevent polyps and colon cancer in these patients. Aspirin has also been tested for prevention of polyps in patients with this condition, with uncertain results and weak effectiveness. COX-2 inhibitors, used for 6 months, at 800 mg per day, was found to reduce the number of polyps among patients with this family predisposition, though it is not know if the risk for colon cancer itself was reduced. Furthermore, nearly one-third of the patients given COX-2 inhibitors experienced rectal bleeding and some preventive trials of these drugs have been halted because of heart attacks. Some physicians now believe *"it is better not to use COX-2 inhibitors to prevent familial colon cancer."* [Prescribe International 15: 13-15, 2006]

A news story sums it all up. COX-2 inhibitor drugs do reduce the risk for colon cancer by up to 33 to 45 % among people who already had polyps removed. But there is no justification for using the anti-inflammatory drugs to prevent colon cancer because they can cause mortal cardiovascular side effects. [Reuters Health, April 3, 2006]

In one study, more than 60 % of those on an inactive placebo developed new polyps, but less than half of those on the COX-2 inhibitor did. However, 3.4% of those taking the drug had heart attacks, strokes or other serious heart-related problems versus 2.5% on the placebo. [National Cancer Institute, Summaries of Newsworthy Clinical Trial Results, Feb. 15, 2005]

In another study, nearly 1,600 people in 32 countries who had previous polyps were given a COX-2 inhibitor and three years later 49 % taking a placebo developed new polyps versus 34 % given the drug. But side effects ranging from heart attacks to chest pain occurred in 7.5% of patients on the drug versus 4.6% taking a placebo. [American Association for Cancer Research conference, Associated Press, April 4, 2006].

Researchers know that anti-inflammatory agents, particularly COX-2 inhibitors, prevent colon cancer, but they also induce serious side effects. A diet high in omega-3 fish oil also reduces inflammation in the colon and in animal studies has been shown to inhibit colon cancer. Researchers have shown that adding a dietary regimen of fish oil, to those taking COX-2 inhibitor anti-inflammatory drugs, synergistically reduces colon cancer in animals. [Cancer Research 65: 8022-27, 2005]

A patient is often prescribed an anti-inflammatory drug after having a non-cancerous polyp removed, meaning the drug will pose a greater threat to life than will the polyp.

Aspirin and colon cancer

Aspirin, like the COX-2 inhibitor drugs, is often recommended for prevention of recurring polyps. One aspirin study showed no reduction in risk for cancerous polyps after 9 years of aspirin use, but the risk was almost cut in half by 20 years of use. What this means to older patients who haven't another 20 years to live, is unknown.

Another study showed that aspirin reduced the occurrence of polyps from 27 to 17 % after 31 months of use. Another study showed little benefit, with aspirin reducing the incidence of polyps from 47 to 45 %. Nevertheless, researchers describe these types of studies as "*encouraging.*" [Postgraduate Medical Journal 81:223-227, 2005]

Aspirin and COX-2 inhibitors may work by causing iron depletion. Aspirin causes a small amount of blood loss and subsequent loss of iron. COX-2 inhibitors also cause blood loss. About 80% of iron in the body resides in the blood circulation. It is iron that is the primary growth factor for colon and rectal tumors.

Of note, aspirin also depletes the body of folic acid and vitamin C, two vitamins known to protect against colon/rectal cancer.

There may be safer COX-2 inhibitors that do not have serious side effects. For example, pomegranate juice has been shown to suppress COX-2 inflammatory enzymes by 79%. [Journal Agriculture Food Chemistry 54: 980-85, 2006]

Lack of follow-up care

An embarrassing, if not distressing, report reveals that many colon cancer patients are not provided adequate follow-up care after treatment. The problem, says a report from the National Cancer Policy Board, the Institute of Medicine, is that there are 10 million cancer survivors who mostly "*go it on their own.*" After treatment patients are sent back to their primary care physicians, often without a plan for follow-up care. The big problem is that doctors are not reimbursed for follow-up care, so it gets neglected. [CA Cancer Journal Clinicians 56: 65-67, 2006] This is puzzling since all it would take to implement follow-up care is to give the patient a list of preventive foods and dietary supplements to take. A pre-printed sheet of paper would suffice. It's no wonder colon cancer recurs with a vengeance – little is done to douse its flames.

What causes colon cancer?

Highest risk groups

In general, patients with a family history of colorectal cancer constitute the highest risk group. Familial adenomatous polyposis, where there is a family predisposition for multiple polyps, receives considerable attention, but accounts for just 1% of all colorectal cancer cases. Adults usually develop this condition in their early 20s and it turns into colon cancer in their fourth decade of life.

Patients with a family history of Crohn's disease or colitis are also at higher risk and often need to undergo more frequent colonoscopy. In ulcerative colitis, the cumulative risk of developing invasive cancer appears to be 2% at 10 years, 8% by 20 years, and 18% by 30 years.

Alcohol and colon cancer

The risk for colon cancer doubles for alcohol drinkers versus non-drinkers. [Journal Epidemiology 15: 173-79S, 2005]

Alcohol and stomach acidity

Studies show that alcohol consumption increases acid secretion and high alcohol intake slows the passage of food through the digestive tract, which may increase symptoms of heartburn (esophageal reflux). [American Journal Gastroenterology 95: 3374-82, 2000] However, wine has components that mildly inhibit stomach acid and is known to kill off *Helicobacter pylori*, the bacterium implicated in gastric cancer. [American Journal Gastroenterology 98: 1440-41, 2003]

Earlier onset of colorectal cancer appears to be associated with alcohol use, tobacco use and male gender. The data showed that alcohol and tobacco users developed cancer an average of 7.8 years earlier than those who had never drank or smoked. Those who had never smoked but drank or who had never drank but smoked were each an average of 5.2 years younger at cancer diagnosis than those who neither smoked nor drank. The effect of smoking appeared to be particularly greater for women. Women who smoked but never drank developed cancer 6.3 years earlier than those who never drank or smoked, compared with 3.7 years in men. Also, current alcohol and tobacco consumption was associated with an increased likelihood of distal (spreading) colorectal cancer, although women in all categories were less likely to have spreading cancer than men. [Archives of Internal Medicine 166: 629-34, 2006]

Smoking and colon cancer

Smoking for 20 years or more increases the risk of dying of colon cancer by more than 40%. [Journal National Cancer Institute, Dec. 6, 2000]

Paradoxically, a 7-8 year study of nearly 60,000 adults in Japan could not find a clear link between smoking and colon cancer. [Journal Epidemiology 13: 323-32, 2003] But the duration of the study was called into question.

There are many studies that do not show a correlation between smoking and colon cancer. If colorectal cancer emerges only after a 35-year induction period, an association would unlikely be detected in studies where exposure assessment is of shorter duration. Most previous studies do not examine smoking of such duration and therefore do not account for the hypothesized 35-year induction period. A 30-year study of over 17,000 twins in Sweden found a 3-fold increased risk of colon/rectal cancer compared to those who never smoked. [International Journal Cancer 91: 585-87, 2001]

Antacids and colon cancer

Use of antacids also increases the risk for colon/rectal cancer. However, they do prevent some forms of cancer such as cancer of the esophagus. [Alimentary Pharmacological Therapy 23: 727-33, 2006] Proton-pump inhibitors (Pepcid, Zantac, Prilosec, Nexium) were first introduced in 1988 and they have become very popular for use in combating common stomach ailments such as heartburn and indigestion. There are no long-term safety data available. One study found that proton-pump inhibitors can also cause tumor cells to become more vulnerable to cancer drugs, overcoming drug resistance. [Expert Opinion Pharmacotherapy 6: 1049-54, 2005]

Users of proton-pump inhibitors will probably be hooked on them for life since initially they induce excessive acidity, which makes a user more dependent upon them. [Expert Opinion Drug Safety 1: 29-38, 2002]

Researchers are concerned that long-term use of antacid drugs, which shut down stomach acid production, may result in polyps and intestinal infections that increase the risk for colon cancer. [Alimentary Pharmacological Therapy 22: 55-63S, 2005]

Omeprazole (Prilosec) reduces vitamin C levels in gastric juice and blood serum. Vitamin C is a protective agent against colon cancer, detoxifying the effects of nitrites in the diet. The vitamin C levels in saliva decline by four times when omeprazole is used and nitrite levels rise by six times when eating a meal with nitrites. [Gastroenterology 116: 812-22, 1999] It is therefore recommended that habitual antacid and proton pump users take vitamin C supplements daily.

NUTRIENTS AND COLON CANCER

Diet and colon cancer:

Fats

Obviously, foods pass through the colon and many cases of colon cancer are believed to be related to diet.

An animal study reveals that consumption of a high-saturated Western-style diet has a four-fold higher potential to promote colon cancer than does ingestion of a diet with an equivalent amount of fat derived from fish oil or a low-fat diet that includes corn oil. [Cancer Research 61: 1927-33, 2001]

Omega-3 oil

Researchers at the American Health Foundation in Valhalla, New York, conducted an experiment among three equal groups of 120 mice to determine the effect of various dietary fats on colon cancer formation. Various studies suggest the composition of dietary fats is more critical to colon cancer risk than the total amount of fat. The consumption of a western-type diet of mixed fats (omega-3s as in fish oil, omega-6s as in corn oil, and saturated fats) was evaluated in mice. The western-style diet had a four-fold (400%) increase in the number of tumors compared to the diets with corn or fish oil. [Cancer Research 61 1927-33, 2001]

Chemically-induced colon tumors in mice after 38-weeks, per group of 120 mice

Diet	% of tumors	Invasive tumors
Corn-oil diet	63%	15.8%
Fish oil diet	69%	23.6%
High-saturated fat	100%	47.4%

Cancer Research 61: 1927-33, 2001

An intriguing study was conducted among fishermen living on the West Coast of South Africa compared to urban Cape Town residents. The fishermen smoked more cigarettes and had higher rates of tuberculosis. The fishermen were black, while the city dwellers were Caucasian. About a third of the urban dwellers took vitamin supplements while none of the fishermen did. The fishermen also consumed fewer vegetables and less fiber than did the urban dwellers. Yet, about six times more urban dwellers in Cape Town developed colon cancer than did coastal fishermen. The consumption of omega-3 oils was six times higher among the fishermen (about 700 mg compared to just 140 mg for the Caucasian urban dwellers). Omega-3 oils appear to provide striking protection against colon cancer. [South African Medical Journal 87: 152-58, 1997]

The Nurses Health Study, considered one of the most authoritative studies available for analysis, found no association between omega-3 oils and prevention of colon cancer. [Cancer Epidemiology Biomarkers Prevention 14: 835-41, 2005] However, Americans consume so little omega-3 oil (10 times less than the Japanese) that the highest consumption doesn't even reach the lowest intake level of people in Japan. With consumption of omega-3 oils almost nil in America, it would not be likely to exert a preventive effect. [Cancer Epidemiology Biomarkers Prevention 15: 406-07, 2006] Studies like these contribute to the growing body of pseudoscience being published to disparage nutritional approaches to cancer prevention.

Omega-6 oil, such as provided in corn and safflower oil, is known to enhance the growth of tumor cells, whereas omega-3 oils, such as from fish or flaxseed oil, has the opposite effect. This has also been found specifically for colon cancer. [Pharmacotherapy 83: 217-44, 1999]

Omega-3 oils have been shown to inhibit colon cancer, but dietary intake or low-dose supplements may have little effect. [Japanese Journal Clinical Oncology 28: 762-65, 1998] Nonetheless, a 24-nation European study found fish and fish oil reduced the risk for colon cancer in men. [European Journal Cancer Prevention 4: 329-32, 1995]

Mice that are genetically prone to develop intestinal polyps, a precursor of colon cancer, hardly develop them at all when given omega-3 oil. [Carcinogenesis 18: 1905-10, 1997

While it is frequently said that dietary supplements interfere with cancer treatment, omega-3 oils have been found to be a useful additive to chemotherapy. [In Vivo 18: 543-57, 2004; Cancer Chemotherapy Pharmacology 55: 12-20, 2004]

Olive oil also appears to cut the risk for colon cancer in half. [Gut 46:191-9, 2000] An antioxidant within olive oil called hydroxytyrosol is believed to provide the colon-cancer preventive effect in olive oil. [European Journal Cancer Prevention 11: 351-58, 2002]
Hydrogenated fats, usually found in baked goods, also increase the risk for colon cancer and should be avoided. [Nutrition & Cancer 39: 170-75, 2001]

Omega-6 oil, such as provided in corn and safflower oil, is known to enhance the growth of tumor cells, whereas omega-3 oils, such as from fish or flaxseed oil, have the opposite effect. This has also been found specifically for colon cancer. [Pharmacotherapy 83: 217-44, 1999]

In animal studies, omega-3 oil from flaxseed has been shown to prevent colon tumors compared to corn oil which is rich in omega-6 oil. [Nutrition & Cancer 51: 52-58, 2005]
Both fish and flaxseed oil have omega-3 and omega-6 oils, but flaxseed oil has a much higher ratio of omega-3 to omega-6, making it the ideal oil for colon cancer prevention and therapy.

Fiber

There is considerable scientific debate over whether fiber in the diet prevents colon cancer.

Studies have demonstrated a reduced risk of colon cancer when populations with diets high in total fat switched to diets high in total fiber and certain whole-grain foods. Researchers, however, indicate the source of fiber needs to be considered. [Proceedings Nutrition Society 62: 63-65, 2003] Bran appears to inhibit colon cancer more consistently than do other sources of fiber. [American Journal Medicine 106: 16-19S, 1999] Refined grain intake actually increases the risk for colon cancer. [Nutrition Cancer 34: 49-55, 1999]

The following paragraphs reveal more about the role of fiber in relation to colon cancer.

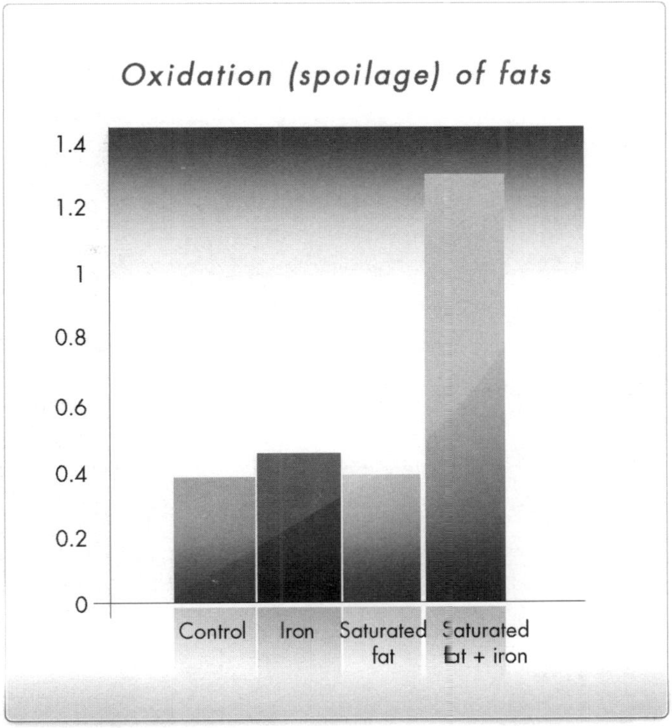

Iron

A long-standing theory has been that iron plays a central role in colon cancer, but studies don't always confirm this notion. Now researchers think they know why. Iron, whether consumed from the diet or from supplements, is better absorbed when the stomach is more acidic. The stomach is lined with good acid-forming bacteria to protect against pathogenic bacteria that enter the digestive tract every day. However, there is variability in the acid state of the digestive tract. The more dietary fiber that is consumed, the more bacterial fermentation that occurs and this mildly increases acidity, enough to increase absorption of iron. Generally, iron from plant foods is less soluble and not as easily absorbed as is iron from red meat. Even small shifts in acidity can significantly increase iron absorption, particularly from iron pills. This suggests that iron supplements combined with certain forms of fiber intake may actually increase the absorption of iron which is a *"rusting agent"* and cancer risk factor when it is unbound. [Nutrition & Cancer 48: 1-5, 2004]

Fiber from bran contains a potent iron chelator (attaching agent) called phytate (IP6) which would negatively affect the increased acidity and iron absorption by binding the iron so it cannot create free radicals that damage tissues and create gene mutations. [Nutrition Cancer 19:11-9, 1993; Anticancer Research 9: 1477-82, 1989]

It is interesting to note that beef induces, while bran prevents, the formation of intestinal polyps, as demonstrated in an animal study. [Carcinogenesis 21: 1167-73, 2000] Phytate (IP6) protects cells in the colon from iron-induced damage. [Proceedings Experimental Biology Medicine 221: 80-86, 1999] Phytate from bran not only protects, but reverses, the tumor-growing effect of iron. [Anticancer Research 9: 1477-82, 1989] Green tea has a synergistic effect with phytate. [Carcinogenesis 18: 2023-26, 1997]

Animal-based foods are associated with higher risk for stomach and esophageal cancer. Not only does meat not provide folic acid, vitamin C and fiber, which are protective factors against gastric tract cancer, but meat is rich in iron that is readily absorbed whether the body needs it or not. By comparison, iron from plant foods is absorbed on an as-needed basis, and is associated with a reduced risk for colon cancer. [Cancer Research 59: 5704-09, 1999]

The dangerous combination of iron and saturated fat

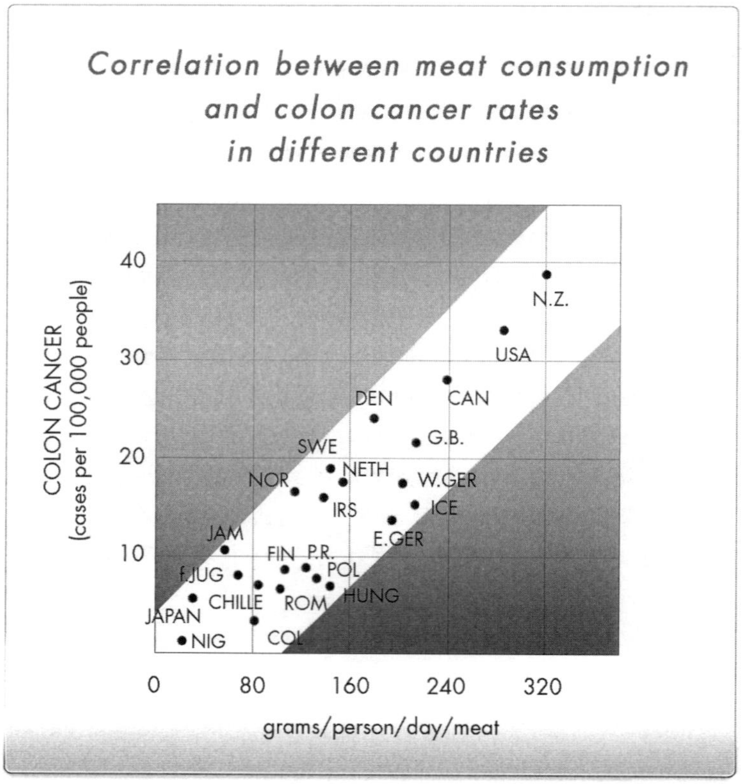

For years researchers have wondered how iron is able to move into living cells and trigger oxidation, cell dysfunction, DNA mutation and eventual cell death. The results of a recent study are revealing.

When iron is separately added to laboratory cell dishes, or when saturated fat is added to living cells, little effect is noted. But when both saturated fats and iron are provided to living cells, iron is able to rapidly enter cells, and cell bodies called mitochondria, in a destructive manner.

Normally iron is bound to proteins as it enters living cells and is detoxified. But when saturated fats are combined with iron, iron rapidly passes through the cell membrane and there is an abrupt increase of iron into cells that results in toxicity.

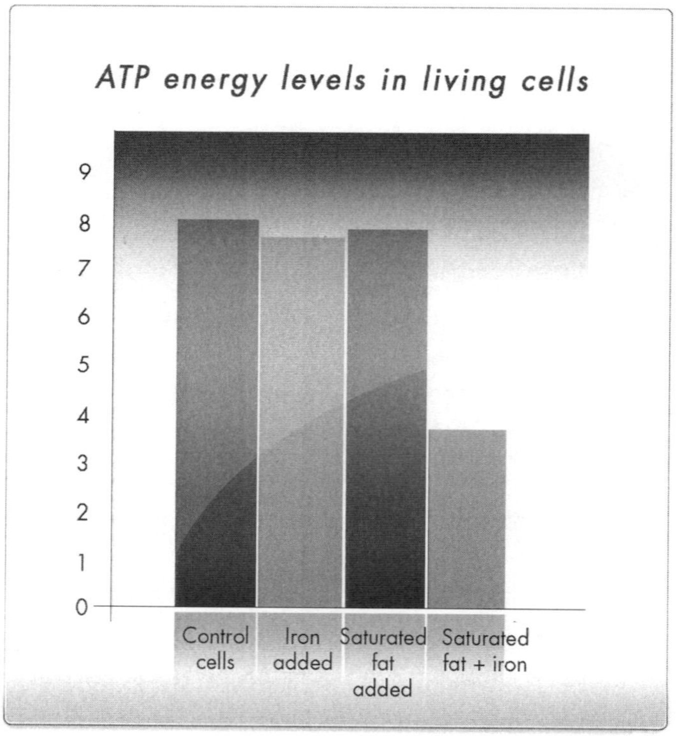

Living cells have small bodies inside them that perform various functions. Mitochondria are cell bodies that produce energy. There are a few hundred mitochondria outside the nucleus of human cells. Mitochondrial function is measured by how much adenotriphosphate (ATP) energy they produce.

Examine the chart nearby. Mitochondria in the control group produce sufficient amounts of ATP. When the cells are provided iron or saturated fat (palmitic acid- a ource of saturated fat commonly found in palm oil), there is only a slight drop in ATP cell energy. But when iron and saturated fats together are administered, the ATP cell energy is cut in half. This is troublesome because a characteristic of cancer cells is low ATP levels in the mitochondria. [Free Radical Biology Medicine, in press, 2005]

The risk for colon cancer increases with dietary consumption of fat. [International Journal Cancer 80: 693-98, 1999] The combination of iron and fat in the diet increases the risk for rectal cancer by 330%! [European Journal Cancer Prevention 8: 501-08, 1999] The combination of fat plus high-dose iron from red meat or iron pills may be problematic.

AGENT	% tumor inhibition
COX-2 inhibitor drugs	93%
Bifidobacteria (probiotics)	93%
Omega 3 oil +beta carotene	91%
Indole 3 carbinol (cruciferous vegetables)	91%
Folic acid	86%
Pectin	82%
Magnesium	81%
Glucarate (fruits)	80%
Quercetin	76%
Bran	76%
Aspirin	75%
Olive oil	72%
Calorie restriction	70%
IP6 phytate from bran	70%
Vitamin D	70%
Vitamin A	67%
Fish oil	64%
Calcium	53%
Selenium	53%
Miso	52%
Green tea	51%
Lemon grass	42%
Lutein	42%

Red meat

In a study conducted in Japan, it was found that red meat increases the risk for colon cancer in men and in women, while daily coffee drinking reduces the risk for colon cancer. [Cancer Letters, March, 3, 2006 online] The bioflavonoids in coffee bind to iron. Red meat is rich in highly absorbable iron while coffee has molecules that bind to (chelate) iron. More adenomas occur when people consume fried or well-done grilled red meat. [Cancer Causes Control 8: 175-83, 1997; Cancer Research 59: 4320-24, 1999]

While red meat is a risk factor for colon cancer, fish consumption appears to protect against colon cancer. [Journal National Cancer Institute 97: 906-16, 2005]

Calcium

For a number of years now the public has been advised that calcium from dairy products reduces the risk for colon cancer. But is it the calcium? Careful dissection of studies now reveals that it may be the vitamin D in dairy products, and not the calcium, that prevents colon cancer. Even earlier studies concluded that *"available evidence does not warrant an increase in calcium intake to prevent colon cancer."* [Journal National Cancer Institute 88: 1375-82, 1996] If there is a preventive effect from calcium, 1,400 mg a day need to be consumed from the diet or supplements, which is higher than current dietary intake levels. [American Journal Clinical Nutrition 83: 527-528, 2006]

There is not sufficient evidence that calcium supplementation will prevent colon cancer. [Cochrane Database System Review 20:CD003548, 2005]

PREVENTION

Preventive agents against colon cancer

Cancer researchers have made a list of the most promising agents against colon cancer. Among 186 agents tested, here is how some of them ranked as colon cancer inhibitors.

Vitamin C

Vitamin C is a powerful protective agent against colon cancer. An animal experiment reveals vitamin C's potent action against colon cancer. The laboratory experiment involved 24 rats, 12 in each of two groups. Gastric cancer was intentionally induced in the laboratory rats. Rats in group 1 received no supplemental vitamin C. Rats in group 2 received the human equivalent of 2,100 mg of vitamin C (based on 160-pound adult). All of the animals developed cancer in the non-vitamin C group compared to just 3 of 12 rats in the supplemental vitamin C group. [World Journal Gastroenterology 9: 446-48, 2003]

Low intake of vitamin C from foods is generally associated with gastric cancer. [International Journal Cancer 73: 684-89, 1997] However, variations in vitamin C blood concentrations, found among various populations around the world, do not reveal that vitamin C protects against colon cancer. [International Journal Cancer 73: 684-89, 1997]

But dietary intake levels are so low in the U.S, around 110 mg per day, that it is unlikely the diet provides sufficient amounts of vitamin C to prevent colon cancer. Also, it should be noted that risk factors for colon cancer, such as *Helicobacter pylori* infection and low stomach acid secretion, inhibit vitamin C absorption.

This was evidenced in a study of patients with low stomach acid secretion and gastric inflammation who were given 1,000 mg of vitamin C per day. DNA damage to the cells in the gastric mucus lining was decreased in 28 of 43 patients. The effect was variable and may point to the need for more vitamin C to produce a preventive effect. [Carcinogenesis 15: 291-95, 1994]

Decades ago supplemental vitamin C was shown to reduce polyps among patients who are genetically prone to colon cancer (familial polyposis). When 3,000 mg of vitamin C was given to five patients who had rectal adenoma polyps following surgery rectal polyps disappeared in two patients, regressed partially in two and increased in one. [Surgery 78: 608-12, 1975]

One report suggests there is no difference in colon cancer risk among individuals regardless of whether vitamin C concentrations in blood serum are high or low. But what they considered "*high*" was still low. [American Journal Epidemiology 142: 608-11, 1995]. There is no way the diet alone can produce optimal blood concentrations of vitamin C. For comparison, most mammals other than humans produce anywhere from 2,000-13,000 mg of vitamin C (human equivalence per pound of body weight) within their own bodies. This is accomplished by enzymatic conversion of blood sugar to ascorbate (vitamin C). For example, colon cancer is extremely rare in dogs, who synthesize vitamin C throughout the day. However, cotton-top tamarin monkeys have a high rate of spontaneous colon cancer. They develop colon cancer in a way very similar to humans. Monkeys do not produce vitamin C as do most other animals.

Health authorities have for a long time erroneously suggested that 60 mg of vitamin C, the amount in a glass of orange juice, is sufficient to meet health needs. The newly updated Recommended Daily Allowance, 200 mg, is certainly not adequate to prevent colon cancer, particularly among smokers and drinkers whose health habits deplete vitamin C. The false notion that high-dose vitamin C is rapidly excreted from the body and creates nothing more than "*expensive urine*" should be dispelled. Recent studies conducted by National Institutes of Health researchers show three times greater concentration of vitamin C can be achieved through oral supplementation than previously thought possible. [Annals Internal Medicine 140: 533-37, 2004] Humans should consume at least 2,000 mg of supplemental vitamin C per day, preferably in divided doses, to prevent colon cancer. Smokers, people at high risk such as those who have had polyps removed or have undergone colon cancer surgery, and people with a genetic predisposition for colon cancer, should probably supplement their diet with more than 2,000 mg of vitamin C per day.

Vitamin E

In animals, a vitamin E deficiency increases cellular markers of pre-cancerous conditions in the colon. [Biochemical Society Transactions 32:979-81, 2004]

In an experiment with rodents, half the animals were given a normal level of iron in their diet and the other half had eight times more iron added to their diet. Cell studies, from cells removed from the colon of these animals, revealed that normal iron intake did not reduce vitamin E levels in blood plasma, liver or feces, but high iron intake depleted vitamin E from these tissues. Gamma tocopherol worked better than alpha tocopherol in lowering measured oxidation within cells. Vitamin E appears to counter the deleterious effects of high iron intake in the colon. [Annals New York Academy Science 1031: 223-33, 2004]

A revealing study was published in 1993. It involved a survey of 35,215 women in Iowa aged 55-69 years without a history of cancer. Women either acquired vitamin E from their diet, about 6-10 IUs per day, or from multivitamins, about 30 IU per day, or from singular dietary supplements providing 100-400 IUs per day. The vitamin E supplement users experienced strong protection against colon cancer, an 84% relative decrease, while those who obtained vitamin E from dietary intake or low-dose multivitamins received no protection. Also, the protective effect provided by supplemental vitamin E only delayed colon cancer in women up until age 65, and then the protective effect dissipated. This could be because of the slow progressive iron overload after menopause. [Cancer Research 53: 4230-37, 1993]

Vitamin D

There is great promise in preventing colon cancer with supplemental vitamin D. The relationship between vitamin D and colon cancer is compelling.

The geographical colon cancer belt in the world is located in the northern hemisphere, where natural vitamin D production in the skin from sun exposure is diminished. In winter months people living in northern climates produce virtually no vitamin D from sun exposure, a shortage that cannot be made up by dietary sources of vitamin D. [European Journal Clinical Nutrition 55:1091-7, 2001]

The lowest rate for colon cancer in the United States is in New Mexico where only 36 per 100,000 adults develop this disease, while Connecticut has a rate of 57 per 100,000, which is the highest in the world. [Cancer 44: 27-42, 1994] Residents in Alaska have substantially higher colon-rectal cancer rates than do Americans living in the state of Washington. [International Journal Epidemiology 27: 388-96, 1998]

The lowest global rate of colon cancer is in Poona, India, 2.8 per 100,000 persons. Poona, India is located near the equator where people are exposed to intense solar ultraviolet radiation that produces vitamin D, a known protective factor against colon cancer, and where the diet is largely vegetarian. [Prevention's Giant Book of Health Facts, Rodale Press, 1991, pp. 118-19]

Vitamin D deficiency is a widespread phenomenon in adults of Central and Western Europe and in North America, especially in dark-skinned adults who produce less vitamin D with sun exposure. Geographically this is where colon cancer rates are the highest in the world. [Journal Nutrition 136: 561-64, 2006]

In 1980, it was proposed that vitamin D was a protective factor against colorectal cancer. Yet advice from dermatologists has likely frightened the public away from sun exposure. The message to get exposed to some solar UV radiation was drowned out by the call to prevent skin cancer.

Several large studies plus a review of all previous studies have shown there is a link between low vitamin D levels and colon cancer. A 50% reduction in colon cancer risk can be achieved by adults who maintain adequate blood levels of vitamin D, but for most adults in North America and Europe this means vitamin supplementation will be required. [Journal Steroid Biochemistry Molecular Biology 97: 179–94, 2005].

Researchers writing for the Medical University of Vienna and the Strang Cancer Research Laboratory at Rockefeller University, reveal that colon cancer cells can produce vitamin D when they are functioning optimally, and thus prevent malignancy. But enzymes can literally degrade vitamin D and create a shortage. [Journal Nutrition 136: 561-64, 2006]

These same researchers note that vitamin D is intertwined with calcium and folic acid to optimally produce vitamin D in the colon. While high-dose calcium helps to normalize cells that line the colon, this only works when there is a sufficient amount of vitamin D. [European Journal Clinical Investigation 35:290–304, 2005] This is just now being understood.

When these same researchers gave a typical western diet (low in vitamin D, low in calcium, low in folic acid and high in fat) to rodents, this diet led to the formation of precancerous cells and eventually colon tumors without any exposure to a carcinogen! [Carcinogenesis 22: 1871–75, 2001]

The new discovery that vitamin D production in the colon is regulated by calcium and folic acid is of great interest. Optimal nutrition, achieved via a multivitamin, would decrease the enzymatic degradation of vitamin D in the colon and enhance the ability of cells to produce vitamin D. Provision of sufficient amounts of folic acid can compensate for shortages of calcium or dietary vitamin D. [Journal Nutrition 136: 561-64, 2006] This is a remarkable discovery!

It is known that night-shift workers have a higher risk of colon cancer, which corroborates with the theory that a vitamin D deficiency is involved in the onset of this form of cancer. [Neuro Endocrinology Letters 27, 2006]

The genetic risk: skin color

Medical researchers know that blacks have much higher rates of colon cancer than do Caucasians, but continue to suggest genetic differences play a role, which obscures the link to vitamin D. There IS a genetic link – blacks genetically produce more melanin in their skin which impairs vitamin D production upon sun exposure. Furthermore, many blacks avoid exposure to sun rays because it blackens their skin. Colon cancer is 1.5 times greater among blacks compared to Caucasians. [Clinical Cancer Research 9: 1112-17, 2003]

Racial differences in colorectal cancer survival have been observed. The 1983 to 1989 five-year relative survival for colon cancer was 61% among white men, 59% among white women, 48% among black men, and 49% among black women. Analysis of the National Cancer Institute's Black/White Cancer Survival Study found that black men and women with colorectal cancer had a 50% greater probability of dying of colon cancer than did white men and women. These differences in survival rates are likely related to diminished vitamin D synthesis in the skin of dark-skinned people.

The best diet only provides a few hundred units of vitamin D, even when fortified milk is consumed. The highest blood levels of vitamin D in most populations is still very low next to what could be accomplished by taking 2,000-3,000 IU of vitamin D daily from dietary supplements.

There is no drug that can potentially reduce the risk for colon cancer by 50%. The possibility that vitamin D may accomplish this speaks for the strong bias in the medical community against dietary supplements. It appears thousands of patients are needlessly dying due to the lack of instruction to supplement their diet with vitamin D. The vitamin D Council now suggests 2,000 IU per day, which is five times greater than most multivitamins provide .

Vitamin D supplementation should be mandated for human populations of blacks, those living in northern latitudes, smokers, over-consumers of alcohol, and all other high-risk groups for colon cancer.

Patients will likely ask their physicians about the potential for vitamin D overdose and are likely to receive mistaken advice. Most physicians have been trained that high-dose vitamin D causes excessive buildup of calcium in cells. This only occurs in a small number of people, and is reversible, while thousands die needlessly of colon cancer.

Studies reveal 10,000 units of vitamin D are typically produced during an hour of summertime sun exposure among Caucasians living in an equatorial area without sun poisoning or side effects. The toxic level for vitamin D from dietary supplements does not begin until 40,000 units are consumed for many months. [American Journal Clinical Nutrition 69:842-56, 1999] Intake of 4,000 units per day has been shown to be safe. [American Journal Clinical Nutrition 73: 288-94, 2001] The current Recommended Daily Allowance for vitamin D (about 200-600 IU for adults), is antiquated and in need of revision. [Journal Steroid Biochemical Molecular Biology 89-90:575-9, 2004]

Folic acid

Folic acid, a B vitamin, is yet another nutrient that exhibits strong protection against colon cancer and yet goes underutilized for lack of physician recommendation.

Cancer is believed to arise as a result of DNA damage that is inadequately repaired. Folic acid is required for DNA repair. [Mutation Research 578: 317-26, 2005] Consumption of at least 700 mcg per day of folic acid has been proposed to adequately maintain DNA repair mechanisms. [Mutation Research 475: 57-67, 2001]

There is about a 40% reduction in colon cancer risk among people who consume the highest amounts of folic acid from their diet. The preventive effect is greatest among smokers. The study that showed this was conducted in Sweden between 1987 and 1990 among 61,433 women. Greater protection was noted among women who smoked cigarettes. [Cancer Epidemiology Biomarkers Prevention 14: 740-43, 2005]

An increase in folic acid intake from 200 mcg or less per day to 400 mcg or more per day produces about a 19% relative reduced risk for colon cancer. The effect is more prominent among adults with a family history of this type of cancer. [Cancer Epidemiology Biomarkers Prevention 11: 227-34, 2002]

The greatest reduction in colon cancer with folic acid supplements appears to be among people with a family history of the disease and people who over-consume alcohol. [Cancer Epidemiology Biomarkers Prevention 11: 227-34, 2002]

When high alcohol intake is combined with low folic acid consumption there is a striking increase in risk for colon cancer, 330%. [Journal National Cancer Institute 87: 265-73, 1995] Nearly 14 million Americans–one in every 13 U.S. adults–abuse alcohol or are alcoholic. There are 40 million alcoholics in Latin America. Millions more often binge drink or drink more than they should. How can colon cancer be prevented without addressing alcoholism? Patients want, or will need, a quick fix. Even hefty doses of vitamins cannot overcome health habits like smoking and over-consumption of alcohol.

People who want to reduce their risk for colon cancer need to take folic acid supplements throughout their lifetime. Among nurses taking folic acid supplements, only insignificant reductions in colon cancer risk were found after nine years of use. However, nurses who consumed folic acid for 15 years experienced a 75% reduction in their risk for colon cancer. [Annals Internal Medicine 129: 517-24, 1998] It is highly unlikely there will ever be a 15-year controlled study to see if supplemental folic acid will prevent colon cancer. This is the best type of study that can be expected.

Folic acid food fortification

With the increase in the population of older adults, there should have been an explosion in the incidence of colon cancer by now. Substantial amounts of folic acid were not available in multivitamins till 1973. Reductions in colon cancer are not expected until 15 years of use. In 1988, it became apparent there was a small decreased risk for colon cancer among folic acid supplement users, more so among those who drank alcohol. [Cancer Causes Control 12: 927-34, 2001] There was a sharp unexplained decline in colon/rectal cancer incidence in the late 1980s, which could be explained by the increase in folic acid in multivitamins in the 1970s. [Journal National Cancer Institute 86: 997-1006, 1994] This benefit would have only gone to the users of dietary supplements.

Modest changes in folic acid intake, within the range of what is considered normal, can have a significant impact upon colon cancer risk. [Journal Nutritional Biochemistry 5: 170-74, 1994] Prior to food fortification, about 9 in 10 Americans consumed less than 400 mcg of folic acid daily. However, folic acid added to foods may spoil due to heating and processing of foods.

Since folic acid supplementation may hide symptoms of a vitamin B12 deficiency, folic acid supplements should be accompanied by vitamin B12. [Journal American College Nutrition 22: 1-8, 2003]

While consumption of folic acid-rich foods such as orange juice, dark green leafy vegetables, asparagus, strawberries and legumes, should be encouraged, these foods will not likely provide adequate amounts of folic acid to optimally prevent colon cancer, particularly among high-risk groups.

Folic acid is much better absorbed from dietary supplements than from foods. [Journal American College Nutrition 17: 625-30, 1998] Some people are unable to utilize folic acid due to genetic predisposition and require greater intake from supplements.

Blood tests for folic acid levels have fooled physicians for many years. A common mistake is to rely upon blood plasma tests to determine folic acid deficiency. Folic acid accumulates 30-40 times more in red blood cells than in blood serum. A decrease of folic acid in blood plasma and red cells is apparent in cancer patients. [Biomed Pharmacotherapy 50: 303-05, 1996]

There should be an urgent demand to fortify foods with more folic acid and to consume high-dose (800 mcg) supplements. Dr. Godfrey P. Oakley Jr, of Emory University, characterizes the foot dragging by public health authorities to fortify the diet with more folic acid as *"public health malpractice."* [Teratology 66: 44-54, 2002]

Does folic acid promote cancer?

There is a paradox in regard to folic acid and cancer. While, folic acid reduces the risk for cancer to develop within the colon, supplementation has the effect of promoting the progression of established colon tumors. [Journal Nutrition 133: 3731-39s, 2003] This is why the first anti-cancer drugs were designed to interfere with folic acid. [Journal Nutrition 133: 3731-39S, 2003]

However, anti-folic acid drugs only increase survival by about 2%, and there are serious side effects and significant costs involved in this form of chemotherapy, usually given following surgery for colon cancer. [Internal Medical Journal 33: 119-24, 2003] The idea of avoiding folic acid during chemotherapy appears flawed. When folic acid is added to chemotherapy drugs, levamisole and 5-FU, it increases survival by about 12%. [Annals Surgery 242: 178-87, 2005]

While folic acid is widely recognized as a preventive agent against colon cancer, malignant cells in the colon, but not healthy cells, exhibit low folic acid levels. Many colon cancer patients have normal blood levels of folic acid. The depletion of folic acid in cancerous tissue appears to be a local problem. [Gastroenterology 112: 1163-68, 1997]

Other B vitamins and colon cancer

Data from the Iowa Women's Health Study shows that the risk for colon cancer declines with intake of foods and supplements that contain folic acid, vitamin B6 and B12. Women with high folic acid intake and low consumption of alcohol appear to be at the lowest risk for colon cancer. [Nutrition & Cancer 43: 152-58, 2002]

Colon cancer patients are known to have lower circulating blood plasma concentrations of vitamin B6. [Journal National Cancer Institute 97: 684-97, 2005]

A study conducted in Japan found that dietary supplementation with vitamin B6 inhibits colon cell proliferation from its earlier stage and that a high-fat diet markedly enhances [Bill, correct?] the inhibitory effect. [Oncology Reports 14: 265-69, 2005]

Zinc

The blood serum ratio of copper over zinc is very high among patients with digestive cancer. [Archives Medical Research 28: 259-63, 1997] Zinc competes with copper for absorption. Zinc also affords protection for the gastric lining against damage caused by non-steroidal anti-inflammatory drugs (example: ibuprofen). [Digestive Diseases and Sciences 38: 1882-84, 1994] It makes sense for cancer patients to supplement with zinc.

Selenium

We know that when animals are given foods with selenium compounds added to them and then given a chemical that causes colon cancer, there are fewer polyps and pre-cancerous cells in the selenium-fed animals. [Nutrition & Cancer 11:11-20, 1988]

Adults with low blood plasma selenium levels are 3-4 times more likely to develop one or more adenomatous polyps. [Cancer Epidemiology Biomarkers Prevention 2: 41-46, 1994] Vitamin C appears to work synergistically with selenium in this regard. [Biomed Environmental Science 15: 223-32, 2002]

We also know that selenomethione, a common form of selenium in food supplements, does not significantly reduce abnormalities in the colon. Food forms of selenium may be more desirable, such as selenium derived from yeast (SelenoExcel). [Biofactors 14: 191-96, 2001]

Since colon cancer takes years to progress into malignant tumors, it is unlikely that nutrients such as B vitamins (folic acid, B6, B12) and selenium will ever conclusively be shown to prevent this type of cancer. It is known that people with adenomatous polyps have low blood serum levels of selenium. Based upon the best available evidence, selenium supplementation is something that should be encouraged given the widespread evidence that this trace mineral protects against a wide variety of tumors. [Nutrition & Cancer 46: 125-30, 2003]

Butyrate

Butyrate is a short-chain fatty acid formed within the gut as fiber ferments. It is a detoxifier and cancer inhibitor. [Carcinogenesis 26: 1064-76, 2005] A number of scientific studies confirm that butyrate could effectively inhibit colon tumor growth. [Molecular Carcinogenesis 43: 207-14, 2005]

Overuse of antibiotics can thwart natural defenses against cancer in the colon. Mucus is the protective lining that buffers the digestive tract against damage by stomach acid. Butyrate is a normal product of gastric fermentation. When butyrate is added to laboratory dishes with cells from gastric linings, mucus production increases. [Gut 36: 93-99, 1995] The overuse of antibiotics kills off the beneficial bacteria in the digestive tract which nourish the mucus lining. The mucus lining then is starved and the digestive tract becomes vulnerable to infection. [Journal Parenteral Enteral Nutrition 19: 410-15, 1995]

There are many mechanisms by which butyrate inhibits colon cancer:

- → One of the mechanisms by which butyrate inhibits colon cancer is its ability to promote transforming growth factor (TGF) which suppresses tumor formation in the gut. [Annals Surgery 243: 619-25, 2006]
- → Another mechanism by which butyrate thwarts colon cancer is its gene-signaling capabilities. Butyrate works like a gene-targeted drug, similar to the way widely heralded drugs like Erbitux and Herceptin work. Butyrate causes a coil-like structure called histones to tightly wrap around genes, switching genes that control cancer growth *"off."* Butyrate is gene therapy. [Oncological Research 14: 427-38, 2004]
- → Butyrate also works as a natural COX-2 inhibitor, working in a similar fashion to COX-2 inhibiting drugs, but without the cardiovascular

side effects. [Biochemical Biophysical Research Communications 317: 463-71, 2004]

→ Butyrate reduces the metastatic properties of colon cancer cells so they won't easily spread to the liver, which is a highly mortal sign. [Clinical Experimental Metastasis 21: 331-38, 2004]

Published reports on the effectiveness of butyrate in inhibiting colon cancer are mixed. Experiments conducted in lab dishes may not produce the same results as those performed on animals and in clinical studies. Furthermore, the type of fiber used to induce the fermentation that naturally produces butyrate in the gut, is of importance. Fiber sources such as guar gum, pectin and oat bran are highly fermented and convert to butyrate, whereas other sources of fiber found in cereals and wheat bran may be poorly fermented and thus may not convert to butyrate. The combination of fish oil plus fermentable sources of fiber such as pectin protects against colon cancer. [Journal Nutrition 134: 479-82, 2004]

Butyrate plus vitamin D appear to work synergistically to prevent colon cancer. Laboratory experiments indicate butyrate and vitamin D in combination offer a new therapeutic approach for the treatment of colon cancer. [World Journal Gastroenterology 11: 7136-41, 2005]

Butyrate is available as a dietary supplement. Probiotics (friendly bacteria such as acidophilus) that encourage fermentation of fiber, and fermentable sources of fiber (pectin, guar gum) are also available as dietary supplements and should be utilized following and in between courses of antibiotics.

Resveratrol

Resveratrol, commonly known as a red wine molecule, is the most promising drug/natural therapy for colon cancer because of its widespread biological action. (The Food & Drug Administration classifies resveratrol as a drug, though it is available as a dietary supplement.)

At the Louis Pasteur Institute in France researchers demonstrated that resveratrol added to the drinking water of mice who are genetically predisposed to intestinal tumors resulted in a 70% reduction in tumor formation. Resveratrol accomplishes this by switching off genes involved in tumor growth. [Nutrition & Cancer 39: 102-07, 2001]

COX-2 inflammatory enzymes are highly involved in colon cancer, and resveratrol is a strong COX-2 enzyme inhibitor. [Carcinogenesis 21: 959-63, 2000]

Resveratrol has been found to be more powerful than butyrate in inhibiting tumor cells growth in the colon. [Journal Nutrition 132: 2082-86, 2002]

The main mechanism of action of resveratrol in intestinal lining is induction of chloride secretion, which can result in diarrhea. This can be suppressed by butyrate. Butyrate and resveratrol may be combined to reduce undesirable side effects in the colon. [Clinical Cancer Research 11: 5651-56, 2005]

Antioxidant supplements and colon cancer

A researcher at Purdue University made a chance discovery that human feces, even when diluted 10,000 times, still generate high levels of free radicals, which produce oxidizing, tissue-damaging oxygen species. The amount of cellular damage was equivalent to receiving 10,000 rads of gamma radiation per day. High levels of iron in feces along with bile pigments may generate the most dangerous hydroxyl radical. The combination of fat and iron in the diet, as provided in red meat, increases hydroxyl radical formation in stool. This may be an important factor in the development of colon/rectal cancer. [Free Radical Biology Medicine 8: 191-200, 1990]

Antioxidants protect tissues from iron and/or oxygen molecules that can be harmful. The body makes some of its own antioxidants, like catalase, superoxide dismutase and glutathione from sulfur, copper, zinc or manganese, and acquires antioxidants from the diet, such as vitamin C and vitamin E.

What the above study means is that antioxidants would be a logical antidote to the formation of oxygen-free radicals in the digestive tract that lead to colon cancer. Unfortunately, modern medicine has chosen to ignore antioxidant therapy.

Doctors argue there isn't sufficient evidence to use antioxidant supplements. For example, a four-year study, where subjects took 25 mg of beta carotene, 1,000 mg of vitamin C and 400 units of vitamin E on a daily basis, did not prevent colon cancer. [New England Journal Medicine 331: 141-47, 1994] But colon cancer is so slow-growing that the study appears to have been designed to fail. The study measured adenomas, not colon cancer itself. Only 2.5% of pre-cancerous adenomas develop into cancers after 5 years, and only 8 to 10% after 10 years. [Gastroenterology 93: 1009-13, 1987]

Patients already diagnosed with colon cancer experience extended survival, up to two years longer, when taking high doses of vitamin C. [Proceedings National Academy Sciences 75: 4538-42, 1978] An antioxidant combination of 9 mg of beta carotene and 750 mg of vitamin C was found to reduce cancerous polyps in the colon. [Gut 34: 963-67, 1993]

Reports that antioxidant nutritional supplements can shrink or erase intestinal polyps were published as early as 1975. [Surgery 78: 608-12, 1975]

Two nutritional supplements that can be acquired in stores, quercetin and rutin, have been shown to inhibit formation of pre-cancerous changes in the colon regardless of the fat content of the diet. [Nutrition & Cancer 20: 199-204, 1993]

Selenium and folic acid also prevent intestinal polyps. [Medical Tribune, April 8, 1993; Journal Nutritional Biochemistry 5: 170-75, 1994]

Individuals taking vitamin A, C and E supplements experience a lower rate of intestinal polyps. [Annals N Y Academy Science 889:152-6, 1999]

A modest protection against colon cancer is afforded by multivitamins after 15 years of use, more so among heavy alcohol drinkers. [Cancer Causes Control 12: 927-34, 2001]

The regular consumption of 200 units of vitamin E has been shown to reduce the risk for colon cancer by 57%. [Cancer October, 1997]

In lab dish studies, both butyrate and dimethylsulfoxide (DMSO), a sulfur antioxidant, increased the time it took for cancer cells to double in number from 18% to 660%. [Cancer 45: 1185-92, 1980] In a human study, the use of DMSO produced improvements in five-year survival of colon cancer patients, equal to the drug allopurinol. [Tumor Biology 14: 9-17, 1993]

An animal experiment in 1988 showed that the addition of a sulfur antioxidant (MSM (methylsulfonylmethane) to drinking water delayed the onset of tumors after colon cancer cells were injected into the animals. [Cancer 62:944-8, 1988]

Most antioxidant studies show modest colon cancer prevention with antioxidants. [Cancer Causes Control 8: 786-802, 1997] However, if colon cancer is initiated by an infectious agent, then the antioxidants would only protect against the inflammation and oxidation germs produce and wouldn't address the cause of the problem.

Only long-term studies will reveal whether supplement antioxidants can prevent adenomas. Knowing this, researchers used another strategy. Twenty patients with rectal adenomas were given supplemental vitamin A (30,000 units), C (1000 mg) and E (70 mg) for six months following removal of polyps and another 21 patients with polyps were not given supplemental antioxidants. Biopsy specimens from all the patients were sent to laboratory and results revealed undesirable cellular changes among the tissue specimens of patients who did not receive antioxidants and far fewer abnormal changes among the tissues obtained from patients who took antioxidants. Six months after the study was completed and the patients were no longer taking supplemental antioxidants, more tissue specimens were obtained from these patients and showed that the protective effect of antioxidant therapy had vanished. This should be sufficient evidence for every physician to recommend antioxidant therapy to patients when adenomas are discovered. [Journal National Cancer Institute 84: 47-51, 1992]

Abnormality of cells obtained from rectal tissues before, during and when antioxidant therapy was stopped.

[Journal National Cancer Institute 84: 47-51, 1992]

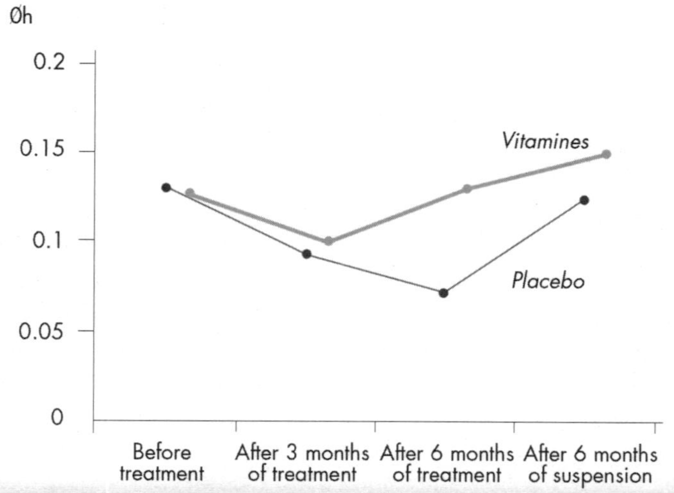

This study alone is sufficient evidence to indict the entire medical profession for lack of interest in true prevention of disease. Other, similar studies corroborate this study. [Gut 34: 963-67, 1993] Yet, researchers continue to debate the issue of antioxidant therapy.

A review of 14 different studies concludes antioxidant therapy does not reduce colon cancer mortality rates. But the antioxidants are intended to prevent, not treat disease, and the studies analyzed were short-term in duration. The analysts rigged the study to pre-drawn conclusions. [Cochrane Database System Review 4:CD004183, 2004]

When prevention is analyzed, the researchers tend to translate statistically insignificant increases into meaningful increases in mortality. [Lancet 364: 1219-28, 2004] In fact, to heighten the appearance that antioxidant vitamins may pose some mortal threat, they make the claim that 900 in every 100,000 users of antioxidant supplements will die prematurely. This comes to 9/10th of one percent increased risk of death, hardly a statistically significant number when pooling data from many studies that used different doses, patient groups, etc. In fact, other analysts claimed that these types of study are unconvincing and do not reach statistical significance. [Lancet 364: 1193, 2004] Yet the alleged dangers of antioxidant supplementation have been widely reported in the news media with no contrary opinions voiced by news reporters. The public is caught in the middle of the debate, not adept enough to know who is telling the truth.

Collagen

Matthias M. Rath, MD, former Linus Pauling Institute scientist, continues to document the ability of antioxidants and collagen-forming food supplements to prevent and treat of cancer. A recent animal study employed collagen-forming nutrients (proline, lysine, vitamin C) along with an antioxidant (green tea). The animals had colon cancer cells injected into their colons. The animals that received the nutrient mix had smaller and slower-growing tumors. [Oncology Reports 13: 421-25, 2005]

Garlic

A garlic diet given to animals subjected to chemically induced colon cancer was found to reduce tumor size and prolong survival. [World Journal Surgery 19: 621-25, 1995]

Dietary consumption of garlic protects against colon cancer. The protection depends upon the species of garlic used, quantity and duration of use. [Journal Nutrition 136: 852-54S, 2006]

Animals subjected to chemically induced colon cancer that were given diallyl sulfide, a sulfur molecule found naturally in garlic, directly into their digestive tracts experienced a 74% reduced incidence of cancer. [Carcinogenesis 8: 487-89, 1987]

Pure, laboratory-grade allicin, and allicin from crushed garlic, have been shown to inhibit colon cancer cell growth in laboratory experiments. Allicin inhibits growth by causing a decline in a critical antioxidant (glutathione) that protects tumor cells. [Nutrition & Cancer 38: 245-54, 2000]

A study conducted in the Netherlands among 120,852 men and women, found that while garlic in the diet conferred a modest reduction in risk for colon cancer, the use of garlic supplements was not associated with a reduction in colon and rectum cancer in men and women. [Carcinogenesis 17: 477-84, 1996] There is good reason for this finding.

Fresh-crushed garlic cloves produce allicin, the primary active ingredient in garlic. Garlic pills must produce allicin within the acidic stomach. Stomach acid destroys the enzyme that initiates the production of allicin, therefore rendering most garlic pills ineffective despite their label claims for allicin delivery. [Planta Medica 67:13-8, 2001] A new type of alkaline-buffered garlic pill (Garli-Eze®, Nutra Products) which counteracts stomach acidity has now been shown to reliably produce allicin, equivalent to a fresh-crushed clove of garlic.

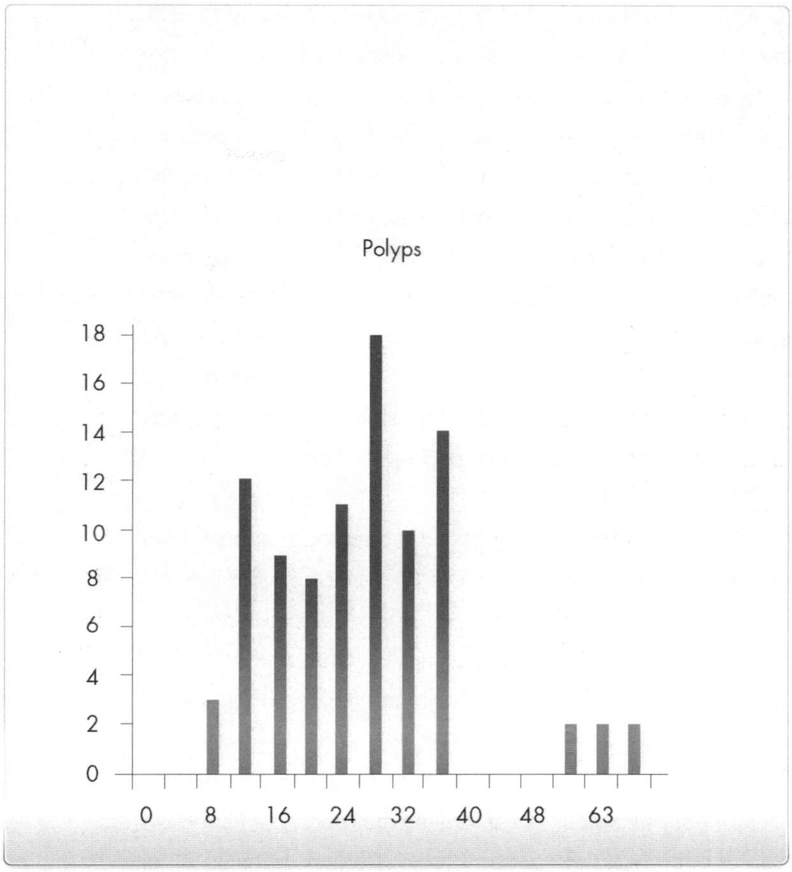

Curcumin (turmeric), quercetin (onions)

Curcumin is found in turmeric, a common kitchen spice. Quercetin is commonly found in onions. The combination of curcumin (480 mg) and quercetin (20 mg) given to patients with familial adenomatous polyposis 3 times a day reduced the number and size of polyps by 50-60% with minimal side effects. The effect was equivalent to that achieved by non-steroidal anti-inflammatory agents without the drawback of bleeding gastric ulcers or adverse cardiovascular events. [Clinical Gastroenterology Hepatology, June 4, 2006 online]

Estrogen

There is also considerable evidence for a protective effect of estrogens against colorectal cancer incidence. At all ages, women are less likely than men to develop colon cancer, and postmenopausal hormone replacement therapy (HRT) even further reduces colon cancer risk by up to 25%. In colon cancer animal models, male rodents had more tumors than females. There are fewer adenomatous polyps when hormone replacement is utilized. Colon/rectal cancer is one of the three most common types of cancer in women, but is very rare during pregnancy when hormone levels are high. [Clinical Colorectal Cancer 5: 247-56, 2005]

This evidence is consistent with the reduction in hormone-related tumors among individuals who consume an Asian diet containing soy products, which provide mild estrogen-like molecules. [Journal Nutrition 136: 561-64, 2006]

The case of Mary, a 12-year old, draws great interest. Mary's father has familial adenomatous polyposis (predisposition to cancerous polyps). So Mary was admitted into a study of anti-inflammatory drugs for this condition. Every four months patients in the study were examined by flexible endoscope evaluation and biopsy of affected tissues. Mary fortunately was in the placebo group (the one not receiving anti-inflammatory drugs), but strikingly polyps appeared, then disappeared over the 60+ months of the study. By the 28th month of the study doctors found 18 polyps. But beginning with the 40-month examination, Mary's polyps completely disappeared, an effect the lasted for16 months and coincided with the use of estrogenic contraceptives. Later Mary was switched to a different contraceptive and a small number of polyps appeared. This striking report suggests estrogen may exert control over polyp formation

Hormone replacement therapy has repeatedly been shown to inhibit colon cancer. [Cancer Epidemiology Biomarkers Prevention 5: 779-84, 1996; 7: 329-33, 1998; American Journal Medicine 106: 574-82, 1999] The same holds true for oral contraceptives. [Epidemiology 9: 295-300, 1998]

Postmenopausal women are likely to be reticent to resume hormone replacement therapy given the reports of increased risk for other types of cancer (breast, uterine), but mild plant estrogens may be an alternative.

Quercetin, an estrogen-like molecule found naturally in onions and other plant foods as well as provided in dietary supplements, competes for the estrogen-binding site on cell surfaces and therefore inhibits colon cancer. [International Journal Cancer 50: 486-92, 1992] Furthermore, Cimetidine, a histamine-blocking drug, inhibits new blood vessel growth (angiogenesis) that feeds colon/rectal tumors, and works in a similar manner to Avastin. [Biomed Pharmacotherapy 59: 56-60, 2005] Quercetin has similar properties to Cimetidine.

Flaxseed lignans, which have similar properties to soy, have also been shown to protect against colon cancer. [Carcinogenesis 17: 1343-48, 1996; Journal Nutrition 135: 598-602, 2005] One study found that when animals were switched from corn oil to flaxseed oil diets the incidence of tumors was reduced from 100% to 54% [Nutrition Cancer 51: 52-58, 2005]

Lesser known risk factors for colon cancer

There are a number of lesser known risk factors and preventive measures for colon cancer.

1. Drinking water reduces the risk of colon cancer in men. Men who consume the most water have a 92% lower risk of rectal cancer compared to men who drink less water. [International Journal Cancer 82: 484-89, 1999]

2. Long-term exposure to chlorinated drinking water (30-40 years) increases the risk of colon cancer. [Cancer Epidemiology Biomarkers Prevention 9:813-8, 2000]

3. Foods with refined sugars confer a three-times increased risk for colon cancer. [Nutrition & Cancer 21: 233-46, 1994]

4. It has long been known that blood clots are common among cancer patients. Researchers now suggest patients admitted to the hospital for blood clots in their legs be screened as they exhibit a three times greater risk for colon cancer. [Cancer 106: 923-30, 2006]

5. Chronic constipation may increase the risk for colon cancer. [Epidemiology 9: 385-91, 1998]

6. In genetically susceptible mice, infection of the colon increased the number of adenomas four times by six months of age. [Journal Infectious Disease 184: 227-30, 2001] *H. pylori* infection has been shown to increase the number of polyps in the digestive tract. [International Journal Cancer 117:1058-9, 2005] Crohn's disease, which increases the risk for colon cancer, is associated with paratuberculosis infection. [American Journal Gastroenterology 100:2724-9, 2005]

7 The weight-loss drug orlistat (Xenical) causes deleterious changes in the lining of the intestines that can lead to polyp formation. Public Citizen has petitioned the FDA to recall this drug.

SUMMARY

Summary and recommendations

It is obvious that the state of colon cancer care today is deplorable. Much that can be done to prevent colon cancer either from occurring in the first place, or from re-occurring is not being put into practice. To survive colon cancer, patients must learn how to navigate around the cancer care system now in place.

There appears to be a concerted effort to confuse the public over otherwise safe and proven methods of colon cancer prevention, such as vitamin C and vitamin D supplementation and dietary measures. Colon cancer patients need to find information, such as that provided in this chapter, in a timely manner, and be able to put the measures described here into practice, sometimes over and above the objection of their physicians. Hopefully, some patients will question the medical establishment and chart a different course for their own survival.

Preventive measures for colon cancer

Diet and health habits

Here are factors which are believed to increase the risk for colon cancer.

- 2 glasses of bottled (non-chlorinated) water daily
- Water-rich foods: grapes, watermelon, peaches, nectarines
- Fresh crushed garlic (not cooked)
- Fiber in the form of guar gum, fruit pectin to encourage fermentation and synthesis of butyrate
- Fiber in the form of bran which provides IP6 (phytate) that binds to loose iron
- Vitamin C-rich fruits and vegetables (citrus, kiwi, papaya, bell peppers)
- Dark-green leafy vegetables for folic acid (kale, spinach)
- Flaxseed meal (1-2 tablespoons) for phytoestrogens, fiber and omega 3 oil
- Reduction in red meat
- Avoidance of tobacco and excessive alcohol (red wine may be OK in moderation)
- Sunlight exposure on a daily basis for vitamin D; supplement in winter months if living in northern latitudes
- Avoidance of corn oil; use of virgin olive oil, rice bran oil

Prevention: dietary supplements

- Vitamin C, 2,000 mg or more per day (divide this into 2-3 doses); Smokers will require much more; quercetin + vitamin C is preferred
- Vitamin E 200 IU, including alpha and gamma tocopherol
- Folic acid, 800 mcg
- B complex vitamins, 25 mg
- Vitamin D, 2,000 IU; 4,000 IU or more for high-risk groups such as dark-skinned individuals, people with inherited risk factors.
- Zinc, 15-25 mg
- Selenium (SelenoExcel) 200 mcg
- Avoidance of copper and iron supplements by full-grown males and post-menopausal females; obtain iron and copper from the diet.
- Omega-3 oils, preferably as flaxseed oil, 1,500-3,000 mg per day; and/or as fish oil 1,500-3,000 mg per day
- Garlic pill, buffered (Garli-eze® garlic powder, Nutra Products, made by Purity Products)
- Periodic rice bran cleanse (IP6), 1,000-2,000 mg with water on empty stomach (if not anemic)

Treatment of active disease: dietary supplements

- All of the above supplements suggested for prevention, plus:
- Butyrate, as directed on bottle
- Resveratrol, 40-200 mg
- Intravenous vitamin C with 5 mg oral vitamin K
- High-dose omega-3 flaxseed oil, 12,000 mg per day
- Chondroitin sulfate to rebuild damaged tissues, 1,000 mg
- Proline and lysine to rebuild collagen, 500-2,000 mg; vitamin A, 5,000 IU
- IP6 rice bran extract, if not anemic (cold hands and feet); 2,000-4,000 mg per day on empty stomach with water, to chelate (remove) iron.
- Nattokinase enzymes to keep cancer cells from sticking in small blood vessels

Case Study: Lonnie, irritable bowel and colon cancer sufferer

Lonnie had irritable bowel (colitis) for years. Diarrhea was so frequent that she couldn't travel very far, almost tethered to a bathroom because of the need for frequent bowel movements. As most irritable bowel patients, she began to develop nutrient deficiencies. Her fast bowel transit time made it more difficult for nutrients to be absorbed from foods and she developed anemia that was detected only after she fainted while watching her son play baseball. Her cold hands and feet, fatigue and pale skin should have alerted doctors to her condition prior to this.

Her doctor demanded that she undergo a colonoscopy and based upon the results gave her digestive tract a clean bill of health. He prescribed iron pills, but her anemia persisted. This should have alerted the doctor that supplemental iron either wasn't being absorbed or wasn't getting to bone marrow to make new red blood cells. This could have been due to an intestinal parasite that feeds off of iron, or to an underlying infection or tumor that uses up great amounts of iron and may cause the body to store and withhold iron rather than deliver it to bone marrow. Her doctor referred her to a hematologist, who prescribed more iron, even intravenous iron therapy.

A year later, with unbearable pain and fatigue, Lonnie returned to her doctor and another colonoscopy was performed. Her digestive tract was overwhelmed with cancer. Just three months earlier, no cancer had been found. A year later her innards were riddled with tumors. Surgery and chemotherapy was required. A small external pouch (colostomy bag) would now accumulate her waste.

The surgeons advised her to avoid antioxidants and vitamins that might interfere with chemotherapy. She followed doctor's orders. Scans showed tumors had spread to the liver, so a liver re-section was performed. More chemotherapy followed. Three months later another scan revealed that lymph glands and the lungs were now cancerous. The tumors were spreading rapidly, so she began to question the idea of withholding antioxidant and herbal therapy. Pain near her surgical sites became unbearable. Pain pills were ordered. What an ordeal. Lonnie didn't have much longer to live.

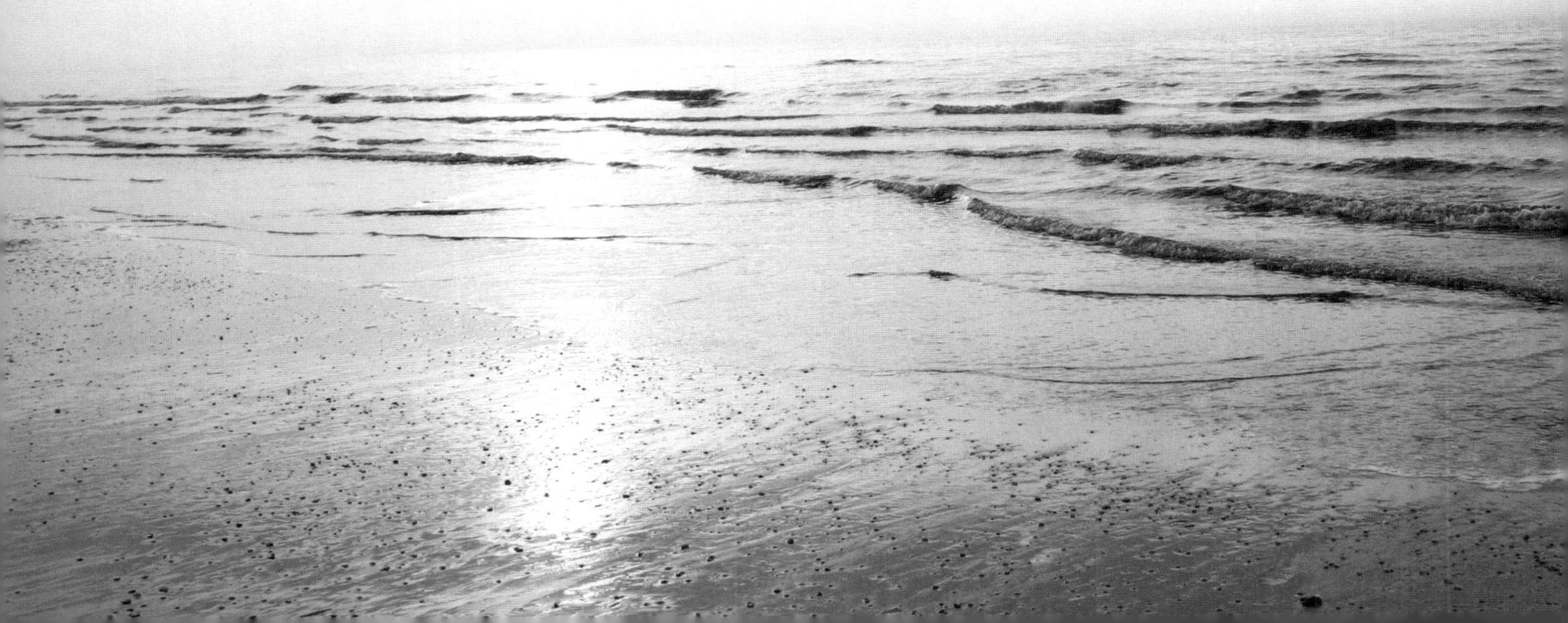

CHAPTER 10

Antioxidants

p 328 - 338

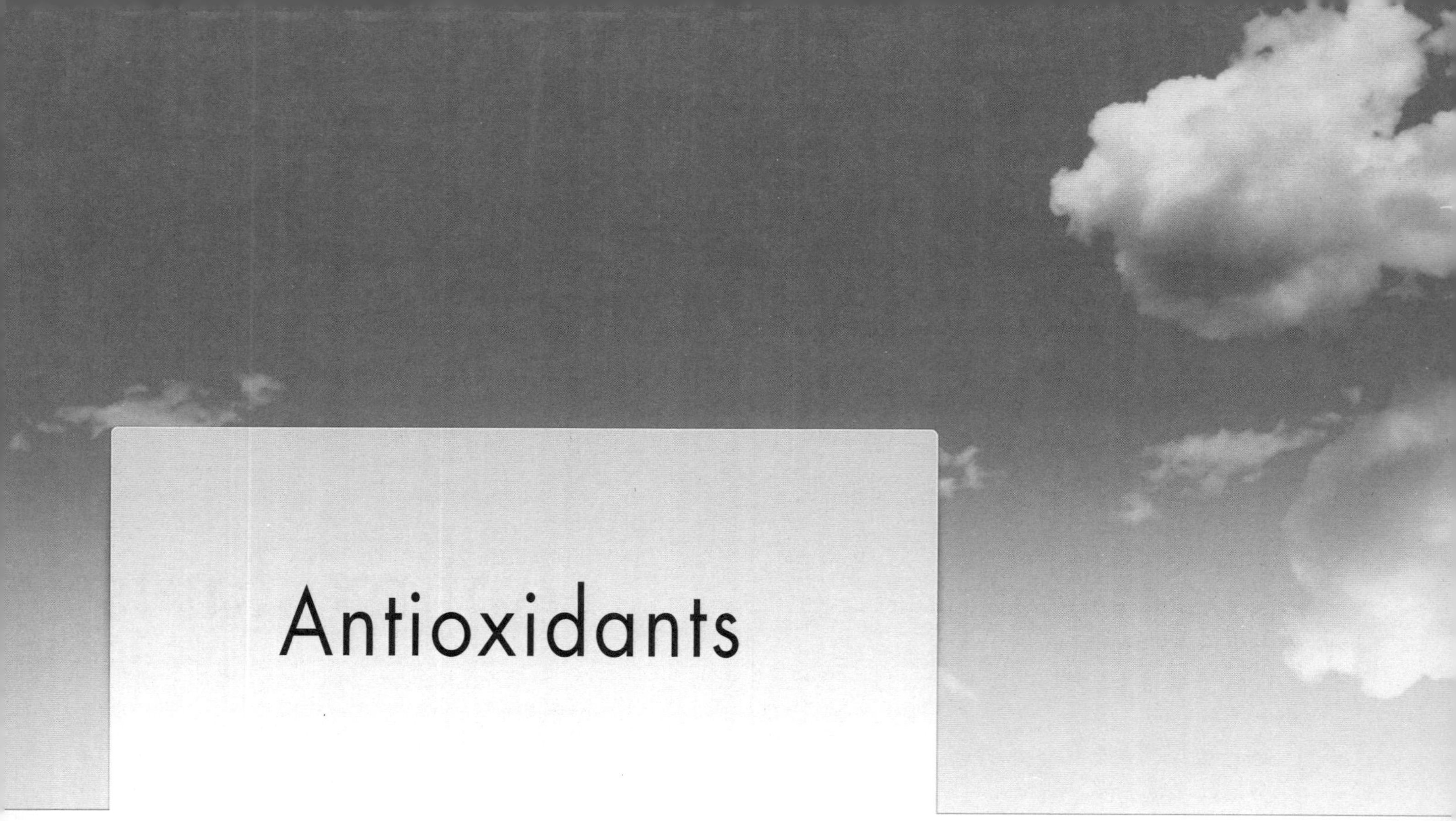

Antioxidants

INTRODUCTION

Americans hear a lot about antioxidants (vitamins A, C, E, beta carotene, CoQ10, and others) these days.

The National Cancer Institute promotes its 5-a-day plant food regimen, but it has failed to prevent cancer. In the largest study of its kind, involving more than 100,000 nurses and physicians, total fruit and vegetable intake did not reduce the risk for cancer. [Journal National Cancer Institute 96: 1577-84, 2004]

Experts estimate that there are approximately 10 million Americans in some phase of cancer development that will eventually result in their early demise. This group has no overt signs of cancer, just pre-cancerous cells. The best prevention suggested has been to consume antioxidants and hormone-controlling molecules found in plant foods. [Cancer Research 53: 5890-96, 1993] But do antioxidants really prevent cancer?

A study involving more than 12,000 adults in France did find that low-dose supplementation with antioxidants (120 mg of vitamin C, 30 mg of vitamin E, 6 milligrams of beta carotene, 100 mcg of selenium, 20 mg of selenium, daily) reduced the risk for cancer among middle-aged males, but not among females. The protective effect was observed primarily among males who had low antioxidant levels to begin with. [British Journal Nutrition 94: 125-32, 2005] Some studies which show that antioxidant supplements prevent cancer are conducted in foreign countries where antioxidant consumption from foods is low. It cannot be assumed that since antioxidant consumption prevents cancer among people living in China that the same will occur among people living in North America. [Journal National Cancer Institute 85: 1448, 1993] The segments of human populations that consume the least amount of fruits and vegetables exhibit the highest rates of cancer and are the most likely to benefit from antioxidant supplements.

How much antioxidant power do your foods plus dietary supplements provide?

In order to answer this question it helpful to gain an understanding of the need for antioxidant protection, which varies from individual to individual. Also, it is important to keep in mind that there is a big difference between prevention and treatment. Most of the data concerning antioxidants and cancer deal with prevention, not treatment. Certainly, antioxidants can allay the many side effects associated with radiation or chemotherapy. So they should not be dismissed outright for use once cancer is diagnosed.

What generates *"rusting"* free radicals in the body?

First, we need to understand what generates oxidation in the body. The oxygen you breathe, the fat and iron/copper content of your meals, the frequency and calorie content of meals, and your age, to a large extent determine the amount of "*rusting*" going on in your body. Exercise, infection and exposure to radiation (solar, x-rays) also increase oxidation.

> A 1993 issue of the Journal of the American Medical Association conceded that *"all human disease has some relationship with free radical species."*
> *Source: J Am Med Assoc 270: 2024, 1993*

Oxygen is a necessary and good thing in the human body, but also a potentially harmful factor. While much is made of toxins in the air, ranging from smog to radon gas, it is oxygen itself that is the primary toxin in the body. About 4 % of the oxygen humans breathe converts into a toxic byproduct called free radicals. These free radicals are the "*rusting agents*" of the body. Exposure to greater than 21% oxygen can produce injurious side effects. Pure O_2 for as little as six hours can cause chest soreness, cough and sore throat. High oxygen levels in incubators produces blindness in babies. [Nutrition Reviews 52: 253-65, 1994] The faddish *"oxygen bars"* where people would come into a bar to inhale oxygen through a nasal tube, improved oxygenation of tissues but also could have been problematic. That is why antioxidants (anti-rusting agents) found in plant foods and dietary supplements are widely promoted to counter aging, improve immunity from disease and to promote health.

While oxygen (O_2) and naturally produced hydrogen peroxide (H_2O_2) are sources of rusting in the human body, they are not very reactive until they are brought into contact with unbound metals such as iron and copper which then generate the most powerful of all rusting agents, the dreaded hydroxyl radical which attacks and damages almost everything found in the human body. [Nutrition Reviews 55: 44-52S, 1997] The hydroxyl radical is believed to be the toxicant that triggers genetic mutations that lead to cancer.

Since DNA damage is considered to be the initial event in producing cancer, the importance of protecting DNA from oxidative damage becomes paramount. Supplementation with 100 mg of vitamin C, 100 mg (~ 00 IU) of vitamin E, 6 mg of beta carotene and 50 mcg of selenium has been shown to reduce breaks in chromosomes by half, with an even greater effect in smokers. [Mutagenesis 18: 371-76, 2003]

Researchers at the University of California at Berkeley estimate that the number of oxidative hits to DNA per cell per day is about 10,000 in humans. Enzymes can repair most, but not all, of the breaks in strands of DNA in human cells. DNA damage accumulates with advancing age. Therefore, there is a greater need for antioxidants with advancing age. The "*flame*" of oxidation in the body increases with advancing age and is associated with unsuccessful aging (disability, disease). [J Am Geriatrics Society 44: 823-27, 1996] In old age there are about 2 million DNA breaks per cell per day! [Proceedings Nat'l Academy Sciences 90: 7915-22, 1993] Think of this as bullets riddling your cells with destruction. The cells can rebuild, but the repair process may not be able to keep up with the pace of destruction.

The antioxidant defense force

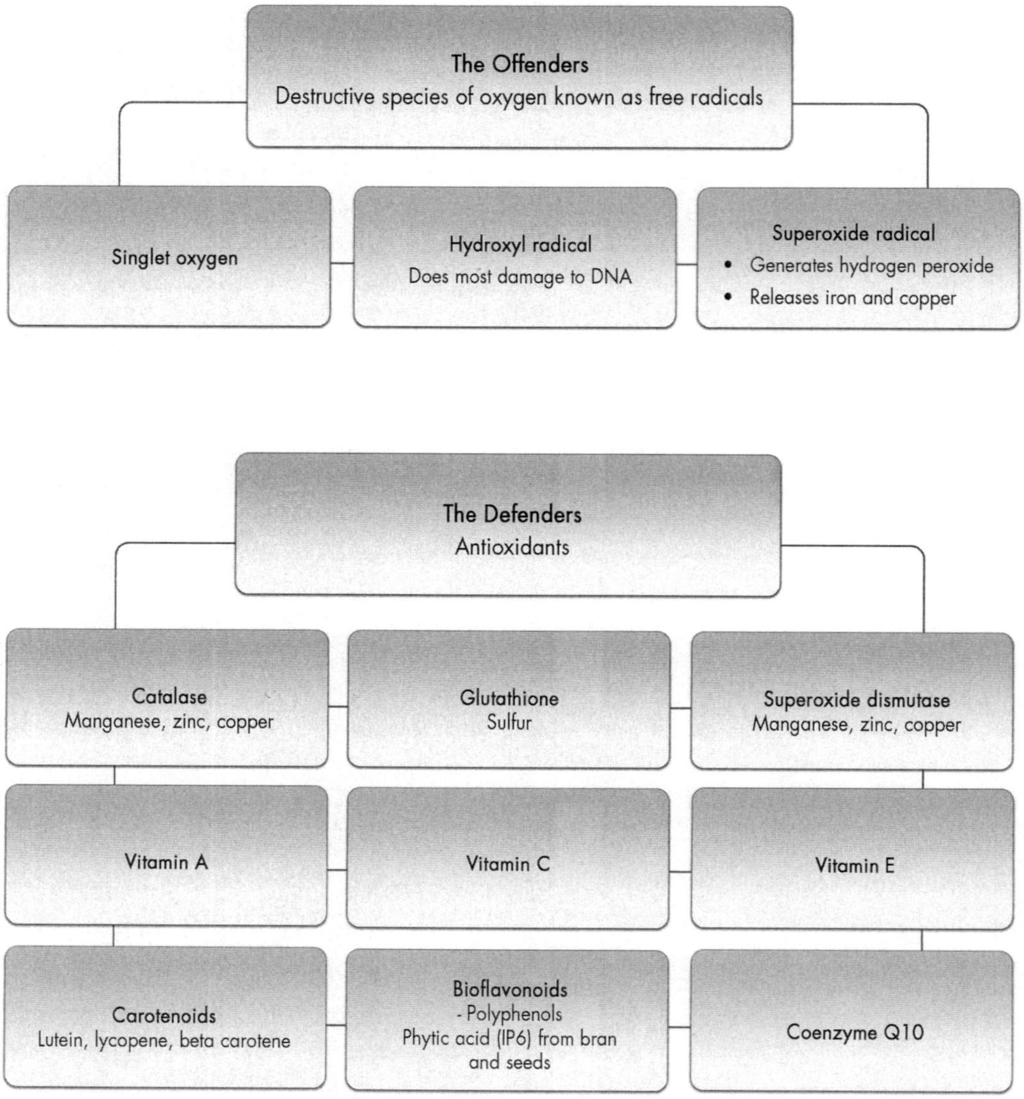

How the human body defends against oxygen free radicals that damage DNA and are believed to promote cancer

Your body makes some of its own antioxidants in the form of enzymes (glutathione, catalase, superoxide dismutase, coenzyme Q10), and also acquires antioxidants from your diet.

Think of *"free radicals"* as an opposing football team called The Offenders, that you must defend against. The major *"players"* on the opposing team are *"free radicals"* known as singlet oxygen, hydrogen peroxide, superoxide and hydroxyl radical. Here's how they line up, and how the human body defends against them.

The antioxidant defense force works as a team. A gap in the defense force, just like a player missing on a football team, means there is a weakness that can result in damage to DNA and eventually cause cancer. The antioxidant team has three layers of defense. The first line of defense against DNA damage is composed of enzymes (catalase, glutathione, superoxide dismutase) produced in the body. These are derived from minerals, as shown in the chart above. The second line of defense is antioxidant vitamins. These vitamins also regenerate each other. For example, vitamin E donates an electron to vitamin C so it can get back onto the field and perform its job. Vitamin C donates an electron to vitamin A so it can become an active antioxidant once it is used up. The third line of defense is the carotenoids, CoQ10 and bioflavonoids, which back up the vitamins. In case there is not enough vitamin A stored in the liver, beta carotene can be summoned from storage in the skin, or from the daily diet, and convert into more vitamin A. In case vitamin E is in short supply, coenzyme Q10 will take its place. Bioflavonoids help to prolong the action of vitamin C. They all work together as a team.

To prove this point, examine the chart below. When hamsters were exposed to a cancer-causing chemical that was applied inside their cheeks and then given antioxidants, it was found that a mixture of antioxidants provided the most protection against cancer.

Treatment	Number of animals	Number of tumors
None	10	17
Vitamin C	10	15
Vitamin E	10	7
Beta carotene	10	7
Glutathione	10	6
Mixture (all of above)	10	2

Source: Nutrition & Cancer 20: 145-51, 1993

Reducing the need for antioxidants by limiting food

Calorie-restricted diets, or fasting, have been found to reduce the "*flame*" of oxidation in living tissues. The way this works is, the less food you eat, the fewer antioxidants you need to counter adverse effects of free radicals. [Arch Biochem Biophysics 333: 189-97, 1996] Even brief fasts are said to be beneficial.

Food stokes the fires of free radical production and Americans generally eat a lot of food, on average 3,700+ calories per day. For comparison, the long-lived Japanese consume about 2,800 calories and the Japanese on Okinawa consume only about 1,100-1,500 calories per day. (Okinawa is where many are living beyond the age of 100 years in good health.) With about 40% of the U.S. population consuming fat-laden fast foods on a daily basis, there is a great need to counter the adverse effects posed by over-consumption through the use of antioxidants. [J Am Dietetic Assn 103: 1332-38, 2003]

The best advice is to take antioxidant supplements with meals, when the "*flame*" of oxidation is high. The provision of high dose vitamins C and E has been shown to counter the adverse effects of consuming a sugar- or fat-laden meal. [University at Buffalo, American Diabetes Association, June 16, 2002]

A high-fat meal impairs the ability of blood vessels to widen (control blood pressure) for at least four hours after a meal. One study found the provision of a powdered fruit-vegetable concentrate can reverse this effect. [J Am College Cardiology 41: 1744-49, 2003]

This is in contrast to another study which showed that 1,000 mg of vitamin C and 800 IU of vitamin E did <u>not</u> improve blood flow following consumption of a high- or low-fat meal. [Journal Am Med Assn 278: 1682-86, 1997]

Why didn't the high-dose antioxidant vitamins work while the plant-food concentrate did?

Here is an important point. According to the U.S. Department of Agriculture, the iron- and copper-binding molecules called polyphenols in some foods (particularly grapes, berries, cherries, olives, cocoa, tea and citrus rind) account for most of the antioxidant capacity of fruits and vegetables. [J AOAC Int 83: 950-56, 2000] A plentiful supply of polyphenols (sometimes called bioflavonoids) may not be provided in the best plant food diet or supplement regimen. Interestingly, it was found that a major measure of oxidation was not reduced among vegetarians compared to non-vegetarians. [European J Epidemiology 11: 207-11, 1995] Even dedicated herbivores may not get enough antioxidants.

Most multivitamins do not provide a significant amount of polyphenols either. Even multivitamins containing mega doses of vitamins C and E, just don't have enough antioxidant punch. In comparative studies, vitamin E did not affect markers of DNA damage in liver cells, but green tea, which contains polyphenols, did. [Free Radical Research 25: 57-74, 1996]

Certainly most Americans consume a diet low in antioxidant-rich plant foods. The most popular plant-based foods consumed by Americans (in order of consumption) are iceberg lettuce, tomatoes, French fries, orange juice and onions.

The mixed message

So just when you are all set to load up on antioxidants, especially the polyphenols, the current advice you are likely to find in the lay press is to forget about pills and capsules. For example a Los Angeles Times article published in 2003 said: *"Several larger research studies have found that people who took antioxidant supplements received no greater protection from chronic diseases than those who didn't... They (antioxidants) are no longer considered the miracle cure they once were."* [LA Times Oct 27, 2003] The LA Times article cited a study of more than 20,000 British adults who took antioxidant supplements but showed no difference in heart attack, stroke or cancer rates compared to people who took a worthless placebo tablet. The LA Times concluded by saying *"For now, many doctors and scientists agree that you're better off consuming antioxidants in their natural form – by eating fruits and vegetables – than by taking a vitamin pill."* Melanie Polk, director of nutrition education at the American Institute of Cancer Research was cited at the end of the article saying: *"We should be spending our money in the produce department, not the vitamin aisle."*

There is always an element of truth in these news reports. Could it be that antioxidant supplements, in particular multivitamins, simply don't provide enough antioxidant power? Are the vitamin supplement nay-sayers correct?

Run to the vegetable stand?

OK, OK, so we're all headed to the vegetable stand. The impetus to increase fruit and vegetable consumption arose over a decade ago when a review of over 200 scientific studies revealed plant food consumption decreases the risk of cancer. That's when the American Cancer Institute developed its 5-a-day program. [J Am Dietetic Assn 94: 32-36, 1994] However, human compliance has been low. A study of 15,000 U.S. adults revealed only 17% consumed 5 or more servings of fruits and vegetables a day. [J Am Dietetic Assn 99: 1241-48, 1999]

But, horrors, the 5-a-day program has met failure also. It's now a decade later and the National Cancer Institute (NCI) can't report its 5-a-day program has dented the rate of cancer. We know that low dietary intake of fruits and vegetables doubles the risk for most types of cancer. [Proceedings Nat'l Academy Sciences 90: 7915-22, 1993] But high consumption of plant foods has not been found to necessarily lower the risk of cancer either.

One study found that when 25 men consumed 5-7 servings of fruits and vegetables or an equivalent in plant food concentrates, their antioxidant blood levels rose, but a chemical marker of oxidation was not affected. [British J Nutrition 85: 459-64, 2001] Does this mean humans need far more antioxidants than most optimal diets and supplement regimens provide? Just how many servings of antioxidant-rich plant foods do we need to consume per day?

The NCI has now updated its plant food campaign to 9-a-day. Five servings is *"just the bare minimum,"* the NCI is now saying. But, only 4 % of U.S. males consume 9 servings a day! [British Medical Journal 326: 1003, 2003]

While vegetables provide important antioxidants like folic acid (required for DNA repair), lutein, beta carotene and lycopene, it is certain fruits that provide the all-important, iron-binding antioxidants, the polyphenols. [J Nutrition 130: 3063-67, 2000]

In the battle of foods versus supplements, a tell-tale study, involving over 12,000 adults in Europe, found that middle-aged males (45-60 years of age) taking a supplement regimen (120 mg vitamin C, 30 mg vitamin E, 6 mg beta carotene, 100 mcg selenium and 20 mg zinc daily) experienced a significant reduction in cancer mortality. [Archives Internal Medicine 164: 2335-42, 2004] Females, however, did not experience a benefit. This most likely was due to the high iron levels in males which increase their need for antioxidant protection. During their fertile years, females derive protection against oxidation and subsequent disease by estrogen and their much lower iron levels.

The males who most benefited from antioxidant supplementation were those who began the 7.5 year study with low antioxidant blood levels. [British Journal Nutrition 94: 125-32, 2005] Smokers, diabetics, and others with poor health habits were the most likely to have low antioxidant blood concentrations and the least likely to be taking supplements or eating a healthy diet.

High antioxidant foods

To help sort out which foods have the most antioxidant power, the U.S. Department of Agriculture developed a measure of the combined antioxidant power of foods and supplements. It's called the Oxygen Radical Absorption Capacity (ORAC). Throw all the plant foods you eat into a pile and how much "*anti-rusting*" or ORAC power do you get? The consumption of five servings of plant foods yields about 1,750 ORAC units, and nine servings yields about 3,150 ORAC units. Here is a comparison of the ORAC values of various plant foods.

Most health conscious Americans simply are not going to be able to consume nine servings of fruits and veggies a day, certainly not on a consistent basis. Is there any shortcut? Yes, we can juice. But people who juice often use vegetables to make their green drinks rather than polyphenol-rich fruits. Certainly, fresh food should not be shunned for a pill or a greens drink. But there is a crying need for more ORAC anti-oxidant power in multivitamins to make up for shortages in the diet.

Multivitamin antioxidant power

Just how much ORAC antioxidant power do multivitamins provide? Various brands of multivitamins were selected based upon their labels which advertised extra antioxidant potency or inclusion of plant extracts. They were tested for ORAC antioxidant power by Genox, an independent laboratory. Surprisingly, no multivitamin provided more than 350 ORAC antioxidant units, equivalent to about 1 serving of fruits and vegetables. [Personal study]

The addition of antioxidant-rich fruit (polyphenol) extracts to a multivitamin can make a big difference in delivery of antioxidant power, equivalent in one top brand of multivitamins in this case to 15.5 servings of fruits and vegetables (5,450 ORAC units).

Bottom line: eat high ORAC antioxidant-rich fruits (apple peel, grapes, pomegranates, cherries, blueberries). Juicing may be advantageous but poses challenges in having to consume high volumes of food and to maintain fresh stocks in the kitchen. Greens formulas (drinks, powders) may or may not be advantageous and should be labeled for their ORAC values to help consumers evaluate their antioxidant power. The addition of a relatively small amount of fruit extracts to a multivitamin regimen could deliver the ORAC antioxidant power needed when the body is challenged by oxidative stress.

Plant food	ORAC antioxidant values per milligram	Increase in ORAC antioxidant power over broccoli, carrots or barley
Broccoli, carrots, barley	Reference for comparison	---
Garlic, nettles, onion	0.05	1.25 times
Spinach, kale	0.07	1.70 times
Melon seed	0.10	2.50 times
Cherry	0.29	7.25 times
Red wine grape	0.30	7.50 times
Blueberry	0.40	10.00 times
Pomegranate	0.45	11.25 times
Grape seed	8.00	200.00 times
Apple peel	15.0	375.00 times

Consumer note: ORAC power is often mistakenly listed as ORAC per 100 grams or even per 100,000 grams of material. ORAC, as defined by the U.S. Department of Agriculture, is ORAC per 1 gram (1,000 mg). Many companies assign an artificially and misleadingly high ORAC score to their products by fudging on these numbers. One serving of fruits and vegetables equals 350 ORAC units, so a multivitamin or antioxidant supplement equivalent to the National Cancer Institute's recommendation to eat more plant foods should deliver around 3,150-4,550 ORAC units.

Misunderstandings about antioxidants and cancer

Antioxidants are cell protectors. They protect the DNA inside the cell from being damaged. They also counter any threats by toxins or free radicals to cell survival.

It is easy to see why antioxidants are often misunderstood when it pertains to cancer treatment. Some antioxidants are not selective in their protective roles. They protect both healthy and malignant cells. Healthy cells produce glutathione, a universal antioxidant. High glutathione activity levels have been associated with cancer prevention. [International Journal Cancer 88: 702-07, 2000] Consumption of glutathione-rich foods decreases the risk for cancer. But once cancer has started, it may help protect tumor cells, even guarding cancer cells from the toxic effects of anti-cancer drugs. Much higher levels of glutathione are produced by tumor cells, and even more by tumor cells that are metastasizing (spreading). [Tumori 81: 132-34, 1995; Hematology Oncology Clinics North America 9: 383-96, 1995]

This brings up the question: should high-dose antioxidants be employed during chemo or radiation therapy? Some oncologists say no. [CAN Cancer Journal Clinicians 55:

319-2005] Other oncologists say yes, antioxidants can minimize tissue damage to healthy tissues and side effects that patients experience. Antioxidants, especially an array of antioxidants, can influence genes and aid in treatment. [Journal American College Nutrition 18: 13-25, 1999] Why is there such a difference of opinion?

The controversy began in 2005 when Gabriella M. D'Andrea, MD, of Memorial Sloan-Kettering Cancer Center in New York, wrote a scathing directive, scaring both patients and doctors away from the idea of using antioxidants during chemotherapy or radiation treatment for cancer. It was published in the prestigious journal *CA Cancer Journal* for Clinicians as well as in newspapers across the country. [CA Cancer Journal Clinicians 55: 319-21, 2005]

D'Andrea said doctors *"should advise their patients against the use of antioxidant dietary supplements during chemotherapy or radiotherapy. Such caution should be seen as the standard approach for any unproven agent that may be harmful."* The news media never sought out a contrary opinion.

D'Andrea called attention to the usual studies such as the one from the Mayo Clinic that discredited the experiments conducted by Dr. Linus Pauling (which showed that intravenous vitamin C extended the lives of cancer patients by many months beyond what conventional cancer treatment could accomplish), and the flawed beta carotene / lung cancer study conducted with smokers in Finland, a study which didn't even involve patients being treated for cancer.

In fact, Levin cited studies that showed a large percentage of cancer patients, up to 40% in one study, die in a state of malnutrition, not overloaded with antioxidants as her paper claimed. [International Journal Cancer 85:643-8, 2000].

Examine the compelling evidence for yourself.

Recurrence of bladder cancer following treatment is high. The five-year recurrence of bladder cancer treated with immunotherapy ranges from 45-61 %. The provision of conventional immunotherapy is not as effective as high-dose antioxidant therapy in preventing recurrence of bladder cancer. In one study, 91% of bladder cancer patients receiving the Recommended Daily Allowance of an array of supplemental vitamins and minerals experienced recurrence of their tumors compared to 41% receiving mega-dose vitamins and minerals (vitamin A [40,000 IU], vitamin B 6 [100 mg], vitamin C [2,000 mg], vitamin E [400 IU] and zinc [90 mg]) [Journal Urology 151: 21-26, 1994]

The 5-year survival of metastatic breast cancer is only about 15% and the use of drugs like 5-FU are only considered to be a palliative (painkilling) treatment. The addition of a folic acid B vitamin infusion increased remissions by 5-53%. [Anticancer Research 20:1969-75, 2000]

Folic acid has also been found to double survival rates for colon cancer patients. Patients with metastatic colon/rectal cancer given the drug 5-FU (5-Fluorouracil) alone or with folic acid infusions experienced the following results:

D'Andrea's paper was not properly peer reviewed by the journal. It cited studies which drew opposite conclusions from what her paper claimed.

Watchdog Neil E. Levin, a certified nutritionist, scrutinized her report. He showed that D'Andrea failed to cite many published papers that do indeed justify the use of antioxidants and other dietary supplements during cancer treatment.

	5-Fluorouracil	5-Fluorouracil + Folic acid
Complete or partial remission	9%	16%
Arrest of tumor growth	20%	60%
Progression	71%	24%
Survival time	7.2-9.1 months	15.0 - 16.3 months

Source: Schweiz Rundsch Med Prax 87:573-7. 1998

When 32 breast cancer patients, age 32-81 years, were given an antioxidant regimen consisting of 2,850 mg vitamin C, 2,500 IU vitamin E, 32.5 mg beta carotene, 387 mcg selenium, 5,000 mg of essential omega-3 fatty acids, and 90 mg of coenzyme Q10, no patients developed distant tumors, quality of life improved (no weight loss, reduced use of pain killers), six patients showed partial remission and none of the patients expired during the 18-month study period. [Molecular Aspects Medicine 15: 231-40S, 1994]

Here is how Kedar N. Prasad of the University of Colorado describes the problems faced by cancer patients today. He says cancer patients can be divided into two groups, those who are undergoing treatment and those who are in remission but carry the risk for a second new cancer. Surgery, chemo and radiation therapy are utilized for the treatment of the first group, however, *"at present there is no strategy to reduce the risk of a new cancer in the second group."* Cancer patients won't discover this till after they have undergone treatment.

Dr. Prasad proposes high-dose multiple antioxidants for those in remission. The objective is to reduce the risk of recurrence. Prasad says *"most oncologists do not recommend antioxidants during therapy, fearing that they may protect cancer cells against the damaging effect of treatment agents."* [Expert Review Anticancer Therapy 3: 903-15, 2003]

What is not factored in is that the body produces its own antioxidants (glutathione, catalase, superoxide dismutase) when toxic drugs or radiation are used. Long-term treatment eventually leads to cancer cell treatment resistance by virtue of increased production of these internal antioxidants. [Drug Resistance Clinical Oncology Hematology 9: 383-95, 1995] The reason why conventional cancer treatment is often ineffective is because it is on a dead-end street.

Drs. Kedar N. Prasad and Rita Kumar at the University of Colorado, report that multiple high-dose antioxidants are essential for a maximal reduction in cancer incidence among high-risk individuals and that the use of one or two vitamins may be ineffective or even harmful. [Nutrition Cancer 26: 11-19, 1996]

Antioxidants: Cell protectors

Head and neck cancer patients who took 400 units of vitamin E for three years following radiation treatment were at greater risk for secondary tumors (288% increase) compared to patients who did not supplement with vitamin E. [Journal National Cancer Institute 97: 481-88, 2005] This increase in cancer recurrence can be explained by the provision of a sole antioxidant [just vitamin E] rather than a variety of antioxidants, and by the fact that vitamin E is not a selective anti-cancer agent. It protects both healthy and malignant cells. However, vitamin E, 400 units, has been shown to reduce the risk for prostate cancer. [Journal Urology 174: 519-22, 2005] This can be explained by the fact that prostatic tissue is very fatty and vitamin E is an antioxidant stored in, and protective of, fats. Overall, however, researchers have found that high-doses of multiple antioxidants are required for prevention and treatment of cancer. [Cancer Letters 115: 105-11, 1997] The next time you read a report that says this vitamin or that vitamin wasn't effective against cancer, you need to determine whether single doses or an array of antioxidants were used.

Oxidation and cancer

With all of the current emphasis on antioxidants, you might be surprised to learn that, once tumors have formed, oxidation can be used to kill off cancer cells. For example, omega-3 oils can easily oxidize and promote what is called lipid peroxidation. When omega-3 oils are used in conjunction with radiation therapy or with chemotherapy drugs such as tamoxifen, 5FU, or Desferal, cancer cell growth is slowed. Researchers even claim that omega-3 oils, when used alone, *"may be a useful alternative therapy for patients who are not candidates for standard toxic cancer therapies."* [Journal Nutrition 134: 3427-30S, 2004] The use of omega-3 oils does not interfere with, but rather enhances, the effect of toxic cancer drugs. [In Vivo 18: 543-47, 2004]

To further show how this dynamic works, a study was performed in a laboratory dish using human breast cancer cells. Anti-cancer drugs, in combination with oxidant-stimulating omega-3 oils, increased cancer cell death. But when vitamin E, an antioxidant, was added to the lab dish, then the effect was abolished.[Breast Cancer Research Treatment 34: 199-212, 1995] In an animal study, untreated tumor cells grew by 34%. Tumor size shrank by 50% when toxic anti-cancer drugs and omega-3 oils were employed. But when antioxidants were added to the lab dish, tumor size increased by 188%. [Nutrition Cancer 51: 178-83, 2005]

Another animal study confirms that low concentrations of antioxidant vitamins, such as C and E, during chemo or radiation therapy, may help kill cancer cells. [Carcinogenesis 21:909-14, 2000] High-doses have the opposite effect. In another study, patients with head and neck cancer were treated with radiation therapy and simultaneously given high-dose vitamin E. The vitamin E caused a higher rate of secondary tumors (288%), but a lower rate when vitamin E was discontinued. [Journal National Cancer Institute 97: 481-88, 2005] This is predictable. The vitamin E should not be given at the same time as radiation treatment.

The problem with this type of information is that the public misconstrues what they read and mistakenly conclude that vitamin E causes cancer. Vitamin E protects cells from toxins including toxic drugs such as chemo. It does interfere with toxic cancer treatment if given at the same time as treatment. However, it also dulls the toxic side effects of chemotherapy, some which can be mortal.

A landmark report written by researchers at Northwestern University, claims oxidative medicine is a new treatment paradigm in cancer treatment. Other methods to increase oxidation being explored are the use of vitamin C with vitamin K, and other drugs. [Frontiers Bioscience 11: 300-12, 2006]

Coenzyme Q10 and cancer

Cancer cells are cells that do not produce energy by respiration (oxygen burning) but rather by fermentation (sugar). Tumor cells have low levels of ATP (adenotriphosphate), which is the energy molecule of the cell. Without ATP, cells cannot perform their normal functions, such as remove cellular debris, pump out excessive sodium or calcium, etc.

Coenzyme Q10 is an antioxidant naturally produced in the body. Cancer patients are known to have lower CoQ10 levels, particularly those with breast and uterine cancer. [International Journal Clinical Pharmacology Therapy 36: 506-09, 1998; European Journal Cancer Prevention 12: 321-26, 2003]

It follows that CoQ10 supplementation may be helpful in cases of cancer. While not the sole agent that induces regression of tumors, CoQ10 may be of value. Animal studies show CoQ10 enhances their immune system. [Biofactors 9: 365-70, 1999]

This led to some experiments on humans in the early 1990s by Dr. Karl Folkers and associates. Thirty-two (32) patients with breast cancer were treated with antioxidants, omega-3 oils, and 90 mg of CoQ10. Six of the 32 patients experienced partial tumor regression and one of the six cases (given 390 mg of coenzyme Q10) no longer had a lump detectable by touch in her breast one month after initiation of nutritional therapy. Another patient also responded well to high-dose CoQ10 therapy. [Biochemical Biophysical Research Communications 199: 1504-08 1994]

Folkers continued his research using CoQ10 among cancer patients. Numerous metastatic tumors in the liver of a 44-year-old patient *"disappeared."* A 49-year-old patient on a 390-mg dose of CoQ10 revealed no sign of a breast tumor six months after nutritional therapy was begun. A 75-year-old patient, after lumpectomy, had no cancer in the pre-existing tumor bed with the use of 390 mg of CoQ10. [Biochemical Biophysical Research Communications 212: 172-77, 1995]

CoQ10 may also be valuable in protecting the heart from side effects caused by anti-cancer drugs. A recent study suggests CoQ10 is safe and effective in protecting heart tissue from damage caused by chemotherapy. [Integrative Cancer Therapy 4: 110-30, 2005] However, there are an insufficient number of studies to confirm that supplemental CoQ10 may be of benefit. [Cochrane Database System Review CD003917, 2005] Cancer patients can't count on their doctors recommending CoQ10 supplements in conjunction with chemotherapy.

A drawback of CoQ10 dietary supplements is that they have not always produced adequate blood level increases to generate antioxidant protection. Oral CoQ10 supplements that are formulated in an oily base (such as olive or rice bran oil) and placed in a softgel capsule were found to be better absorbed. [Annals Nutrition Metabolism 47: 16-21, 2003]

Given the miserable performance of cancer treatment over the past four decades, with no meaningful improvements in survival rates, a rush to further investigate the promising role of coenzyme Q10 in the treatment of cancer would be anticipated. Instead, over a decade has passed since Dr. Folkers reported his first cases of cancer remissions with CoQ10 therapy, and the National Cancer Institute has no clinical trials underway.

Here is what the National Cancer Institute website has to say about CoQ10:

- CoQ10 has shown an ability to stimulate the immune system to protect the heart from damage caused by certain chemotherapy drugs.

- Low blood levels of CoQ10 have been detected in patients with some types of cancer.

- No report of a randomized clinical trial of CoQ10 as a treatment for cancer has been published in a peer-reviewed, scientific journal.

CHAPTER 11

Vitamins

p 340 - 384

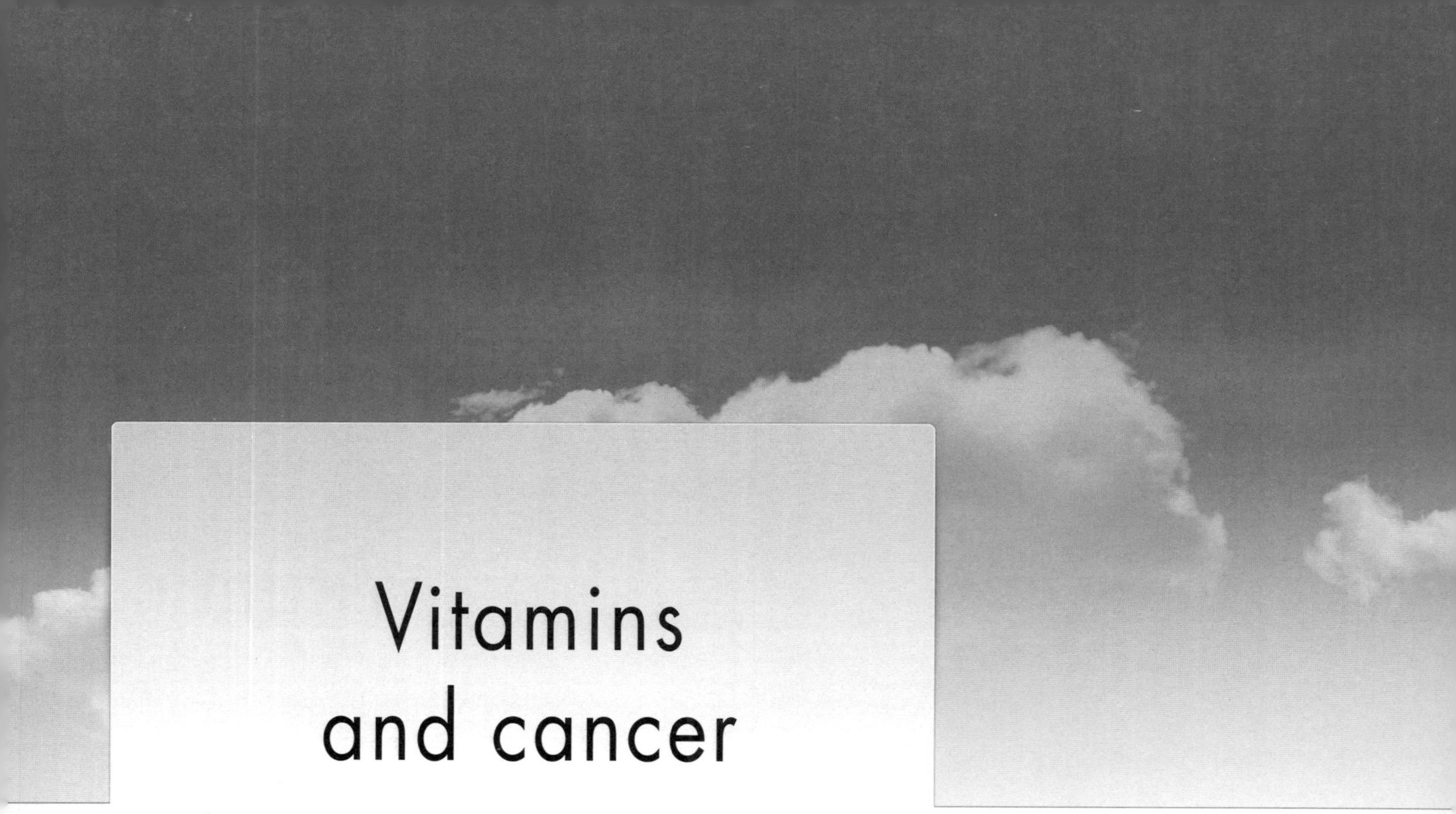

Vitamins and cancer

Beta carotene (vitamin A)

The timing was perfect. The negative study about beta carotene supplements was released to the news media just prior to the vote in Congress on access to dietary supplements. It was April of 1994. The bogus study was published in the most prestigious of medical journals – the New England Journal of Medicine and its lead author was in Helskinki, Finland, where he wouldn't have to face tough questions from skeptics in the U.S. [New England Journal Medicine 330: 1029-35, 1994]

The headlines were startling, especially for dietary supplement users. The study involved male smokers in Finland, a country also known for its high consumption of alcohol. Somehow 20 milligrams of synthetic beta carotene was found to pose a mortal risk to these men while their tobacco use and booze consumption weren't mentioned. Dietary supplements were now and forever more to be regarded as toxic. The amount of beta carotene in a couple of raw carrots was now considered carcinogenic.

Supplemental beta carotene raised the incidence of lung cancer by 18 percent, said the study. But when the hard data, rather than the relative statistics, were carefully analyzed, the concern over beta carotene appeared to be a false alarm. Here is the data, provided from the original report:

	Lung cancer deaths	Rate (%)	Difference
Beta carotene	302 out of 7287	4.144%	
Placebo	262 out of 7287	3.596%	One-half of 1%

Source: Cancer Causes & Control 7: S49-54, 1996

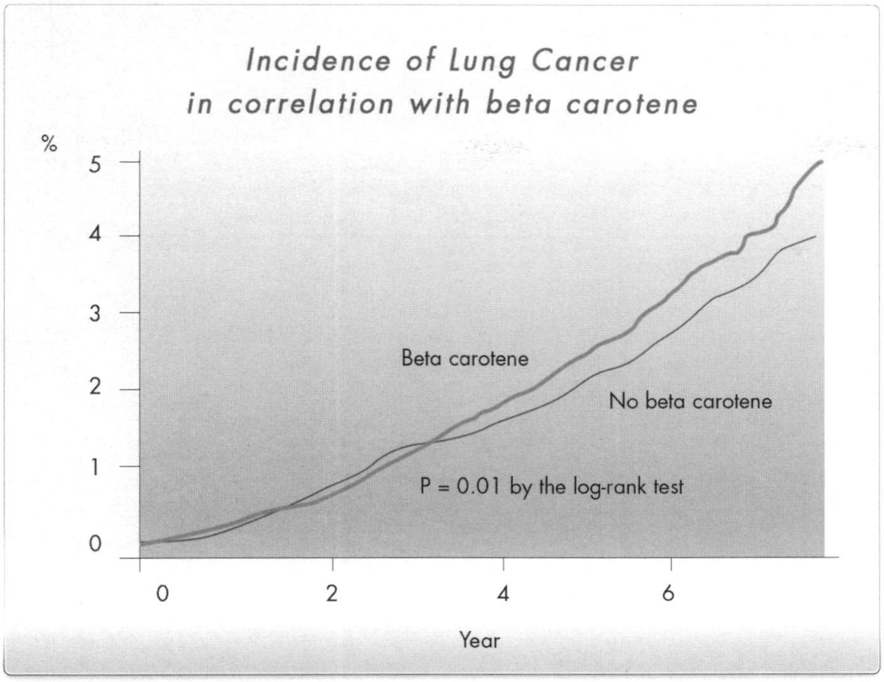

This above chart was extracted directly from The New England Journal of Medicine 1994 report involving beta carotene supplements. Notice that the increased risk between beta carotene and placebo pills is hardly discernible, less than 1 percent. When the incidence of a disease is very low, in this case around 4 percent, any small difference will appear to be significant. The actual difference in risk for lung cancer incidence, in hard numbers, was less than 1 percent, but the relative difference was 18 percent. The newspaper headlines that circled the globe in 1994 made it sound like 18 out of 100 men taking beta carotene supplements would get lung cancer. In fact, the difference was hardly measurable and the risk was only among smokers. Some of these Finnish males had such iron-overloaded livers from the alcohol they consumed that their skin turn yellow during the study, an indication beta carotene wasn't being properly metabolized and converted into vitamin A in their liver.

The dietary supplement industry responded defensively, saying the beta carotene used was synthetic rather than from a natural source, that the dosage was too low, and that the wrong vitamin was employed. But the study itself was misleading, if not an outright deception. It is 20 times more effective to stop smoking than to avoid beta carotene supplements. Yet this study is cited again and again, for over a decade, as evidence that dietary supplements can pose health risks.

Instead of saying that tobacco use overcomes some of the health benefits derived from eating fresh fruits and vegetables and advising men to stop smoking, the study advised men to stop taking dietary supplements There was no major criticism of the study from public or private health authorities. Physicians all bought into the story. Only health reporter Jack Challem reported that beta carotene supplements create no appreciable risk of lung cancer when people smoke less than 20 cigarettes daily and drink little or no hard alcohol. [Nutrition Science News 2: 100, 1997]

In the most recent study, smokers who consumed high-dose beta carotene, mostly from supplements, were reported to experience an increase in their risk for cancer, from 174 to 368 per 10,000 women. [Journal National Cancer Institute 97: 1338, 2005] The advice from the French researchers who conducted the study and the National Cancer Institute (NCI) is that smokers should avoid beta carotene supplements.

But hold on. A critical reviewer reported that the final risk estimates were based on only 12 women smokers who took supplements! The National Cancer Institute is making a recommendation based upon data from only a handful of subjects. [Journal National Cancer Institute 97: 1319, 2005]

Health authorities spend a considerable amount of time and money attempting to steer the public away from dietary supplements. The long war against beta carotene and vitamin A continues. In 2001, the National Academy of Sciences scared people away from vitamin A.

Examine the news release below, issued in 2001, concerning vitamin A.

Too Much Vitamin A Dangerous

January 10, 2001

WASHINGTON (AP) - Don't pop too many vitamin A supplements, because large amounts, particularly megadoses available from health-food stores, can be dangerous, the government says in guidelines that update how much of certain nutrients Americans should consume for good health.

Men need 900 micrograms of vitamin A a day (~3000 IU) and women 700 (~2800 IU), says Tuesday's report by the Institute of Medicine, which slightly lowers the ``recommended daily allowance,'' or RDA, of the nutrient.

Never eat more than 3,000 micrograms a day (~ 10,000 IU), because such high levels can cause severe liver disease and, in pregnant women, birth defects, the panel concluded.

It's easy for most Americans to get enough through diet alone, said Tufts University nutrition professor Robert Russell, who chaired the Institute of Medicine panel.

But vitamin supplements - even a regular multivitamin that contains three times the RDA - can push people over safe levels, the report cautioned. Of most concern are megadoses sold in health food stores, often measured in confusing "international units." Know that 10,000 international units is the same as 3,000 micrograms, a dangerous amount, Russell warned.

The institute is part of the National Academy of Sciences, a nonprofit organization that advises the federal government and has set the nation's RDAs for nutrients since 1991.

β-Carotene content of foods

Food	Content (mg/100 g wet wt)
Carrots, raw	18.3
Mangos, canned	13.1
Sweet potato, cooked	9.5
Carrots, cooked	8
Pumpkin, canned	6.9
Kale, cooked	6.2
Spinach, raw	5.6
Spinach, cooked	5.2
Winter butternut squash	4.6
Swiss chard, raw	3.9
Apricots, raw	2.6
Pepper, red, raw	2.4
Pepper, red, cooked	2.2
Cantaloupe, raw	1.6
Lettuce, romaine, raw	1.3
Tomato paste	1.2

In the USA maybe 50-60 people a year develop vitamin A toxicity in the liver, but this largely occurs in people with existing liver disease. Furthermore, the condition is reversible. Nothing is said of the many millions who are vitamin A-deficient and have diminished night vision. People with night blindness (retinitis pigmentosa) take high-dose (15,000 IU) vitamin A daily without reports of liver toxicity. [Archives Ophthalmology 111:761-72, 1993]

No case of death from a vitamin A overdose has ever been reported, save for one guy who shot a bear in Canada and ate its liver and died because bear liver provides 1 million units of vitamin A. [The Right Dose, Patricia Hausman, Ballantine Books, New York, 1987, p. 25]

According to the National Academy of Sciences, 10,000 units of vitamin A is dangerous — what? That's the equivalent amount of vitamin A from beta carotene provided in a single carrot!!! Look, beta carotene found in carrots converts

Prospective studies on dietary intake or plasma levels of carotenoids and lung cancer			
Exposure measured	Association	Relative risk (high vs low)	Population
Carotenoid intake	Decrease	0.14	Men, US
Green salad and fruit	Decrease	0.56	Men and women, China
Green, yellow vegetables	Decrease	0.79 (men); 1.35 (women)	Men and women, Japan
Carotenoid intake	n.s.	0.68	Men and women, The Netherlands
Carotenoid intake	Decrease	0.72 (men); 0.67 (women)	Men and women, US
Carotenoid intake	Decrease 0.93 (smokers)	0.40 (non-smokers)	Finland
Fruit and green salad	Decrease	0.26 (fruit); 0.65 (salad)	Men and women, California Adventists
Plasma total carotene	n.s.		Men and women, US
Plasma -carotene	Decrease	0.43	Men, US
Plasma β-carotene	Decrease	0.29	Men, Japanese (Hawaii)
Plasma β-carotene	Decrease	0.41	Men, UK
Plasma β-carotene	Decrease	0.56	Men and women, Swiss
Plasma β-carotene	n.s.	1.00	Men and women, Finland
Plasma β-carotene	Decrease	0.45	Men and women, US
Plasma β-carotene	Decrease	0.33	Men and women, US

to vitamin A in the liver, and excesses are stored in the skin. You can't overdose on beta carotene. It's possible, but not likely, you could get too much formed vitamin A (called vitamin A palmitate on your vitamin bottle), if you eat some beef liver every day, but again, some people have weak livers and need vitamin A already formed, unlike beta carotene which must be converted to vitamin A in the liver. Why not ban beef liver along with beta carotene? A 100-gram portion of beef liver provides 35,000 IU of vitamin A. This is the kind of misinformation health authorities distribute, without batting an eyelash.

It turns out that alcohol consumption will cause instability in the beta carotene molecule, and inhibit its ability to convert to vitamin A, which is one likely reason why alcoholics get cancer in the first place. [American Journal Clinical Nutrition 69: 1071-85, 1999] Researchers recommend that individuals who regularly drink alcohol should take beta carotene with vitamins C and E . Smoking depletes vitamin C and therefore beta carotene may also be vulnerable to instability in tobacco users. [Nutrition Reviews 57: 263-72, 1999]

A very revealing experiment was undertaken which may unknot the whole beta carotene controversy. The study was not given any attention in the news media. Researchers in Brazil exposed rats to tobacco smoke and then induced a heart attack. The rats pre-exposed to the smoke had a lower mortality rate than unexposed animals. The tobacco smoke triggered a defensive mechanism from within the body, activating antioxidant enzymes, which were at a higher level in the pre-smoke exposed animals. When beta carotene was given to the animals, it erased the protective adaptive antioxidant enzyme response and the tobacco smoke plus beta carotene animals actually experienced a higher mortality rate than the animals pre-exposed to tobacco smoke only. [Journal Nutrition 135: 2109-13, 2005]

The conclusions that can be drawn from this study are that beta carotene is a powerful antioxidant and is protective in healthy adults, but if a person is going to have a heart attack, he is at better odds to survive the heart attack by avoiding beta carotene. Health-minded individuals will be wise to supplement with beta carotene, and smokers should abandon tobacco. Those are the correct conclusions. If you are still not convinced, after looking at the chart above showing no significant difference between beta carotene and placebo in regard to lung cancer? The very point of this book is to uncover and reveal this factitious representation. Since 1994 all we have heard is that beta carotene can cause cancer.

Another application for high-dose beta carotene supplements might be women who have a suspicious Pap smear. In a study of 30 women who had had an abnormal Pap smear, 30 milligrams of beta carotene was provided for 6 months. At this point, 21 of the 30 patients had a negative Pap smear, with 30% still free of a relapse 6 months after stopping the beta carotene supplementation. [American Journal Clinical Nutrition 62: 1535-40S, 1995] A larger controlled study was proposed at the time, in 1995, but never followed up. Doctors virtually offer nothing to prevent cervical cancer once a Pap smear is abnormal.

Vitamin A versus beta carotene

Beta carotene isn't vitamin A; it converts to vitamin A on an as-needed basis, with excess amounts being stored in the skin. Foods like carrots, squash, pumpkin, cantaloupe and sweet potatoes provide exceptional amounts of beta carotene.

When animal products, such as butter, milk, fish and liver, are consumed, their beta carotene content has already been converted to vitamin A, so it is ready to use, and no liver conversion is necessary.

Unfortunately, the Food & Drug Administration requires that beta carotene be labeled for its capability to convert to vitamin A, so many consumers mistakenly think they are overdosing on vitamin A when they consume beta carotene. Just 3 milligrams (3,000 micrograms) of beta carotene is listed as providing 10,000 IU (international units) of vitamin A, which sounds like a lot. But it's only the amount of beta carotene provided in one-third of a carrot. Since most North Americans consume over 5,000 IU of pre-formed vitamin A from foods per day, supplemental sources of vitamin A should be derived solely from beta carotene which only converts to vitamin A on an as-needed basis.

Vitamin A and cancer

Vitamin A, like its companion fat-soluble vitamin D, works to dull the aggressiveness of tumors. Vitamin A, also known as retinoic acid in scientific terms, promotes the maturation of embryonic cells into any of the 200 types of cells in the body, thus preventing cancer. In a laboratory dish, vitamin A demonstrates the ability to slow cancer cell growth and induce tumor cell death. [Prostate 61: 142-52, 2004]

One of the reasons why vitamin A may have not met its promise to prevent or cure cancer is because it works in tandem with vitamin C. For example, the combination of vitamin A and vitamin C inhibits the growth of breast cancer cells by switching off 30 genes involved in breast tumor cell growth. [Journal Nutritional Biochemistry 17: 454-62, 2006] Since humans don't produce vitamin C within their own bodies as do most animals, and there is a mistaken impression that high-dose vitamin C is worthless or even potentially harmful, vitamin A's cancer fighting properties may be diminished.

The way beta carotene has been mischaracterized by health authorities is likely only a signal of what is to come in the future when more non-prescription anti-cancer agents are discovered.

Vitamin B1 and cancer

Vitamin B1 (thiamine) deficiency frequently occurs in patients with advanced cancer. Vitamin supplementation is often practiced as nutritional support. Thiamine is metabolized into another molecule (thiamine pyrophosphate), which is a co-factor for an enzyme (transketolase) that produces the backbone for DNA, which is necessary for cell duplication. Therefore, the more thiamine in the body, theoretically the more tumor cells can replicate.

One animal study of thiamine supplementation produced interesting findings. Thiamine, in doses ranging from 12.5 to 250 times the recommended daily allowance (RDA), were administered to mice after experimental tumors were implanted. Thiamine had a stimulatory effect at 25 times the RDA (1.9 milligrams). So the human equivalent dose, about 50 milligrams in a 160-pound adult, could be problematic for cancer patients. Of note, super-high doses, 250-times the RDA, inhibited tumor growth. [European Journal Biochemistry 268: 4177-82, 2001]

Since many B vitamin and multivitamin formulas provide this much vitamin B1, and since B vitamins are known to be *"growth"* vitamins, it would be wise not to overdose on thiamine once cancer is diagnosed.

Some researchers believe over-nourished, over-supplemented populations could be a reason why developed countries have higher rates of cancer than do undeveloped nations. [Anticancer Research 20: 2245-48, 2000]

However, deficiencies of Vitamin B1 can prevent the growth of healthy cells. Severe thiamine deficiency leads to a build-up of lactic acid in the blood. Healthy cells rely upon the thiamine-ribose pathway to rapidly reproduce. Low thiamine levels can also predispose people to cancer. [Cancer Letters 202: 125-29, 2003] Thiamine deficiency, which commonly occurs among patients with leukemia (blood cancer), can result in heart failure, nerve damage and other side effects. Alcohol also depletes thiamine. Therefore, a careful balance of thiamine status is recommended for cancer patients. [Postgraduate Medical Journal 77: 582-85, 2001] Probably 10-15 milligrams per day is adequate from dietary supplements.

In an animal study, rats fed low-thiamine diets with simple sugars developed pre-cancerous abnormalities in their colon. A thiamine-fortified diet significantly reduced this occurrence. [Cancer Letters 202: 125-29, 2003]

Then again, there is a report from Louisiana State University Health Sciences Center which describes the direct injection of thiamine into human cancers and masses with complete cures. Two cases of mandibular cysts and 13 out of 15 Baker's cysts behind the knee cap were cured without recurrence for several decades. Just one injection of thiamin into a confirmed case of osteosarcoma reduced its size by 50-75% in 2 days. [Oncology Reports 14: 1589-92, 2005] Could direct supra-high dose injection of thiamine bring about complete prolonged cures of other cancers? .

It is important to supplement the diet with thiamine during and after chemo and radiation therapy, as these treatments induce a severe acidic condition (lactic acidosis) that can be lethal. [Journal Neurosurgery 89: 1025-28, 1998]

Niacin and cancer

There is not an expansive data base concerning the role of niacin and cancer. Niacin is necessary for the production of DNA and is necessary for proper immunity. [Nutrition Cancer 46: 110-18, 2003] Niacin deficiency increases the risk for certain types of tumors. [Mutation Research 475: 45-56, 2001] Niacin blood levels vary by as much as 12 times from individual to individual. [Biochime 77: 394-98, 1995] The topical application of niacin has been shown to prevent skin tumors in mice. [Nutrition Cancer 34: 36-41, 1999] Niacin protects bone marrow cells and may be helpful in preventing side effects caused by chemotherapy drugs. [Mutation Research 508: 83-97, 2002] Niacin counters many of the side effects caused by adriamycin, a commonly-used cancer drug. [Pathology Research Practice 181: 168-74, 1986] A niacin deficiency is associated with carcinoid tumors. [American Journal Gastroenterology 100: 2307-14, 2005] Carcinoid tumors emanate in the neuroendocrine system which is a network of glands that produce hormones and send them into the bloodstream. Most carcinoid tumors occur in the digestive tract.

Niacin, oxygen and tumors

The presence of oxygen in tumors is an essential element for the effectiveness of radiation therapy in the treatment of cancer. Solid tumors grow so fast they literally outgrow their blood supply and are hypoxic, that is, filled with cells that do not utilize oxygen for energy production. Therefore, radiation therapy is of limited use in solid tumors because it requires the production of oxygen free radicals to destroy tumor cells.

Extreme high-dose niacin, injected into tumors, can improve blood flow to solid tumors and enhance radiation treatment. [Journal National Cancer Institute 82: 672-76, 1990]
The use of high-dose nicotinamide (niacinamide), which does not cause flushing and side effects as niacin does, improves oxygen flow to tumors. Patients with advanced cancers given 5,600 milligrams of nicotinamide experienced an increase in delivery of oxygen to tumor cells. [Cancer Research 57: 5261-64, 1997] Co-treatment using niacin and radiation therapy is more promising than radiation alone.

Vitamin B6 and cancer

The available data on the role of vitamin B6 and cancer is limited.

Vitamin B6 is a co-enzyme involved in the biosynthesis of thymidine, a component of DNA. Thymidine deficiency has been reported to increase DNA replication errors and hence increase mutations (abnormal cells). A vitamin B6 deficiency occurring at the same time as contact with carcinogenic agents could well lead to tumor initiation and subsequent cancer development. [Medical Hypotheses 16: 421-28, 1985]

There are recent studies showing that deficiencies of vitamin B6 increase the risk for colon/rectal cancer [Journal National Cancer Institute 97: 684-92, 2005] The protective effect of B6 against colon cancer appears to be more prominent among young women who drink alcohol. [Gastroenterology 128: 1830-37, 2005] Animal studies confirm that B6 prevents colon cancer. [Journal Nutritional Biochemistry 14: 246-50, 2003]

Folic acid and cancer

Folic acid, also known as folate, has such promise both to prevent and treat disease. It's a shame it is not being utilized effectively. It's problem: it doesn't fit into the existing cancer research and development system. As a natural molecule, it cannot be patented and sold for exorbitant profits as most cancer drugs are today.

It is already well established that folic acid supplements reduce birth defects, but the latest studies show fewer and fewer fertile women are adding folic acid to their diet. Will the public take folic acid pills to reduce cancer risks? Public health authorities have such a dim view of vitamin pills that they don't emphasize the importance of supplementing the diet. Folic acid has been fortified in foods, but only in moderate amounts, and it is subject to spoilage during processing and cooking. Furthermore, folic acid in foods is not nearly as well absorbed and bioavailable as folic acid from dietary supplements. [British Journal Nutrition 95:181-7, 2006]

Should everyone supplement with folic acid to prevent cancer? A large body of data indicates this. Folic acid is critical because the first step in the development of cancer is genetic mutation and breaks in genetic material called DNA. Folic acid is required for DNA repair and prevention of DNA mutations. [British Medical Bulletin 55: 578-92, 1999]

Dr. Bruce Ames of the University of California, Berkeley, says :
"a level of folic acid deficiency causing chromosome breaks is present in approximately 10% of the US population, and in a much higher percentage of the poor. Folic acid deficiency causes extensive incorporation of uracil, normally a component of RNA, into human DNA

(4 million per cell), leading to chromosomal breaks. This mechanism is the likely cause of the increased colon cancer risk associated with low folic acid intake." [Mutation Research 475:7-20, 2001]

Folic acid levels decline with advancing age and coincide with an increased risk for colon/rectal cancer. [Carcinogenesis 25: 69-76, 2004] A shortage of folic acid is related to the onset of prostate and breast cancer. [Cancer Epidemiology Biomarkers Prevention 14: 944-48, 2005; British Medical Journal 331: 807, 2005] Low folic acid levels are also associated with cervical cancer. [Cancer Research 64: 8788-93, 2004]

Folic acid conquers one type of cancer

After years of dragging their feet and delaying fortification of foods with ample amounts of folic acid, public health authorities finally took action in 1998. A surprising outcome was a decline in the number of cases of neuroblastoma, the second most common pediatric tumor and the most prevalent solid tumor that occurs outside of the brain in children under the age of five. Neuroblastoma affects one in every 6,000 to 7,000 children in North America. It develops in the womb. The incidence of this type of tumor dropped from 1.57 to 0.62 cases per 10,000 births, a 60 percent reduction, after folic acid food fortification became widespread. [Clinical Pharmacological Therapy 74: 288-94, 2003] The cancer care industry will take credit for this, but it wasn't intended. Cancer prevention remains a stepchild to cancer treatment.

Human studies

Animal studies provide an example of what would happen if humans consumed more folic acid. Beagle dogs were supplied with 20 milligrams (20,000 micrograms) of folic acid along with a cancer-causing chemical. That is the human equivalent dose of 170 milligrams of folic acid. All eight of the beagle dogs that were not supplied folic acid developed gastric cancer. Only 3 of 8 dogs treated with folic acid developed cancer. [Gut 50: 61-64, 2002]

1 In 1997, researchers in Italy reported on the use of folic acid supplements among irritable bowel (ulcerative colitis) patients. These patients have a 10-40 times increased risk of developing colon/rectal cancer. Patients were given 15 milligrams (15,000 micrograms) of folic acid daily, while others received inactive placebo tablets. In just 3 months, cells obtained from rectal tissue of these patients showed beneficial changes. The researchers concluded that these findings *"may be significant for prevention of colon cancer."* [Cancer Epidemiology Biomarkers Prevention 6:469-7, 1997]

2 Another human study was conducted and published in 2002. Eleven patients with recurrent intestinal polyps of the colon, believed to be precancerous growths, were given 2 milligrams (2,000 micrograms) of folic acid per day for three months. The usual dietary intake of folic acid is around 200 micrograms, so this represented a 10-fold increase over their diet. In just 12 weeks researchers were able to measure significant reductions in abnormal cells. [Gut 51: 195-99, 2002] Colon cancer is supposed to arise as the result of a series of genetic mutations, progressing gradually in steps from abnormal cells to polyps and then invasive cancer.

Recognize there is no effective treatment for colon cancer. It is the leading cause of cancer-related mortality in western countries. Recurrent or metastatic disease occurs in half of the new cases within one year of diagnosis and median survival does not exceed 18 months. [Technology Coloproctology 8:S248-52, 2004] The prognosis of patients with advanced colon/rectal cancer is dismal, with estimated 5-year survival rates of 5%. The world is desperate for a way to prevent this form of cancer since treatment is so disappointing.

Folic acid and cervical cancer

When women undergo a Pap smear and abnormal cells are detected, the question arises, what to do now? For many physicians, the recommendation of surgical hysterectomy is often posed to the patient. In 1992 doctors took 235 women with early-stage abnormalities on their Pap smear and provided them with 10 milligrams (10,000 micrograms) of folic acid. Other women received inactive placebo tablets. Six months later 16% of the folic acid supplement group exhibited Papilloma virus infection versus 37% in the unsupplemented group. Folic acid supplements prevent, but don't alter the course of, cervical cancer. [American Journal Obstetrics Gynecology 166: 803-09, 1992]

It is no secret that millions of women take birth control pills that contain estrogen, which in turn depletes the body of folic acid. It's just that women are never informed their birth control pills deplete an important vitamin. This means millions of women are taking a contraceptive pill that potentially can induce cervical cancer. In 1982, doctors reported that abnormal Pap smears among women taking birth control pills were reversed with 10 milligram folic acid supplements. [American Journal Clinical Nutrition 35: 73-82, 1982]

Women march in the streets, calling for a cure for breast cancer. Yet 17 million American women take birth control pills that deplete folic acid and increase their risk for breast and cervical cancer, as well as increase the number of children born with birth defects. A March of Dimes survey indicates women who don't take a daily multivitamin would be more likely to take a folic acid supplement if encouraged by their physician. [AWHONN Lifelines 8: 12-13, 2004] Why there is no mandate to place folic acid in birth control pills goes unexplained.

Folic acid and viral-induced cancer

There is a relatively new discovery involving folic acid and cancer. It involves a relationship between Epstein-Barr virus, cancer and folic acid.

Epstein-Barr is a herpes family virus that is responsible for mononucleosis. Epstein-Barr is also associated with the development of several malignancies, namely nasal/pharyngeal cancer, Burkitt's lymphoma and some cases of Hodgkin's lymphoma, as well as some of the AIDS-related lymphomas. [Journal Virology 73: 9959-68, 1999] A process called methylation can inhibit genes that trigger latent viruses from becoming active. Folic acid is involved in methylation. A shortage of folic acid can facilitate the activation of cancer-causing viruses like Epstein-Barr.

Since Epstein-Barr virus is transmitted through saliva, it often infects the oral cavity. It can travel to the gastric tract and cause infection there. Viruses remain dormant, hiding in nervous tissue from the immune system. Years later they can erupt. Herpes Papilloma Virus shuts off gene-controlled immune responses to herpes infections. [Journal Virology 73: 9959-68, 1999] The provision of adequate amounts of folic acid may prevent cervical cancer caused by this virus. [Cancer Research 64: 8788-93, 2004]

Researchers are attempting to temporarily use methylation inhibitors to uncloak hidden Epstein-Barr in tumor cells. Countering methylation will, however, raise homocysteine levels, which is also problematic. A class of drugs known as histone deacetylase inhibitors could potentially be used to treat Epstein-Barr related tumors by de-methylating tumor cells only, not healthy cells, which would render them more susceptible to the immune system. [Clinical Immunology 109: 53-63, 2003] Dietary supplements such as curcumin from turmeric, N-acetyl cysteine from sulfur and resveratrol from red grapes, have the same biological action and could potentially inhibit the Papilloma virus. [Biochem Pharmacology 68: 1255-67, 2004]

The first long-term prospective study involving women at high-risk for infection by the Herpes Papilloma Virus found folic acid significantly reduces the risk of cervical cancer. [Cancer Research 64: 8788-93, 2004]

This should be sufficient evidence for women to supplement with folic acid throughout life.

How much more evidence is needed?

An investigation involving 88,756 female nurses showed a reduction of 75% in the numbers getting colorectal cancer among those taking a vitamin supplement containing more than 400 micrograms of folic acid for more than 15 years compared to non-supplement users. [Annals Internal Medicine 129: 517-24, 1998] The benefits of dietary supplementation have been clearly established, but public health authorities continue to drag their feet.

The researchers at the University of Bologna in Italy who conducted the study employing high-dose folic acid among ulcerative colitis patients have practically begged the cancer care community to consider folic acid as prevention against colon cancer for all patients with this disease. [European Journal Cancer Prevention 14:395-8, 2005]

A number of other short-term human studies, involving a small number of subjects, using up to 10 milligrams (10,000 micrograms) of folic acid have been conducted with positive findings. However, public health authorities will only take action when large long-term studies are conducted, which is years away. Several trials are underway but they may not be conclusive for a variety of reasons. Most of the trials involve high-risk groups (adults with surgically removed polyps), who may not be characteristic of the population at large. Some of the trials are only 3-5 years in duration, probably not long enough to show significant benefits. Furthermore, adenomas do not always turn into full-blown colon cancer. These studies may mislead.

In the laboratory, the diet and environment of animals can be completely controlled. This may be the best way to examine the potential of folic acid to prevent colon cancer. When rodents are completely deprived of folic acid in their diet, 100% of these animals will develop small microscopic colon tumors after 20 weeks of being subjected to a cancer-causing chemical. In rodents given a super-high dose of folic acid (the human equivalent of thousands of milligrams), only 29% develop microscopic tumors. [Cancer Research 52: 5002-06, 1992] It's clear: folic acid-deprived individuals are at greater risk to develop colon/rectal cancer.

How much folic acid?

The Recommended Daily Allowance for folic acid, which solely addresses the nutritional needs for perfectly health people, is only a paltry 400 micrograms (4 tenths of one milligram), with an additional 100-200 micrograms for lactating and pregnant women. [Journal Nutrition 129: 779-82, 1999] Smokers require an additional intake of 250 micrograms of folic acid per day to raise their levels to be comparable with that of nonsmokers. [American Journal Clinical Nutrition 60: 559-66, 1994] Aspirin, alleged to decrease the risk for colon cancer, depletes folic acid, as do many other commonly used drugs such as ibuprofen, prednisone, estrogen replacement, the anti-diabetic drug metformin and the heartburn drug cimetidine (Tagamet). Aging impairs absorption of folic acid exactly when the risk for cancer rises and higher doses are therefore needed for older adults. Yet no increase in the Recommended Dietary Allowance for folic acid is suggested among older adults. What an oversight.

A few years ago Dutch researchers provided 5 milligrams (5,000 micrograms) of folic acid to healthy adults whose folic acid levels were adequate, and their homocysteine levels dropped further. [Ned Tijdschr Geneeskd 142: 782-86, 1998] It was noted then that the RDA for folic acid is inadequate. Adults who consume the most folic acid from diet and supplements are at a 40 percent lower risk of developing colon cancer compared with adults who consume the lowest amounts of this B vitamin. [Journal Nutrition 133: 3731-39S, 2003]

Why no action?

Health authorities have been reluctant to fortify foods with folic acid because folic acid can mask a vitamin B12 deficiency, which is prevalent among older adults who have poor absorption. [Journal American College Nutrition 22: 1-8, 2003] Oral absorption of folic acid ranges from 10 to 45 percent, which is a wide range. [Annals Clinical Lab Medicine 11: 516-24, 1981] But the simple answer to this concern is to supplement folic acid and B12 together. [Drugs Aging 13: 415-20, 1998]

By age 50, about 25% of people in the US have intestinal polyps (adenomas). Men over age 50 have an even higher incidence of polyps: as high as 60%. So there is concern that excessive folic acid could accelerate the growth of colon/rectal tumors. [Journal Nutrition 133: 3731-39S, 2003]

Folic acid reversal

Once colon tumors have been established, very high folic acid intake can actually promote the growth of the tumors. But, before you back away from taking folic acid, keep in mind that only very high doses of folic acid produce this undesirable effect. In experimental studies, 140 to 500 milligrams (140,000-500,000 micrograms) of folic acid increases abnormal growths in the colon once they are already established.

Supra-high doses folic acid don't always promote tumors if given prior to development of cancer. A study of mice that were provided supplemental folic acid at the time of weaning (21 days), before colon tumors could possibly develop, was conducted. At 3 months, the mice receiving the human equivalent of 1,400 milligrams (1,400,000 micrograms) of folic acid experienced a 68-78% reduction in small intestinal tumors. [Cancer Research 60: 5434-40, 2000]

However, once tumors are established, a folic acid deficiency inhibits the growth of tumor cells. This was reported in the 1940s and subsequently shown among children who had leukemia and were given folic acid, which accelerated the growth of the cancer. [Blood 4: 160-67, 1949]

What these studies indicate is that it is all important to start folic acid supplementation prior to the onset of cancer. Young-In Kim, of the University of Toronto, suggests modest folic acid supplementation, 4-10 times above common dietary intake, will suppress colon cancer. That would be about 800 to 2,000 micrograms per day from supplements. The National Academy of Sciences set the Tolerable Upper Limit at 1,000 micrograms per day for adults, which tends to inhibit consumers from taking seemingly high doses. A study using 700 micrograms of folic acid in cereal, which is greater than the recommended 400 microgram intake, significantly lowered homocysteine and raised red-blood cell folic acid levels. [Carcinogenesis 18: 1320-36, 1997]

Folic acid and natural killer cells

Folic acid is also known as a cancer fighter by virtue of its ability to raise natural killer cell activity among individuals who are deficient in folic acid. [Journal Nutrition 132: 1361-67, 2002]

However, there is justified concern over provision of too much folic acid. At about 200 micrograms per day, folic acid will begin to overwhelm the enzymatic metabolism of folic acid to methylfolate. At 400 microgram intake there is saturation and much of the folic acid enters the blood circulation without being metabolized. In a study of postmenopausal women, among the 54% who took multivitamins, 78% were found to have unmetabolized folic acid in their blood serum and experienced about a 23% reduction in natural killer cell activity. [Journal Nutrition 136: 189-94, 2006] Health authorities are concerned that this may cause symptomless, undetected micrometastatic cancer to begin to grow and spread.

A study of postmenopausal women taking high-dose folic acid found a very slight increased risk for breast cancer (about 2/10ths of 1 percent difference between women whose intake of folic acid was less than 335 micrograms compared to those whose intake was over 853 micrograms). While not alarming, it does show a trend that is of concern. [American Journal Clinical Nutrition 83: 895-904, 2006]

But don't become too alarmed, another study found a benefit to high dose folic acid. When 5,000 micrograms (5mg.) of folic acid was given 3 times a day to 43 subjects at risk for laryngeal (throat) cancer for six months, at the end of the study, 12 patients (28%) no longer had pre-cancerous lesions, and 19 patients (44%) had the size of their lesions reduced by half or more. The remaining 12 patients experienced no change in the size of their lesions. [Institute of Otolaryngology, Universita Cattolica del Sacro Cuore, Rome, Italy, 2006]

While high intake levels of folic acid are desirable, the drawback of diminished natural killer cell activity needs to be addressed. The answer is to use a type of folic acid supplement called Metafolin (Merck) that is pre-metabolized. It is widely available as a dietary supplement.

Up to 40% of adults are genetically flawed so that they are unable to convert folic acid to its active form. [Journal Nutrition 129: 919-22, 1999] These individuals may be at increased risk for micrometastases. However, high-dose folic acid supplementation may exacerbate the problem, not improve it. The new understanding that high-dose supplemental folic acid may caused unmetabolized folic acid to enter the blood circulation and impair natural killer cell-derived immunity, may explain why some individuals who take dietary supplements are observed to have difficulty controlling cancer while others are able to maintain dormant tumors that never cause symptoms during their lifetime.

Anti-folate treatment

But conversely, since folic acid is needed for repair and growth of healthy cells, it is also utilized by tumor cells. So while a shortage of folic acid may induce cancer, once tumors have been established, folic acid can actually feed tumor cells. Therefore, oncologists have attempted to intentionally inhibit the action of folic acid in order to starve cancer cells. The first antifolate drug was described in 1947 and the drug methotrexate was developed in 1949.

The chemo preparation, 5-FU (5-fluorouracil), an anti-folate drug, has been the mainstay of treatment for colon/rectal cancer for more than 40 years. Yet it produces a response in fewer than 15% of patients with metastatic colon/rectal cancer, with survival ranging from 6 to 9 months. [Cancer Medicine, 6th edition, Folate Antagonists, BA Kamen, et al, BC Decker, Chp. 49, 2003] This is all part of the nonsensical modern treatment of cancer. Why treat with a drug that doesn't work?

Methotrexate is the other commonly used anti-folate drug. But, it produces serious side effects, such as nausea, loss of appetite, ulcers, and kidney damage. Methotrexate does not solely target tumor cells and produces toxicity to healthy cells as well. Because of these side effects, cancer doctors employ a special prescription type of folic acid called leucovorin to selectively rescue the healthy tissues exposed to methotrexate toxicity. But treatment of cancer with methotrexate and leucovorin has not been shown to be superior to methotrexate alone. In 1987, researchers reported that methotrexate therapy is "*cumbersome, costly and of unproven benefit.*" [Journal Clinical Oncology 5: 2017-31, 1987] By 2002, cancer doctors realized anti-folate drugs produced such toxic side effects that they were forced to search for antidotes. Pre-treatment of patients receiving methotrexate with vitamin B12 and folic acid "*led to a marked reduction in toxicity and the abolition of treatment-related deaths with apparent preservation of anticancer activity.*" [Seminars Oncology 29: 3-7, 2002]

Vitamin E and cancer

One's impression on whether vitamin E effectively prevents or treats cancer may depend upon the most recent medical journal report you have read on this topic. Reports are sometimes confusing and misleading.

Vitamin E is an essential nutrient. North Americans get about 10 milligrams of vitamin E in their daily diet, a dose not considered sufficient for optimal health. Almost 27% of US adults have low blood levels of vitamin E, which may put them at increased risk for cancer and other diseases, suggests a federal survey. [American Journal Epidemiology 150: 290-300, 1999] Only 8.0% of men and 2.4% of women meet the watered-down Estimated Average Intake levels from foods for vitamin E. [Journal American Dietetic Assn 104: 567-75, 2004] The recommended intake (Dietary Reference Intake) level is 15 milligrams for adults.

So, most Americans need more vitamin E than they get from their diet. In a survey of nearly 5,000 US adults, about 11% took 400 IU supplements of vitamin E. [Annals Internal Medicine 143: 116-20, 2005] A study of male smokers in Finland reveals that only men who took vitamin E supplements achieved high blood levels of vitamin E that reduced their risk for death from cancer by 30% compared to men with low blood concentrations of vitamin E. [American Journal Clinical Nutrition 84: 1200-07, 2006] About 100 IU supplement of vitamin E would confer protection from cancer. Better than 9 in 10 Americans consume less than the 15 milligram Recommended Daily Allowance for vitamin E. [American Journal Clinical Nutrition 959-60, 2006]

Now, with that said, do high-dose vitamin E supplements provide greater cancer prevention than do low-dose supplements? Do vitamin E supplements help or hinder cancer treatment? Do vitamin E supplements help prevent side effects caused by cancer treatment?

A revealing study was conducted in 1982. Rodents that were fed a diet of low-dose corn oil, which enhances the growth of cancer, and given a cancer-causing chemical were placed on a low-dose regimen of vitamin E, about the human equivalent of 500 IU. This was found to be minimally effective in stopping cancer from developing. When the rodents were then given higher amounts of corn oil, the tumors grew wildly. High-dose vitamin E, a human equivalent of 70,000 IU, was able to block tumor development, but only when selenium levels were adequate. . This indicates animals which consume high levels of polyunsaturated fats require more vitamin E to prevent cancer. Selenium and vitamin E combine to produce an antioxidant enzyme in the body called glutathione peroxidase. [Carcinogenesis 3: 1453-56, 1982] This study utilized doses of vitamin E that are not practical in humans. But it did reveal that vitamin E protects fats from turning rancid and that the more fat a person consumes the more vitamin E he requires.

Now, with this knowledge in mind, where are the fattiest tissues in the human body? They are found in the female breast, the male prostate and testes and in the brain and liver of both sexes. So it is not surprising to find that vitamin E is cited as a nutrient that prevents cancer in these tissues. For example, vitamin E levels are about seven times lower in breast tissue taken from cancer patients than from healthy patients. [International Journal of Cancer 67: 170-75, 1996]

But figuring out how much, and what form of supplemental vitamin E to take, is not easy to ascertain. Prostate cancer serves as an example. Studies suggest vitamin E may decrease the risk of prostate cancer. But when 400 IU of vitamin E was given to males with high PSA levels, it was found to have no effect on their PSA or testosterone levels. Obviously, vitamin E has little to do with hormone levels. A physician is likely to dismiss the use of vitamin E supplements among males solely because it doesn't bring down their PSA levels. [Journal Urology 174: 519-22, 2005] But that doesn't mean vitamin E supplements are of no value. In contrast, vitamin E supplementation in women was found to inhibit estrogen induced cell growth in breast tissues by 30 percent. [Nutrition Cancer 52: 43-48, 2005]

The National Cancer Institute and the National Public Health Institute of Finland conducted a study that showed that long-term use of a moderate-dose vitamin E supplement substantially reduced prostate cancer incidence and deaths in male smokers. Men age 50- to 69 years who took 50 milligrams (100 IU) of a synthetic form of vitamin E (dl-alpha-tocopherol), for 5 to 8 years, had 32 percent fewer diagnoses

Two families of vitamin E molecules

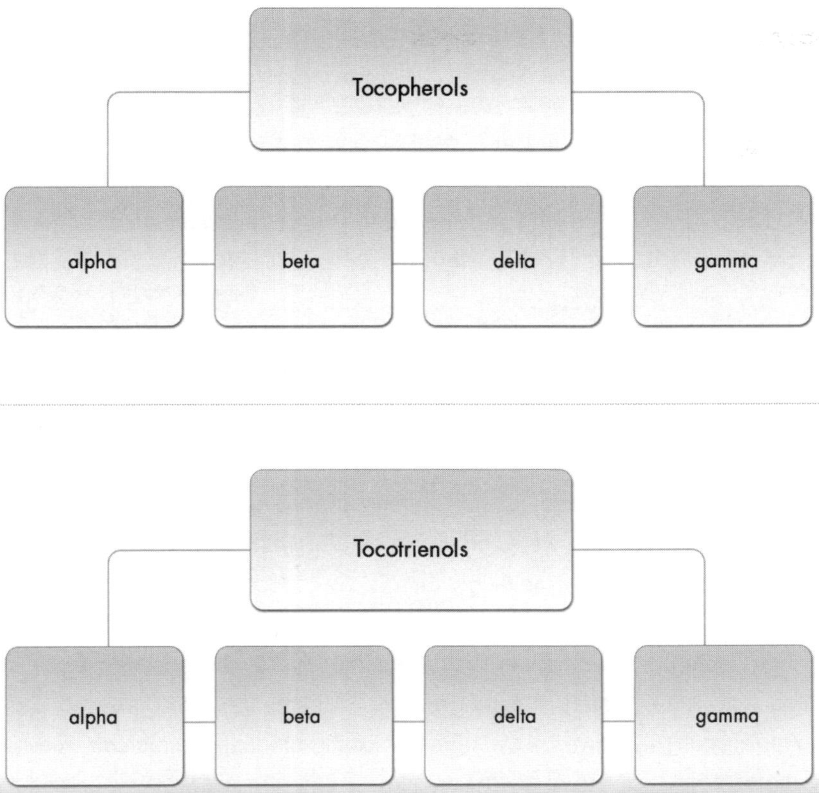

of prostate cancer and 41 percent fewer prostate cancer deaths compared to men who did not receive vitamin E.

In hard numbers, the incidence of prostate cancer declined from about 1.4% to 0.9% by the 8th year of the study. This means about 1.4 men in 100 who did not take vitamin E supplements developed prostate cancer during the 8 years, compared to just under one man in 100 among vitamin E supplement users. [Journal of the National Cancer Institute 1998; 90:440-446]

To project these figures from Finland to the US male population, which has about 50 million men over the age of 45, only about 4.5 million males taking a vitamin E supplement would develop prostate cancer in an 8-year period versus 7.0 million males who did not take vitamin E supplements. It's a significant difference if the figures are applied to the entire population. However, it is still not a knockout punch. Prostate cancer still occurs in large numbers.

The greatest anti-cancer effect is seen among males who supplement with vitamin E who initially have low antioxidant levels. The effect of vitamin E supplementation appears to be concentrated among males with low dietary intake of antioxidants. [British Journal Nutrition 94: 125-32, 2005]

Furthermore, the benefits of vitamin E supplementation become more evident with long-term use. For example, regular use of vitamin E supplements significantly reduces the risk for bladder cancer when taken for 10 years or more. [American Journal Epidemiology 156: 1002-10, 2002]

Furthermore, at least for the prostate gland, a form of vitamin E called gamma tocopherol has been found to be superior in lab dish and human studies in regard to inhibiting prostate cancer growth. [Seminars Urology Oncology 17: 85-90 1999] In 1982, it was established that alpha tocopherol succinate is the most effective form of vitamin E in regard to cancer cell inhibition. [Journal American College Nutrition 22: 103-17, 2003] Since then, cancer researchers have learned more about vitamin E's cancer fighting properties.

Gamma tocopherol, the dominant form of vitamin E in foods, has been found to have a powerful effect at inhibiting prostate cancer too, so much so, that experts now suggest dietary supplements provide both alpha and gamma tocopherol. [Journal National Cancer Institute 92: 2018-23, 2000] Not all studies involving vitamin E conclude that supplements reduce the risk for prostate cancer. [Cancer Epidemiology Biomarkers Prevention 13: 378-82, 2004] Whether this is because both forms of vitamin E were not given is unknown.

In females, the evidence that vitamin E supplements prevent breast cancer is lacking. However, animal experiments do indicate other forms of vitamin E, called tocotrienols, have potent anti-cancer effects that would be expected to reduce the risk for breast cancer. [Journal Nutritional Biochemistry 13: 2-20, 2002]

In a 6-year study of adults over age 55 with diabetes or blood vessel disease, the incidence of cancer fell from 12.3% to 11.6% among users of 400 IU natural-source vitamin E. [Journal American Medical Assn 293: 1338-47, 2005] Still, not a knock-out punch against cancer, but millions would avoid a cancer diagnosis by taking a vitamin E pill.

Bottom line, what can we conclude from the above studies? Probably that everyone benefits from vitamin E supplementation in regards to cancer prevention, more so for people who smoke or have low-antioxidant diets. How much supplemental vitamin E should you take? The study of males in Finland mentioned earlier showed that 50 milligrams (100 IU) reduced the risk for prostate cancer. A study of women in the US shows that 75 milligrams (approximately 150 IU) of vitamin E significantly reduced the risk for ovarian cancer. [Nutrition Cancer 40: 92-98, 2001] The major point here is that levels of vitamin E beyond the US Recommended Dietary Allowance (15 mg) lowers cancer risk. Consumers are going to have to ignore food and supplement labels which mislead. One-hundred percent of the RDA does not produce optimal cancer prevention. Moderate-dose vitamin E supplementation, 50-200 IU, lowers the risk for cancer, especially over the long term. Furthermore, the provision of the full array of vitamin E molecules (alpha, beta, delta and gamma tocopherols and tocotrienols) in a vitamin E supplement is advised.

Vitamin E and cancer treatment

So while it is agreed that vitamin E prevents cancer, what about it's effect during cancer treatment?

Vitamin E is an anti-oxidant, that is, it counters the effects of oxidation (a process that utilizes uncontrolled oxygen to break down tissues). Fatty tissues oxidize much quicker. For example, an avocado, a very fatty fruit, when cut open and exposed to the air, will rapidly spoil (oxidize). But the addition of an antioxidant, such as lemon juice, will preserve the avocado for hours.

It is known that omega-3 polyunsaturated fish or flax oil can selectively kill tumor cells by increasing oxidation while causing little or no harm to normal cells. This has been demonstrated in the laboratory many times. However, if vitamin E is added to the tumor cells after the fish or flaxseed oil is administered, it will completely block the cancer-killing effect of the oil. [Cancer Letters 98: 207-11, 1996] The addition of vitamin E to mice with tumors that are fed a fish oil diet will result in an increase in tumor growth! [Carcinogenesis 12: 1231-35, 1991]

A study sought to examine the growth of tumors in rodents that were fed a fish oil diet with an antioxidant (vitamin E) or a chemical that induces oxidation. Tumors were allowed to grow to a predetermined size. Then an anti-cancer drug was given to the animals. In the anti-cancer drug-only animals, tumors grew by 34 percent. In the group of animals given a fish oil diet plus the oxidizing chemicals, tumor size shrunk by 50 percent. So the fish oils work when combined with chemotherapy. However, in the group given fish oil plus vitamin E as an antioxidant, tumors grew by 188 percent! [Nutrition Cancer 51: 178-83, 2005] So it may be wise to limit the simultaneous use of vitamin E during chemotherapy. However, its use after therapy may be of great value in limiting the side effects of treatment.

Should vitamin E supplements be taken during cancer chemotherapy? Well, if the sole objective is to kill as many cancer cells as possible, the answer is no. But if the objective is to kill as many cancer cells as possible and survive the toxic effects of treatment, then the answer is yes. Killing cancer cells can be very toxic to the body and lead to the early demise of the patient. This is why many patients succumb to the effects of treatment rather than cancer itself.

For example, the anti-cancer drug cisplatin is very toxic to nerve tissues. When patients are pre-treated with vitamin E supplements prior to cisplatin treatment, the incidence of nerve damage is reduced from 85 to 31 percent without inhibiting the effect of the drug. [Journal Clinical Oncology 21: 927-31, 2003] In another study, vitamin E (600 mg/day) reduced nerve damage caused by chemotherapy from 73% to 25% of patients. [Neurology 64: 26-31, 2005]

When vitamin E and another antioxidant (N acetyl cysteine) is given to cancer patients prior to treatment with adriamycin, a very toxic chemotherapy agent, liver damage is prevented. [Clinical Chemistry Lab Medicine 43: 834-40, 2005]

Vitamin E prevents damage to heart muscle by the anti-cancer drug doxorubicin. [Basic Clinical Pharmacology Toxicology 97: 311-19, 2005]

Vitamin E enhances the activity of 5-FU, a commonly used chemotherapy agent. [Nature Medicine 3: 1233-41, 1997]

Vitamin E consumed during radiation therapy for cancer may improve the effectiveness of treatment and protect healthy cells. [Journal American College of Nutrition 21: 339-43, 2002] However, a contrary study, widely reported by the news media, indicates high-dose vitamin E (400 IU) combined with radiation treatment for head and neck cancer almost doubled the number of patients likely to develop a new cancer over time. Actually, the percentage of patients that developed a new cancer taking a vitamin E was 23.0%, versus 18.7% among the placebo users, a difference of only 4%. Patients with head and neck cancer have a 60-90% 5-year survival rate, but 15-20% will develop second tumors. [Journal National Cancer Institute 97: 481-88, 2005] Vitamin E supplementation didn't significantly change this pattern. Yet the study drew wide attention in the news media. [New York Times, April 12, 2005]

Recently The Cancer Treatment Centers of America sponsored a study that conclusively found antioxidant therapy does not interfere with radiation treatment. [3rd Annual Conference, Society for Integrative Oncology, Boston, Nov. 12, 2006]

Researchers at Ohio State University report that a derivative of vitamin E causes the death of cancer cells. Vitamin E succinate, available as a dietary supplement, causes cancer cells to die off without toxicity or harm to healthy cells. This has been known for some time, but now the mechanism is better understood. Vitamin E has a long, coiled, protruding tail that keeps the molecule from fitting tightly into the groove in the Bcl-xL protein which controls cancer growth. Vitamin E succinate is a different vitamin E molecule that lodges into the groove in the protein and increases its ability to kill cancer cells by 5 to 10 times. Vitamin E succinate may help reduce the risk for prostate, colon and other cancers, say researchers. [Journal Biological Chemistry 281: 11819-25, 2006]

Vitamin D and cancer

A 65-year old woman in Japan is among the first to report remission of an advanced form of thyroid cancer which involved both lobes of the thyroid, blood vessels, trachea and esophagus. Despite the severity of her condition, provision of high-dose oral vitamin D "*stalled both tumor growth and further increases of growth hormones and led to a good preservation of quality of life for the last two years,*" her doctors report. - Endocrinology Journal 52: 613-16, 2005

Cancer Defeated:
Vitamin D Pill For All
Economical Pill Would Cut
Cancer Rates In Half!

December 28, 2005: The world is waking up to astonishing news today .... the risk for most cancers can be cut by 30 to 50 percent with use of an economical vitamin D pill. Widespread use of vitamin D supplements would be expected to reduce colon cancer by 50%, and breast and ovarian cancer by 30%.

Researchers at the University of California San Diego caught the cancer industry by surprise with their stunning review of 63 published papers, revealing cancer rates can be dramatically reduced by raising blood levels of vitamin D beyond dietary levels with the use of vitamin pills. Large portions of human populations, especially in northern latitudes and people with darkly-pigmented skin, have very low circulating levels of vitamin D.

Surprisingly, the report did not emanate from the National Cancer Institute, which issued a report that same week saying unproven nanotechnology and genetically-targeted drugs could *"eliminate the suffering and death due to cancer by 2015."* Nor was the report on the front pages of the New York Times that chose instead to extol Gleevec, a disappointing anti-cancer drug that costs $2,500 for a month of treatment. Instead, the media ignored this report which said that a 5-cent pill, heralded by independent researchers, appears to be the biggest cancer breakthrough in history.

The report, published in the February 2006 issue of the *American Journal of Public Health*, did not reveal anything new, but rather tabulated results from scientific reports conducted over the past 40 years that public health authorities had ignored. [American Journal Public Health 96:252-61, 2006]

Repeat of earlier study

Over 15 years ago the same doctors who wrote this recent report documented that the mortality rate for breast cancer in the US is 17-19 per 100,000 women in sunny southern states where vitamin D levels are high, compared to 33 per 100,000 in northern climates where vitamin D levels are low. [Preventive Medicine 19: 614-22, 1990] No action was taken then to advise the public to get more vitamin D. This time lead researcher, Professor Cedric F. Garland of the University of San Diego, is appealing to *"leadership from the public health community to provide the best hope for action."* But will public health authorities break from their long-standing complacency in the face of undeniable scientific evidence?

Two years ago researcher William B. Grant, PhD reported that a shortage of vitamin D due to lack of sun exposure is a major cause of cancer, but public health authorities largely shunned his report as well. [Recent Results Cancer Research 164:371-7, 2003] Dr. Grant has shown that cancer survival rates are 20-50% higher in sunny southern areas of the U.S. (below 50 degrees North latitude) for many forms of cancer. [Anticancer Research 26: 2605-14, 2006] In a paper published in 2002, Grant estimated the annual number of premature deaths from cancer due to low vitamin D/sunlight levels was 23,600. [Cancer 94:1867-75, 2002] *"It's the great cancer cover-up. Panicked into avoiding sunlight by health experts, we are now dying by the thousands from diseases linked to deficiencies of vitamin D. But still the exaggerated warnings come,"* says Dr. Grant.

Here are some examples of how vitamin D deficiency raises the risk for cancer:

- Prostate cancer mortality is lower in the southeast (14-22 deaths per 100,000 yearly) compared to the northwest (24-48 per 100,000 annually). Adequate winter time vitamin D could prevent 10,000 cases of prostate cancer and 1,300 premature deaths in the US annually. [International Journal Cancer 111: 470-71, 2004]

- Even in cases of dreaded melanoma, sun exposure cuts the death rate in half. [Journal National Cancer Institute 97: 195-99, 2005]

- Hodgkin's lymphoma is related to vitamin D. There is a 20 percent reduction in mortality for cases of Hodgkin's lymphoma that are diagnosed in autumn versus winter. [British Journal Cancer 93: 571-74, 2005]

- Mortality rates from ovarian cancer are much higher in northern than in southern climates. [International Journal Epidemiology 23: 1133-36, 1994]

- Higher rates and aggressiveness of prostate and breast cancer are reported among people with darkly pigmented skin who produce far less vitamin D from sun exposure than do Caucasians. [Cancer Research 55: 4014-22, 1995]

- Higher levels of vitamin D are associated with less breast density in women. [Cancer Epidemiology Biomarkers Prevention 13: 1466-72, 2004]

- A study conducted by researchers at St. George's Hospital Medical School in London finds local production of vitamin D in breast tissue reduces the risk for breast cancer. For women with low breast tissue levels of vitamin D the risk for breast cancer rose by 354%! [Anticancer Research 26: 2573-80, 2006] This study suggests women sunbathe with breast tissue exposed to the sun to enhance local vitamin D production.

- The provision of 400 IU of vitamin D per day has been found to reduce the risk of pancreatic cancer by 43%. [Cancer Epidemiology Biomarkers 15:1688-95, 2006]

- Annual age-adjusted breast cancer mortality rates in the US range from a low of 17-19 per 100,000 in sunny areas (southwest) to 33 per 100,000 in cloudy areas (northeast). [Preventive Medicine 19: 614-22, 1990]

- A vitamin D deficiency develops in a significant percentage of patients with advanced prostate cancer. With vitamin D treatment, pain scores drop among prostate cancer patients. [Journal Urology 163: 187-90, 2000] PSA (prostate specific antigen) scores also drop when supplemental vitamin D is provided to early recurrent prostate cancer patients. [Journal Urology 159: 2035-39, 1998] In one study, 81% of prostate cancer patients experienced a 50% drop in their PSA with vitamin D therapy. [Urological Oncology 21: 399-405, 2003]

- There is a 50 to 80 percent decrease in rates of colon cancer in sunny southern areas of the US compared to cloudy northern areas. [Cancer Causes Control 3: 95-99, 1992]

- Vitamin D inhibits cancer cells from forming and multiplying, inhibits the formation of new blood vessels, called angiogenesis, that feeds tumors, and inhibits the spread of cancer, called metastasis. [Journal Urology 160: 247-51, 1998; Anticancer Research 1A: 321-24, 2001; Cancer Letters 120: 65-69, 1997] That's three drugs in one.

- Lung cancer patients who undergo surgery during the summer exhibit a 5-year survival rate of 56% compared to 23% for patients who undergo surgery in the winter. [Cancer Epidemiology Biomarkers Prevention 14: 2303-09, 2005]

- Surprisingly, vitamin D (as a metabolite, calcitriol) has been found to reduce blood clotting in a wide variety of cancers. Blood clots facilitate the spread of cancer. [American Society Clinical Oncology meeting, June, 2006]

Researchers say the *"newly recognized association with risk of several types of cancer is receiving considerable attention. A deficiency of vitamin D may account for several thousand premature deaths from colon, breast, ovarian and prostate cancer annually."*

Professor Garland says: *"A preponderance of evidence from the best observational studies... has led to the conclusion that public health action is needed. Primary prevention of these cancers has been largely neglected, but we now have proof that the incidence of colon, breast and ovarian cancer can be reduced dramatically by increasing the public's intake of vitamin D. The easiest and most reliable way of getting the appropriate amount is from food and a daily supplement."* [American Journal Public Health 96:252-6, 20061

The geographic cancer belt

There is a cancer belt in the world. Ever hear of it? Probably not. It's where the sun doesn't shine, in northern climates. The rates of colon, breast, uterine and prostate cancer are much higher in sun-deprived areas of the world.

Vitamin D3 Level Achieved Among Canadians in Summertime *Source: American Journal Clinical Nutrition 73: 288-94, 2001*	
Amount supplemental vitamin D3	Blood concentration achieved
No supplemental vitamin D3	46.7 nanomole/liter
1000 IU vitamin D3/day (25 micrograms)	68.7 nanomole/liter
4000 IU vitamin D3/day (50 micrograms)	96.4 nanomole/liter

For example, the highest rate of colon cancer in the world is in New Jersey, in the most developed country in the world, while the lowest rate is in Punna, India, a third-world country. The chief reasons are Punna, India is closer to the equator where vitamin D-producing sun rays are more intense, and the people there eat plant foods rather than meat.

Health authorities certainly know what the chief reason for increased rates of cancer is in northern climates – it's the lack of vitamin D. Exposure to the sun's ultraviolet rays produces vitamin D in the skin. Vitamin D is so essential for life that a few months' supply is stored in the liver.

One researcher estimates the annual number of premature deaths due to inadequate sun exposure (vitamin D production) is nearly 22,000 in the US. [Cancer 94: 1867-75, 2002] Another researcher estimates 30,000 US cancer deaths could be averted by moderate sunning. [Preventive Medicine 22: 132-40, 1993] The world death rate from all causes rises in winter, when vitamin D levels are low. [Age Ageing 25: 343-48, 1996]

Sunscreens and cancer

But since excessive exposure to the sun increases the risk for skin cancer, there has been a royal battle over whether to protect or expose the skin to more sunlight. For comparison, researchers estimate 50,000-63,000 Americans die prematurely from cancer annually due to insufficient vitamin D, while only about 9,800 Americans die of skin cancer yearly. [Photochemistry Photobiology January 1, 2005] The death rate from sun/skin induced cancer is 0.3% versus 20-65% for the type of cancers prevented by sunlight exposure. [Preventive Medicine 22: 132-40 1993]

Yet each summer the public is bombarded with warnings about skin cancer and advised to use sunscreen lotion while there is no equal public awareness created for the massive public deficiency of vitamin D. More than 40% of the American population is at higher risk for cancer due to shortages of vitamin D.

The shocking revelation came in 2005 from researchers at the Melanoma and Skin Cancer Research Institute, Sydney Cancer Centre, Sydney, Australia. Both UV-A and UV-B sun rays promote skin cancer. [Photochemistry Photobiology 81:3-8, 2005] Sunscreen lotions typically only block the vitamin D-producing UV-B rays while allowing UV-A rays to reach the skin. Sunscreen lotions block the cancer-preventing effects of vitamin D while allowing the deeper penetrating UV-A rays to bombard human skin, all the while giving consumers a false sense they are protected from the sun. As sales of sunscreen lotion have soared, so have the rates of melanoma, the most dangerous form of skin cancer. Colon cancer is rising too. Frankly, sunscreen lotion promotes cancer more than it prevents cancer.

Attorneys have filed lawsuits on behalf of the public against sunscreen manufacturers for misleading labels that falsely claim their products block UV-A and UV-B sun rays. [Los Angeles Times March 30, 2006] Sunscreen products that contain microfine titanium dioxide exhibit greater protection from both UV-A and UV-B sun rays. [British Journal Dermatology 124: 258-63, 1991] However, total blockage of solar vitamin D production is not advised. A few minutes of unfiltered sunlight offers obvious health benefits.

Call for action

Recently the Vitamin D Council has been calling for public health officials to take urgent action, given the growing body of data linking low levels of vitamin D with a wide list of health problems in addition to cancer, such as rickets, hypertension, diabetes, autoimmune disease, heart failure, bone deterioration, urinary incontinence, heart failure, thyroid problems, loss of muscle tone and weakened immunity.

The researchers conservatively recommend 1,000 international units (IU) of vitamin D daily, which by weight is only 25 micrograms, or 1/4th of one milligram, to prevent cancer. Public health authorities could easily fortify foods with this much vitamin D, but there is no impetus to do so. Most Americans, including health professionals, mistakenly avoid "*high-dose*" vitamin D because of unfounded concerns over toxicity.

Nay sayers confuse the public

A recurring theme in this book is that there are proven ways to prevent or treat cancer, more effectively than what is currently practiced, but such measures go unused. The denials and unfounded warnings are already being issued by health authorities who have spread misinformation about vitamin D for decades.

In the case of vitamin D, thousands of cases of cancer could be prevented and mortality from cancer delayed, but this vitamin is ignored. There are many reasons why.

First, physicians have been misinformed. They have had the idea drilled into them that high-dose vitamin D is toxic to the liver and poses other side effects. "*Large doses of the vitamin must be treated with caution. More than 2,000 IU a day can lead to the body absorbing too much calcium, and possible damage to the liver and kidneys,*" says a report by CNN [Dec. 28, 2005].

For healthy adults, this is absolutely untrue. It has become such a widespread falsehood that a group of leading vitamin D researchers formed The Vitamin D Council just to correct the misinformation about this vitamin.

Toxicity from oral-dose vitamin D doesn't begin till 40,000 IU are consumed daily for many months. [American Journal Clinical Nutrition 69:842-56, 1999] The National Academy of Sciences says 2,000 IU is a perfectly safe limit. There are reports of side effects at lower doses, but these involve synthetic vitamin D2 used to fortify milk, not vitamin D2 used in dietary supplements.

A representative of the American Dietetic Association said 200 IU is sufficient, but apparently didn't read the research paper which showed there was no cancer preventive effect at this low intake level. [CNN Dec. 28, 2005]

Americans typically ingest 200-250 units a day of vitamin D from foods, which prevents a frank deficiency but does not provide enough vitamin D to prevent bone loss or cancer. Dietary sources are limited – a glass of milk, for instance, contains only 100 IU of the vitamin, and provides synthetic vitamin D2, not the vitamin natural-source D3 reported to prevent cancer in the study. Vitamin D2 is many times less effective than D3. [American Journal Clinical Nutrition 68: 854-58, 1998; Journal Clinical Endocrinology Metabolism 89:5387-91, 2004] Vitamin D intake from milk and/or common multivitamins does not prevent low vitamin D nutritional status of young women in winter. [European Journal Clinical Nutrition 55: 1091-91, 2001]

Sun exposure will produce vitamin D An hour of total body exposure to midday summer sun at a southern latitude produces about 10,000 IU of vitamin D in the skin without causing toxicity. So fears of overdosing from supplements appear to be ill founded Depending upon the season and latitude, 30 minutes of sunning at midday could produce a significant amount of vitamin D, though blacks would need 5 times more sun exposure to produce the same amount as Caucasians. However, because of concerns over skin cancer from exposure to solar UV rays, the most practical option is vitamin D pills.

The Vitamin D Council says most multivitamins provide only the Recommended Daily Intake of 400 IU, which is only about 10% of the body's daily need.

One of the ways the public is misled concerning the cancer preventive properties of vitamin D is to cite studies which show circulating levels of vitamin D are not always related to the development of cancer. But unless dietary supplements are being consumed, paltry amounts of vitamin D in the diet never measurably raise circulating vitamin D levels. The diet may provide 150-400 IU of vitamin D, which is only about 10% with the rest coming from sun exposure. [Nutrition Cancer 48: 115-23, 2004] Most vitamin D researchers now recommend intake of vitamin D from food and supplements should exceed 600-800 IU, and probably reach 1,000 IU per day. [Journal Internal Medicine 247: 260-68, 2000] This is beyond what the diet plus modest sunlight and common dietary supplementation provides. A rise in blood levels cannot be detected till 4,000 IU is consumed from supplements.

Another reason why vitamin D often falls short of preventing cancer is that people in sunny areas are not advised they need vitamin supplements. The small amount of vitamin D produced by marginal sun exposure, 200 IU, may not be enough to prevent cancer.

Vitamin D deficiency has even been noted in sunny areas. [New England Journal Medicine 340: June 10, 1999] Americans living in sunny Florida commonly experience low vitamin D levels. [Nutrition Reviews 63: 203-09, 2005]

Vitamin D Intake Levels and Health Benefits

Vitamin D is measured in IUs, international units. 40 IUs equals 1 microgram of vitamin D. So the Vitamin D Council now recommends 4,000 IU per day, which is only 100 micrograms, or just 1/10th of one milligram. It's difficult to imagine such a small amount by weight could cause major side effects that are falsely alleged.

One microgram vitamin D3 per day (cholecalciferol) increases circulating vitamin D levels by about 1 nmol/L (0.4 ng/mL) Synthetic vitamin D2 (ergocalciferol) is what is used to fortify milk.

200-250 IU

Amount consumed from the average daily diet

200 IU (5 micrograms/day)

At least 20% of women will still have low circulating levels of vitamin D at this level of intake. [European Journal Clinical Nutrition 55: 1091-97, 2001]

400 IU (10 micrograms/day)

Current Recommended Daily Intake Leve

800-1000 IU (20-25 micrograms/day)

Amount required for most adults to reach 75 nanomolar/liter. [Osteoporosis International 16: 713-16, 2005] Intake of less than 800 IU vitamin D per day has never been shown to prevent hip fractures. [Annals Medicine 37:278-85, 2005]

1,000 IU (30-45 nanograms/liter blood concentration)

Minimum blood concentration required to prevent cancer

2,000 IU (50 micrograms/day)

Safe upper limit established by National Academy of Sciences. 2000 IU of vitamin D3 has been shown to reduce or stabilize PSA in some prostate cancer patients. [Nutrition Cancer 51:32-6, 2005]

2,200 IU (55 micrograms/day)

Required for optimal calcium absorption to prevent bone loss (60 nanomolar/liter blood concentration). [Journal Steroid Biochemistry Molecular Biology 97: 13-19, 2005]

4,000 IU

Safe daily intake level proven in recent study. [American Journal Clinical Nutrition 73:288-94, 2001] This dosage is probably the minimum that blacks and people living in northern climates should consume daily in winter months. Eventually 4000 IU is expected to be recommended universally for all adults.

40,000 IU (1000 micrograms/day)

Produces toxicity after many months

Therapeutic use of vitamin D in active cases of cancer may employ even greater amounts of vitamin D.

Most vitamin D pills provide 400 IU, a few brands offer 1,000-2,000 IU. Vitamin D in 5000 IU and 50,000 IU pills are also available now.

Based upon the facts presented so far, a person would think that public health authorities would call for a re-evaluation of the Recommended Daily Allowance for vitamin D and universal food fortification, especially for people living in northern climates and blacks who produce far less vitamin D from sun exposure. In fact, a minimal amount of synthetic vitamin D is added to milk to prevent rickets in children, and even this is not sufficient for black children. Vitamin D food fortification or supplementation has the advantage of not damaging the skin as does solar ultraviolet radiation. Vitamin D pills represent *"sunlight in a bottle."* [reference? Photochemistry Photobiology 81: 1287-90, 2005]

Title 21 of the Code of Federal Regulations sets standards for the optional addition of moderate amounts of vitamin D in enriched grain products, a provision that is not utilized. Researchers now suggest vitamin D grain fortification be mandated in the US with the specific goal in mind of reducing cancer rates over time. [American Journal Clinical Nutrition 80: 264-70, 2004] It is the Food & Drug Administration that limits the dosage of vitamin D in supplements. That one agency is keeping the lid on an undeniable way of preventing thousands of cases of cancer.

If readers get one message out of this book it is that public health authorities and physicians are remiss in preventing cancer. You will have to take matters into your own hands, you can't rely upon physicians or dieticians who were educated years ago and whose reference books are now outdated.

Cancer Rates, age-adjusted by race/ethnicity (1992-2002)			
Cancer site	Caucasian	Black	Asian/Pacific Islander
Lung/bronchus	56.9	66.9	28.6
Colon/rectum	21.1	28.6	13.5
Breast	28	36.2	12.9
Prostate	31.2	73.7	14.1
Liver	4.1	6	10.8
Leukemia (blood cancer)	7.9	7	4.3
Esophagus	4.1	7.3	2.1

Some cancer researchers claim vitamin D therapy may herald a *"new era in the treatment of various malignancies."* [Onkologie 24: 128-33, 2001] When will this occur? Don't wait for public health authorities to appear on television and confirm what you have already learned here. Every reader of this book can significantly reduce his or her risk for cancer by taking supplemental vitamin D. Patients battling cancer or needing to prevent recurrence, vitamin D should be at the top of their list of helpful measures.

Estimated cancer mortality rate per 100,000 (all sites excluding non-melanoma skin), males, 2002

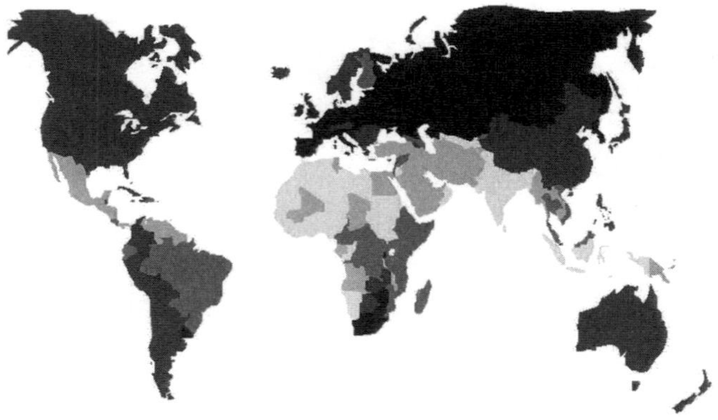

Notice cancer rates are lower near the Equator.

Do buildings cause cancer?

Well, some people think so. From time to time reports appear in the news media regarding cancer clusters associated with people who work in the same building. This was the case in 1991 when 15 cancer cases were reported among 65 workers at the Pacific Bell office in Garden Grove, California. Researchers suggested the cancers might be caused by electromagnetic fields emitted by office equipment. So far, no association has been made between these cancer clusters and electrical devices, radon gas or any other carcinogen. The problem is that cancer investigators often search for factors that are present, not ones that are absent.

Cancer Incidence Among African Americans And Whites Source: SEER Cancer Statistics Review, 2003

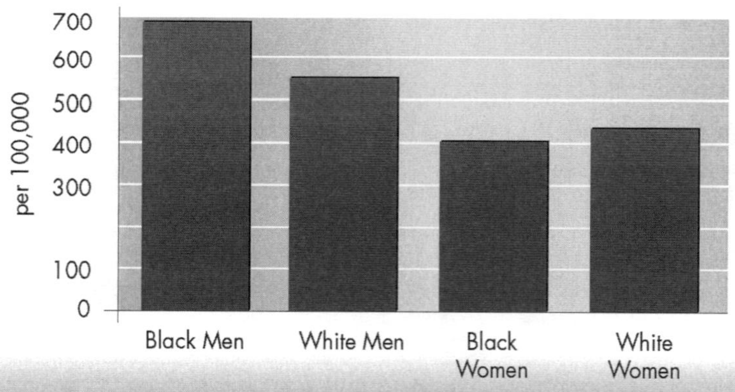

Overlooked in the Associated Press story was the fact the 65 workers labor in a basement office. It's likely that these workers, driving to work early in the morning, and leaving by automobile late in the afternoon, never obtained sufficient exposure to the sun's rays to produce enough vitamin D that prevents cancer. The current mindset is to sue an employer for a discovered carcinogen rather than really ascertain the actual cause of work-related cancer. What these workers need are roof breaks.

Should cancer patients die vitamin D deficient?

Here is a reprint of a report from the Vitamin D Council Online Newsletter. It is re-printed here in its entirety, so you can recognize the full effect of Dr. John Cannell's persuasive argument for more research concerning vitamin D and cancer

Should Cancer Patients Die Vitamin D Deficient

Dr. John Cannell of the Vitamin D Council asks: *"Should cancer patients die vitamin D deficient?"* [The Vitamin D Newsletter April 24, 2005] Most cancer patients will die in a state of vitamin D deficiency,claims Dr. Cannell.

He says, *"An impressive science now connects vitamin D deficiency with increased risk of developing cancer. Dozens of studies also suggest, but do not prove, vitamin D may be helpful in cancer treatment as well."*

Dr. Cannell points to two studies which indicate vitamin D may be a remarkably effective cancer treatment. The first was a study of 15 male patients given 2,000 units of vitamin D3 daily. In 9 of the 15 patients, the PSA levels (a prostate cancer marker) decreased or remained unchanged, an effect which was maintained for nearly two years. [Nutrition & Cancer 51:32-6, 2005]

The second study, from Harvard Medical School, announced that vitamin D obtained from sunshine, diet and supplements almost tripled the 5-year survival of patients with lung cancer. The five-year survival rate was 72 percent in the group with the highest vitamin D intake compared to 29 percent with the lowest. [Cancer Epidemiology Biomarkers Prevention 14:2303-9, 2005]

Vitamin D and hypercalcemia

Researchers are dragging their feet concerning vitamin D for cancer prevention and treatment because they say that high doses cause calcium overload (hypercalcemia), particularly among cancer patients. So pharmacologists are attempting to re-design vitamin D into what are called analogs, patentable versions of the vitamin. [Onkologie 24: 128-33, 2001]

Between 10 and 20% of patients with cancer develop hypercalcemia (high blood calcium levels) at some point in their disease. The parathyroid glands normally control calcium. Hypercalcemia that occurs with cancer is associated with suppressed parathyroid hormones and normal vitamin D levels. Also, extensive bone degradation can cause cancer-related hypercalcemia, such as in cases of myeloma.

Hypercalcemia of malignancy results primarily from increased bone breakdown (called resorption) by cells called osteoclasts. In healthy adults before midlife, bone formation and resorption are in dynamic balance primarily through the activity of osteoblasts (bone-forming cells) and osteoclasts (bone-reabsorbing cells). In many cases of cancer, parathyroid hormone is excessively secreted which produces growth factors that results in the circuitous expansion of tumors. [American Journal Health Systemic Pharmacology [58: S4-7, 2001]

There is interest in using vitamin D to treat cancer, but physicians are reticent because vitamin D increases the absorption of dietary and supplemental calcium. However, vitamin D also suppresses parathyroid hormone and blunts the production of growth hormone (insulin growth factor 1). [Medical Hypotheses 54: 475-82, 2000]

When vitamin D is provided with vanadium, a mineral that blocks the entry of calcium into cells, cells do not overload with calcium (hypercalcemia). [Chemico Biological Interactions 128: 1-18, 2000]

The co-administration of vitamin D with vanadium, a mineral that blocks entry of calcium into cells, would be a desirable way to treat cancer with vitamin D and avoid hypercalcemia. [Chemical Biological Interactions 128: 1-18, 2000] A vegetarian diet also would inhibit parathyroid hormone secretion. [Medical Hypotheses 61: 543-60, 2003] The provision of vitamin D with IP6 rice bran extract (phytic acid) remedies hypercalcemia and elevates the circulating concentration of vitamin D. [British Journal Nutrition 66: 251-59, 1991]

Vitamin D and multiple myeloma

Multiple myeloma is bone marrow cancer. Multiple myeloma remains an incurable disease for most patients, with a median survival of 4 to 5 years. High-dose chemotherapy followed by bone marrow transplantation has resulted in improvement in response rates and survival compared with conventional therapy, but relapse is nearly universal and not all patients are candidates for such aggressive treatment.

A remarkable study involving multiple myeloma patients reveals the shortcomings of modern cancer treatment. A group of 75 patients were treated immediately following diagnosis with multiple myeloma. Another group of 70 patients were not treated untill their disease progressed. Many multiple myeloma patients do not initially report symptoms, so this allows for such a study. Surprisingly, the patients who initially received no treatment following diagnosis lived about 92 months (7.6 years) versus only 56 months (4.7 years) for patients undergoing conventional treatment (steroids, chemotherapy). [British Journal Cancer 82: 1254-60, 2000]

Hypercalcemia and bone fractures are common in cases of multiple myeloma. Physicians commonly prescribe drugs called bisphosphonates (Fosamax, Actonel) in cases of multiple myeloma to decrease bone pain and fractures. However, vitamin D facilitates bone healing and regeneration while elevating immunity. Supplemental vitamin D has been shown to be superior to bisphosphonates in multiple myeloma patients. [American Journal Medicine Science 318: 61-66, 1999]

What causes multiple myeloma?

A study conducted in Yugoslavia reveals factors that increase the risk to develop multiple myeloma. [Neoplasma 50: 79-83, 2003]

Cigarette smoking	→	670% increased risk
Rheumatoid arthritis	→	420% increased risk
Yogurt consumption	→	310% increased risk
Vegetable consumption	→	60% reduced risk

Vitamin K and cancer

Vitamin K is the vitamin that young babies are given after birth so they won't hemorrhage. It is known as the blood-clotting vitamin. Since vitamin K is abundant in dark-green leafy vegetables, this is one of the reasons why greens are recommended in the daily diet. Researchers are calling for the Recommended Daily Allowance for vitamin K (80mcg) to be re-evaluated. [Hemotology Concology Clinics North America 14: 339-53, 2000] Average daily intake is only about 64 and 72 micrograms for females and males respectively. [Nutrition Bulletin 25: 125-34, 2000] Only small amounts of vitamin K are actually absorbed, and since this is a fat-soluble nutrient, it is better absorbed with sources of fat or oil. Even milligram quantities (1 milligram = 1000 micrograms) are safe.

Oddly, while it can be claimed that vitamin C prevents scurvy, vitamin D prevents rickets, vitamin B1 prevents beri beri, and vitamin B3/niacin prevent pellagra, the US Food & Drug Administration forbids food or vitamin companies from claiming that their vitamin K-rich products promote healthy blood clotting. [Federal Register 63: 34115-17, 1998]

Vitamin K is the cancer-destroying vitamin. It can virtually obliterate cancer cells, splitting them in half, especially in combination with vitamin C. [Anticancer Research 21: 3439-44, 2001] Vitamin C/K cancer treatment, unlike conventional treatment, is non-toxic, can overcome drug resistance, and is additive to radiation treatment. [Current Medicinal Chemistry 9: 2271-85, 2002]

This anti-cancer agent seems so promising, as it is non-toxic to healthy cells, yet it never seems to enter human clinical studies. After over a decade, a human study was finally undertaken using intravenous vitamin K. It was only an initial safety study. [Investigative New Drugs 23: 235-39, 2005]

Here is what cancer researchers are saying about vitamin K:

- Researchers indicate that *"data strongly suggests the possibility of using vitamin K for the treatment of patients with lung cancer."* [International Journal Oncology 23: 627-32, 2003]
- Researchers are also calling for vitamin K treatment for ovarian cancer. [Microscience Microanalysis 9: 311-29, 2003]
- Vitamin K is particularly effective against liver cancer, more so when vitamins C and K are used simultaneously. [International Journal Oncology 26: 1337-44, 2005; Apoptosis 9: 223-33, 2004]
- More recently researchers in Japan have called for vitamin K's use with anti-cancer drugs for the treatment of lung cancer because it is a *"safe medicine without prominent adverse effects."* [International Journal Oncology 26: 33-40, 2005]

Given that currently used anti-cancer drugs are so toxic as to produce mortality ahead of the cancer it is intended to treat, the foot-dragging involved in the human study of this vitamin is inexplicable.

Vitamin K and blood thinners

The problem is that anti-blood clotting drugs are often used in cancer treatment because of the risk of blood clots in the legs. So anti-clotting drugs such as warfarin are often employed. Vitamin K, being a blood clotting agent, runs counter to the use of blood thinners. [Current Opinion Hematology 11: 187-91, 2004]

Physicians have been too quick to place cancer or cardiovascular disease patients on anti-vitamin K/anti-clotting drugs and have made many patients phobic over an essential vitamin that does more than clot blood. Vitamin K is needed to prevent calcifications throughout the body and to prevent bone loss.

Some physicians are changing their minds and prescribing low-dose vitamin K to their patients on blood thinners. Patients on warfarin need about 65-80 micrograms of vitamin K per day. [Nutrition Reviews 57: 288-96, 1999] Doctors often don't follow guidelines to prescribe low-dose vitamin K to their patients on blood thinners. [Archives Internal Medicine 162: 1893-96, 2002] High doses of vitamin E may antagonize vitamin K levels. [American Journal Clinical Nutrition 80: 143-48, 2004]

Vitamin K and metastasis

Animal studies certainly indicate vitamin K is promising. In one study, rodents were administered oral vitamin C and K and then tumor cells were injected into the animals' thighs. Among untreated animals 42% experienced spread of cancer to the lung and 27% spread to lymph nodes, whereas only 24% of vitamin-treated animals exhibited lung tumors and 10% had spread to lymph nodes. [Life Sciences 75: 955-67, 2004]

This is a striking finding because anti-clotting drugs like warfarin are often prescribed for cancer patients and may block the adherence of roaming cancer cells to the walls of small capillaries where they can start a colony distant from the original tumor site. Anti-clotting drugs prevent metastasis

– the spread of tumors. [Journal National Cancer Institute 91: 22-36, 1999] But conversely, even though it is a pro-clotting agent, vitamin K does this too.

Vitamin K promotes oxidation

Whereas antioxidants are often suggested for cancer therapy and prevention of treatment-induced side effects, vitamin K in an alkaline environment is toxic to cancer cells, destroying them by oxidation. [Anticancer Research 21: 2387-92, 2001; 3439-44, 2001]

Both high-dose vitamin C and vitamin K are toxic to cancer cells. Vitamin C-treated tumor cells decrease in diameter by 23% while vitamin C/K-treated tumor cells decrease in diameter by 66%. [Scanning 25: 137-49, 2003] Tumor-bearing animals treated with vitamin C/K live longer. [Current Medicinal Chemistry 9: 2271-85, 2002]

There is hope that some day vitamin K will be used in conjunction with other existing treatments. In a lab dish, the combination of vitamin K with two anti-cancer drugs (vinblastine, 5-FU), exhibited *"remarkable synergy."* [International Journal Oncology 17: 323-28, 2000]

Vitamin K's real potential will be seen when physicians begin to employ intravenous vitamin C with vitamin K to treat cancer.

The case of an 85-year old man with liver cancer (tumor was 13 centimeters in diameter – about 5 inches) who received no other treatments but vitamin K is reported in Japan, with total remission of his tumor within 3 months. This remarkable case was reported by doctors at the Hiroshima City Hospital in Hiroshima, Japan. [World Journal Gastroenterology 11: 6722-24, 2005]

Vitamin C and cancer: mutant humans

The chronic malnourished state of Americans creates a false sense of health. All human beings are vitamin C deficient when compared to most animals that continually produce vitamin C through the enzymatic conversion of blood sugar in their livers or kidneys. For comparison, a 160-pound goat produces 13,000 milligrams of vitamin C per day, while humans don't produce vitamin C at all, that's why it is considered an essential vitamin.

It is believed that long ago humans produced vitamin C in their liver. It would have been a hormone rather than a vitamin then. But a universal genetic mutation many generations ago caused the liver to cease production of a key enzyme (gulonolactone oxidase) that converts sugar to ascorbate, the scientific name for vitamin C. [Journal Nutrition 2:7, 2003] Scientists have located the mutant gene once used to produce gulonolactone oxidase, but it is defective. Therefore, all subsequent human generations must make up for this lost capacity to produce vitamin C.

A few animals are in the same predicament as humans – they don't internally produce their own vitamin C. Among these non-vitamin C producing animals are fruit bats, primates and guinea pigs. For example, long-term dietary deficiencies of vitamin C in guinea pigs result in esophageal and gastric cancer. [IARC Science Publication 41: 665-77, 1982]

Americans produce no vitamin C internally, and obtain all their vitamin C from their diet, about 110 milligrams per day. Hunter gatherers long ago consumed as much as 600-700 milligrams of vitamin C daily, so the sparse amount consumed in modern times appears historically low.

Americans believe, since they do not have overt signs of scurvy, they don't need any additional vitamin C. They simply don't understand they need to take vitamin C supplements to make up for their lost capacity to produce vitamin C. Most Americans have been taught to believe that the amount of vitamin C in a glass of orange juice is sufficient to prevent disease. Public health authorities, primarily from the National Institutes of Health, are to blame for this misdirection.

Most humans are in a state of sub-marginal vitamin C deficiency and aren't aware of it. Cancer rates rise, particularly with advancing age and among males and smokers, who have the lowest blood levels of vitamin C. This creates a condition in cancer patients who waste away as if they had scurvy. The bleeding, bruising, fatigue, weight loss and pain associated with advanced cancer are the same symptoms as seen in cases of scurvy. This fact never dawns upon cancer patients and their families because they falsely believe scurvy was cured many decades ago. In fact, many Americans exhibit overt signs of scurvy. About 4 in 10 Americans don't even consume the amount of vitamin C found in one orange.

Cancer cells utilize much more vitamin C than do healthy cells, up to 26 times more. The body only has a pool of about 1,500 milligrams of vitamin C on hand, and tumor cells use this up quickly. Vitamin C also enhances absorption of iron from foods. Iron is also a growth factor for tumor cells. The fact that cancer cells utilize more iron has often been used to mischaracterize vitamin C, as if vitamin C is being used to "*feed*" cancer cells. Actually, vitamin C blocks cancer by a variety of mechanisms.

1 Vitamin C elevates the production of macrophage cells that literally digest cancer cells. Macrophages are part of the immune system.

2 Vitamin C is required for collagen production in the body. Collagen (also called connective tissue), is the "*goo*" in between living cells. Collagen is a barrier against the spread of cancer.

3 Vitamin C, by virtue of its ability to generate collagen production, helps to maintain smooth cells (called endothelium) which prevent cancer cells from sticking to the inside of blood vessels. Weak artery walls can collapse and create blood clots in small capillaries, trapping roaming tumor cells that can then begin to invade surrounding tissues. Strong artery walls prevent blood clots and thwart the spread of cancer.

4 Vitamin C is an anti-inflammatory agent. Anti-inflammatory drugs, like aspirin, are known to reduce the risk for cancer.

5 Vitamin C inhibits the production of hypoxia inducible factor, a type of protein that puts tumor cells in a state of oxygen deprivation and triggers the undesirable formation of new blood vessels (called angiogenesis).

Timeline of events and scientific reports

Both high intake levels of dietary and supplemental vitamin C can prevent and treat cancer. Intravenous vitamin C can achieve much higher concentrations of vitamin C and can effectively be used to treat cancer.

Vitamin C as a treatment for cancer has gone through stages of acceptance and rejection since its discovery in 1922. First, early reports showed promise that vitamin C could be used as a preventive agent against cancer. This was followed by the discovery that intravenous vitamin C is a potent treatment against existing cancer by Drs. Ewan Campbell, Linus Pauling and colleagues. Then pseudo-science was manufactured to disprove vitamin C's important role as an anti-cancer agent. Finally, recent modern scientific studies vindicate vitamin C as a potent weapon against cancer cells, yet modern medicine inexplicably ignores its irreplaceable role in cancer prevention.

Linus Pauling era

The validity of the use of high-dose vitamin C to treat cancer has almost solely been pegged to research conducted by Drs. Ewan Cameron of Scotland and Nobel laureate Dr. Linus Pauling in the mid-1970s. But there were both animal and human studies dating back to the 1930s which revealed unusual reports of remissions and prolonged survival associated with vitamin C therapy. These other reports are almost never referred to.

In the late 1960s and early 1970s there were seminal studies published by European researchers which suggested vitamin C played an important role in the prevention of bladder cancer. By the mid-1970s Cameron and Pauling had published two papers reporting on prolonged remissions from cancer with use of intravenous vitamin C therapy.

Three follow-up studies using oral-dose vitamin C performed by Mayo Clinic researchers between 1979 and 1985 then misled the scientific community and the public and vitamin C was dismissed as an anti-cancer agent. The Mayo Clinic doctors failed to make a distinction between oral and intravenous vitamin C treatment.

The flawed RDA

Mixed in with the research on cancer and vitamin C were studies conducted by National Institutes of Health scientists that falsely claimed that high-dose oral vitamin C is excreted and produces nothing more than "*expensive urine.*" Data from two studies involving only 7 and 15 healthy subjects was used to establish a Recommended Daily Allowance of 90 milligrams for vitamin C. An upper limit of 1,000 milligrams of oral-dose vitamin C was proposed to avoid alleged side effects. Public health authorities failed to disclose to the public that the demand for vitamin C is dynamic and increases with biological stress (infection, inflammation, malignancy). Millions of Americans who have greater need for vitamin C (growing children, pregnant females, smokers, diabetics, the elderly, and those who take vitamin C-depleting medications such as aspirin, steroids, birth control pills and estrogen) are all likely to be in a state of semi-scurvy and falsely believe their diet or low-dose vitamin pills provide sufficient amounts of vitamin C. This is due to the misinformation distributed by the National Institutes of Health.

New research

Recent studies conducted 28 years after Drs. Ewan Cameron and Linus Pauling first proposed that vitamin C can prolong survival among cancer patients, now confirm that intravenous vitamin C therapy can reach blood concentrations 70 times greater than oral doses and that vitamin C is a powerful, selective anti-cancer agent. Unlike chemotherapy, intravenous vitamin C is not toxic to healthy cells. The same study also shows that high-dose oral vitamin C can achieve blood concentrations three times higher than previously thought possible, therefore refuting the "*expensive urine*" contention put forth by the Mayo Clinic scientists. [Annals Internal Medicine 140:533-7, 2004; Proceedings National Academy of Sciences 102: 13604-09, 2005]

Enter Drs. Hickey and Roberts

In 2004, Drs. Steve Hickey and Hilary Roberts, pharmacology graduates of Manchester University in England, published their book, *Ascorbate: The Science of Vitamin C*, showing previous studies conducted by the National Institutes of Health failed to calculate for the degradation rate (half life) of vitamin C and were therefore flawed. Hickey and Roberts call for a re-evaluation of the RDA for vitamin C. Noted antioxidant researchers from around the globe then joined Drs. Hickey and Roberts in petitioning the US Food & Nutrition Board and the US National Institutes of Health to revise the RDA for vitamin C. The petition was ignored by public health officials and the news media.

Sadly, many cancer patients fail to hear of the benefits of intravenous vitamin C therapy, and others fail to increase their intake level of vitamin C to optimal levels that may prevent cancer, because of this misleading information.

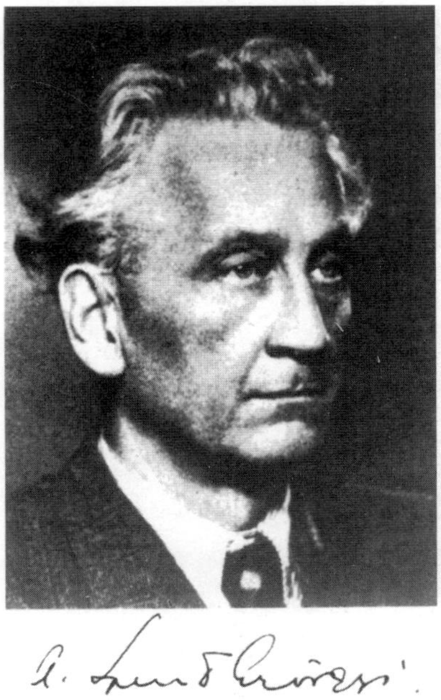

Albert Szent-Györgyi

There is no more revealing way to tell of the exasperation surrounding vitamin C/cancer story than to provide a timeline of events that have transpired over the past three-plus decades. Notice there were a flurry of research reports in one year (12 in 1982) and then very few thereafter. There have been very few research grants from the National Cancer Institute to conduct experiments involving vitamin C as cancer therapy. Dr. Linus Pauling submitted applications for research grants four times to the National Institutes of Health, all of which were rejected. Here is the timeline:

1926: Vitamin C is first isolated in 1926 by Albert Szent-Györgyi. Its structure is determined in 1932 and it is synthetically produced in 1933. Gyorgy receives the Nobel Prize in 1937 for his discovery.

1936: Plum and Thomsen inject 200 milligrams of vitamin C per day in patients with myeloid leukemia and obtain remissions in two cases.. [Ugeskrift for Laeger 98: 1062-67, 1936]

1940: Deucher in Europe reports on the use of up to 4,000 milligrams of oral vitamin C per day to treat cancer patients. He reports that it had a *"remarkably favorable effect on their general condition and increased their tolerance to X rays."* [Strahlentherapie 67: 143-51, 1940] (Oral or IV? And what's tolerance to X ray mean, strange]

1948: Goth and Littmann find cancers most frequently originate in organs whose ascorbic acid levels are below 4.5 milligram % and rarely grow in organs containing ascorbic acid above this concentration. Fully corrected individuals should have tissue levels of ascorbic acid in excess of 4.5 mg %. [Cancer Research 8: 349-51, 1948]

1952: Russell reports on the use of vitamin C with guinea pigs, an animal that does not produce vitamin C whereas most other animals do. He shows that cancers develop sooner in guinea pigs that are fed a diet deficient in vitamin C and then exposed to carcinogens as compared to guinea pigs exposed to the same carcinogens but on an adequate ascorbic acid diet. [Cancer Research 12: 216-18, 1952]

1954: Schneider reports on the use of 1,000 milligrams of vitamin C in combination with vitamin A. This combination was said to *"arrest"* cancers. [Deutsche Medizinische Wochenschrift 79: 584-86, 1954]

1954: W. J. McCormick writes a series of papers describing cancer as a *"collagen disease secondary to a nutritional deficiency"* and as a *"preventable disease secondary to vitamin C deficiency."* [Archives Pediatrics 71: 313-22, 1954; Clinical Physiology 5: 198-204, 1963] Says McCormick: *"We maintain that the degree of malignancy is determined inversely by the degree of connective tissue resistance, which in turn is dependent upon the adequacy of vitamin C status."*

1954: Greer reports on the successful treatment and complete remission of a case of myelogenous leukemia with high-dose vitamin C therapy. Twice the vitamin C treatment was withdrawn, with the patient falling ill each time, showing cause and effect. [Medical Times 82: 765-68, 1954]

1958: Food and Nutrition Board of the National Academy of Sciences sets the Recommended Daily Allowance for vitamin C at 75 milligrams per day.

1961: Further progress is reported on a possible connection between vitamin C and the genesis of cancer. [Geneeskd Gids 39:227-9, 1961].

1968: The Food and Nutrition Board of the National Academy of Sciences lowers the Recommended Daily Allowance for Vitamin C to 60 milligrams.

1969: Dean Burk and colleagues at the National Cancer Institute reports that vitamin C is highly toxic against cancer cells. [Oncology 23: 33-43, 1969] The researchers mention that: *"The great advantage that ascorbates (vitamin C) ... possess as potential anticancer agents is that they are, like penicillin, remarkably nontoxic to normal body tissues, and they may be administered to animals in extremely large doses (up to 5 or more grams per kilogram) without notable harmful pharmacological effects."*

"In our view, the future of effective cancer chemotherapy will not rest on the use of host-toxic compounds now so widely employed, but upon virtually host-nontoxic compounds that are lethal to cancer cells, of which ascorbate ... represents an excellent prototype example."

1969: Doctors in Germany report on the role of ascorbic acid in the prevention of bladder tumors. [Transactions American Association Genitourinary Surgery 61: 85-89, 1969; Proceedings Society Experimental Biology Medicine 131: 522-24, 1969]

1969: An almost immediate confirmation of Dean Burk's proposals was contained in the research conducted at Tulane University School of Medicine by Schlegel and coworkers. They claimed that vitamin C prevented bladder cancer due to smoking and other causes. Tulane researchers recommended 1,500 milligrams of ascorbic acid a day to avoid the recurrence of bladder tumors. [The Journal of Urology 101: 317-24, 1969]

1970: German doctors file their third report on the use of vitamin C in the prevention of bladder cancer. [Journal Urology 103: 155-59, 1970]

1972: Dr. Ewan Cameron reports on *"Ascorbic acid, cell proliferation and cancer"* in The Lancet. [The Lancet 1: (7749), 542, 1972]

1972: Irwin Stone, a member of the American Chemical Society and New York Academy of Sciences, publishes his landmark book, *The Healing Factor* (Grosset & Dunlap, New York) about the history of vitamin C. His book claims humans suffered a genetic mutation at some time in past generations which left *Homo sapiens* unable to synthesize vitamin C as most other animals do. His book describes the promise of vitamin C for cancer therapy.

> Stone writes: *"The National Institutes of Health researchers bring out the amazing fact that in the screening program that has been going on for years to find new cancer-killing materials at the Cancer Chemotherapy National Service Center, ascorbic acid has been bypassed, excluded from consideration, and never tested for its cancer-killing properties. The reason given for not screening ascorbic acid is even more fantastic – ascorbic acid was too nontoxic to fit into their program!"*

1973: Dr. Ewan Cameron and Dr. Linus Pauling publish a conceptual report on vitamin C as an *"orthomolecular approach to cancer."* [Oncology 27: 181-92, 1973]

1974: Dr. Ewan Cameron and Dr. Linus Pauling again report on the orthomolecular treatment of cancer and the *"role of ascorbic acid in host resistance."* Fifty consecutive advanced cancer patients are administered large doses of vitamin C. Pauling and Cameron do not use a placebo group for comparison because the cancer cases are deemed to be *"hopeless"* and untreatable and it would be ethically wrong to withhold treatment given other early favorable impressions using vitamin C therapy. One could hardly claim there would be some placebo effect that would prolong survival, and even if so, modern medicine should attempt to capitalize upon it if true.

Each of the 50 patients received high-dose (10,000 milligrams) intravenous vitamin C. Some patients received 45,000 milligrams per day. No patients experienced kidney stones, which has been all alleged risk of mega-dose vitamin C therapy. A portion of the patients experienced a severe worsening of their condition, not due to vitamin C. Seventeen patients experienced no response to treatment.

50 consecutive patients,
intravenous vitamin C therapy:

- Tumor hemorrhage: 4
- No response: 17
- Minimal response: 10
- Static condition: 3
- Tumor regression: 5

[Chemical Biological Interactions 9: 273-83, 1974]

This pilot study showed that mega-dose vitamin C therapy prolonged survival times in some patients and ameliorated symptoms in others. Given that the study was confined to end-stage cancer patients, it was encouraging. Doctors would later learn to start with low doses of IV vitamin C and then work up to larger doses in order to reduce side effects.

1975: The Food and Nutrition Board of the National Academy of Sciences lowers the Recommended Daily Allowance for vitamin C to 45 milligrams.

1975: Dr. Ewan Cameron reports on the case of a 42-year-old truck driver with malignant lymphoma who was given 10,000 milligrams of vitamin C intravenously for 10 days and then 10,000 milligrams thereafter orally. His appetite returned, night sweats disappeared, and this man returned to normal activity levels. The patient had a relapse a month after initial treatment, returned for more intravenous vitamin C treatment, and months later was normal and active in his job as a truck driver. [Chemical Biological Interactions 11: 387-93, 1975]

1975: Doctors report on the use of high-dose vitamin C to induce regression of rectal polyps. [Surgery 78: 608-12, 1975]

1976: Drs. Ewan Cameron and Linus Pauling publish their hallmark study using high-dose intravenous vitamin C among 100 terminal cancer patients compared to 1000 conventionally treated cancer patients. Vitamin C therapy (10,000 milligrams) prolongs survival 4.2 times greater than conventional cancer treatment alone (210 days versus 50 days). For a subgroup of patients, a 20-times greater survival rate was experienced. [Proceedings National Academy Sciences 73: 3685-89, 1976]

1977: Quotation by T.W. Anderson: *"The risk/benefit ratio relative to the severity of the disease as well as to other available treatments in cancer is so heavily weighted in favor of vitamin C in this situation (terminal cancer) that validation or refutation by other groups will presumably occur quite quickly."* [Nutrition Today 12: 6-13, 1977]

1978: Drs. Ewan Campbell and Linus Pauling publish another study, this time to make up for deficiencies in their first study involving terminal cancer patients. Some of the data in the control group in the previous study was questionable. So a fresh selection of 1,000 control subjects was produced and data from some vitamin C-treated patients were replaced by data from patients with more reliable survival times. Vitamin C-treated patients survived, on average, 300 days longer than untreated patients. One-year survival was experienced by 22% of vitamin C-treated patients versus only 0.4% of the untreated patients. Eight of the 100 vitamin C-treated cancer patients were still alive 3.5 years following treatment versus zero for untreated subjects. [Proceedings National Academy Sciences 75: 4538-42, 1978]

1979: Dr. Allan Campbell describes two cases of Hodgkin's disease and a case of bronchial cancer where intravenous vitamin C treatment was associated with the development of potentially dangerous symptoms. Slow increases in dosage are recommended to avoid untoward symptoms. [Scottish Medical Journal 24: 151-53, 1979]

1979: Conventional medicine mounts opposition to the vitamin C cancer therapy. Mayo Clinic doctors publish a study in the New England Journal of Medicine that involves 150 patients with advanced cancer who were given 10,000 milligrams of oral vitamin C (not intravenous vitamin C as used by Drs. Cameron and Pauling in their studies). There were no appreciable changes in symptoms and median survival was about 7 weeks in both treated and untreated patients. [New England Journal Medicine 301: 687-90, 1979]

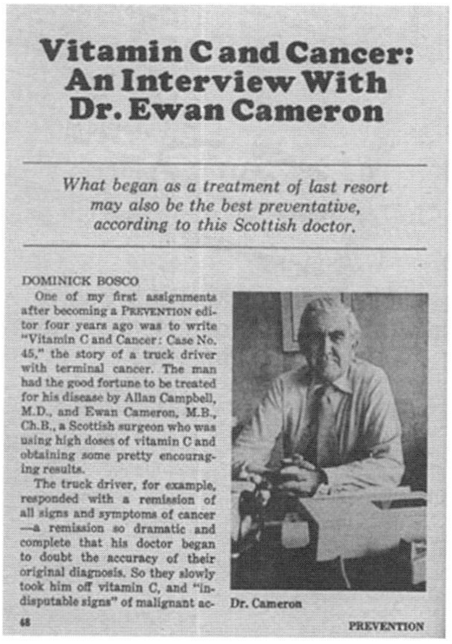

Vitamin C and Cancer: An Interview With Dr. Ewan Cameron

What began as a treatment of last resort may also be the best preventative, according to this Scottish doctor.

DOMINICK BOSCO

One of my first assignments after becoming a PREVENTION editor four years ago was to write "Vitamin C and Cancer: Case No. 45," the story of a truck driver with terminal cancer. The man had the good fortune to be treated for his disease by Allan Campbell, M.D., and Ewan Cameron, M.B., Ch.B., a Scottish surgeon who was using high doses of vitamin C and obtaining some pretty encouraging results.

The truck driver, for example, responded with a remission of all signs and symptoms of cancer—a remission so dramatic and complete that his doctor began to doubt the accuracy of their original diagnosis. So they slowly took him off vitamin C, and "indisputable signs" of malignant ac-

Dr. Cameron

68 PREVENTION

Dr. Ewan Cameron

1979: Drs. Ewan Campbell and Linus Pauling are joined by researcher Brian Leibovitz in explaining the rationale for vitamin C therapy in the treatment of cancer. The ability of vitamin C to develop immune resistance against cancer is described. The report cites 358 other published reports. [Cancer Research 39: 663-81, 1979]

1970s-1990s: Linus Pauling applies four times for research grants from the National Cancer Institute (NCI). His requests are all denied. The NCI initially insisted upon animal studies before human testing could be performed. Pauling applied for research grants for animal studies, and these were rejected. Dr. Pauling is reported to have said: *"In recent years I have reached the conclusion that the National Cancer Institute is not operated in such a way as to favor the discovery of new methods of controlling cancer."* Pauling went on to say: *"It is my opinion, which has grown stronger and stronger during the past four years, that the use of ascorbic acid in controlling cancer may well turn out to be the most important discovery about cancer that has been made in the last quarter century. Ewan Cameron deserves the credit for having made this discovery. The National Cancer Institute has not contributed to it."* [David M. Rorvik, The Alicia Patterson Foundation year?]

1981: Higher concentrations of vitamin C are found in leukemia cells than in healthy cells. Cancer cells use more vitamin C. [Proceedings National Academy Science 78: 6481-84, 1981] This type of study is mistakenly interpreted by some biologists to mean that vitamin C *"feeds"* tumor growth.

1981: Quotation from Dr. Louis Lasagna of the University of Rochester Medical School: *"It seems indefensible not to at least try substantial doses of vitamin C in these cancer patients."*

1981: A study conducted in New York showed that greater dietary vitamin C intake (108 mg) significantly reduces the risk for cervical cancer compared to women who consume low levels of vitamin C (~80 mg or less). The report stated that 29% of women with cervical cancer were found to consume less than 50% of the Recommended Daily Allowance for vitamin C compared to just 3% of healthy women. Approximately 35% of young women consume less than 30 milligrams of vitamin C daily and 68% have intake levels below 88 milligrams per day. [American Journal Epidemiology 114: 714-24, 1981]

1981: Immunological studies show that vitamin C can induce immunity against some cancers in mice. Vitamin C accomplishes this by altering the cancer cell surface structure and the immune response. [Physiological Chemistry Physics 13: 325-33, 1981]

1982: Hairless mice exposed to ultraviolet light develop skin cancers, but the incidence decreases and onset is delayed when increasing amounts of vitamin C are added to their diet. Dr. Linus Pauling is a co-author of this study. [Proceedings National Academy Sciences 79: 7532-36, 1982]

VITAMIN C (Ascorbate) and cancer survival			Mean survival times, days				Increased survival times of ascorbate-treated patients, days*		
			From first hospital attendance		From date of untreatability				
Primary tumor type	Patients, no.		A	B	C	D	E	F	G
	Test	Controls	Test	Control	Test	Control	A-B	C-D	G
Colon	17	170	458+	316	352+	33	142+	319+	324
Bronchus	17	170	219+	118	186+	31	101+	155+	184+
Stomach	13	130	286+	159	182+	32	127+	150+	134+
Breast	11	110	1396+	1020	487+	52	376+	435+	378+
Kidney	8	80	77+	492	381+	39	282+	342+	348+
Bladder	7	70	1669+	420	355+	21	1249+	334+	226+
Rectum	7	70	634	336	270	43	298	227	247
Ovary	6	60	884	366	183	69	518	114	157
Others	14	140	706+	279	278+	37	427+	241+	189+
All	100	1000	681+	360	293+	38	321+	255+	234+

Source: International Journal Vitamin Nutrition Research 23: 115-27, 1982

1982: High doses of ascorbic acid averaging about 540 milligrams per day, administered to rodents orally in drinking water, did not inhibit the growth of implanted breast cancer cells nor did oral vitamin C improve survival times. [Cancer Letters 17: 67-73, 1982] It was known in 1982 that oral-dose vitamin C doesn't effectively treat cancer, but Mayo Clinic doctors continued to conduct studies using oral rather than intravenous vitamin C.

1982: Blood plasma samples obtained from lung cancer patients reveal 64% had such low levels of vitamin C as to be considered to have scurvy. Cancerous lung tissues were found to have vitamin C concentrations double that of healthy tissues. Vitamin C was found to be essential for the production of immune cells (phagocytes) that digest tumor cells. Researchers call for further human studies. [British Journal Cancer 46: 354-67, 1982]

1982: Japanese researchers reported that supplemental vitamin C fed to rodents did not reduce the incidence of gastric cancer, but had a "*remarkable effect*" in maintaining the physical integrity of surrounding tissues which inhibited the spread of tumors. [Cancer Letters 16: 57-63, 1982]

1982: Long-term dietary deficiencies of vitamin C in guinea pigs result in esophageal and gastric cancer. Guinea pigs are in the same predicament as humans in that they cannot produce vitamin C as most other animals do. [IARC Science Publication 41: 665-77, 1982]

1982: Vitamin C is shown to "*completely inhibit*" growth of tumor cells implanted into mice. [Experimental Cell Biology 50: 34-38, 1982]

1982: Vitamin C was given to mice and guinea pigs with leukemia that were being treated with the anti-cancer drug Adriamycin. The vitamin C-treated animals survived longer and had less heart damage caused by the drug. Cancer doctors continue to resist the use of antioxidants when employing toxic anti-cancer drugs like Adriamycin. [Cancer Research 42: 309-16, 1982]

1982: An evaluation of the mega-dose vitamin C studies conducted by Drs. Cameron and Pauling and the contrary studies published by Mayo Clinic doctors, fails to note Pauling and Cameron used intravenous vitamin C whereas the Mayo Clinic studies used oral doses. [Medical Hypotheses 8: 49-84, 1982]

1982: Skin tumors were observed on toads after application of a cancer-causing chemical, while injectable vitamin C inhibited tumor formation. [Oncology 39: 399-400, 1982]

1982: Dr. Ewan Cameron reports that supplemental vitamin C should be of some therapeutic value in the treatment of cancer. It is predicted that in the not-too-distant future, supplemental ascorbate will attain an established place in all comprehensive cancer treatment regimes. [International Journal Vitamin Nutrition Research 23: 115-27, 1982]

1982: While a scientific battle ensues between the Linus Pauling pro-vitamin C camp and the skeptical Mayo Clinic camp, Japanese researchers conducted their own study. During a 4-year period (1973-77) 99 patients with terminal cancer at the Fukuoka Torikai Hospital were examined and monitored. Forty-three (44) of these patients who had low vitamin C levels survived an average of 43 days compared to 55 patients with high vitamin C levels who survived an average of 246 days. A similar experience was reported at the Kamioka Kozan Hospital where 31 patients with terminal cancer were monitored from 1975-79. The average survival for patients with low vitamin C levels was 48 days compared to 115 days for patients with high vitamin C levels. One patient survived 215 days. [International Journal Nutrition Research 23: 103-13, 1982]

1983: Vitamin C, added to the drinking water of mice that had been inoculated with melanoma cancer cells, resulted in a delay in the appearance of visible tumors (2-4 weeks) and increased the survival time, by 12-50% at the 3-month post-inoculation period. [Life Sciences 32: 1559-64, 1983]

1983: Ewan Cameron and Allan Campbell are joined by L Moffat in reviewing their published papers on cancer treatment involving high-dose intravenous vitamin C. It is noted that there is a significant increase in survival for patients with stomach, colon and bladder cancers and no significant difference in the survival rates of those with lung and breast cancers. [Protective Agents in Cancer 1983 missing data]

1985: In a repeat of their earlier study, Mayo Clinic doctors report that high-dose oral vitamin C therapy (10,000 milligrams) *"is not effective against advanced malignant disease regardless of whether the patient has had any prior chemotherapy."* [New England Journal Medicine 312: 137-41, 1985]

1987: Researchers in Belgium report that the combination of vitamin C and vitamin K increases survival of tumor-bearing mice and that the effect is only reproducible when both agents are used. [International Journal Cancer 40: 575-79, 1987]

1990: A report in the Journal of Orthomolecular Medicine states: *"So little interest being shown in the past by granting agencies such as the National Cancer Institute and the American Cancer Society, and by medical researchers in carrying out studies of the value of vitamin C and other nutrients in the prevention and treatment of cancer, in spite of impressive results of Cameron and his associates."* [Journal Orthomolecular Medicine 5: 143-49, 1990] Incidentally, the National Library of Medicine refuses to list reports published in the Journal of Orthomolecular Medicine, many of them authored by Linus Pauling.

1991: Drs. Cameron and Campbell examine records of hospitalized patients in Scotland over a 4.5 year period (1978-82). Among 2,804 cancer cases, 1,826 were judged to be incurable and 294 of these incurable cases were treated with intravenous vitamin C. The overall survival time of the vitamin C-treated patients was 343 days compared to 180 days for the untreated patients. [Medical Hypotheses 36: 185-89, 1991]

1991: Drs. Ewan Cameron and Allan Campbell report on the remarkable case of a 42-year old man who in 1975 was shown to have reticulum cell carcinoma as proven by a pathology report. The patient experienced two remissions of cancer over a period of years that coincided with the administration of high-dose intravenous vitamin C treatment. The man was alive 17 years later. [Oncology 48: 495-97, 1991]

1991: Researchers at Mercyhurst College in Pennsylvania, report that vitamin C combined with vitamin B12 prolongs the survival of mice with leukemia by three times (19 days for untreated mice, 60 days for 50% of vitamin-treated mice). [American Journal Clinical Nutrition 54: 1261-65S, 1991]
1991: University of Texas (Galveston) researchers report that vitamin C can decrease estrogen-induced tumor growth by 50% in hamster kidneys. [American Journal Clinical Nutrition 54: 1256-60S, 1991]

1992: German researchers report that vitamin C protects against liver cancer in rats caused by nitrosamine in drinking water. The rate of liver cancer was reduced from 90 to 55 percent when Vitamin C {ok?? OK] was administered.. [European Journal Surgical Oncology 18: 275-81, 1992]

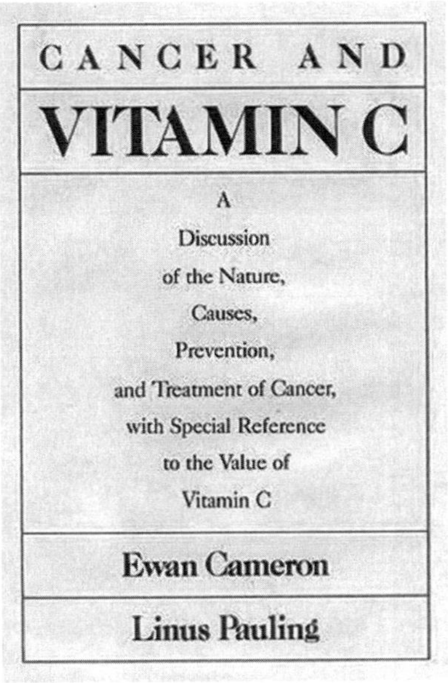

1993: The book entitled *Cancer and Vitamin C: A Discussion of the Nature, Causes, Prevention, and Treatment of Cancer With Special Reference to the Value of Vitamin C*, by Linus Pauling and Ewan Cameron, is published.

1995: Drs. James A. Jackson and Hugh D. Riordan of Wichita, Kansas, describe a case involving a 68-year old male with inoperable pancreatic cancer with metastasis to one lymph node. Vitamin C levels in blood serum were very low. Intravenous vitamin C was administered. After four 8-hour infusions, plasma levels of vitamin C exceeded 158 mg/deciliter. The patient received 39 IV vitamin C treatments in all over a 13-week period. A CAT scan failed to note any progression of the tumor at 6 months. The patient survived 12 months and received no radiation or chemotherapy. [Journal Orthomolecular Medicine 10: 2nd quarter, 1995]

1995: Hugh Riordan MD and colleagues report that vitamin C is potentially toxic to cancer cells if a high concentration is achieved in tissues. Unlike modern chemotherapy, vitamin C selectively kills cancer cells and not healthy ones. [Medical Hypotheses 44: 207-13, 1995]

1996: Researchers in Wichita, Kansas report that vitamin C alone or in combination with vitamin K, lipoic acid or an anti-cancer drug (doxorubicin) can effectively kill cancer cells. [British Journal Cancer 84: 1544-50, 2001] This report confirms that high-dose vitamin C works to kill cancer cells by oxidation.

1996: Drs. Neil and Hugh Riordan and James Jackson report the case of a terminal breast cancer patient who was bedridden and in considerable pain and underwent intravenous vitamin C therapy. The patient experienced a startling recovery, despite a hospital nurse who exclaimed to the patient that *"you are going to die"* from vitamin C treatment. Within one week of vitamin C therapy the patient was walking and able to be discharged from the hospital. The patient survived a few months. [Journal of Orthomolecular Medicine Volume 11, 1996]

1996: The current recommended dietary allowance (RDA) for vitamin C, as proposed by the Food and Nutrition Board/ National Research Council in 1980, and reconfirmed in 1989, is a paltry 60 milligrams per day for nonsmoking adult males. Based on a study of vitamin C dynamics in just seven healthy men, National Institutes of Health (NIH) researchers propose that the RDA be increased to 200 mg daily. NIH researchers incorrectly claim that at single doses of 500 milligrams and higher, bioavailability declines and the absorbed amount is excreted. Vitamin C supplements are ignored in favor of 5 servings of fruits and vegetables which can provide ~200 milligrams of vitamin C. NIH researchers claim that safe doses of vitamin C are below 1,000 mg daily, and that daily doses above 400 mg have no evident value. [Proceedings National Academy Sciences 93: 3704-09, 1996]

1997: Using data from just 7 healthy adults, researchers mistakenly claim that blood plasma becomes saturated at low intake levels (~200 milligrams) of vitamin C. [Pharmacological Research 14:1133-9, 1997] The data is flawed because it does not take into consideration the half-life (degradation rate) for vitamin C. The data also does not apply to adults or children who are ill or have factors that deplete the body of vitamin C.

1999: National Institutes of Health researchers errantly propose the tolerable upper intake level for vitamin C, the highest daily level of nutrient intake that does not pose risk or adverse health effects to almost all individuals in the population, is "*less than 1,000 milligrams of vitamin C daily. Physicians can tell patients that 5 servings of fruits and vegetables per day may be beneficial in preventing cancer and providing sufficient vitamin C intake for healthy people, and that 1000 milligrams or more of vitamin C may have adverse consequences in some people.*" [Journal American Medical Assn 281:1415-23, 1999]

1999: Dr. Stephen Barrett, MD, of QuackWatch, publishes his report entitled "*High Doses of Vitamin C Are Not Effective as a Cancer Treatment,*" which dismisses high-dose vitamin C therapy and characterizes Nobel Prize laureate Dr. Linus Pauling as a "*health quack.*" Despite later revelations that vindicate intravenous vitamin C as having potential for cancer treatment, Barrett continues to dismiss Dr. Pauling's achievements.

2000: A review of the Pauling-Cameron vitamin C/cancer studies and the three contrary Mayo Clinic studies is published in *Nutrition Forum*, but again never mentions the main difference in the studies: intravenous therapy used in the Cameron/Pauling treatment versus oral vitamin C pills in the Mayo Clinic studies. [Nutrition Forum 17: 3-5, 2000]

2001: National Institutes of Health researchers publish a study suggesting the Recommended Daily Allowance for Vitamin C be increased slightly to 90 milligrams for young women and that 400 milligram doses completely saturated blood plasma and mega-doses are of no value. [Proceedings National Academy Sciences 98:9842-6, 2001]

2001: National Institutes of Health Researchers incorrectly claim the highest blood plasma concentration of vitamin C from vitamin C pills ranges from 70-85 micromole per liter. [Biofactors 15:71-4, 2001] Prior studies show blood concentrations can exceed 140 micromole per deciliter, but these studies are ignored. [Acta Ophthalmologica 63: 277-80, 1985; Current Eye Research Aug; 10:751-9, 1991; Epidemiology 9: 316-21, 1998]

2001: Ian Blair, a researcher at the Center for Cancer Pharmacology, at the University of Pennsylvania, is the lead author of a report published in *Science Magazine*, stating that high-dose vitamin C (human equivalent of about 200 milligrams) in a test tube has been shown to cause the same genetic mutations that have been found in tumor cells. His report alarms the public and receives worldwide attention. Dr. Blair claims the public should limit their intake to 200 milligrams of vitamin C per day. He skips out of the country so as not to be available for immediate questioning by reporters. Blair's argument is not against vitamin C-rich foods, but rather high-dose supplements. The Center for Cancer Pharmacology, at the University of Pennsylvania is sponsored by pharmaceutical companies. [Science 292: 2083-86, 2001] A rebuttal by this author is published in *Science Magazine* which reveals that five human studies employing up to 5,000 milligrams of vitamin C had previously been published and showed vitamin C does not cause genetic mutations. Dr. Blair overlooked these studies, which he did not cite in his paper. [Science 293: 1993-95, 2001]

2002: Researchers report that high concentrations of vitamin C accompanied by copper can effectively stop cancer cells from replicating in a lab dish. [Puerto Rico Health Science Journal 21: 21-23, 2002]

2002: A reexamination of vitamin C cancer treatment shows that intravenous treatment can achieve blood concentrations that are proven to be toxic to tumor cells. The inclusion of lipoic acid with vitamin C reduces the amount of vitamin C that is needed to accomplish effective tumor treatment. [Orthomolecular Oncology 21: March 2002]

2004: Antiinflammatory drugs like Vioxx and Celebrex are COX-2 inhibitors and are widely purported to reduce the risk for cancer. Researchers in Korea now show that high-dose vitamin C exerts anti-tumor activity by inhibiting markers of inflammation, such as COX-2. [Journal Cell Biochemistry 93: 257-70, 2004]

2004: Researchers in Germany show that high-dose intravenous vitamin C is not toxic to healthy adults and that it transiently produces free radicals that are eliminated efficiently. [European Journal Clinical Nutrition 58: 1151-58, 2004]

2004: National Institutes of Health researchers publish a paper showing intravenous vitamin C can produce much higher concentrations than oral doses and that *"the role of vitamin C in cancer treatment should be reevaluated."* It took 28 years for medicine to discover that intravenous vitamin C produces 70 times greater concentrations of vitamin C than oral doses, levels that are toxic to cancer cells. Slowly increasing intravenous vitamin C in healthy volunteers did not produce side effects. This study invalidates the Mayo Clinic studies which used oral-dose vitamin C. For unknown reasons, this striking report, which vindicates Dr. Linus Pauling and Dr. Ewan Cameron's seminal studies using intravenous vitamin C in the 1970s, went unreported by the news media. [Annals Internal Medicine 140: 161, 2004]

2004: Drs. Steve Hickey and Hilary Roberts, pharmacology graduates of Manchester University, England, publish their landmark text, *Ascorbate: The Science of Vitamin C*, which proposes a dynamic flow model to determine the need for vitamin C. Hickey and Roberts reveal the NIH studies which determined the RDA for vitamin C never considered the degradation rate (half life) of vitamin C and the need to re-supply via oral or intravenous doses. Repeated oral dosing is suggested throughout the day to achieve optimal blood concentrations of vitamin C. [www.lulu.com/ascorbate]

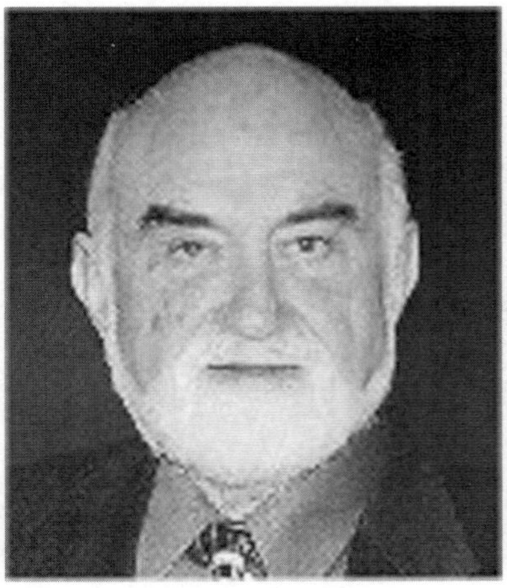

Dr. Hugh Riodan

2005: Dr. Hugh Riordan reports that efforts to kill cancer cells should be accompanied by efforts to heal damaged tissues or cancer therapy will be unsuccessful. [Medical Hypotheses Nov. 13, 2005] Vitamin C is a collagen-boosting nutrient that is required for tissue repair.

2005: A lab dish study shows that vitamin C when combined with commonly used chemotherapy drugs, such as 5-Fu or cisplatin, exert a *"significantly enhanced toxic effect on cancer cells compared to both drugs individually."* [Journal Chemotherapy 17:539-49, 2005] Should vitamin C have been used along with chemotherapy all along?

2005: National Institutes of Health researchers report that vitamin C concentrations that can be achieved through intravenous therapy are capable of inducing cancer cell death but are not toxic to healthy cells. Lymphoma cells are killed off especially well. This report concludes: *"vitamin C, at concentrations achieved only by intravenous administration may produce hydrogen peroxide which is toxic to cancer cells. These findings give plausibility to intravenous ascorbic acid in cancer treatment."* [Proceedings National Academy Sciences 102: 13604-09, 2005]

2005: Researchers in Great Britain report that vitamin C in a lab dish inhibits the production of a gene-controlled enzyme (hypoxia inducible factor) involved in inducing a state of hypoxia (a deficiency of oxygen) characteristic of tumor cells. This state of hypoxia, induced when vitamin C concentrations are low, then triggers the formation of new blood vessels, a process called angiogenesis, that facilitates the feeding and growth of tumors. The level of vitamin C required to inhibit this enzyme is achievable through dietary supplementation. [Cancer Research 63: 1764-68, 2005]

2005: Drs. Steve Hickey and Hilary Roberts publish their book, *Cancer Nutrition & Survival*, which thoroughly describes the biochemical basis of vitamin C therapy for cancer.

2005: The results of a survey of 957 Americans, published in the August 1 issue of *Cancer*, found more than 27 percent think that the *"cure"* for cancer is known but is being withheld by a profit-hungry conspiracy of drug companies, doctors and hospitals. [Cancer 104: 653-60, 2005]

2005: The parents of Katie Wernecke a 13-year old Texas girl with Hodgkins lymphoma, elect to send their daughter for high-dose intravenous vitamin C therapy rather than harsh chemotherapy. The story makes news headlines when child protection workers take Katie away from her parents.

Later, a judge rules that Katie's parents can make all her medical decisions.

To show how indoctrinated the public is with mistaken information about vitamin C as cancer therapy, an online blogger writes of Katie's struggle with cancer. *"Katie's only hope is that the chemotherapy she has received thus far is adequate to save her. However, without high dose chemotherapy and stem cell transplantation, her odds have dropped even more, because intravenous vitamin C is useless for treating cancer. Studies from the 1970's and 1980's show that it does no better than placebo, and there is certainly no evidence that it will kill the cancer or 'strengthen her immune system'."*

2006: Three well-documented cases of advanced cancers, confirmed by biopsy, where patients had unexpectedly long survival times after receiving high-dose intravenous vitamin C therapy, have been reported. These case reports *"indicate that the role of high-dose intravenous vitamin C therapy in cancer treatment should be reassessed."* [Canadian Medical Association Journal 174:937-42, 2006]

2006: The Vitamin C Cancer Cure breaks into the news on WCCO-TV in Minnesota with a report that cancer patients are electing to undergo intravenous vitamin C treatment. Helen Kwak, a Minnesota resident, reports that vitamin C infusions saved her mother's life from stomach cancer. Her mother had lost 70 pounds in less than 2 months but after a few vitamin C treatment she began gaining weight back. Her mother has now been declared cancer free. [WCCO TV Sept. 17, 2006]

Mounting evidence

Most oncologists are not aware of the scientific about face underway regarding vitamin C and cancer. Researchers note these were unexpected.

Vitamin C has recently been shown to:

- Enhance the action of anti-cancer drugs like adriamycin. [Anticancer Research 21: 3439-44, 2001]

- Inhibit the production of hypoxia inducible factor, a protein that deprives tumor cells of oxygen and therefore inhibits {ok?] the undesirable formation of new blood vessels (a process called angiogenesis) that delivers food for tumor cell growth.
  Cancer Research 63: 1764-68, 2003

Does vitamin C prevent cancer?

There has been a lot of attention focused on the debate over whether vitamin C is an effective treatment for existing cancer, but the larger question remains, does vitamin C prevent cancer?

Gladys Block, a University of California researcher, conducted the most exhaustive study to date to address this question. Of the 90 epidemiological studies which examined the role of vitamin C or vitamin-C-rich foods, the vast majority were found to indicate a statistically significant protective effect. [American Journal Clinical Nutrition 54: 1310-14S, 1991]

Range of vitamin C intake and Blood Levels Related to Cancer Deaths in US Males			
Vitamin C groupings	Lowest (1,478 men = 17%)	Mid-range (2,755 men = 36%)	Highest (4,220 men = 50%)
Ascorbic acid intake/day	50 mg	76 mg	129 mg
Serum ascorbic acid, (milligrams per deciliter)	0.3	0.8	1.4
Cancer deaths	5.7%	-	4.8%

Source: Journal of the American College of Nutrition 20: 255-263, 2001

** 45 subjects who had unusually high blood plasma levels of vitamin C (greater than 2.7 milligrams per deciliter, or 9 times greater than the lowest group of males), were not included in the above data because researchers deemed them to be inaccurate.*

University of California at Los Angeles researchers examined the relationship between vitamin C intake and mortality among 12,000 US adults over a period of about 10 years. The group of adults in the highest intake of vitamin C, both from the diet and supplements, had the lowest mortality rates for all cancer, with greater protection exhibited among males. [Epidemiology 3: 194-202, 1992]

University of Toronto researchers examined 12 studies involving diet and breast cancer and concluded that there is a statistically consistent reduced risk for breast cancer among groups who consume more vitamin C. The researchers report that consumption of more vitamin C-rich foods could prevent 24% of breast cancers among postmenopausal and 16% among pre-menopausal North American women. [Journal National Cancer Institute 82: 561-69, 1990]

How many have low vitamin C intake levels and are at increased risk for cancer?

A study conducted by researchers at Arizona State University reveals that 42% of Americans don't even consume 60 milligrams of vitamin C, about the amount in one orange. [European Journal Clinical Nutrition 54: 573-78, 2000] All would be at increased risk for cancer during their lifetime.

Vitamin C measured by blood plasma concentration

The Third National Health and Nutrition Examination Survey found that vitamin C deficiency is common, with 23% of adults exhibiting true deficiency based on blood serum levels, and 17% in a depleted state. Smokers who did not use supplements had higher rates of deficiency. [American Journal Public Health 94: 870-75, 2004]

Intake and blood concentrations of vitamin C	Lowest	Low	Higher	Highest
Blood plasma concentrations for males -mean 49.4 micro-mole/liter	Below 28.4	28.4–51.0	51.1–73.7	Above 73.7
Estimated daily dietary intake of vitamin C, males	52.4 mg	70.1 mg	117.1 mg	146.9 mg
Gross percentage who died of cancer	8.9%	-	-	6.5%
Number of cancer deaths avoided if all males achieved highest intake/blood levels of vitamin C (Based on 2000 US Census, ~70 million American men age 30-75 years)	Estimated 1,680,000 Cancer Deaths Prevented			

Source: Data from the NHANES II Mortality Study, part of the second National Health and Nutrition Examination Survey (1976–1980) drew blood samples from over 7,000 US adults 30–75 years of age at examination.

In one study, 16.9% of hospitalized patients were vitamin C deficient and 47.3% had low vitamin C levels. [European Journal Internal Medicine 14: 419-25, 2003]

A study conducted among 350 US adults found the mean blood plasma vitamin C concentration was low (32.4 micromole per liter of plasma). Six percent were in a true state of deficiency (below 11.4 micromole per liter). [Journal American College Nutrition 17: 366-70, 1998] Vitamin C deficiency is also prevalent in up to 2% [correct?? YES] of young adults, with up to 16% exhibiting marginal levels. [Journal American College Health 46: 209-13, 1998]

In a study of over 8,000 US males, age 30-75 years of age, over a 4-year period, those who consumed 4 times as much vitamin C from diet or supplements experienced a decline in cancer deaths from 5.7 to 4.8% (a relative 30% drop). The researchers in this study removed data obtained from 45 subjects because their blood levels of vitamin C were deemed to be too high (above 2.7 milligrams per deciliter, or 9 times greater than the low intake/blood level group!).

Using an estimate of 70 million American males in the 30-75 age group (2000 US Census), a crude estimate of the number of cancer deaths among US males over a 4-year period of time that would be prevented with higher intake of vitamin C would be 630,000. This study hides the fact that much higher vitamin C blood concentrations can be achieved and are likely to produce an even greater drop in cancer death rates.

In another study, it was found that American men who have low blood plasma concentrations of vitamin C (less than 28.4 micromole per liter of blood) have an increased risk of cancer death from 6.5% to 8.9% (relative 62% difference) compared to males whose vitamin C plasma levels are higher (above 73.8 micromole/liter). [American Journal Clinical Nutrition 72: 139-45, 2000] If the estimated 70 million American males (2000 US Census) all achieved the highest blood plasma concentration of vitamin C as measured in this study, the cancer deaths would drop from 8.9 to 6.5 percent, a difference of 1,680,000 over a 12-16 year period!

Cancer patients generally exhibit lower blood plasma concentrations of vitamin C than the above healthy populations. In a sample of cancer hospice patients, 30% had blood levels so low as to be classified as truly deficient (less than 11 micromole per liter of blood plasma). Another 42% of cancer patients had marginally acceptable vitamin C levels (11-23 micromole per liter).

Survival of cancer patients in hospice care		
	Low blood plasma vitamin C (below 11 micromole/liter)	Normal blood plasma vitamin C [above 11 micromole/literinsert normal level]
Survival, mean	29 days	121 days

Source: Palliative Medicine 19: 17-20, 2005

	Cancer Patients Hospice Care	Normal Average US males, age 30-75 years	Maximum Recorded Blood Concentration of Vitamin C Possible
Blood plasma vitamin C concentrations, mean	42% have blood concentrations below 23 micromole per liter of blood plasma	49.4 micromole per liter of blood plasma	220 micromole per liter of blood plasma

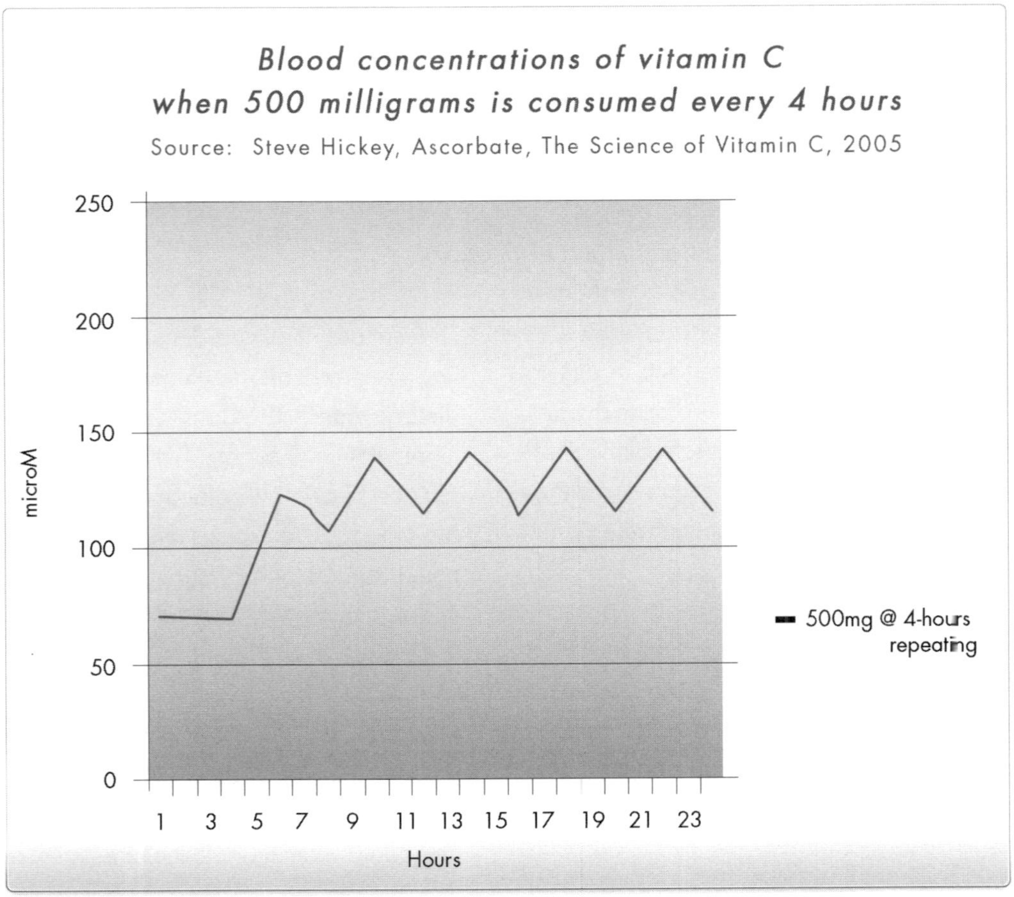

Researchers noted in this hospice study that it is likely that cancer survival is related to vitamin C levels. The cancer patients with low vitamin C levels survived an average of 29 days versus 121 days for the patients with *"normal"* vitamin C levels. [Palliative Medicine 19: 17-20, 2005]

Why are cancer patients dying in a vitamin C-deficient state? It's a crime that Americans aren't being told their vitamin C levels could reach even higher levels, further reducing their risk for cancer. They are misled by food and dietary supplement labels that claim 60 milligrams of vitamin C is *"100% of the Daily Value,"* or by reports emanating from the National Institutes of Health that high-dose vitamin C creates nothing more than *"expensive urine."* In fact, a study conducted by National Institutes of Health researchers shows that blood concentrations can safely reach 2.58 times higher (220 micromole per liter of blood plasma) than previously believed possible (70-85 micromole per liter). [Annals Internal Medicine 140:533-7, 2004]

American males age 30-75 are at much greater risk to die from cancer than are females due to a shortage of vitamin C. Drs. Steve Hickey and Hilary Roberts, pharmacologists trained at Manchester University in England, report that consumption of 500 milligrams of vitamin C taken at timed intervals, 5 times a day, will produce maximal blood concentrations.

What has been documented here is an American travesty. Millions of lives are needlessly lost due to a shortage of vitamin C. We are in the midst of a failed war against cancer with no significant advancements in survival time through the use of surgery, chemo or radiation therapy, no accountability for these failures by public health authorities, the intentional creation of contrary science to confuse the public against vitamin C, and a persistent rejection of the evidence.

The newly published evidence that calls for the use of high-dose intravenous vitamin C therapy has not as yet taken hold. It is not likely oncologists will embrace IV vitamin C therapy. The public will have to demand it, or seek alternative health practitioners who can perform IV vitamin C therapy.

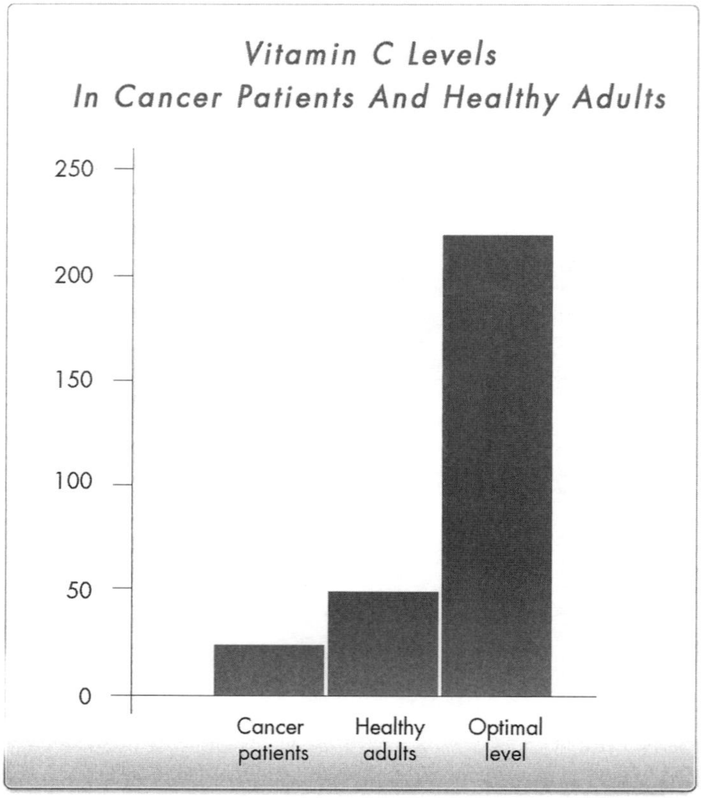

Blood concentrations commonly found among North American cancer patients, healthy adults, compared to the optimal level that can be achieved by oral vitamin C supplementation.

Sources: How to Get Intravenous Vitamin C Given to a Hospitalized Patient: http://www.doctoryourself.com/strategies.html
Preparation of Sodium Ascorbate for IV and IM Use http://www.orthomed.com/civprep.html

Furthermore, the Food & Nutrition Board shows no inclination to re-evaluate the Recommended Daily Allowance for dietary vitamin C. Don't expect foods to be fortified with more vitamin C either. The public is going to have to embark on its own self-guided vitamin C supplement regimens. Most doctors, dieticians and pharmacists are so indoctrinated against dietary supplements, and vitamin C in particular, that they are not reliable sources of information on this topic.

Most patients shirk any confrontation with their doctors and wince at the idea of defying their doctor's instructions. Only patient-driven changes will force cancer doctors to capitulate and adopt vitamin C into their treatment regimens. Whether there will be meaningful adoption of vitamin C therapy by physicians, or only the appearance of approval, remains to be seen.

Furthermore, the public is likely to anticipate more false and misleading news reports about vitamin C and cancer.. The news media is complicit in hiding the truth about vitamin C from the public and has failed o take responsibility for airing erroneous reports about vitamin C and cancer over the past decades. The public can categorically assume any further negative reports concerning vitamin C to be nothing more than planted misinformation.

Only when the public catches onto the compelling data behind vitamin C will meaningful advancements in cancer survival be achieved.

CHAPTER 12

Minerals

p 386 - 402

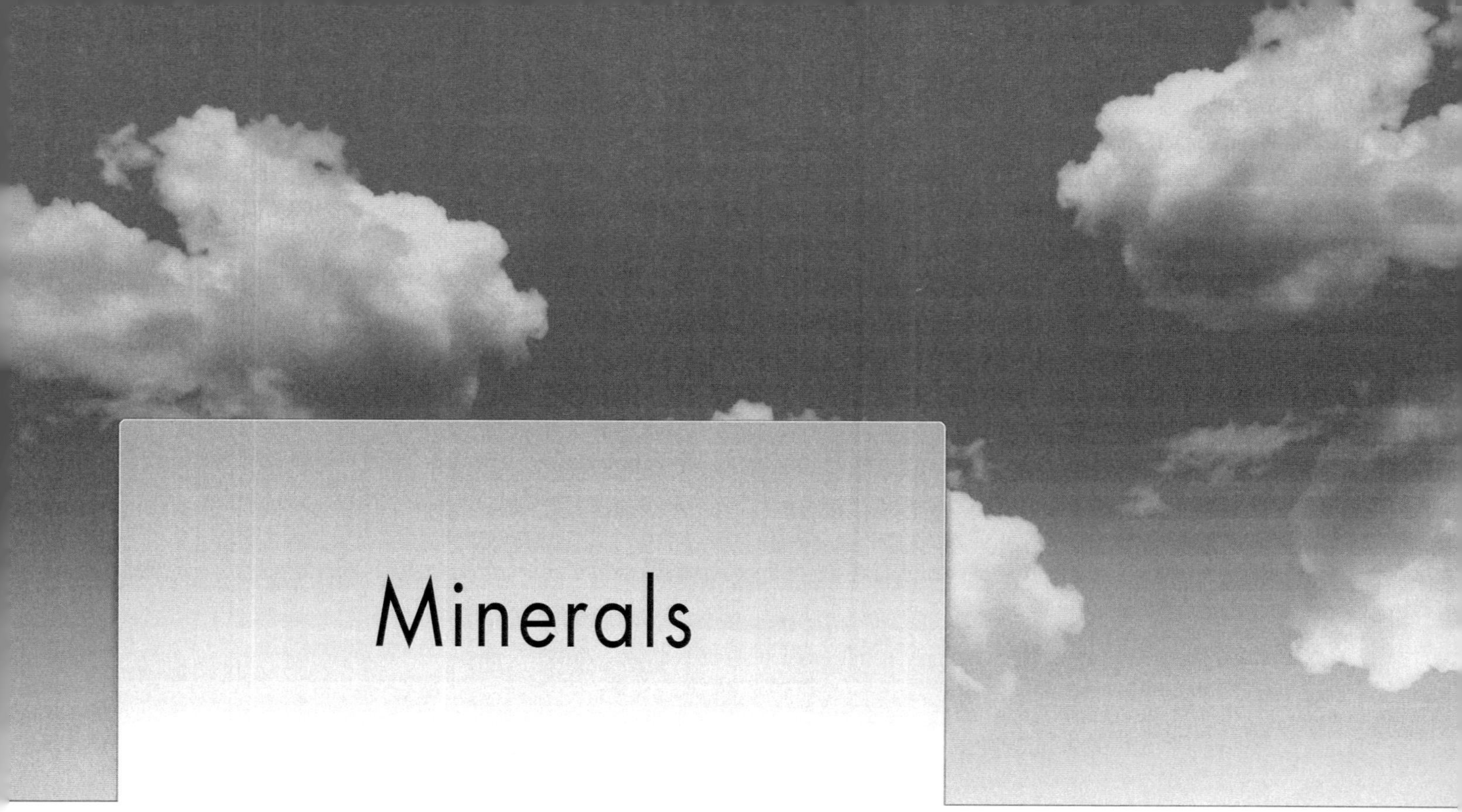

Minerals

Selenium and cancer

It was a stunning report. A government health researcher said: *"If it's real, it's the most important discovery for cancer prevention in my lifetime."* An astonishing 50 % reduction in total cancer mortality and a 63% reduction in the occurrence of cancer were reported after the 10-year use of a single trace mineral supplement – selenium. The risk for lung, prostate and colon/rectal cancer were significantly reduced. Lead researcher Larry C Clark had found the first proven dietary agent to prevent cancer. [Journal American Medical Assn 276: 1957-63, 1996] The study, which involved 1,312 adults, began in 1983 and was published in 1996. The study met every requirement that scientists like to see, long-term, controlled, compared against placebo, patients were randomized to receive selenium.

If this were a drug it would be called a blockbuster. Consumption of selenium increased 40-fold after the study was published. Because of such striking data, the study results were released early. The nay-sayers claimed the results were inconsistent, that adults can overdose on selenium, and the typical call for more studies was heard. Furthermore, the study didn't reduce the risk for skin cancer. [Journal National Cancer Institute 95: 1477-81, 2003] The study was done in the Southeast where many people don't get much selenium from their diet, so this may have heightened the response.

This was the first controlled cancer prevention trial to test whether a nutritional supplement could reduce the risk for cancer.

That was 1996. Nearly a decade later, health authorities stand in disbelief. Walter Willett of the Harvard School of Public Health said there was nothing wrong with the study, but *"It's almost too good to be true."*

Even six years later, when the results of the resumed study (the study was stopped temporarily to report the wonderful news, then continued on) were published, the data held true. [Cancer Epidemiology Biomarkers Prevention 11: 630-39, 2002]

One would think there would be a national mandate to fortify foods with selenium as is the case for iodine.

The cancer preventive effect of selenium was later seen in an animal study. When mice were fed broccoli enriched with selenium they experienced a significant drop in intestinal tumors versus un-enriched broccoli. [Journal Nutrition 132: 307-09, 2003] The cancer preventive effect of garlic is attributed to its selenium content rather than garlic per se. [Carcinogenesis 16: 2649-52 1995]

Gerald F Combs, Jr., of Cornell University, says most animal studies show selenium reduces cancer risk. There is ample evidence to indicate the same is true for humans.

In China, selenium treatment eliminated liver cancer incidence among hepatitis carriers reducing the incidence from 414 to 175 per 100,000 persons. Selenium-fortified table salt has been shown to lower the incidence of liver cancer from 54.8 to 34.5/100,000 in China.

In 1969, it was first observed that cancer mortality rates are higher in soil areas low in magnesium. It's taken a long time to prompt public health authorities to take any action on this beyond the recommendation to eat five servings of plant foods a day.

The health benefits of selenium go way beyond cancer prevention. Selenium is useful in preventing the side effects caused by chemotherapy. [Journal Environmental Pathology Toxicology Oncology 17: 291-99, 1998] Selenium aids cancer drugs in overcoming drug-resistance. [Clinical Colorectal Cancer 5: 132-35, 2005] It even enhances the action of certain anti-cancer drugs. [Medical Hypotheses 64: 1162-65, 2005] Selenium inhibits a chemical that promotes the growth of tumors (thioredoxin). [Oncology Research 9: 303-12, 1997] More importantly, selenium inhibits tumor metastasis (spread), the factor that results in most cancer deaths. [Anticancer Research 19: 1337-42, 1999]

With the cancer care industry inclined to treat rather than prevent disease, it's understandable why selenium remains in the shadows. If you are at high risk for cancer due to familial or genetic history, or you are attempting to prevent recurrence of a tumor, then selenium supplements should be at the top of your list of anti-cancer measures.

There are two basic types of selenium selenium bound to organic proteins in foods and some supplements, (selenomethionine, selenocysteine) and inorganic selenium, or selenite, which does not support higher tissue concentrations. Furthermore, one study showed that inorganic selenium (selenite) was ineffective when combined with vitamin C, whereas the organically bound form (selenomethionine) had a strong anti-cancer effect in the presence of vitamin C. [Journal National Cancer Institute 77: 299-303, 1986] Therefore, organically bound selenium is preferred.

Potential side effects from selenium are often overstated. Usually reports of overdose involve exceptionally high intake levels from areas where mining has laid bare selenium deposits. Cases of selenium over-dosage are mostly limited to mistakes by manufacturers who provided excessive dosage beyond what product labels indicated. Most side effects from selenium involve skin problems at intake levels exceeding 1,000 mcg per day. Dr. Combs could not detect adverse effects from chronic daily use of a 400 mcg selenium supplement in those who also consumed an additional 100 mcg from their diet. [Selenium and Cancer Prevention, Gerald F Combs, Jr. Cornell University, 1997]

Iron and cancer

Understanding how to control levels of iron in diseases like cancer may lead to increased survival and/or improved quality of life, complete remission, or even to a cure. Iron is THE dominating factor in the control of cancer. [In Vitro Cell Developmental Biology Animals 31: 625, 1995] Iron is the most abundant metallic metal in the body and it is iron that is the primary growth factor for tumor cells. Iron removal (chelation) suppresses the gene that causes cancer cells to become hypoxic, that is, unable to use oxygen to produce cell energy. [Experimental Neurology 195:407-15, 2005]

The search for an iron chelator is a prime example of how the medical community puts "*profiteering*" over "*life saving*" in its pursuit of cancer cures. Cancer researchers keep saying they are searching for a safe iron chelator that penetrates into tumors and deprives them of the iron they require for growth. [Current Topics Medicinal Chemistry 4:1623-35, 2004] But only man-made molecules that can be molecularly arranged, patented and made into a drug are being considered. Safe, natural chelators, such as IP6 from rice bran, are dismissed or ignored. [Complementary Medicine Therapy 10:229-34, 2002] (More information about IP6 can be found in Chapter 13 and other parts of this book.) While denigrating alternative physicians who practice chelation therapy using more natural means, conventional medicine practitioners disingenuously utilize conventional iron depletion methods such as blood letting and iron-chelating drugs (Adriamycin, Desferal) to treat cancer.

Iron chelators work by inhibiting the formation of new DNA needed to produce new tumor cells, and inhibiting the development of new blood vessels (angiogenesis) that feed tumors, thus preventing tumor spread (metastasis). [Current Medicinal Chemistry 12: 2711-29, 2005]

It is interesting to note that in study after study, whole grain consumption has been unequivocally found to reduce cancer risk. [British Journal Cancer 92:1803-7, 2005] Whole grains contain an iron-binding molecule called IP6 phytate. [Proceedings Nutrition Society 62:129-34, 2003]

Researchers at the Department of Biology at the University of Indiana explain the link between iron and cancer quite succinctly. Iron favors cancer cell growth. Excessive metal is carcinogenic due to its ability to form hydroxyl radicals, a type of undesirable by-product of cellular respiration (oxygen metabolism) that causes oxidation (rusting of tissues) and tissue destruction. In both animals and humans, tumors initially develop at, or spread to, sites of excessive iron stores (liver, colon). The body makes an all-out attempt to withhold iron from the cancer sites by forming a storage protein called ferritin. Furthermore, there is an attempt to extract iron by macrophages (immune-fighting cells) which produce a gas called nitric oxide. Researchers at the Department of Biology at Indiana University report that "*pharmaceutical methods for depriving cancer cells of iron are being developed in experimental and clinical protocols.*" [European Journal Cancer Prevention 5: 19, 1996]

Here are some more compelling findings on cancer and iron.

- Cancer patients with higher serum iron levels are at a greater risk for mortality. [Annals Epidemiology 14: 195-201, 2004]

- High iron stores increase the risk of disease. In one study of patients with lung cancer, longer survival times were exhibited by those with the lowest serum iron levels. [British Journal Cancer 64: 895, 1991]

- Following administration of a chemical that induces mammary (breast tissue) tumors, 96 percent of mice develop tumors between the 7th and 9th month of life. A low-iron diet reduces tumor growth to 64 percent compared to 112 percent growth in the normal iron group. Low iron consumption does not prevent the development of tumors, but it does impair the growth of tumors. [Cancer 68: 2407, 1991]

- Cancer cells behave like invading microorganisms in that both require iron. Iron both promotes genetic mutations which initiate cancer, and provides "*food*" to stimulate tumor growth. The iron-rich liver is a frequent site of new cancer colonies (metastasis). [Environmental Health Perspectives 37: 291, 1990]

- The risk of liver cancer increases by 400 percent among Americans with high iron stores in their liver. [Hepatology 27: 1563, 1998]

- Blood transfusion increases the risk of cancer recurrence due to additional iron loading among cancer patients undergoing surgery. [Biology Trace Element Research 34: 123, 1992] A unit of blood carries about 200-250 milliliters of iron.

- Habitual blood donors have a significantly lower risk of developing cancer than do non-donors. [International Journal Epidemiology 19: 505, 1990] Blood contains 80% of the iron in the body. [Pathology International 46: 311, 1996]

- The incidence of testicular cancer has increased considerably in the past century. Various hypotheses are offered for this increase which includes exposure to environmental estrogens in plastics, though the data provided to support this thesis is inconsistent. A more consistent theory is that of iron overload. [Medical Hypotheses 51: 129, 1998]

- "*Iron oversupply in cancer patients might enhance tumor growth and adversely affect cancer therapy.*" [Cancer Research 48: 4168, 1988]

- "*Free iron may be the most important factor that can lead to oxidative DNA damage and thus is potentially carcinogenic.*" [Pathology International 47: 203, 1997].

- Iron overload disease (hemochromatosis) and asbestosis are two iron-induced disorders associated with cancer. Free unbound iron is both mutagenic and carcinogenic. [Free Radical Biology Medicine 20: 553, 1996]

- Freely circulating copper and iron, unbound to protective proteins, are involved in DNA damage and the genesis of cancer. [Pathology International 47: 203, 1997]

- Anemia is common among cancer patients, restricting the physical activity and quality of life in 20-50 percent of patients requiring transfusions. [Tumori 84: S3, 1998] However, cancer doctors may mistakenly misdiagnose this type of anemia and prescribe supplemental iron, thus "*feeding*" any existing tumors all the more. In cancer, slow loss of blood, rather than low iron consumption or absorption, may induce anemia. Anemia (low ferritin) and low hemoglobin is the body's way of depriving iron from the tumor cells. In true anemia (lack of red blood cells) related to cancer, the administration of a hormone (erythropoietin) improves about 60 percent of the cases of cancer-related anemia. [Seminars Oncology 25: 27, 1998]

- It is not a surprise that cancer does not occur in bloodless tissues, such as the clear cornea of the eyes, the vitreous jelly of the inner eye, and cartilage in the joints. The idea of providing shark cartilage to treat cancer stems from this observation, though it doesn't cure cancer. [Pharmacological Therapy 63: 265, 1994]

- Cancer researchers intentionally caused kidney tumors in rats with the use of iron and then divided the rats into two groups, one group receiving only adequate amounts of vitamin E and another group receiving supplemental vitamin E. Among the rats that received low levels of vitamin E, 44 percent develop kidney tumors while among the rats receiving supplemental vitamin E only 5 percent developed tumors. This study suggests iron is a carcinogen and vitamin E is an antidote. [Cancer Research 57: 2410, 1997]

Iron, occupation and cancer

People who work with metals, particularly individuals who may inhale airborne iron particles, have been found to be more prone to develop cancer and other diseases.

- In 1936, it was reported that children who polished clock screws with iron oxide developed lung cancer in adulthood by way of inhalation of iron oxide powder. [Journal Free Radical Biology Medicine 4: 185, 1988]

- In China, long-term steel workers were found to have a 40 percent increased risk to develop both lung and stomach cancer. [American Journal Industrial Medicine 30: 7, 1996]

- A Swedish study reveals that among workers in aluminum foundries and smelters there was no overall increased risk of cancer among male or female workers. However, when specific cancer sites were analyzed, there was a significantly increased risk for lung cancer, anal/rectal cancer and sinus-nasal cancer among male workers. [American Journal Industrial medicine 32: 467, 1997] Males have higher iron levels than females.

- Exposure to metallic minerals such as steel, iron, nickel and lead, has been shown to double the risk of prostate cancer. [British Journal Cancer 74: 1682, 1996]

A 320 percent increased risk for brain tumors has also been reported among welders and iron and steel workers.
Source: British Journal Industrial Medicine 48: 597, 1991

Iron and colon cancer

The colon is an iron-rich tissue.

- The majority of patients with a new diagnosis of colorectal cancer are iron deficient at presentation. [Colorectal Diseases 7: 398-402, 2005] This is because the tumor is taking all the dietary iron before it can reach the bone marrow to produce new red blood cells.

- Adults with high blood iron storage levels (plasma ferritin levels greater than 289 mcg/ liter) have a 1.5 times greater risk of developing colorectal polyps, which are believed to be the precursors for colon cancer. [American Journal Epidemiology 144: 34, 1996] A review of 14,407 patients with colorectal polyps reveals that elevated iron consumption increases the risk of cancer by 1.51 times for both men and women. [Cancer Epidemiology Biomarkers Prevention 5: 503, 1996]

- In rat studies, high concentrations of iron in the diet increased chemically induced colon/rectal tumors [Journal Nutrition 128: 175, 1998]. Rats fed a diet with extra iron exhibited 23% more pre-cancerous growths in the colon. [Journal Nutrition 129: 1060, 1999]

- Low serum albumin levels were found to increase the risk of digestive tract cancer by a factor of 14 and may be used to predict colon cancer. [European Journal Clinical Nutrition 52: 271, 1998] Albumin is an iron-controlling protein.

- Body iron stores and dietary iron intake are associated with an increased risk of colon cancer. As iron storage levels increase (ferritin levels) the risk of colon cancer increases by 500 percent or more. [Journal National Cancer Institute 86: 455, 1994]

- Some reports indicate iron supplementation does not increase the risk for colon cancer. For example, the use of iron food supplements has not been found to increase the risk of colon cancer. [Cancer Epidemiology Biomarkers Prevention 6: 1029, 1997]. Another study of iron-fed rats did not show an increased risk for colon cancer. [Journal Nutrition 128: 764, 1998] Iron consumption does not appear to increase the recurrence of colorectal polyps, either. [Cancer Epidemiology Biomarkers Prevention 6: 1029, 1997] However, in two groups of rats fed iron, one group receiving ten times as much iron as the other, the high-iron group showed increased changes in the nucleus of mucus cells of the colon and decreased levels of protective antioxidants (superoxide dismutase). [Food Chemistry Toxicology 36: 819, 1998]

- Furthermore, these studies don't consider the type of iron consumed. The greater the consumption of heme iron, from meat products, the greater the risk for cancer. [International Journal Cancer 117: 643-47, 2005]

- Iron and saturated fat appear to work in concert to promote colon cancer. In one study, researchers chemically induced colon tumors in rats. Then they fed rats lean beef with or without extra iron. No significant differences were found in the total number of colon tumors or the incidence of tumors between rats fed lean beef with iron and rats fed beef without added iron. When lean beef is consumed the risk for colon cancer is not increased. [Cancer Letters 112: 87, 1997]

- In a human study, patients with colon cancer actually had lower blood serum iron concentrations than patients with intestinal polyps or healthy patients. Malignant tissues had higher levels of iron than healthy tissues. So blood serum levels may not be an accurate indicator of the risk posed by iron for colon cancer.

- Patients with colon cancer will exhibit blood serum iron levels that are half that of healthy individuals because the tumor is taking away the iron. [Biological Trace Element Research 95: 19-28, 2003]

- Most dietary iron is not absorbed and is excreted in the feces. Iron levels are ten times greater in feces than in other tissues and thus can expose the colon and rectal tissues to more iron-induced oxidation. In one study, a 250-percent increased risk for colon cancer was observed among adults who consumed high amounts of fat in addition to iron. Researchers have recorded high iron stores (elevated serum ferritin) among colon cancer patients, which decreased the risk for colon cancer. [International Journal Cancer 80: 693, 1999]. In states of disease, the body moves iron from availability to storage. So high levels of stored iron (ferritin) often fool investigators into thinking high iron levels somehow reduce the risk of cancer. The body stores iron away in states of disease so it cannot be used to fuel abnormal cell growth such as tumors and undesirable microorganisms.

- About 50 percent of colorectal cancers are attributed to dietary factors. Presenting symptoms are rectal bleeding and iron-deficiency anemia. [Medical Journal Australia 169: 493, 1998] The anemia commonly found in colon cancer patients is explained by the fact that most of the iron in the body is in the blood circulation and loss of blood due to rectal bleeding reduces iron levels. Treating the *"anemia"* caused by rectal bleeding may fuel tumor growth. A slight anemia is desirable with cancer.

- High levels of stored iron (ferritin) are commonly reported in liver and pancreatic tumors whereas with colorectal cancer both high and low levels have been reported. Decreased iron levels can indicate chronic gastrointestinal hemorrhage, high fiber intake (which inhibits iron absorption) or low iron consumption. These dynamic factors may confound the use of iron storage levels (ferritin) as a marker in colon cancer. [Scandinavian Journal Gastroenterology 32: 233, 1997]

- In a study of dietary risk factors for colon cancer, all of the foods that contain highly-absorbable iron or that increase iron absorption from other foods (red meat, alcohol and refined grains), were found to increase the risk of colon cancer. All the factors that limit the provision or absorption of iron (whole grains, vegetables, citrus fruit, coffee and garlic) were found to decrease the risk. [British Journal Cancer 79: 1283, 1999] A similar study of factors that promote pancreatic cancer revealed that iron-rich meats and alcohol that enhances iron absorption increased the risk while iron-poor foods (fruit, olive oil) were protective. [European Journal Cancer Prevention 7: 455, 1998]

Iron and sarcoma

- Sarcomas are highly malignant tumors made of cells similar to connective tissue. Iron compounds were first reported to induce sarcomas in rats in 1959. [Free Radical Biology Medicine 20: 553, 1996]

- It is interesting to note that the medical literature contains a few reports of sarcoma associated with metal orthopedic implants. [Schweiz Med Wochenschr 126: 607, 1996]

- A specimen from an amputee with osteo sarcoma revealed higher levels of iron, copper, zinc, calcium and magnesium compared to tumor-free normal bone tissue. [Z Orthopedic 122: 848, 1984]

- The growth of Kaposi's sarcoma cells accelerate in an iron-rich medium, but their growth is inhibited by iron-chelating drugs. [International Journal Cancer 78: 720, 1998]

	Growth Years	Years of Fertility	Change of Life
Males	High iron needs	Markedly lower iron needs	Lower iron needs
Females	High iron needs	High iron needs (unless hysterectomy)	Markedly lower iron needs

Iron and breast cancer

- The injection of iron into breast tissue exposed to a toxic carcinogen doubles the frequency of tumors observed in rats. Tumors in iron-injected rats were also larger. [Carcinogenesis 18: 1757, 1997]
- Japanese researchers have found that progesterone increases the serum iron levels among breast cancer patients. [Ganko To Kagaku Ryoho 18: 983, 1991] Progesterone helps to mobilize and transport iron away from the tumor site.
- Dietary iron increases the incidence and severity of estrogen-induced tumors. [Carcinogenesis 19: 1285, 1998].
- Iron-carrying transferrin is a growth factor for tumor cells. Breast cancer cells display 5 to 15 times more transferrin receptors than do normal breast tissue. The body responds to cancer by sequestering the available iron and storing it (nutritional immunity). [Medical Oncology Tumor Pharmacotherapy 8: 229, 1991]

While the etiology of breast cancer is linked to high lifetime exposure to estrogen, there are disparities in studies that attempt to establish this association. [J Steroid Biochem Mol Biol 80: 163-74, 2002] Estrogen alone is not the sole governing factor in breast cancer.

If estrogens alone were the primary factor in breast cancer, then why don't more women get this form of cancer during their fertile years when hormone levels are very high?

One answer to this question is that these high hormone levels occur when iron levels are low and metallic minerals like iron are either being lost in the monthly menstrual flow or being donated to a developing baby.

Widely overlooked is that fact that the risk for breast cancer dramatically increases as females cease menstruation and thus lose their ability to control iron via blood loss. About 80 percent of the iron in the body is found in red blood cells. The increased stores of iron in postmenopausal females are linked to an increased mortality from cancer. [Int J Epidemiology 24:665-70, 1995] The parallel rise in heart disease in postmenopausal females can also be attributed to an increase in iron stores due to cessation of menstrual blood loss. [Arteriosclerosis Thrombosis 14:857-61, 1994] Menstruating females exhibit half the stores of iron compared to middle-aged men and have half the rates of heart disease, diabetes and cancer. [Lancet Jun 13; 1: 1293-4; 1981; Iron Time Bomb, B Sardi, 2001]

It should not be surprising that precisely when women lose their ability to control iron, when monthly blood loss with accompanying iron depletion ceases, is exactly when the risk of breast cancer rises dramatically. For example, the liver stores iron and iron stores in the liver are higher among women in whom menstruation has stopped before the age of 50. [Annals Internal Med 127: 105-10, 1997]

When women are still having monthly cycles in their fertile years the likelihood of developing breast cancer is only 1 in 231 up to age 39. But there is an abrupt elevation in risk from age 40 to 59 years to 1 in 25 women, and from 60-79 years of age to 1 in 15 women, [Breast Cancer Family Foundation] which coincides with the buildup of iron.

It is well established that the iron content of cells increases the risk of cancer. [Environmental Health Perspectives 87: 291-300, 1990; Pathobiology 60: 2-9, 1992] One report says: *"Iron has not received much attention in discussions of estrogen-induced carcinogenesis and human hormone-asso-*

ciated cancer." An elevated dietary intake of iron enhances the incidence of breast tumors in animals. The buildup of iron in the body has been specifically linked to higher mortality rates due to cancer among postmenopausal women. [International J Epidemiology 24: 665-70, 1995

RISKS FOR BREAST CANCER	REGULATION OF IRON
Menopause; advanced age	Loss of menstruation and blood loss of iron
Alcohol	Increases dietary absorption of iron
Plant food diets	Iron more difficult to absorb from plants
Red meat consumption	Contains highly absorbable form of iron

Estrogen administration (estrogen pills, birth control pills) increases iron accumulation. [Current Medical Chemistry 8: 839-49, 2001] Metabolites of estrogen can induce release of iron from its carrier molecule (ferritin) to generate the dreaded hydroxyl radical, the rusting agent that contributes to the initiation of breast tumors via DNA mutation. [Archives Biochemistry Biophysics 346: 180-86, 1997; Mutation Research 475: 153-59, 2001]

The accumulation of iron among postmenopausal women also contributes to other common health problems among postmenopausal women such as high cholesterol and coronary heart disease. [Arteriosclerosis Thrombosis 14: 857-61, 1994]

While iron is necessary for the production of hemoglobin in red blood cells, when it is unbound from its carrier proteins (what is called *"free iron"*), it becomes a rusting agent that can induce the hydroxyl radical which is the primary *"culprit in cancer."* [Stem Cells 12: 289-303, 1994] Metastatic (spreading) breast tumors exhibit a two-fold increase in hydroxyl radical damage compared to non-spreading tumor cells. [Proceedings Natl Academy Science 93: 2557-63, 1996]

The role of iron in cancer was demonstrated by experiments in which animals were given estrogen supplements along with an iron-fortified diet. The incidence of kidney tumors was two to four times higher with an estrogen + iron regimen than when estrogen was given with an iron-poor diet. No tumors were observed in animals treated with low or high-iron diets Estrogen is needed to loosen the iron to promote tumors, circulating levels of iron are not meaningful because most iron in the blood circulation is bound to proteins and will not promote cancer growth. Circulating levels of iron are much higher in animals given a high-iron diet plus estrogen. [Carcinogenesis 19: 1285-90, 1998]

Transferrin is the transport molecule or delivery truck for iron in the blood circulation. Transferrin carries iron back to the liver for storage and transferrin receptors permit transferrin to carry iron into cells. Malignant cells have more transferrin receptors. It would make sense that estrogen increases transferrin receptors in female tissues so as to facilitate the delivery of iron as a growth factor for a developing baby. [Proc Annual Meet Am Soc Clinical Oncology 11:A75, 1992] Of particular interest is the fact that breast cancer cells exhibit 5 to 15 times more receptors for iron deposition (transferrin receptors) than normal cells. Iron-carrying proteins like transferrin are growth factors for breast tumors. [Med Oncology Tumor Pharmacotherapy 8: 229-33, 1991]

The removal of iron via chelation is believed to be a viable method of preventing and treating cancer.

The removal of iron via chelation is believed to be a viable method of preventing and treating cancer. [European J Cancer Prevention 5: 19-36, 1996] Bran obtained from whole grains, which contains the iron-binding molecule called IP6 phytate, has been shown to inhibit the growth of breast tumors in laboratory experiments and in animals. [Archives Latinoamerica Nutrition 49: 309-17, 1999] IP6 phytate, found in relatively high amounts in flaxseed, sesame seed and rice bran, reproducibly inhibits experimental breast tumors in laboratory animals. [Carcinogenesis 16: 1055-58, 1995]

Conventional medicine is not unaware of the important role

iron plays in breast cancer. It's just that researchers would like to develop patentable molecules for use as drugs to treat existing cases of breast cancer rather than study natural nutrients such as flaxseed which could potentially be used for prevention on a widespread basis. For example, researchers are studying an iron-binding drug to treat mammary tumors. [Anticancer Research 22: 2685-92, 2002]

It is interesting to note that alcohol consumption is associated with increased risk for breast cancer. Alcohol increases the absorption of iron from the diet and "*accumulation of iron coupled with diminished antioxidant defenses in breast tissue with advancing age*" contribute to breast cancer. [Free Radical Biology Medicine 26: 348-54, 1999]

Another widely known risk for breast cancer is the increased consumption of animal meat combined with a decrease in the consumption of plant foods. Animal meat provides iron in a form (heme iron) that is more readily absorbed than in plant foods (non-heme iron). [Oncology Reports 6: 865-70, 1999]

The body attempts to withhold iron when tumors, infection or chronic inflammation arise. This appears to be a survival mechanism. [Blood Rev 9: 33-45, 1995] So the withholding or iron via dietary binding or chelating factors like IP6 phytate would also inhibit the growth of tumors.

Widely overlooked is that fact that the risk for breast cancer dramatically increases as females cease menstruation and thus lose their ability to control iron via blood loss.

Iron and leukemia

Leukemia is cancer of the blood. The blood carries 80% of the body's iron. Iron-overloaded males and metal workers develop leukemia more frequently than do females. Iron chelators are employed to treat leukemia. [Advances Experimental Medicine Biology 509: 231-49, 2002] Iron reduction by blood letting is also employed to reduce risk of recurring cases of leukemia. [Transfusion 44: 833-37, 2004]

The problem is that leukemia patients develop low hemoglobin levels and require blood transfusions, but donor blood will infuse as much as 250 milligrams of iron into their system, again fueling tumor growth.

Furthermore, chemotherapy releases a toxic form of iron which not only produces side effects, but also feeds tumor cells. This is one of the major reasons why tumors recur following chemotherapy. The chemotherapy drugs killed the tumor cells but release more iron for remaining tumor cells to feed off of. The co-administration of iron-chelators can minimize the adverse effects of chemotherapy. [Cancer Letters 94: 219-26, 1995]

Leukemia patients often develop fungal infections which, like tumor cells, feed off of iron. [Journal Clinical Oncology 4: 216-20, 1986]

Kidney (renal) tumors and iron

- In 1995, researchers noted there is no accurate chemical marker for renal tumors and suggested iron storage molecules (ferritin) as a marker. (A marker is an indicator, usually some chemical substance present in abnormal amounts in the blood or urine that serves to inform the doctor that an illness is present.) Some 20 percent of kidney tumor patients experience anemia, which spontaneously corrects itself following surgical removal of the kidney. This provides evidence that tumors soak up a lot of iron. [European Urology 28: 131, 1995] About 80 percent of iron circulates in the blood stream. The kidneys filter the blood and thus may be exposed to, or accumulate, high levels of iron.

- Iron levels help to predict recurrence of kidney cancer. One study found that after kidney removal surgery, the circulating iron levels (ferritin) returned to normal among patients who experienced no spread of their tumor, while those who experience recurrence indicated low ferritin levels. [British Journal Urology 58: 617, 1986] The body responds to iron overload, inflammation, infection and disease by binding iron to a storage protein called ferritin.

- Some 35 to 50 percent of patients with renal cell tumors experience recurrence after surgical removal. The larger the tumor, the higher the serum ferritin levels. Thus serum ferritin (iron storage) may be a marker for the recurrence of renal tumors. [Urology 45: 211, 1995]

- When nickel, a heavy metal, was used to induce cancer in the kidneys of male rats, the addition of iron resulted in tumors in 60 percent of rats over a two-year period. The addition of magnesium reduced the incidence of tumors to just 20 percent. [Toxicology 90: 129, 1994].

Blood and iron dynamics in cancer

- In healthy individuals, the transferrin iron saturation ranges from 20-35 percent, but patients with malignancies, particularly leukemia, exhibit diminished capacity to bind to iron. Thus unbound iron is free to destroy cells and tissues through oxidation. Since cardiac tissue is particularly vulnerable to oxidation the heart may be damaged during cancer therapy. Chemotherapy appears to increase unbound iron levels. Iron chelators are proposed to counter this undesirable effect. [The Lancet 347: 342, 1996] However, researchers have been unable to confirm that transferrin saturation is consistently related to increased risk for cancer. [American Journal Epidemiology 142: 692, 1995]

Iron deprivation, iron chelating (removing) drugs and cancer

- Various iron chelators are being investigated for the treatment of cancer. [Blood 86: 4295, 1995]

- Scientific reports concerning the link between iron and cancer are not always consistent. In 1981, an experiment with rats did *not* confirm that an iron-deficient diet helps to inhibit chemically induced tumors [Anticancer Research 1: 293, 1981]. This inconsistency may be explained by the type of iron consumed (heme from meat versus non-heme iron from plant foods). However, the vast majority of the data confirms that low iron levels inhibit tumor quantity and tumor growth.

- However, a study in the Netherlands shows that, under some circumstances, iron-chelating drugs increase the production of growth chemicals that enhance the growth of tumors. [Cancer Research 56: 3747, 1996]

- Iron depletion can lead to the inhibition of an essential enzyme (ribonucleotide reductase), thus preventing new DNA synthesis and inhibiting tumor-cell growth. [Journal Biological Chemistry 27 : 20291, 1996]

- Bleomycin, an antibiotic that binds to and damages DNA by virtue of its ability to attract iron, copper and other metals, is often used as a cancer treatment. [Cancer Research 43: 1049, 1983]

- Copper is companion to, though not as abundant as, iron. Reducing copper levels has been proposed as a strategy to prevent cancer. [Endocrinological Related Cancer 11: 255-63, 2004] Copper withheld from the diet of rats with brain tumors results in a reduction in tumor weight and fewer blood vessels to feed the tumor. The use of a copper chelator (D-penicillamine) reduces tumor size. [Neurosurgery 37: 287, 1995] Copper chelation is known to inhibit angiogenesis (abnormal blood vessel formation that feeds tumors). [Oncological Research 14: 529-39, 2004] The use of a copper-chelating drug completely prevented the development of visible breast cancers in mice. [Current Cancer Drug Targets 5: 195-202, 2005]

- Adriamycin (doxorubicin) is an excellent iron binder, and it is used to treat leukemia by stopping cancer cells from making new DNA. This prevents them from dividing, but it produces serious side effects, particularly heart damage. [Antioxidants in Nutrition, Health and Disease, J.M. Gutteridge, B. Halliwell, Oxford University Press, 1994]

- Iron chelators also stimulate the production of a hormone (erythropoietin) that controls the growth of red blood cells, and thus helps to overcome *"anemia of cancer."* [British Journal Haematology 95: 241, 1996]

- Iron chelators have been shown to block the reproduction of breast cancer cells. [Experimental Cell Research 229: 60, 1996]

- Iron chelators inhibit melanoma cell growth. [Cancer Research 54: 685, 1994]

- Canadian researchers confirm that iron chelators have potential for controlling tumors. [Biochim Biophys Acta 1320: 45, 1997].

- Cisplatin, an anti-cancer drug, is highly toxic to the kidneys by way of its ability to increase the iron content in kidney tissues. The use of an iron-chelator protected against the side effects caused by cisplatin. [Kidney International 53: 394, 1998]

- In 1996, Italian researchers concluded that the anti-tumor effect of an iron-chelating drug (deferoxamine) is *"very promising."* [Acta Haematology 95: 66, 1996].

- Iron chelators or toxic metals that bind to the iron transport protein (transferrin), can inhibit tumor growth. Animal studies have found that when an iron chelator (deferoxamine) was injected intravenously into rats on a low iron diet, there was a significant reduction in the growth of breast tumors. Metals, such as gallium, indium, and the anti-cancer drug cisplatin, cling to the iron-binding site of transferrin, thus replacing the iron, and inhibiting malignant cell growth. [Advances Enzyme Regulation 37:147, 1997]

- An example of an iron-chelator that elevates oxidation is found in nature. Artemisia is a Chinese herb (qing hao) which has been used for centuries, particularly for the treatment of malaria. An ingredient in artemisia forms free radicals when combined with iron which leads to the death of the parasite that causes malaria. Since cancer cells hunger for iron more so than normal cells, cancer cells are more susceptible by up to 100 times to the toxic effect of artemisia when iron levels are high. In animal tests, tumors still grew when animals were given a high iron diet and artemisia, but at a 30 percent lower rate of growth. [Cancer Letters 98: 83, 1995]

- It is no surprise that adriamycin, an antibiotic, is used for the treatment of cancer. Adriamycin is an iron chelator, though it doesn't bind to iron as effectively as it should and is very toxic in clinical use.[Biological Trace Element Research 56: 295, 1997]

Adriamycin (doxorubicin) is an anti-cancer drug that often induces heart failure and eventual demise of the patient. This drug binds strongly to iron and stimulates oxidation. These undesirable side effects are successfully countered by iron-binding bioflavonoids. The beating force of the heart was reduced by 50 percent with the anti-cancer drug but only 18 percent with the drug and bioflavonoids combined. [Cancer Chemotherapy Pharmacology 37: 55, 1995]

- Anemia is common in cancer patients, as well as patients with chronic infection or inflammation. Since iron is a growth factor for tumor cells, the body withholds it from tumors in a survival effort, but iron is so tightly bound that it then can't be released into the bone marrow to produce new red blood cells, resulting in anemia. Inflammation accompanying cancer also shuts down the production of a kidney hormone (erythropoietin) that controls the production of red blood cells. Cancer-fighting cells called phagocytes bind up iron. Cancer doctors can prescribe replacement erythropoietin hormone and savvy doctors now recognize hemoglobin levels (an indicator of red blood cells) should

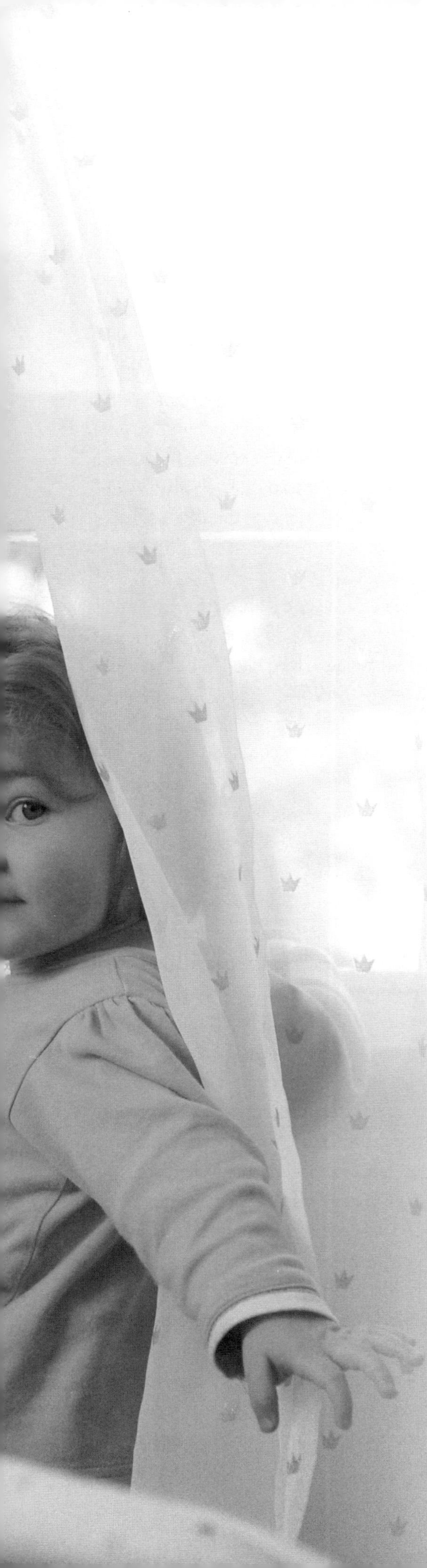

A woman calls

A woman calls......... she has liver cancer. A mother of two children, the youngest is a 5-year old, so she wants to live. She refuses treatment, doesn't want toxic treatment.

I ask, what has she been doing to fight the cancer? She is taking a lot of dietary supplements....... a liver formula, acidophilus good bacteria, coenzyme Q10, an herbal blend, a multivitamin. I ask her to examine the label on the liver formula. Does it have iron in it? What about the multivitamin? Both provide supplemental iron. I ask who recommended those products? She says a nutrition counselor. I inform her that iron is the problem in the liver. Iron grows tumor cells. I suggest she eliminate all supplemental sources of iron, even though she is a bit anemic. She will get iron from her diet.

But she says she is not eating much, has lost her appetite, and weighs about 60 pounds less her diagnosis in May. She needs protein, she may soon be wasting away.

I ask her, what happened to trigger liver cancer in a woman of her relatively young age? She mentions that she had a pregnancy that ended up in a miscarriage in March and the tumor was diagnosed thereafter. I informed her that hormone levels are high during pregnancy and that frees up iron to be released for a growing baby. Once the pregnancy was terminated, the hormone levels remained high, but there was no baby to donate the iron to, and loose iron in the liver could then cause genetic mutations that lead to cancer.

I asked her if she ever drank alcohol or had a liver virus. She said no virus, but she did drink modest amounts of alcohol over the years. Alcohol increases the absorption of iron from foods.

Her sister has hepatitis, she adds. I'm thinking she has had hepatitis and didn't know it.

She now faces a dilemma. She is anemic, but if she takes more supplemental iron to remedy the anemia, it will encourage the growth of the tumor.

She has a limited income. She wants to live. She wonders if a liver transplant would work, but knows the transplant list is long. She wonders if she can get a new liver outside the country. She obviously has no idea what a liver transplant would cost.

She is fatigued now. If she elects to undergo chemotherapy, she will likely experience terrible side effects that make it impossible for her to take care of her children. She has little understanding of what lies ahead. She hasn't begun to even think of not being there for her children.

be kept in the range of 10 grams per 100 milliliters rather than 14 as is commonly practiced. [Medical Hypotheses 13: 119-21, 1984; European Journal Internal Medicine 15: 481-86, 2004]

- An estimated 50% of North Americans harbor a bacterium in their digestive tract called Helicobacter pylori, a parasite that feeds off of iron. H. pylori infected individuals generally have lower blood serum iron levels, which may reduce their risk for tumors, however H. pylori itself is a risk factor for gastric cancer. [Digestive Liver Diseases 36: 455-60, 2004]

Magnesium, zinc, copper and cancer

Care to reduce your risk for cancer by 50%? A study conducted at the Pasteur Institute in France, among 4,000 men aged 30-60 years over a period of 18 years, found that high levels of magnesium in blood serum reduces the risk for cancer by as much as 50%. High copper and low zinc and magnesium levels had an opposite effect, increasing the risk for cancer death significantly. [Epidemiology 17: 308-14, 2006]

There is a growing body of evidence that magnesium and zinc are protective against cancer, while copper promotes cancer growth, particularly the spread of cancer (metastasis).

The evidence for this is compelling.

Magnesium

→ A prospective study among Swedish women suggests a relationship between reduced risk for colon/rectal cancer and high dietary levels of magnesium. The study was conducted over a period of 17 years and involved 35,196 women in Iowa, age 55-69 years of age. [American Journal Epidemiology 163: 232-35, 2006]

→ High levels of magnesium in drinking water were found to protect against ovarian cancer among women living in Taiwan. [Magnesium Research 17: 28-34, 2004]

→ A shortage of magnesium in drinking water in Poland was found to increase the risk for liver cancer morbidity. [Central Europe Journal Public Health 10: 157-62, 2002]

→ Polish researchers report that the lowest blood serum levels of magnesium increased the risk of cancer spreading to the liver. [Przegl Lek 59: 267-68, 2002]

→ Magnesium supplements vary by absorption and mineral content. Magnesium oxide is the most widely sold magnesium supplement, but only 4% is absorbed. [Magnesium Research 14:257-62, 2001] Suggested daily supplementation with magnesium is 200-400 mg. Excessive magnesium may cause loose stool – reduce dosage if this occurs.

Copper

→ It has long been known that breast cancer patients have high blood serum levels of copper. [Oncology 39: 38-41, 1982]

→ While copper, manganese or zinc are utilized to produce antioxidants (superoxide dismutase) within the body, unbound copper enables tumor growth, invasion of surrounding tissues and development of new blood vessels to feed tumors (angiogenesis). Copper-removing drugs (chelators) are being explored to treat cancer. [Current Cancer Drug Targets 5: 543-49, 2005]

→ A high copper over zinc ratio has been linked to gallbladder cancer. [Journal Surgical Oncology 91: 204-08, 2005]

→ The formation of new blood vessels (angiogenesis) is the initial step in progressive tumor development and metastasis. The first stage in tumor angiogenesis is the activation of endothelial cells. Copper ions stimulate proliferation and migration of endothelial cells. It has been shown that serum copper concentration increases as cancer progresses. Copper ions also activate several growth factors. [Journal Trace Elements Medical Biology 18: 1-8, 2004]

Zinc

→ In a rodent experiment, animals were fed normal chow or chow plus supplemental zinc. Only the animals who received no zinc supplements developed liver cancer. Zinc supplements reduce copper levels in the liver. [Biology Trace Element Research 105: 117-34, 2005]

→ Low blood levels of zinc are often noted in acute lymphocytic leukemia, but zinc is not administered as part of any modern chemotherapy regimen. In a case involving a 3-year old girl with leukemia, zinc administered during chemotherapy and through 3 full years of therapy produced a remission (blast cells reduced to zero) with remarkable return to normal red blood cell production. Identical results were reported among 13 other children with leukemia who were given supplemental zinc. Zinc (3.18 milligrams per kilo of body weight) with magnesium (8.0 mg per kilogram of body weight) are suggested by researchers for leukemia patients. [Medical Hypotheses 64: 1124-26, 2005]

→ A study was conducted to examine the relationship of minerals to cancer mortality rates in the US. The study involved over 6,000 men and women. Cancer mortality increased for incremental increases in blood serum iron and copper and decreased for increases in zinc concentration. [Annals Epidemiology 14: 195-201, 2004]

→ Since zinc competes with copper for absorption and counters its effects, this would explain the reduced cancer deaths rates associated with zinc, and the elevated death rates with copper. [Experimental Biology Medicine 226: 665-73, 2001]

Percent Magnesium Content In Oral Supplements

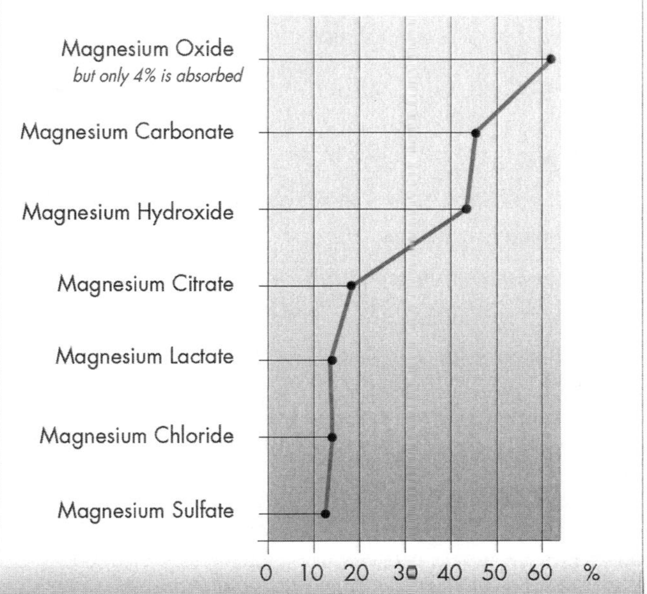

→ Remarkably, 10% of the U.S. population consumes less than half the recommended dietary allowance for zinc and are at increased risk for zinc deficiency. [Journal Nutritional Biochemistry 15: 572-78, 2004] Most Americans are also deficient in magnesium.

Does calcium prevent cancer?

Two decades ago researchers hypothesized that calcium neutralizes the toxic effects of fats and bile acids in the large bowel by forming soaps and mineral-fat complexes. Animal experiments followed and seemed to show that calcium inhibits colon cancer.

Population studies suggest little or no protective association between calcium and colon/rectal cancer. [Journal National Cancer Institute 96: 893-94, 2004] Some studies of calcium supplement users do not confirm that calcium prevents colon cancer. [Cancer 78: 723-28, 1996]

When researchers examined patients four years after they had polyps surgically removed from their bowels, they could not find any protective relationship between calcium consumption, either from the diet or supplements, in regards to preventing a recurrent polyp. [Journal Nutrition 135: 252-59, 2005]

Researchers set out to settle the issue of whether calcium prevents cancer or not. They provided 1,200 milligrams of supplemental calcium carbonate to 930 patients in addition to the calcium they consumed in their diet (estimated at ~600-800 milligrams per day). Four years later the patients were examined for polyps in their colon/rectum. High calcium intake was only effective in preventing larger polyps and adenomas rather than other types of abnormal growths. Nineteen patients with adenomas would need to be treated with calcium supplementation for 4 years to prevent one advanced polyp or adenoma. [Journal National Cancer Institute 96: 921-25, 2004]

A review of 10 controlled studies found dietary calcium intake slightly reduces the risk for colon cancer, but the protective effect was only significant among those with the highest vitamin D intake. [Journal of the National Cancer Institute 96: 1015-1022, 2004] So was it the calcium or the vitamin D?

A collaboration of scientists weighed in on the issue of calcium and colon cancer risk by analyzing all available published data. They concluded: *"Although the evidence from two studies, using 1,200 and 2,000 milligrams of calcium per day, suggests that calcium supplementation might contribute a moderate degree to the prevention of colorectal polyps, this does not constitute sufficient evidence to recommend the general use of calcium supplements to prevent colorectal cancer."* [Cochrane Database System Review 20; (3):CD003548, 2005] Despite advertising claims that milk prevents cancer, *"available evidence does not warrant an increase in calcium intake to prevent colon cancer."* [Journal National Cancer Institute 88: 1375-82, 1996]

The idea of drinking milk to prevent cancer is such a mixed bag. On the one hand, it is alleged calcium in milk slightly reduces the risk and the added vitamin D does too. But milk harbors paratuberculosis bacterium (Para-TB) that often escapes pasteurization. Para-TB infection may trigger cancer. Modern milk also contains growth hormones that may enhance tumor growth and whole milk is fatty, making it unsuitable for cancer prevention.

The fact that there is a three-fold higher death rates from colon cancer in the northeastern US compared with sunnier southern regions, has caused researchers to lean towards vitamin D deficiency rather than calcium as a more plausible preventive factor for colon/rectal cancer. Researchers believed vitamin D, which helps the body absorb and utilize dietary calcium, is the key factor in colon cancer prevention. [Cancer Epidemiology Biomarkers Prevention 5: 897-900, 1996; Cancer Letters 127: 43-53, 1998]

High intake of calcium is also being linked to prostate cancer. Harvard Medical School researchers have linked prostate cancer with high intake of milk. The association is particularly strong for advanced prostate cancer. Calcium from milk or supplements exceeding 1,500 milligrams per day increased the risk for prostate cancer by more than two-fold. [Cancer Epidemiology Biomarkers Prevention 15: 203-10, 2006]

Boron and cancer

Boron is an overlooked mineral that is often used as a dietary supplement to promote bone hardness. Supplemental boron has also been reported to allay symptoms of arthritis. More recently, an animal study reveals that supplemental boron inhibits growth factors and prostate specific antigen (PSA) which was shown to reduce the size of tumors in animals by 25-38% and reduce PSA by 86-88%. This may be a promising treatment for males with prostate cancer. [Toxicology Pathology 32: 73-78, 2004]

Typical dosage range of minerals for adults

- 200 mg Selenium (organically bound) selenomethione or SelenoExcel
- 15 - 25 mg Zinc
- 200 - 400 mg Magnesium (citrate, glycinate, gluconate, others); not mag oxide which is poorly absorbed
- 5 - 10 mg Boron

CHAPTER 13

Specialized Nutriens (nonvitamin)

Specialized Nutrients
(nonvitamin)

IP6 Rice Bran Extract

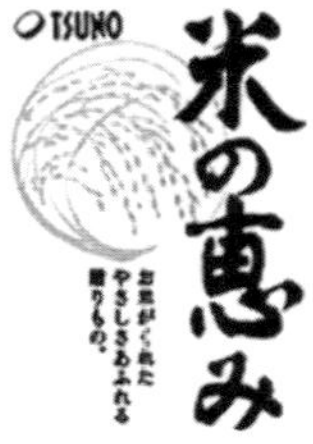

The Overlooked Cancer Cure From Japan

Nature provides an anti-cancer molecule found in rice bran that exceeds the effectiveness and safety of most anti-cancer drugs. Yet it goes unutilized by modern medicine.

Most drugs are modeled after molecules found in nature. Nature's molecules are then re-arranged so as to acquire a patent. Pharmaceutical companies can then justify the expense of conducting studies to prove the safety and efficacy of their pharmaceutical compounds. But frequently, nature cannot be improved upon. This is the case of rice bran extract.

Given that tumor cells utilize iron as a primary growth factor, cancer researchers are searching for a drug that would be able to attach to (chelate) iron molecules and remove them from the body, thus producing an effective anti-cancer drug. Researchers at Wake Forest University Health Sciences state that "*iron chelators (pronounced key-lay-torz) may be of value as therapeutic agents in the treatment of cancer. They may act by depleting iron, a necessary nutrient, and limiting tumor growth.*" [Current Topics Medical Chemistry 4: 1623-35, 2004]

> Another report says: *"There is therefore an urgent need for an orally active, inexpensive iron chelating drug, because the only currently available iron chelator cannot be administered orally, is expensive and side effects have raised doubts about its safety."* [Current Opinion Hematology 2: 153-58, 1995]

Toxicity of iron chelating drugs

The primary iron chelator utilized in anti-cancer studies, Desferal (desferrioxamine), can retard tumors. [Current Medicinal Chemistry 10: 1021-34, 2003] However, Desferal has a modest effect because of its poor ability to get inside tumor cells and remove iron. [Critical Review Oncology Hematology 42: 267-81, 2002]

Adriamycin (doxorubicin), an antibiotic drug often used for cancer treatment, is an iron binder. One of the major drawbacks of Adriamycin is that it often results in severe damage to the heart. In certain circumstances this drug can release iron from its storage protein (ferritin), resulting in heart damage. [Arch Biochem Biophysics 248: 684-89, 1986] The beating force of the heart is reduced by 50 % with Adriamycin. [Cancer Chemotherapy Pharmacology 37: 55-62, 1995] Even if Adriamycin cures cancer, the patient is likely to die of a heart problem.

Recently, an oral drug that can remove iron from the body was introduced. Ferriprox (deferiprone) is the world's first and only orally active iron chelating drug, which is effective and inexpensive to produce, but has similar toxicity to other chelating drugs. [Current Med Chemistry 11: 2161-83, 2004]

I've gone to the trouble of citing these many scientific reports to make this undeniable statement – that iron-sequestering molecules are currently utilized to treat cancer and less toxic iron chelators are being sought. Many of the drugs and alternative therapies for cancer already involve iron chelation.

Rice bran extract (IP6)

Nature's most effective iron-chelating molecule is inositol hexaphosphate (IP6), found naturally in seeds and bran. IP6 phytate (also known as IP6 phytic acid) is a selective agent against cancer cells. Because cancer cells are high in iron content, IP6 directs most of its attention to abnormal cells. IP6 selectively removes iron from tumors cells, which deprives them of their primary growth factor. IP6 does not remove iron from red blood cells which are tightly bound to hemoglobin. Unlike cancer drugs, healthy cells are not affected by IP6, so IP6 has very low toxicity. [British J Haematology 117: 577-87, 2002]

There have been numerous lab dish and animal studies that conclusively prove IP6 is an effective and nontoxic, anti-cancer molecule. But the National Cancer Institute(NCI) has never seen fit to conduct a human trial even though IP6 made it on a list of promising anti-cancer agents. [Complementary Therapy Med 10: 229-34, 2003]

As an alternative to chelating drugs, IP6 has been shown to desirably alter the expression of proteins produced by the p21 and p53 genes that control cancer growth, but goes unused as a cancer treatment. [Anticancer Research 18: 1479-84, 1998]

IP6 enhances the anti-cancer effects of Adriamycin and Tamoxifen, two commonly used cancer drugs. [Breast Cancer Research Treatment 79: 301-12, 2003] However, it goes ignored by cancer doctors.

While Desferal, an iron chelating cancer drug, has only a modest effect because of its poor ability to get inside tumor cells and remove iron, IP6 is found in every cell in the body and is essential for life. By virtue of its ubiquitous presence in living human cells, it is nontoxic. [Critical review Oncology Hematology 42: 267-81, 2002]

In 2001, Food and Drug Administration researchers reported that 8 of 12 chelating agents tested were mutagenic (caused gene mutations). Among the four nontoxic chelators was IP6. [Environmental and Molecular Mutagenesis 38: 347-56, 2001]

The obvious choice among available iron chelators is IP6. IP6 meets all the requirements for a safe iron chelator to treat cancer. It penetrates inside cells. It is nontoxic, and inexpensive, and very effective. It's just not a drug.

Rice bran extract from Japan

In my many investigations involving cancer cures I traveled to visit the Tsuno Foods & Rice Company of Wakayama, Japan (near Oscka). This company sends trucks to rice processing plants in Japan to pick up rice husks. From rice bran, Tsuno Foods extracts many useful nutrients such as inositol used in baby formulas, tocotrienols used in dietary supplements, ferulic acid, a natural sunscreen agent, rice bran oil (which has twice the antioxidants as virgin olive oil), and inositol hexaphosphate (called IP6), which is nature's most potent iron chelator.

A few years ago Tsuno Foods & Rice Company sponsored a worldwide symposium on the role of IP6 rice bran extract and cancer. Researchers from around the world attended and extolled its potential as a cure for cancer. [Anticancer Research 19:3633-808, 1999] [http://www.tsuno.co.jp/e/06/mcin.htm] Sadly, efforts by Tsuno Foods & Rice Company to educate the world about the potential anti-cancer properties of IP6 rice bran extract have been ignored by cancer treatment specialists.

Tsuno Foods, founded in 1947 by Masaji Tsuno, is now managed by his daughter, Fumi Tsuno, an exception in the male-dominated Asian business world.

About 70% of the IP6 made by Tsuno Foods is available to chelate (attach) to iron (as well as heavy metals), which are primary growth factors for tumors. IP6 as an extract from rice bran is a far more effective anti-cancer agent than rice bran or bran cereal alone. [Nutrition Cancer 28: 7-13, 1997]

The safety record of IP6 is long standing. First, it is a normal dietary component and is found in every living cell of the body. Second, extensive studies have been conducted to confirm its lack of toxicity. In 1987, phytic acid researcher Ernst Graf reported that only 4 of 22 chelating agents studied, including IP6, block hydroxyl radical production. Only IP6 was found to be economical, nontoxic, and effective. [Journal Biological Chemistry 262: 11647-50, 1987]

Does it work? Case reports

I've received numerous reports of dramatic cancer remissions involving this dietary supplement. Some of them notably stand out.

- An 80-year-old man with terminal liver cancer took IP6 for a few weeks prior to a scheduled rescue procedure where an anti-tumor drug was to be injected directly into the liver. A cat scan performed just prior to the procedure revealed the liver tumor was completely necrotic – the tumor was a ball of dead cells.
- A middle-aged woman, whose husband worked for a prominent member of Congress, who had stage 4 breast cancer, experienced a rapid and complete remission following the consumption of IP6.
- A 70-year-old man was diagnosed with lung cancer. Radiologists had missed a lung tumor the size of a golf ball in an earlier x-ray. A year later it was the size of a softball. Chemotherapy reduced the tumor by 75 %. In 1999, the man began taking IP6. By 2004, the lung tumor had completely disappeared, which was confirmed by bronchoscopy and x-ray.
- A man with recurrent bladder tumors submitted to surgical removal in 1999, 2000 and 2001. He then embarked upon the use of IP6 as a dietary supplement and has not experienced a return of bladder tumors in 38 months.

Cancer Patients Talk

I wrote to you a while ago and you suggested I use some various things for Lymph Gland cancer, while I was trying to locate some IP6 made by Tsuno Rice Co. in Japan; I've been using IP6 now for twelve weeks, and just got my blood test results this morning- all gone!! I'm clean clean clean clean!! I thank the living Lord in Jesus name for seeing your report The overlooked cancer cure from Japan. Bless you for your service to help people out of a good heart.

– DK, South Africa
Email received November 2005

I have been taking IP6 powder for about three months. It has taken two calcium bumps off my forearm and I hope it is doing the same to the tumor on my lung. I told the doctors that have been practicing on me to take the chemo and radiation and stick it! I will die on my own terms and for a heck of a lot less money and inconvenience.

- Garfield
Email received October, 2005

I found your information on IP6 and cancer and told my brother because he had just been diagnosed with non-Hodgkin's lymphoma. He immediately began taking IP6, stopped eating beef and took other supplements. Now, some 4-months later, his lympohoma is gone. His cancer doctors are all standing around with their mouths open, scratching their heads.

- Dave, Southern California
Telephone call received 2004

I bought IP6 rice bran extract for an 80-year old friend with liver cancer. The doctors scheduled him to have a drug injected directly into his liver because the tumor had grown to the size of a softball. He had a few weeks to take IP6 before the procedure. The doctors had laying him on a procedure table ready for the injection, and a recent CAT scan in the viewing box. The doctor walked in, examined the scan, turned off the light box and said there was nothing more that needed to be done. The cancer cells were all dead and the tumor had stopped growing.

- Maria, Northern California

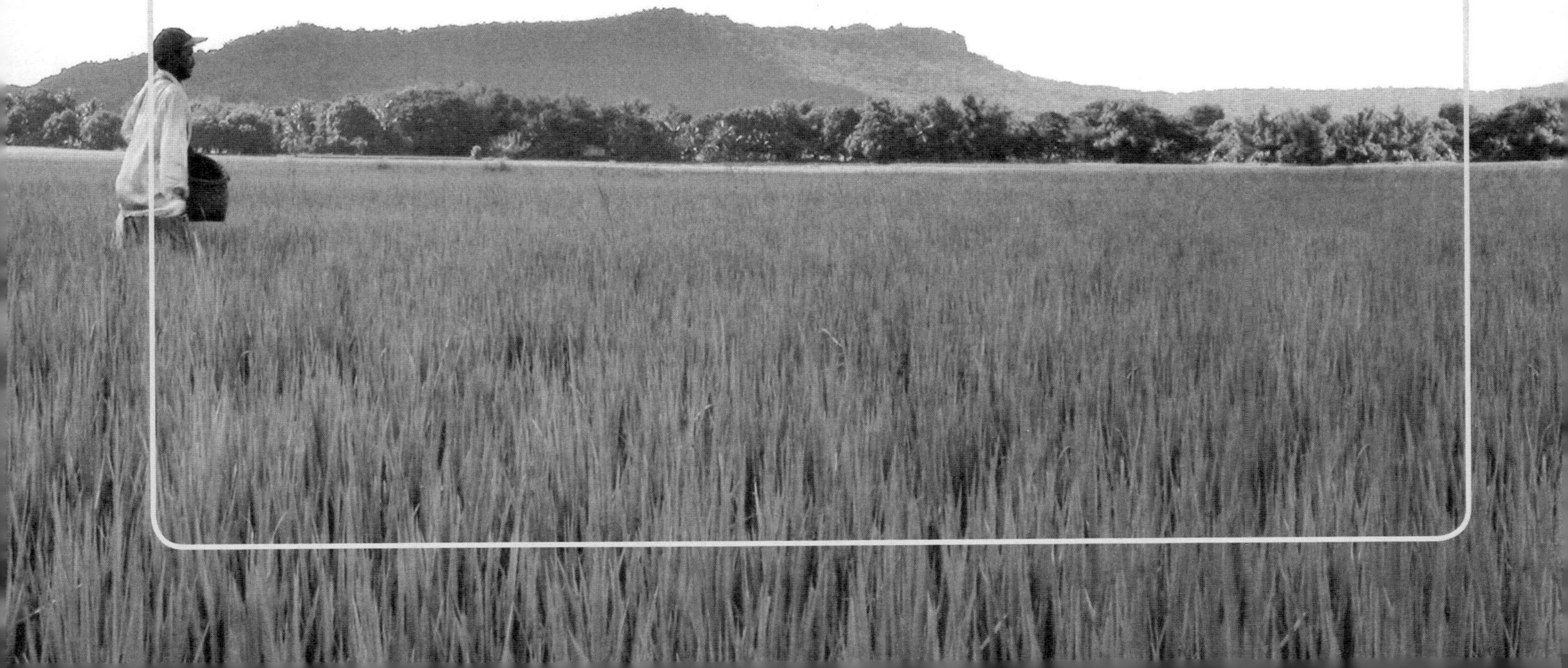

Reports continue to mount regarding the therapeutic potential of IP6 in the treatment of cancer. Researchers indicate IP6 is *"potentially useful in human breast cancers."* [Breast Cancer Research 91: 35-45, 2005] IP6 works alone or in tandem with other anti-cancer drugs (tamoxifen, adriamycin), so there is little excuse not to begin clinical use of this potential anti-cancer weapon. [Breast Cancer Research Treatment 79: 301-12, 2003] IP6 is also considered a strong anti-prostate cancer agent. [Anticancer Research 23: 3855-61, 2003] Tumors interfere with the p53 tumor suppressor gene, but IP6 restores its function. [Anticancer Research 18: 1479-84, 1998] IP6 also boosts natural killer cell activity. [World Journal Gastroenterology 28: 5044-46, 2005]

IP6 rice bran extract, made by Tsuno Foods of Wakayama, Japan, is available under different brand names (Purity Products, Source Naturals, Jarrow) as a dietary supplement in health food stores throughout the U.S. The National Cancer Institute (NCI) only makes brief mention of IP6 as *"a substance found in many foods that come from plants, including corn, wheat, rice, and soybeans, and in large amounts in cereals and legumes. It is being studied in the prevention of cancer."* According to its website, there are no current or planned human clinical studies of IP6.

Many cancer patients have begun to take IP6 rice bran extract, both preventively and during cancer treatment. Its only drawback is that the body withholds iron and induces anemia on its own, to slow down the growth of tumors. Anemic individuals (usually have cold hands and feet) may feel weak, sleepy or faint when taking IP6. The best way to take IP6, for optimal removal of metallic minerals, is with water on an empty stomach. IP6 is an excellent chelator (remover) of excessive amounts of iron, copper, cadmium, mercury and calcium. [Journal Agriculture Food Chemistry 47:4714-7, 1999]

The claim that extra inositol is required to produce optimal anti-cancer effects is not born out by scientific evidence. Researchers at Seoul National University in Korea compared IP6 (which contains inositol), IP6 plus extra inositol and inositol only in animals given chemicals to intentionally produce liver cancer. IP6 or inositol produced similar results, reducing size and number of tumors by more than 50%, while IP6 plus extra inositol offered no significant additional benefit. [Asian Pacific Journal Cancer Prevention 6: 41-47, 2005]

Enzymes

Enzyme therapy is yet another overlooked weapon against the spread of cancer. Modern medicine utilizes enzyme treatment in the form of drugs such as urokinase or tissue plasminogen activator, so this approach should not be considered far-fetched. These drugs are usually used to treat blood clots that occur after a heart attack or for other clotting problems.

Cancer is often accompanied, or preceded by, blood clots. Blood thinning drugs only now are being considered *"an attractive strategy in cancer therapy,"* even though the association between blood clots and cancer was observed decades ago. [Haematologica 90: 1258-66, 2005]

Once cancer cells have grown into detectable tumors, and new blood vessels have formed to nourish them, some malignant cells escape into the blood circulation where they are assaulted by the immune system. Most cancer cells are literally digested by white blood cells known as macrophages. But some tumor cells escape detection, find their way into the smallest of blood vessels, called capillaries, where the walls are thin and tumor cells can easily invade surrounding tissues. But tumor cells must remain stagnant for about 20 minutes for a distant tumor, called a metastasis, to occur. This is facilitated by blood clots. Either the cancer cells adhere to sticky blood platelets (a clotting factor) like fly paper, or the clot completely blocks the capillary and halts movement of blood cells and tumor cells. The tumor cells are nourished by the iron that is released from smashed red blood cells, and a colony of malignant cells begins to form and invade through the wall of the capillary.

An animal experiment was conducted that demonstrated how this occurs. [Journal Cancer Research Clinical Oncology 114: 507-08, 1988] The neck (carotid) artery of a rodent was chemically damaged by acid. The smooth endothelial cells that line the inside of arteries were thus disrupted and in need of repair. The blood platelets began to stick to the wall of the capillary in the same way as platelets accumulate to seal a wound when a person cuts his finger. Cancer cells passing by adhered to the clotty material and the process of metastasis began.

It must be emphasized that to survive, cancer patients must stop metastasis. Localized tumors in the breast, prostate, brain, while painful and damaging, usually do not threaten life. Prevention of metastasis should be the first objective in any cancer treatment program.

This is why enzyme therapy is valuable. Oral enzyme therapy can effectively break up clots, averting the development of metastatic tumors. In 1988, the Journal of Cancer Research Clinical Oncology published a report that documented the ability of bromelain, a pineapple enzyme, to prevent metastasis. [Journal Cancer Research Clinical Oncology 114: 507-08, 1988]

Even doctors at Memorial Sloan-Kettering Cancer Center in New York reported favorably on bromelain enzyme treatment for patients suffering from inflammatory disease. [Pathobiology 64: 339-46, 1996] Investigators in Germany more recently confirmed that bromelain can inhibit metastasis. [In Vivo 19: 483-85, 2005]

In 1990, researchers in Japan found that nattokinase, a traditional fermented soy food, had anti-clotting activity. When natto capsules were given to dogs with chemically induced blood clots, the degradation of the clots was observed by arterial photographs (angiography). [Acta Haematology 84: 139-43, 1990]

In 1995, a study conducted in Japan, showed that nattokinase was far more effective than traditional drugs in breaking up clots. [Biological Pharmacology Bulletin 18: 1387-91, 1995] In fact, natto was shown to have the highest clot-busting activity of 200 foods tested in Japan.

It doesn't take long to recognize that the consumption of natto among Japanese may be a reason for their longevity. The prevention of blood clots is crucial in preventing and surviving heart attacks and strokes. Natto can also hinder the development of clots in the legs that can be released into the brain or lungs and threaten life, prevent bacteria from adhering to tissues, and halt the spread of undetected tumors.

Dr. Hiroyuki Sumi, MD, PhD, a professor at the Kurashiki University of Science and the Arts, was the first to identify the properties of natto. His discovery was reported in 1986. A packet of natto (about 100 grams) has the same effectiveness as the drug urokinase, which only has anti-clotting activity up to 20 minutes, whereas nattokinase maintains activity for 4-12 hours. Nattokinase was deemed safe over 15 years ago. [Acta Haematologica 84: 139-43, 1990]

For skeptics, it has been confirmed that nattokinase is orally absorbed from the intestinal tract and that it cleaves to blood clotting factors. [Biological Pharm Bulletin 18: 1194-96, 1995]

Other enzyme products may also be useful. For example, a commercial brand enzyme product, Wobenzym, was found to break up lymph congestion in cancer patients. [Wien Med Wochenschr 146: 67-72, 1996]

In conclusion, enzyme therapy is considered safe, may improve the absorption of anti-cancer drugs, may elevate the immune response, does not interfere with chemotherapy and is absorbed orally despite claims to the contrary. [Cell Mol Life Science 58: 1234-45, 2001]

Calcium D-glucarate: Detoxifying cancer

Everything that enters the gastric tract is subject to the detoxification process. Digested food particles are ushered to the liver where they are further complexed with molecules that couple up and render them unavailable to interact with other molecules in the body. This detoxification process involves the production of sulfur and sugar-like molecules (glucaric acid), in processes called sulfation and glucuronidation, that conjugate with toxins, knocking them out of action. For example, glucaric acid will link with toxins from poisonous mushrooms to help dull their poisonous effect. [Integrative Cancer Therapy 2: 139-44, 2003]

Glucaric acid, found abundantly as a calcium salt in fruits and vegetables, especially apples, Brussels sprouts, broccoli, cabbage, and bean sprouts, is one of the likely reasons why plant food diets prevent cancer. [Alternative Medicine Review 7: 336-39, 2002] Glucaric acid inhibits the production of an uncoupling enzyme called glucuronidase. This enzyme is abundant at the site of tumors, infection and inflammation. Elevated beta-glucuronidase activity is associated with an increased risk for various cancers, particularly those that are hormone-dependent, such as breast, prostate, and colon cancers. Glucaric acid helps to detoxify various carcinogenic molecules that invade the body. [Cancer Detection Prevention 21: 178-90, 1997] Calcium D glucarate is widely sold as an anti-cancer dietary supplement. Manufacturers recommend 200-400 mg doses. Extremely high doses of calcium D glucarate have been shown to reduce tumor incidence and multiplicity by about 60% in animals. But it is not known if more practical doses are as beneficial. [International Journal Oncology 16:43-8, 2000]

On the other hand, glucarate may have the undesirable effect of coupling with anti-cancer drugs, and ushering them out of the body via urination, thwarting cancer treatment. [Neoplasma 31:649-53, 1984]

There is more theoretical benefit attributed to calcium D glucarate supplements than is demonstrated by actual human experience. Calcium D glucarate may not be appropriate during chemotherapy.

Glucuronic acid and cancer

At the end of a woman's monthly menstrual cycle estrogen is dumped into the gut. Estrogen then couples up with glucuronic acid in the liver and excretes it in the bile. Certain bacteria in the gut produce an enzyme, glucuronidase, which breaks the bond between estrogen and glucuronic acid, thus enabling estrogen to be reabsorbed back into the body. Calcium D-glucarate inhibits the glucoronidase enzyme, facilitating normal rather than elevated estrogen levels. In one animal study, two groups of rodents were studied. The rodents were bred to develop breast cancer. The animals were split into two groups, one of which received calcium D-glucarate. Only 56% of the animals in the treated group developed breast tumors compared to 100 % in the untreated group. Among the animals that did develop breast tumors, there were fewer tumors than normal. The number of tumors was reduced by 90%. The recommended consumption of calcium D-glucarate is 200-400 mg per day and more for individuals with existing breast cancer. [Israeli Journal Medical Science 31; 101-05, 1995]

Omega-3 oils

In one lab experiment after another, the provision of omega-6 oil (such as corn oil) enhances the growth of tumor cells, while omega-3 oil (such as from fish or flaxseed) inhibits tumor cell growth. [Nutrition Cancer 37:119-27, 2000; Neoplasia 8:112-24, 2006] While both of these oils are essential for life, omega-3 oils are in such short supply in Western diets as to favor tumor growth. Omega-3 oil is virtually absent in tissues of many human beings.

Use of omega-3 oils should be considered one of the most powerful ways to prevent or treat cancer. Evidence continues to mount for omega-3 oils in the battle against cancer. There are many examples.

A remarkable investigation was conducted among Eskimos, known as Inuit. An autopsy of 61 Inuit males who died in 1990-94 found only one invasive prostate cancer. There were no latent or early-stage tumors.

The mean weight of the 60 benign prostate specimens was 23.2 grams, versus 112 grams in the one cancerous gland. The cancerous prostate gland, obtained from a 73-year-old male, was very low in omega-3 oils (0.9%) versus the other specimens (1.79%). Omega-6 oil (such as that found in corn oil) was 12 times greater than omega-3 oil in the one cancerous prostate gland versus just five times greater in the other specimens.

Prostate cancer incidence

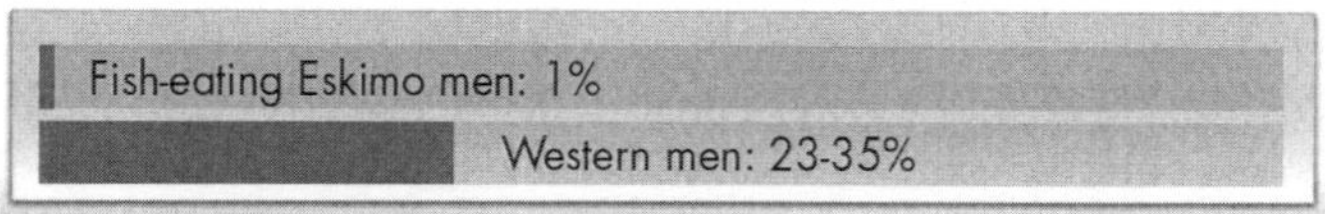

The very low incidence of prostate cancer among the Inuit (less than 1% or about 7.8 per 100,000) is in stark contrast to the 23-35 % incidence in Western populations. This is attributed to the Inuit diet which is rich in omega-3 fish oil and the trace mineral selenium. [Cancer Epidemiology Biomarkers Prevention 12:926-7, 2003]

South African researchers found that Cape Town fishermen who consume a greater amount of fish containing omega-3 fatty acid are less likely to develop colon cancer than are non-fishermen who consume less fish, even though the fishermen smoke more tobacco and consume fewer fruits and vegetables. Cape Town fisherman developed colon cancer at the rate of 0.00005%, while 0.00034% of mainland adults developed tumors during a five-year period, nearly a 700% difference. [South African Medical Journal 87: 152, 1997]

In 1995, researchers at the American Health Foundation in Valhalla, New York, suggested that omega-3 oils be provided to women with breast cancer to prevent recurrence. [Journal National Cancer Institute 87: 587-92, 1995] Omega-3 oils can be used to both prevent and treat cancer. But most cancer patients will have to find this information on their own. A minority of oncologists prescribe fish or flaxseed oil for their cancer patients. It's not like this information is new. As early as 1961, it was proposed that cancer is an omega-3 oil deficiency. [Physiology Review 41: 1-51, 1961]

In rodents, the provision of pure omega-3 oil from microalgae has been shown to reduce the number of blood vessels that feed breast tumors by 43%. [Clinical Cancer Research 12:5879-86, 2006]

A man recovers from lung cancer

Armed with the knowledge that omega-3 oils drastically reduce the risk for cancer, Ron Pardini, a professor of biochemistry at the Nevada Agricultural Experiment Station in Reno, decided to treat his cancer patients with omega-3 oil. A 78-year-old with terminal lung cancer, with only a few weeks to live, was given pure omega-3 fish oil from microalgae, and corn oil (containing omega-6 oil) was withdrawn from his diet. Five years later he was still alive. The lung tumors were still there, though they had shrunk a little. Pardini's patient was actually a two-year-old mouse (the equivalent of an 78-year-old human) [Science Daily Nov. 14, 2005] Dr. Pardini found that tumors in mice fed corn oil grow faster and become larger. [Cancer Letters 187: 169-77, 2002]

Omega-3: halts metastasis

Another stark fact is that with all of the cancer treatments that have been developed in the past decades, none address metastasis, the spread of cancer to other organs that is responsible for 90% of the mortality among cancer cases. Yet, omega-3 oils have been shown to inhibit the adhesion of roaming tumor cells to the wall of small blood capillaries where most metastatic tumors form. [Nutrition Cancer 31: 143-50, 1998]

Omega-3: halts breast cancer

The drug Herceptin is widely used to treat breast cancer. Herceptin®, is advertised as the only FDA-approved therapeutic for HER-2 protein. This drug is quite expensive and only adds a few months to the life of a woman with advanced-stage breast cancer. HER protein is human epidermal growth factor receptor 2 that is overly abundant in metastatic breast cancer. Omega-3 oils inhibit HER-2 protein. Researchers conclude that omega-3 oils have a "*strong suppressive effect on HER-2 protein.*" [Journal Nutrition 135: 983-88, 2005]

More evidence

- The following are a sample of studies showing a definite link between omega-3 oil consumption and favorable outcomes of cancer patients:
- Just two servings of fish a week reduce the risk for all types of cancer. [American Journal Clinical Nutrition 70: 85-90, 1999]
- Among patients with colon polyps who are at high risk to develop colon cancer, the provision of omega-3 fish oil (8,000 mg per day) reduces the multiplication of abnormal cells. [Nutrition Reviews 51: 241-43, 1993]
- The level of DHA from omega-3 oil in fatty tissues of the breast among patients with complete or partial remission in response to anti-cancer drugs is higher than in patients with no response or progression of tumors. [Lipids 34:S109, 1999]
- A study shows the omega-3 oils do not interfere with anti-cancer drugs. [Journal Nutrition 134: 3427-30S, 2004]
- One report suggests an omega-3 oil supplement "*may be a useful alternative therapy for patients who are not candidates for standard toxic cancer therapies.*" [Journal Nutrition 134: 3427-3430S, 2004]

How much fish oil?

The maximum tolerated dose in one study of cancer patients was determined to be 21,000 mg for a 160 pound patient (300 mg per 2.2 pounds). [Clinical Cancer Research 5:3842-3947, 1999]

Another study employed 12,000 mg of fish oil per day, which produced a favorable weight gain in pancreatic cancer patients. [Journal Nutrition 12:S27-S30, 1996]

Fish oil during cancer treatment

An analysis of available studies shows that oral omega-3 supplements increase appetite in cancer patients and improves survival. Tube feeding with omega-3 oils results in shorter hospital stays, and a lower incidence of infections and complications. [International Journal Oncology 28: 5-23, 2006]

Source of omega-3 oil

Dr. Johanna Budwig of Germany has been successfully prescribing flaxseed oil to treat cancer patients since 1956. [Hippokrates 27: 605-12, 1956] Dr. Budwig utilizes flaxseed oil for many reasons.

Omega-3 oils emanate from two primary sources: fish and plant foods. Fish eat phytoplankton to obtain omega-3 oils. Plant sources of omega-3 oils are flaxseed, perilla seed, purslane, and to a lesser extent almonds and walnuts. Flaxseed has the highest concentration of omega-3 oil (known as alpha linolenic acid) and the highest concentration of omega-3 over omega-6 oil of any source.

Composition of oils	Omega-3 Oil	Omega-6 Oil
Fish oil (salmon)	30%	20%
Flaxseed oil	60%	20%

Flax provides more than oil. Flaxseed is loaded with weak estrogen-like molecules called lignans (about 1/1000th the strength of natural estrogen produced in the body). Phytoestrogens (estrogens obtained from plants) have a dual nature. Phytoestrogens normalize hormone levels. If estrogen levels are low, soy and flax molecules can act as substitutes. If estrogen levels are high, soy and flax molecules can dull the effects of natural estrogen. So it follows that human populations that consume more plant estrogens have lower rates of cancer, particularly hormone-related (breast, prostate) cancer.

An intriguing study was conducted adding flaxseed to the diets of women with estrogen-dependent breast cancer who were taking tamoxifen, the anti-estrogen drug. At low estrogen levels, flaxseed shrunk pretreatment tumor size by 74 %. Tamoxifen alone initially reduced tumor size, but later tumor size increased and then reverted to about the same pretreatment size. Flaxseed plus tamoxifen shrunk tumors 53% more than tamoxifen alone. When estrogen levels were high, tumors shrunk by 22% with flaxseed, 41% with tamoxifen and 53% with flaxseed plus tamoxifen. [Clinical Cancer Research 10: 7703-11, 2004]

In mice with estrogen-positive breast cancer, the provision of flaxseed not only slowed tumor growth, but reduced the incidence of tumors spreading to the lung by 34%, meaning flaxseed yields meaningful protection from tumor spreading to other organs. [Nutrition Cancer 43: 187-92, 2002]

Flaxseed inhibits a growth factor for cancer (vascular endothelial growth factor). [Cancer Letters 185: 31-37, 2002]

A study was conducted to determine if it is the flax oil, flax lignans or both that inhibits breast cancer. Estrogen-negative breast cancer cells were injected into mice and the animals were fed a regular diet with or without flaxseed, flax oil or flax lignans. Tumor growth rate was significantly lower in the flaxseed, flax oil and lignans groups. Spread of cancer to the lung was inhibited by all three forms of flax. Flax oil and flax lignan components inhibit cancer, not by inducing oxidation to kill cancer cells, but by other mechanisms. [International Journal Cancer 116: 793-98, 2005]

The flaxseed conundrum and prostate cancer

Flaxseed, flax oil and flax lignans sound like major cancer fighters, except there has been a pause in the enthusiasm for flax when it comes to prostate cancer. So much so that Harvard Men's Health Watch published a report in 2002 entitled: *"Good for the heart but not for the prostate? The alpha linolenic acid dilemma."*

While flaxseed, its omega-3 oil and lignans are heralded for their many healthy properties, a number of puzzling population studies appears to show an opposite effect for prostate cancer. The more alpha linolenic acid (omega-3 oil) consumed, the greater the risk for prostate cancer. This has caused a great stir among men with prostate cancer. Many males elect to forgo treatment (watchful waiting) and are certainly concerned about any dietary component that might exacerbate their condition. Since flax and flax oil as a source of omega-3 oil is often promoted for heart health, it poses a conflict for health-conscious males, particularly vegetarian males.

A confusing part of this debate is that most of the arguments center around markers of prostate cancer such as PSA count, or even tumor size, but not survival, which in the end is the final arbiter. Furthermore, studies do confirm that low levels of fat, regardless of type, help to prevent prostate cancer. [Anticancer Research 16: 815-20, 1996]

Enter Charles E. Myers Jr., MD, who at age 55 faced prostate cancer himself. He altered his diet and elected to undergo radiation treatment plus an unproven treatment called brachytherapy (radiation seed implant) followed by estrogen hormone therapy to further shrink or retard growth of prostate cancer. Dr. Myers gained the attention of males since he firmly does not recommend flaxseed oil, the richest source of omega-3 oil, for men. He prefers fish oil

Dr. Myers said he reviewed the existing medical literature published on the topic of fats and oils related to prostate cancer and found six studies that positively linked increased consumption of alpha linolenic acid (omega-3 oils) with prostate cancer. That was enough evidence for him. He decided to recommend omega-3 fish oil instead of flax oil to his patients, and to all other males facing prostate cancer via his now infamous website.

According to Dr. Myers: *"Clinical studies that are available suggest that alpha linolenic acid may actually be dangerous for prostate cancer patients."*

Dr. Myers refers to *"six epidemiology (population) studies that have examined the association between dietary alpha linolenic acid and risk of prostate cancer. Five out of six of these studies found an increase in the risk of prostate cancer associated with alpha linolenic acid. I should also note that our laboratory, as well as others, found that alpha linolenic acid is one of the most powerful growth stimuli for human prostate cancer cells. ...It is the most powerful stimulus we know of for prostate cancer cells."*

Dr. Meyers refers to a study conducted in Uruguay, where there is a very high rate of prostate cancer, which found that the consumption of alpha linolenic acid from both red meat and vegetable sources increased the risk for prostate cancer. [Cancer Epidemiology Biomarkers Prevention 9: 335-38, 2000] This looks bad for flax. Except it is unlikely there is any consumption of flaxseed whatsoever in Uruguay where the intake of red meat is among the highest in the world. How flaxseed got bunched in with this data is puzzling. Furthermore, while there are six population (epidemiological) studies linking alpha linolenic acid intake with prostate cancer risk, there are other studies that do not show such a relationship. [Bulletin Cancer 92: 670-84, 2005]

At the time Dr. Myers wrote his paper, in 2000, he said there was *"no evidence that flaxseed slows or prevents the growth and spread of prostate cancer."* [Prostate Forum, August 5: 7-8, 2000]

But a year later researchers at Duke University provided flaxseed to patients awaiting prostate cancer surgery and found it lowered their testosterone and PSA and that combined with a low-fat diet, flaxseed beneficially altered the markers for prostate cancer. [Urology 58: 47-52, 2001]

In 2002, Duke University researchers also confirmed their earlier work by demonstrating that flaxseed inhibits the growth of prostate cancer. Table below shows the results of that animal study.

The same researchers followed up with another study in 2004, this time providing flaxseed to males on a low-fat diet and reported that their PSA and proliferation rates, as proven by biopsy, dropped significantly. [Urology 63: 900-04, 2004]

This is very puzzling because Dr. Myers himself takes estrogen to slow down the growth of his prostate tumor, yet flax oil, which provides a small amount of mild estrogen-like molecules, called lignans, is said to cause prostate cancer risk to rise dramatically, as much as 350%. [Cancer Epidemiology, Biomarkers & Prevention 5: 889-95, 1996]

	Regular diet	Flaxseed diet
Percent developed prostate cancer	100%	97%
Tumor weight, grams	3.6	1.9
Lung or lymph metastases	13% / 16%	5% / 12%
Proliferation rate (multiplication)	38.1	26.2

Source: Urology 60: 919-24, 2002

	Whole Flaxseed	Crushed Flaxseed	Flaxseed Oil	Flax Lignan Extract
Omega-3 oil	Not as available	Available 1,500 mg per tbsp**	Highest	None
IP6 Phytic acid (iron binder)	Not available	Highly available 160 mg per tbsp**	None	None
Lignans	28% available*	43% available* 25 mg per tbsp**	Small amt	Highest

** Journal Nutrition 135: 2812-2816, 2005 ** Barlean's Forti-Flax*

Researchers at the RMIT University in Melbourne, Australia, have stepped in to examine this controversy. They report that there has been a mistaken assumption that blood serum levels of alpha linolenic acid (omega-3 oils) are indicative of levels in prostate tissues. When prostate tissues, not blood levels of alpha linolenic acid, were measured, much lower levels of alpha linolenic acid (omega-3) were found.

Alpha linolenic acid is found in such low concentrations in most foods (meat, milk, dairy products, fish) that it is often less than 1% of total fats and oils consumed. It is unlikely such a small amount would have any effect upon cancer compared to the high amounts of saturated fat consumed. Even in blood tests this type of fat is no more than 2% of total fatty acids, which means there is not much room for error. Many males have no detectable levels of alpha linolenic acid.

These studies also rely upon estimates of alpha linolenic acid in foods which are highly variable, particularly from one country to another.

Researchers recommend all future studies be confined to the study of actual fatty acid levels within prostate tissue rather than blood serum levels and that animal studies use appropriate models, such as canines where prostate cancer occurs spontaneously rather than by use of chemicals. [Journal Urology 171: 1402-07, 2004]

Myers jumped the gun and misled many men with prostate cancer away from flaxseed or flaxseed oil.

However, there is a strong argument for the use of whole, crushed flaxseed in addition to flaxseed oil or flaxseed lignans, in the fight against cancer. Flax has three major anti-cancer molecules–omega-3 oils, lignans and IP6 phytic acid--that bind iron. Only the crushed or milled flaxseed meal provides ample amounts of all three.

Omega-3 with chemotherapy

The addition of omega-3 oils enhances the cancer-cell killing effect of chemotherapy drugs. [Free Radical Biology Medicine 39:742-51, 2005]

Omega-3 fatty acids such as derived from fish or flaxseed oil, which are vulnerable to turning rancid, increase oxidation in target cancer cells specifically. This increase in oxidation from omega-3 oils can be utilized in an advantageous manner to kill cancer cells

For example, in a rat study, omega-3 fatty acids were readily incorporated into mammary tumor cells and then iron was added to enhance oxidation, resulting in selective destruction of the tumor cells without killing normal cells. The use of omega-3 fatty acids combined with iron *"might be an effective cancer therapy for humans."* [British Journal Cancer 76: 347, 1997]

Chemotherapy often does not work because of tumor resistance to the drug over time. Omega-3 oils help to reverse drug resistance. [Prostaglandins Leukotrienes Essential Fatty Acids 58:39-54, 1998]

This information adds to the body of knowledge as to how to alternatively use oxidation (cell destruction) and antioxidation (cell preservation) to treat and prevent cancer.

A human body that is devoid of or has low omega-3 tissue levels is a body that is ready to foster tumor cell growth.

Hyaluronic acid and cancer

Collagen is the barrier that limits the spread of disease in the human body. Collagen, also called connective tissue, is likened to mortar between bricks. This is the *"goo"* that surrounds living cells. Healthy and abnormal cells are held in place by collagen and its water-holding gel called hyaluronic acid (HA). In disease states, germs or tumor cells can excite enzymes that break down collagen and HA, facilitating the spread of infection or cancer. It is essential to maintain connective tissue to remain healthy.

Experiments have been conducted over the past decade at Harvard Medical School in Massachusetts and the Lawrence Berkeley National Laboratory in California that expand the current understanding of cancer therapy beyond that of just killing cancer cells. These researchers believe that the connective tissue or collagen that anchors cells in place, much as mortar anchors bricks, is essential to maintaining healthy cells.

The experiments have involved the application of ionizing radiation, like that used to treat cancer, in connective tissues. Scientists call this the *"extracellular matrix."*

The current thinking is that DNA mutations occurring within living cells can lead to abnormal and unstoppable cell replication. The experiments reveal that cells have interaction with their immediate environment and that damage to that environment, such as occurs during exposure to radiation, is what facilitates the DNA mutations inside living cells and frees tumor cells to travel.

What researchers notice is that a gel-like substance, called hyaluronic acid (HA), that resides within connective tissue, is rapidly lost from the mammary gland when it is exposed to radiation. [Journal Mammary Gland Biology Neoplasia 3: 165-75, 1998] Hyaluronic acid is the scaffolding or space filler of the body. It also holds water, up to six liters of water per 1,000 mg of HA. Water is the great dilutor and detoxifier of animal and human tissues. Without HA, tissues shrivel up and dry out.

HA is a long molecule. HA is a di-saccharide, two sugar-like molecules holding hands – glucosamine and glucuronic acid. Now repeat these two molecules, like stringing paper clips together, and you end up with a long strand of HA. HA varies in molecular weight (strand length) from 2 to 6 million.

Beyond cancer cells

The widely held view that radiation induces DNA damage and DNA damage induces mutations, and mutations then cause cancer, is now in question. It is not just the cells, it is also the connective tissue that surrounds cells that must be considered in cancer prevention and therapy. An integral part of connective tissue is hyaluronic acid, which is abundant during youth and pregnancy, when cancer risks are low. High levels of estrogen during pregnancy trigger more hyaluronic acid to be produced, to protect the developing baby.

The revealing experiment

In an animal experiment, supporting tissue that surrounds mammary-gland epithelial cells was exposed to low-dose ionizing radiation. Then healthy non-irradiated breast gland cells were implanted within this matrix. A massive increase in tumors was observed in the non-irradiated mammary cells! More tumors occurred and arose more quickly and grew larger compared to non-irradiated tissue. Only

19% of non-irradiated connective tissue produced tumors versus 81% tumor incidence (larger more frequent tumors) in irradiated connective tissue. The tumors grew so fast in the mammary cells implanted in irradiated connective tissue that by six weeks all of the mammary glands had tumors! Only 39% of the mammary gland cells implanted in non-irradiated connective tissue expressed small tumors and some of these regressed. The study had to be halted because all of the irradiated mammary gland cells were tumorous by the sixth week. Had the study continued, the difference between the two groups would have been greater because of the tumor regression observed in the non-irradiated animals. [Radiation Research 156: 618-27, 2001; Molecular Medicine Today 61: 324-29, 2000]

This experiment reveals something very important. Tumors can arise and then regress and disappear on their own, without treatment!

Experiments have shown that the placement of tumor cells inside developing embryos induces their "*normalization.*" Embryos exhibit gobs of extra connective tissue and hyaluronic acid.

Investigators observe that after radiation treatment to cancerous tissues there is an initial period of a few years where cancer may recur, and then there is another rise in risk in the same tumor area some time later. This is interpreted to mean that tumor cells remain dormant. [Nature Reviews Cancer 5: 867-75, 2005] Some change that occurs later, such as a decline in the immune system, or a degradation of HA, may facilitate these cells waking up from dormancy.

In 1986, O.J. Stone proposed that HA and the entire matrix of connective tissue is an important barrier against the growth and spread of tumors. Stone wrote that anything that helps to retain the viscosity (consistency) of HA increases the body's resistance to tumors whereas enzymes that break down HA, like hyaluronidase, which is stimulated by infection or radiation exposure, encourage tumors. [Medical Hypotheses 20: 117-24, 1986]

Previously the connective tissue was believed to be an uninvolved bystander to cancer. It is now obvious that disrupted connective tissue permits the initial tumor cells to proliferate. As Barcellos-Hoff says, "*Indeed, it has been suggested that cancer may be a physiological response to an abnormal environment.*" Studies reveal there are many more mutated cells produced that can initiate cancer than actual number of tumors that develop. The initiation of cancer appears to be a far more frequent event than the cases of cancer that develop. Radiation upsets the environment surrounding cells and promotes tumors, an effect that lasts for 14 days following radiation exposure. By re-establishing the matrix of supporting tissue, tumors and pre-tumorous cell processes can be reversed, even in the presence of grossly abnormal, genetically-damaged cells. [Cancer Research 60: 1254-60, 2000]

Barcellos-Hoff notes that conventional thought is that the ionizing radiation promotes cancer by its ability to damage DNA. But her experiments clearly show that cells undamaged by radiation, but existing in an environment of connective tissue that has been irradiated, will aggressively grow tumors of large size and numbers. Barcellos-Hoff suggests it is possible to develop blocking agents to interrupt tumor progression. [Journal Mammary Gland Biology Neoplasia 3: 165-75, 1998]

Even more evidence of HA's anti-cancer barrier effect comes from Japan. Researchers at Osaka Medical Center for Cancer and Cardiovascular Disease report that removal of an extended zone of connective tissue in addition to lymph glands surrounding pancreatic tumors increased the five-year survival rate from 8 to 25 %. [Gan To Kagaku Ryoho 29: 364-69, 2002] This is an astounding improvement in survival for a type of cancer that traditionally has a very high mortality rate.

It is for the reasons above that hyaluronic acid presents one of the most promising approaches to cancer therapy and prevention.

Shark cartilage disappointing

The observation that tumors do not grow in cartilaginous tissues led to the idea that shark cartilage taken orally may serve as a treatment for cancer. While shark cartilage added to the diet of animals has been shown to delay the growth of tumors, it does not abolish their progression. [Anticancer Research 21: 10565-69, 2001] Cartilage is tissue that does not contain any blood vessels, and thus it is low in iron content. Iron is required for tumor cells to grow, which explains why tumor cells don't grow in connective tissues. Cartilage inhibits the formation of new blood vessels which are required for tumor growth. But shark cartilage has not been proven in clinical trials to be of much benefit. [Biol Pharm Bulletin 24: 1097-101, 2001]

HA's dual role

HA has a dual nature in regard to cancer. [European Journal Cancer 37: 849-56, 2001] Intact HA can keep tumor cells planted at their site of origin, preventing them from growing and spreading, while broken down HA can facilitate invasion and spread of tumors (metastasis).

Cells adhere to each other. The cells that can move and break away the easiest are found in the epithelia, the surface layers, of the skin, stomach, lungs, mouth and other organs. The majority of tumors begin in the epithelial tissue. In cancer cells the adhesion molecules that keep cells together are partly or entirely missing. Degraded hyaluronic acid binds to the surface of a tumor cell and gives the cell "*roller skates.*" In other words, when HA is broken down it can facilitate slippery movement of the tumor cells. In order to spread (metastasize), tumor cells must be able to avoid adhesion (sticking) to other cells, detach from the tumor mass and pass through barriers in the connective tissue.

Cancer and blood levels of HA

Because HA is broken down in tumor masses, and because cells called fibroblasts make more HA in damaged tissues, cancer doctors know that high amounts of HA being released into the blood circulation could be a marker that there is a tumor somewhere in the body.

Oncologists have been attempting to measure HA in the blood serum as a marker for tumors. However, HA is a poor marker for cancer because serum HA levels are not significantly elevated until the late stage of the disease. One would think as tumors destroy connective tissue that more HA would make its way into the blood circulation. But HA levels are not elevated in all types of tumors.

The concentration of HA in blood serum has not been found to be elevated in patients with sarcomas, lymphomas, brain tumors, breast carcinomas, and other malignancies, but is elevated five-fold among patients with mesothelioma, a form of chest cancer, compared to healthy adults. [Cancer 62: 326-30, 1988] High HA serum levels have also been found in Wilms tumor and in bladder cancer. [Annals Medicine 28: 241-53, 1996]

If the HA breaks down due to exposure to radiation, either x-ray, gamma ray or solar radiation, or due to viral or bacterial infection, or inflammation, then the connective tissue loses its consistency and any existing tumors cells can use the slipperiness of the watery HA to travel to distant locations. For example, the recurrence rate for colon cancer after an operation increases from 20 to 80 % as the levels of HA increase in cancer cells. [Cancer Research 58: 342-47, 1998]

Because HA facilitates the spread of cancer, and it is more abundant at tumor sites, it is sometimes mistakenly thought to contribute to the spread of cancer. There are numerous reports one can find on the internet where health counselors suggest cancer patients avoid hyaluronic acid supplements. This is kind of like blaming the road for auto accidents and then advising drivers to stay off the road. This doesn't mean HA causes cancer, but rather it is a marker of damage and degradation. More HA is then produced in an attempt to heal the tissues. More about this below.

How does HA break down?

Tumor cells can break down the barrier of connective tissue that surrounds them via enzymes, such as hyaluronidase and metalloproteinase. [International Journal Cancer 98: 210-15, 2002]

Hyaluronidase is the same enzyme found in snake and insect venom which causes toxins to spread. Hyaluronidase is produced in tumors such as melanoma, colon carcinoma and certain brain tumors.

Hyaluronidase also enables tumor cells to avoid adhesion, make their way through the connective tissue barriers and release growth factors that promote the development of new blood vessels. The new blood vessels are then used as a conduit to provide nutrients for tumor cells to grow.

Hyaluronidase has been described as one of the "*molecular saboteurs*" that destroy HA. [Proceedings Natl Academy Sciences 93: 7832-37, 1996] The growth and spread of tumors is totally dependent upon new blood vessel formation. The process of new blood vessel formation (angiogenesis) all starts with hyaluronidase, the body's own venom, inducing new blood vessel formation in tumor cells. Hyaluronidase inhibitors can block angiogenesis. [Proceedings National Academy Science 93: 7832-37, 1996]

In prostate tumors there is a high level of the HA breakdown enzyme (hyaluronidase). High-grade tumors have up to 20 times more of this enzyme than low-grade tumors. [Cancer Research 56: 651-57, 1996]

The Gleason (invasion) score is higher among prostate cancer patients who exhibit high hyaluronidase levels. Invasion of a prostate tumor outside the prostate gland was found in 83% of cases with high hylauronidase levels, whereas no invasion was found among specimens with low levels of this enzyme. [Oncology Reports 6: 1431-33, 1999] There is no mortal danger when tumor cells stay inside the prostate gland.

Elevated levels of hyaluronidase correlate with invasive breast cancer. [Oncology Reports 6: 607-09, 1999] Invasiveness of breast cancer is directly related to elevated levels of hyaluronidase. One study found that breast tumors exhibited four times more hyaluronidase than did healthy breast tissue. [Oncology Reports 6: 607-09, 1999] Aging, there is no mortal danger when breast cancer remains within the breast.

Certain hyaluronidase inhibitors completely block hyaluronidase and angiogenesis (new blood vessel formation). A report in the Proceedings of the National Academy of Sciences says "*a number of hyaluronidase inhibitors are readily available.*" [Proceedings National Academy Sciences 93: 7832-37, 1996] For example, a very low dose of green tea bioflavonoids provided in drinking water has been shown to prevent the growth and spread of colon cancer in rodents. [Japanese Journal Cancer Research 84: 1007-09, 1993] A patient with early-stage lung cancer has been reported to be successfully treated with an inhibitor of hyaluronidase. [Japanese Journal Clinical Oncology 7: 85-92, 1977].

New blood vessel formation is enhanced by various growth factors while genestein from soy, heparin, cyclosporine A, and steroids, are among an array of angiogenic inhibitors. [Internal Review Cytology 159: 113-60, 1995]

The native, high-molecular weight HA can only form into small fragments that facilitate the growth and spread of tumors if the HA is broken down by enzymes such as hyaluronidase and metalloproteinase. This is why hyaluronidase blockers such as iron-binders (bioflavonoids, IP6 phytate) are so important. High-dose vitamin C can also play a preventive role by inhibiting the production of hyaluronidase which helps to "*wall off*" tumors. [Alternative Medicine Review 3: 174-86, 1998] HA is part of the vitamin C story in regard to cancer prevention and treatment.

Using hyaluronidase to treat cancer

Like HA, hyaluronidase has a paradoxical nature. A recent report said: "*Paradoxically, both hyaluronic acid and hyaluronidase are involved in malignant transformation and cancer progression.*" Their mechanisms of action are not fully understood. HYAL-1 is the predominant form of hyaluronidase and the loss of HYAL-1 often correlates with tumor progression, particularly tobacco-related cancers. [Cancer Letters 163: 95-101, 2001]

Hyaluronidase can be employed in the treatment of cancer. In studies where human breast cancer cells have been implanted in animals, hyaluronidase given intravenously shrinks the tumors to half their size in just four days. [International Journal Cancer 102:192-7, 2002] In Austria, doctors have used hyaluronidase to treat children with brain tumors and have produced favorable results. [Cancer Letters 131: 101-08, 1998]

In mice where melanoma cells had been implanted, the pre-administration of hyaluronidase before injection of an anti-cancer drug (vinblastine) was shown to produce marked anti-tumor effects. Hyaluronidase by itself did not alter tumor growth or metastasis. [Journal Cancer Research Clinical Oncology 121: 193-202, 1995]

Hyaluronidase is being successfully used to break down HA so that anti-cancer drugs can penetrate into areas of the brain where tumors reside. Children with brain tumors who received hyaluronidase plus chemotherapy faired better and had fewer relapses. [Cancer Letters 131: 101-08, 1998] Hyaluronidase is only available as a drug, not a food supplement.

HA intercepts cancer cells

Another intriguing quality of HA is that it sticks to cancer cells and therefore has the ability to intercept roaming cancer cells in the blood circulation. Cancer cells that metastasize (spread) make their way from the original tumor site through newly formed blood vessels into the blood circulation. These roaming tumor cells have cellular parking spaces for HA. Dr. David C. Baker, Professor of Organic Chemistry at the University of Tennessee, has conducted research on short, low-molecular weight HA that immediately halts metastasis in mice. Short-length HA attracts migrating cancer cells and thus renders them harmless. Think of an elaborate anti-missile defense system whereby incoming missiles (tumor cells) are immediately intercepted by HA before they can develop into a ball of tumor cells at a site distant from their origin.

While degraded HA at the site of a tumor may enable tumor cells to travel to distant locations, short-length, low-molecular weight HA introduced into the circulatory system may completely block the spread of cancer. Inhibition of cancer at 90-100 % effectiveness was achieved in animals with short strands of HA. No toxicity was observed. [Data: David C. Baker, U of Tennessee]

Bladder tumors and HA

HA is involved in bladder cancer. High levels of HA (2.5 to 6.5 fold increase) and hyaluronidase (3 to 7 fold increase) are found in the urine of bladder cancer patients. Measuring the levels of HA and hyaluronidase in urine may help to diagnose bladder cancer. [Journal Urology 163: 348-56, 2000; Urologe 40: 121-26, 2001]

Hyaluronidase levels are five to seven times higher among patients with medium- to high-grade bladder cancer compared to healthy individuals. [Cancer Letters 131: 21-27, 1998] Urinary levels of HA and hyaluronidase may indicate the presence of a bladder tumor. [Miami Nature Biotechnology Short Reports, The Scientific World 106SR, 2001]

In Canada, Bioniche Life Science, Inc. has been licensed to use Cystistat (hyaluronic acid) in Europe for the treatment of radiation cystitis, cystitis caused by infection or trauma, and neoplasia (cancer). Cystistat is injected directly into the bladder where it helps to restore tissues. [Doctor's Guide, Sept. 7, 2000]

Prostate cancer and HA

Three to eight times more HA is found in prostate cancer cells. [Journal Biological Chemistry 276: 11922-32, 2001] Prostate cancer cells often migrate to bone marrow. Increased HA levels apparently enhance the adhesion of prostate tumor cells to bone. [Journal Biological Chemistry 276: 17949-57, 2001]

Skin cancer and HA

Hyal Pharmaceutical Corporation has received a patent for its Solarase product which combines HA and anti-inflammatory agents for the treatment of actinic keratosis, a form of skin cancer. [Doctor's Guide, Jan. 21, 1997]

Breast cancer and chondroitin

A remarkable study using oral chondroitin sulfate (a natural component of human connective tissue) in animals shows that breast tumors can be completely inhibited. Oral chondroitin sulfate has been shown to reduce the incidence and size of mammary tumors in virgin female mice. Chondroitin stimulates the production of HA.

Incidence of mammary tumors after 18 weeks of feeding	
Purified diet	35.0%
Purified diet +	
0.5 % chondroitin sulfate	28.6%
1.0 % chondroitin sulfate	11.4%
2.5 % chondroitin sulfate	0.0

Morrison LM, Schjeide OA, Coronary Heart Disease and the Mucopolysaccharides (glycosaminoglycans), Charles C Thomas, Springfield, Ill, 1974.

Female sex hormones increase HA and collagen production in the mammary glands. In rodents, estrogen and progesterone administered together elevate levels of chondroitin and HA. Estrogen alone elevates HA while progesterone only elevates concentrations of chondroitin sulfate. In animals whose ovaries have been removed, progesterone alone or in combination with estrogen decreases levels of HA. [Acta Physiol Scandinavia 168: 385-92, 2000]

Elevated blood serum levels of HA are not found among breast cancer patients. [Int J Cancer 52: 873-76, 1992]

Size of HA and cancer

Landmark work conducted by Eva A. Turley and associates at the London Regional Cancer Center, University of Western Ontario, Canada, indicates that the size and concentration of HA determines HA's ability to inhibit tumors.

Blocking the cancer receptor site

The Winnipeg Free Press in Canada reported a startling story of widespread interest on July 15th, 1995. The report said Manitoba scientists found they can stop the spread of cancer in mice by turning off a cancer cell's sensing ability. Sensors, called receptor sites, on the surface of living cells, are able to be knocked out and completely block the spread of a tumor. The knocked-out receptors later return to normal when the cancer risk has subsided. It's like pulling blinders over a cell. Tumor cells just die once they are blinded. [Winnipeg Free Press, July 15, 1995]

This is taken from the Winnipeg Free Press, Saturday, July 15, 1995:

This is taken from the Winnipeg Free Press
Saturday, July 15, 1995:

CANCER FIND HAILED

Manitobans stop disease in mice; discovery grabs world's attention

By Bill Redskop (Staff Reporter)

Manitoba scientists have found that they can stop the spread of cancer in mice by turning off a cancer cell's sensing ability.

Testing on animals will continue for about two years before human treatment is tried.

The treatment, hailed as a huge breakthrough in the fight against cancer, involves knocking out a cell's RHAMMs (re ceptors for hyaluronic acid mediated motility.)

The receptors sit on the surface of a cell and act as its eyes and ears.

But when the Manitoba scientists used genetic engineering to knock out those senses, the cancer cells would simply lie inert and not reproduce.

Even more astonishing, the receptorless cancer cells soon turned to their normal, non-cancerous state.

"*If you blind it, the cancer cell just dies,*" said Dr. Arnold Greenberg, one of three molecular biologists making up the research team. "*It surprised us, and everyone else who saw it.*"

"*Researchers never thought of this before. It's quite novel,*" said team leader Dr. Eva Turley, who discovered and named the RHAMM receptor three years ago.

Turley, 45, has been traveling the globe in recent months sharing her findings with other scientists, with stops in Atlanta, Colorado, Hawaii, Australia, Sweden, Switzerland, and London, England. She travels to Japan later this year.

"*When I gave a talk in Colorado, I was the last speaker to talk, and everyone was restless and talking about going out skiing. After I finished, there was stunned silence,*" said Turley, a microbiologist with the University of Manitoba.

Turley cautioned that they only studied the gene called ras, responsible for 20 to 30 per cent of cancers. And experiments have only been conducted on mice so far.

But in theory, the treatment - using high concentrations of hyaluronic acid, which cells generally use in small amounts - should work in humans, she said.

It's hoped the findings will lead to biotechnological treatment of cancer that would be more effective than radiation chemotherapy, and without the negative side effects she said.

Dr. Jim Wright is the third member of the team.

The scientists, who work out of the Manitoba Institute of Cell Biology, are funded by the Terry Fox Program of the National Cancer Institute of Canada.

Turley said all the travel and attention in recent months has been overwhelming.

The discovery was written up in yesterday's edition of Cell Magazine, the most prestigious biomedical sciences journal in the world.

HA is an ideal anti-cancer agent because it is naturally found throughout the body and is therefore nontoxic and is readily available to be harvested from animal tissues. [International Journal Cancer 77: 396-401, 1998]

For example, HA strands can be introduced into the body to bind to cell receptors (called CD44 and RHAMM) and compete with native HA. To determine whether this works, small osmotic pumps were used to slowly administer strands of HA to tumor sites in animals. As much as 80% inhibition of tumor growth was achieved. This was demonstrated over a period of 7-14 days with just 0.5 mcg of the HA strand. [New Frontiers in Medical Sciences: Redefining Hyaluronan, Elsevier Science, 2000, pp. 51-62]

HA drug combo

HA can be combined with anti-cancer drugs to target cancer cells. When HA is injected into rats who have liver cancer, the HA targets and adheres to the cancer cells. Pre-treatment with chondroitin sulfate enhances the targeting effect. This means that HA can be used to selectively deliver certain drugs to cancer cells. [Glyconconj Journal 15: 935-39, 1998] There is an adhesion molecule that creates an affinity between cancer cells and HA. HA is an interceptor of cancer cells that are on the move. Pharmaceutical researchers have successfully combined HA with an anti-cancer drug (Taxol). This helps the drug in targeting the cancer cells. [Biomarcomolecules 1: 208-18, 2000] Other methods of targeting cancer cells, such as monoclonal antibodies, have failed because they only target the outside of the cancer cell but do not enter and destroy it. Because cancer cells utilize the cell receptors for HA in order to spread, the use of HA with an anti-cancer drug can help target the tumor cells better than use of the drug alone. [Pharmaceutical Research, Volume 19, April 2002]

Preclinical studies demonstrate that the addition of HA to cytotoxic drugs results in increased cellular uptake, increased response rates, reduced toxicity and prolonged survival. The addition of HA infused with anti-cancer drugs in a human study reduced the loss of neutrophils (immune-fighting cells), and reduced drug toxicity. [American Society Clinical Oncology Meeting 2002]

Here is how researchers at the Department of Chemistry and Institute of Chemical Biology and Drug Discovery, State University of New York at Stony Brook, New York, explain the way HA intercepts cancer cells. *"Traditional cancer chemotherapy relies on the premise that rapidly proliferating cancer cells are more likely to be killed by a toxic agent. In reality, however, toxic agents have very little or no specificity, which leads to systemic toxicity, causing severe undesirable side effects. Therefore, various drug delivery protocols and systems have been explored in the last three decades. Tumor cells overexpress many receptors and biomarkers, which can be used as targets to deliver cytotoxic agents into tumors. In general, a tumor-targeting drug delivery system consists of a tumor recognition moiety and a cytotoxic warhead connected directly or through a suitable linker to form a conjugate. The conjugate, which can be regarded as 'prodrug', should be systemically nontoxic. This means that the linker (HA) must be stable in circulation. Upon internalization into the cancer cell the conjugate (HA plus the anti-cancer drug) should be readily cleaved to regenerate (release) the active toxic agent."* [Bioorganization Medicinal Chemistry 13: 5043-54, 2005] Hyaluronic acid is one of these cancer interceptors.

Researchers in Italy actually used hyaluronic acid coupled with butyric acid as cancer therapy. The result: 87-100% of animals were metastasis-free using this treatment, which is ten-times more effective than butyric acid alone. [Anticancer Drugs 16: 373-79, 2005]

If hyaluronic acid is a suspected cancer-causing agent, then why is it being used along with other molecules to treat cancer? Researchers in Italy indicate HA combined with other compounds are *"promising"* and responsible for the *"arrest"* of tumor cell growth. [Investigative New Drugs 22: 207-17, 2004]

Summary

In summary, the best strategy to prevent cancer involving HA is to block its degradation. This keeps the cells that have turned cancerous in their place and keeps them from growing and spreading. It also hinders the development of new blood vessels (angiogenesis) that then feed nutrients to tumors that are required for their growth.

Natural iron chelators such as bioflavonoids (extracts from grape seed, bilberry, cranberry, blueberry, cherry, milk thistle, ginkgo biloba, green tea, quercetin, rutin, and others), IP6 rice bran extract, or echinacea, may be consumed from foods and supplements, to inhibit the production of hyaluronidase, the enzyme that breaks down HA.

Once cancer has begun to grow and spread, short-length, low-molecular weight HA taken orally may help to intercept circulating tumors cells.

Use of hyaluronidase to treat cancer should remain under a doctor's supervision.

The primary contraindication for oral HA among cancer patients is the occurrence of lymphedema (leg swelling). Cancer treatments may encourage the onset of lymphedema. Since HA thickens lymph fluid, oral HA supplements may worsen lymphedema.

Does hyaluronic acid promote or accelerate the spread of cancer?

While repetitious, the subject of whether HA promotes the spread of cancer must be re-addressed because of continued concerns expressed by many cancer patients and their families. Internet search engines for hyaluronic acid (HA) have spread poorly founded opinions that hyaluronic acid supplements promote cancer. Because this misinformation alarms so many people, it will be dealt with at length here.

Hyaluronic acid is produced continually throughout life, more so in early childhood and during pregnancy, when cancer rates are almost nonexistent. Yet the opinion prevails that somehow, taking oral HA might cause cancer.

For the naïve viewer of medical literature, there are many reports indicating elevated levels of HA are associated with the spread of tumors, what is called invasion. Tumor cells can mobilize and spread (become metastatic) by using HA as a biological *"slip and slide."* However, ingesting oral HA supplements has little to do with this biological phenomenon. More HA shows up at tumor sites because it is a healing agent. Anywhere there is a wound in your body, cells called fibroblasts, make more HA.

A recent study, conducted by researchers in Finland, investigated the role of hyaluronic acid in squamous cell carcinoma (oral cancer). *"At the end of the follow-up (median 52 months) 43% of patients had died because of this type of cancer. A significant difference in overall survival and disease-free survival was noticed between the patients with the different epithelial staining patterns for HA. The reduction of HA staining was associated with poor survival. These results suggest that HA is a prognostic marker in oral squamous cell carcinoma."* [Oral Oncology 40:257-63, 2004]

Notice the words *"prognostic marker."* Since more HA is produced in tissues that are damaged by trauma, burns, toxic chemicals, or tumors, broken down (degraded) HA can be used to detect or measure the progression of tumors. This is akin to fire fighters who show up at fires. They are *"associated with,"* but not considered a cause, of the fires. The fire fighters are there to put the fire out, just like HA attempts to heal the damaged tissue.

The difference between cause and association is easily understood by the following example. Let's say investigators want to know the causes of childhood pedestrian accidents. They collect data from all cases where children were hit by automobiles and they find that nearly all of the children were wearing tennis shoes. So, can we conclude that tennis shoes caused the accidents? Obviously not. The tennis shoes are only by-standers. So is HA.

Finnish researchers noted that *"hyaluronic acid is involved in the growth and progression of malignant tumors."* The researchers stated that *"a high proportion of HA-positive cells of all cancer cells was significantly associated with deep tumor invasions, spreading to lymph nodes, and is associated with tumor progression and poor survival rate."* Sounds pretty terrible, to the uninformed reader, doesn't it? Notice the report says HA is "*involved*" and "*associated*," but never indicates it was a cause of tumors or increased their severity. [Br J Cancer 79:1133-8, 1999] Hard paved roads are responsible for the severity of trauma when people are thrown out of cars in auto accidents, but we can't say the road caused the accident, can we?

Recently a study examined the role of various components of the connective tissue (the goo in between living cells, like mortar in between bricks). Tumor tissue from 86 patients with breast cancer that had not yet spread to lymph nodes was examined by staining the tissues so that each type of connective tissue component could be identified (versican, chondroitin sulfate, tenascin, and hyaluronan). Researchers at the Hanson Institute in Adelaide, Australia, said: "*analyses indicated that elevated expression of versican predicted increased risk and rate of relapse in this cohort. Elevated expression of tenascin was predictive of increased risk and rate of death only......neither chondroitin nor hyaluronic acid were predictive of disease outcome in this group.*" [Clinical Cancer Research 10: 2491-98, 2004]

In another study, researchers noted that "*cancer patients with a scattered and weak HA staining had a significantly higher probability of recurrent disease and unfavorable outcome.*" [Oral Oncology 40:257-63, 2004] Low HA concentrations in cancer patients are indicative of poor outcomes.

The day is long overdue when oral HA is used to intercept cancer cells.

Melatonin: The sleep hormone that prolongs survival

Cancer is related to sleep. People who sleep less are at greater risk for cancer. Night-shift workers have an increased risk for cancer. Investigators point to melatonin, a brain hormone that is produced during sleep, as the agent that reduces the risk for cancer. Melatonin's production is controlled by light entering the eyes. Upon awakening, as light enters the eyes the pineal gland at the base of the brain ceases production of melatonin.

Melatonin inhibits cancer in many ways. First, it is a powerful antioxidant that increases the production of another antioxidant in the body called glutathione. Second, it calms the production of estrogen that spurs the growth of ovarian and breast cancer. Third, it boosts the immune system, elevating the production of natural killer cells. Four, melatonin inhibits omega-6 fatty acids (linoleic acid), such as from corn oil, from entering tumor cells. Omega-6 oils are widely known to encourage rapid growth of tumors. [Endocrine 27: 179-88, 2005]

Researchers have even developed some concern that the prolongation of "*daylight*" by use of electric lamps increases the risk for cancer. Animals subjected to constant light exhibit increased risks for cancer. [Cancer Research 65: 11174-84, 2005] The pineal gland reaches peak production of melatonin around 2 to 3am. Sleep interruption and exposure to light will certainly result in weakened immunity. [Pathology Biology 53: 265-68, 2005] An animal study found that when the pineal gland was surgically removed from the base of the brain, and then the animals were provided with supplemental oral melatonin, their cancer risk dropped. [Neuro Endocrinology Letters 23: 28-36, 2002]

Tamoxifen is the widely-used anti-estrogen drug for breast cancer. Melatonin is overlooked as a mainline anti-estrogen. [Journal Pineal Research 38: 217-22, 2005] Animals given melatonin, followed by a drug that causes breast cancer, will live longer. [Molecular Cell Biochemistry 268: 25-31, 2005] Melatonin also inhibits testosterone and it is likened to castration as a treatment for prostate cancer. [Prostate 52: 252, 2002]

COMPARISON OF SURVIVAL TIME, BY CANCER, SITE AND AGENT					
Type of cancer	Agent and Cost	Compared with	Increased survival in months, total	Range of increase, in months	Reporting Date
Lung cancer	Iressa ($1,800/month)	Placebo	0.5	5.1 - 5.6	2005
Inoperable Pancreatic	Gemzar & Xeloda	Gemzar alone	1.4	6.0 - 7.4	2005
Brain	Radiation -2 types	Radiation – 1 type	1.6	4.9 - 6.5	2004
Breast	Xeloda + Taxotere ($15,500 course)	Taxotere alone	1.9	4.2 - 6.1	2001
Small cell lung cancer	Tarceva ($2,000/month)	Placebo	2	4.7 - 6.7	2005
Lung	Avastin ($4,400/ month)	Chemotherapy	2.3	10.2 - 12.5	2005
Brain Glioblastoma	Temodar ($9,000/ month)	Radiation only	2.5	12.1 - 14.6	2004
Prostate	Taxotere + chemotherapy ($14,000 course)	Chemotherapy	2	16.0 - 18.0	2004
Colon / rectal	Erbitux (ImClone)+ Campostar (Erbitux $12,000/month)	Campostar + 5-FU	1.9	6.9 - 8.6	2004
Brain, metastatic	Melatonin 20 mg/day	Untreatable	3.7	5.5 - 9.2	1994
Small cell lung cancer	Melatonin ($30 month)	Untreatable	3.8	4.1 - 7.9	1992
Metastatic prostate cancer	Provenge	Placebo	4.5	21.4 - 25.9	2005
Breast cancer	Herceptin + chemotherapy (Herceptin $2,500/ month)	Chemotherapy	4.8	20.3 - 25.1	2001
Metastatic colon/ rectal	Avastin + chemotherapy	Chemotherapy	4.9	15.6 - 20.3	2003
All sites, terminal (Linus Pauling)	Vitamin C, intravenous	Untreatable	5.3	1.9 - 7.0	1976
All sites, terminal (Cameron, Campbell)	Vitamin C (10,000 mg) ($300 /year)	Untreatable	5.4	6.0 - 11.4	1991
All sites, terminal (Murata, Japan)	Vitamin C	Untreatable	6.7	1.4 - 8.2	1982
All sites, terminal -from date of untreatability (Linus Pauling)	Vitamin C	Untreatable	8.4	1.3 - 9.7	1978
Stomach	Chemo + surgery	Surgery alone	9	27.0 - 36.0	2001

Melatonin as cancer therapy

Melatonin production declines with advancing age. [Immunity Ageing 2: 17, 2005] As cancer advances into more severe stages, the secretion of melatonin declines. [Medical Science Monitor 11: CR284-88, 2005] Researchers propose that dietary melatonin supplementation, timed to be consumed at bedtime, inhibits the growth of liver tumors in animals, leading to the speculation that melatonin supplementation with advancing age *"has the potential to be a new preventive/therapeutic strategy."* [Endocrine 27: 179-88, 2005]

Melatonin given to tumor-bearing animals increases their survival time. [Molecular Cell Biochemistry 278: 15-20, 2005] A review of all human studies involving supplemental melatonin and cancer reveals a consistent improvement in survival. The dosage used in most studies was greater than used for jet lag, about 20 mg per day (range 10-40 mg), taken prior to bedtime. [Journal Pineal Research 39: 360-66, 2005] One mechanism by which supplemental melatonin prolongs survival is to inhibit angiogenesis, the formation of new blood vessels that feed tumors. [Neuro Endocrinology Letters 22: 45-47, 2001]

Examine the chart on the left on the track record of supplemental melatonin compared to other cancer treatments in regard to prolongation of survival in all types of cancers.

Why melatonin therapy is resorted to in the final stages of cancer, when other treatments are ineffective, goes unexplained. The prolonged survival documented with the use of supplemental melatonin is comparable with many widely promoted, anti-cancer drugs. Since approximately a third of cancer patients already have secondary tumors that have spread to other locations on the day of diagnosis of their initial tumor, it appears one of the first things that newly diagnosed cancer patients should do is begin to take supplemental melatonin.

Supplemental melatonin helps overcome symptoms during cancer treatment

Supplemental melatonin improves the quality of life of cancer patients.

A study showed the following improvements among cancer patients:

	Without melatonin	With melatonin
Fever	15%	4%
Nausea, vomiting	5%	2%
Anorexia	10%	5%
Depression	8%	2%
Elevated liver enzymes	18%	9%
Anemia	5%	2%
Bruises, bleeding	8%	0%

British Journal Cancer 69: 196-99, 1994

What impairs melatonin production?

A folic acid deficiency may impair the production of melatonin in the pineal gland. It is important for cancer patients with sleep disorders to take supplemental folic acid. [Journal Nutrition 132: 2781-84, 2002]

Non-steroidal anti-inflammatory drugs (such as ibuprofen, aspirin and COX-2 inhibitors) suppress melatonin in humans. [Physiology Behavior 59: 133-39, 1996]

Melatonin and chemotherapy side effects

Melatonin also protects the heart from toxic side effects caused by chemotherapy. [Molecular Cell Biochemistry 282: 31-37, 2006]

Cancer patients and sleep problems

Insomnia affects up to 50% of cancer patients. [Clinical Cornerstones 6: S6-14, 2004] Slow-release melatonin pills may help induce prolonged, deep sleep. [Lancet 346:541-4, 1995]

Magnesium citrate is an excellent nutritional aid to inducing deep sleep. [Sleep Medicine 4: 263-64, 2003] Magnesium oxide, the most common form sold in retail stores, is poorly absorbed and is of little value. A dose of 200-400 mg of magnesium [preferably citrate) should be sufficient. Excessive magnesium may induce loose stool.

Prolonged sleep deprivation can produce nerve damage. Niacin is an antidote. [Medical Hypotheses 34: 275-77, 1991]

Sleepiness during the day (hypersomnia), the opposite of insomnia, is also frequently experienced by cancer patients and is confused with fatigue. It can be corrected with vitamin B12. [Psychiatry Clinical Neuroscience 49: 305-07, 1995]

Melatonin enhancement

The fact that blind people, who produce more melatonin, have lower rates of cancer, and that cancer rates are higher in developed countries where artificial lighting is used during evening hours, stimulates the idea that there must be ways of enhancing melatonin production without taking supplements.

There is evidence that even a night light in the bedroom will alter the production of melatonin by the pineal gland. Researchers believe this may increase the risk for cancer. Sleeping in dark, unlighted bedrooms is recommended.

An experiment simulated night-shift conditions with human subjects wearing goggles that filter out the blue portion of the light spectrum which shuts off melatonin production via ocular exposure. Subjects who wore the blue-filter goggles from 8am to 8pm maintained melatonin levels typically measured at night. Unfiltered light drastically suppressed melatonin production. The goggles did not impair work performance or sleepiness. [Journal Clinical Endocrinology Metabolism 90: 2755-61, 2005]

Or if light is required in a room, yellow light bulbs (blue light filtering) can be used at night to enhance melatonin production. Physicists at John Carroll University have even launched a company to market blue light-filtering bulbs, goggles and night lights with the purpose of reducing cancer risk. The products can be obtained from Lighting Innovations LLC (www.LowBlueLights.com).

Does melatonin enhancement really protect against cancer?

Researchers at the Bassett Research Institute, The Mary Imogene Bassett Hospital, in Cooperstown, New York, set out to test this hypothesis. They obtained blood samples from healthy premenopausal females, collected at three different time periods: during the daytime, at nighttime following exposure to light and at nighttime after complete darkness. Then they infused the blood samples into breast tumors that had been implanted into small animals. The melatonin-rich blood samples (obtained after total darkness) severely slowed the growth of the tumors, while the blood samples taken during the day had no effect on tumor growth. [Cancer Research 65: 11174-84, 2005] This recent study is compelling evidence of the role of light-controlled hormones affecting tumor cell growth.

An animal experiment also backs up the idea that ocular light-control may impair tumor growth. Female birds with implanted ovarian tumors were exposed to short or long daylight periods to enhance or suppress the production of melatonin, or melatonin itself was injected into the animals during the long-daylight periods. Remarkably, short-daylight periods produced complete regression of the tumors, while re-exposure to a long daylight period triggered regrowth of the tumors. Supplemental melatonin delayed the regrowth of tumors. [Neuro Endocrinology Letters 25: 94-101, 2004]

Since melatonin hormone/light control was able to completely manipulate tumor growth, this could be a powerful preventive and therapeutic tool in the war against cancer. It certainly appears to be more powerful than current efforts to kill cancer cells with toxic drugs or radiation.

Zeolites

Zeolites are porous minerals that form naturally where volcanic rocks and ash layers react with alkaline ground water. Zeolites have the unique ability to adsorb (adhere to) molecules by particle size. Ironically, humans exposed to fine particle zeolites in their lungs may develop a form of cancer called mesothelioma. [Journal National Cancer Institute 98: 414-17, 2006]

Zeolites have metal chelating, toxin-removing, even oxygen-removing properties, which means they will act to reduce oxidation of tissues when taken internally. Zeolites have been tested in animals and have performed favorably without toxicity to reduce the number and size of tumors. [Journal Cancer Research Clinical Oncology 128: 37-44, 2002] In animal tests, zeolites worked well with an anti-cancer drug to reduce metastases to the lungs. [Anticancer Research 23: 1589-95, 2003] When used with dogs and mice, zeolites improved overall health, decreased tumor size, and prolonged life span. [Journal Molecular Medicine 78: 708-20, 2001]

The internet carries the report from a supplier of zeolite that its use among cancer patients brought about 78% full remission of stage-4 cancers. However, survival times were not provided.

Natural zeolites, as well as synthetic ones, are considered to be inert and nontoxic, as documented in the Code of Federal Regulations. (CFR 40, Part 180.1001] Zeolites are sold as dietary supplements and are over-promoted as a cancer cure. Why speculate? Whether or not zeolites are a promising cancer therapy is unknown at this time.

Probiotics (beneficial bacteria) and cancer

The gut lining provides a home for more bacteria than there are cells in the human body. These living bacteria, in the trillions, represent 70% of the human immune system and are important in detoxifying the body from incoming carcinogens, cancer-causing bacteria and viruses, and in eliminating heavy metals from the body. Certain fecal enzymes can convert pro-cancerous molecules into full-blown cancer generators. In one study, probiotics reduced the cancer-causing bacterial count from 48% to 16%. [Folia Microbiology 50: 443-47, 2005] [Journal Applied Microbiology 98: 1303-15, 2005] Probiotics promote the production of short-chain fatty acids in the gut, such as butyrate, which has been identified as an inborn cancer-fighting molecule. [Journal Clinical Gastroenterology 40: 235-43, 2006]

Since colon cancer is one of the four major types of human cancers, the residence of beneficial bacteria in the playing field where colon cancer begins, is of importance. In 29 animal studies evaluated, probiotics (beneficial bacteria supplements), 26 showed positive results. Primary benefit was derived from supplementation with probiotics prior to exposure to a cancer-causing agent. [Digestive Liver Disease 38: 2877-82S, 2006] Probiotics may be of particular aid to individuals with inflammatory bowel disease (Crohn's disease, irritable bowel) are at increased risk for colon cancer. [International Journal Food Microbiology 115: 1-11, 2007]

Furthermore, probiotics have been shown to reduce diarrhea that frequently occurs among cancer patients undergoing radiation treatment. Probiotics have been shown to be *"easy, safe and feasible approach to protect cancer patients against radiation-induced diarrhea."* [World Journal Gastroenterology 13: 912-15, 2007]

While there are over 1000 strains of bacteria that reside in the human digestive tract, of particular interest are Bifidobacteria species that represent about 95% of the gut bacterial population in healthy breast-fed newborns. Bifidobacterial bacteria decline during adulthood till they represent only about 3 to 6 percent of the total bacterial count and in old age Bificobacteria decline even further. The initial colonization of the intestine at birth with beneficial bacteria is of critical importance in order for the human immune system to properly develop and mature. [Journal Applied Microbiology 98: 1303-15, 2005] Several studies have shown that consumption of bifidobacteria reduces colon cancer risk in carcinogen-treated animals, suggesting that consumption of certain bacteria has a beneficial effect on the balance of colon bacteria. Probiotics have even been shown to reduce the recurrence of bladder cancer. [European Urology 47: 288-96, 2005]

There are many misconceptions regarding probiotics, the most prevalent being that yogurt delivers beneficial bacteria. In fact, a study shows that yogurt does not confer any significant improvement in immunity in humans. [Nutrition & Cancer 37: 27-35, 2000]

Experts in probiotics emphasize that evidence for health benefits for one strain of probiotic cannot be conferred and extrapolated to other strains. [Clinical Microbiology Infection 11: 958-66, 2005]

Probiotics have not lived up to their promise, primarily because of poor quality products. In a study of probiotic supplements, the labeled strain of bacteria could not be found in 9 of 11 brands. [New Microbiology 2006 Oct; 29(4):281-91] In another study, only two of five probiotics studied produced improvement in gastrointestinal symptoms (indigestion, bloating, and abdominal discomfort). [Digestive Diseases and Science 2006 Dec; 51(12):2134-44]

Bifidobacterium infantis is the strain of bacteria that is abundantly found in breast-fed newborns and affords special protection. Bifidobacterium infantis supplements are available and recommended for infants and adults (Natren Lifestart).

This God-given strain of bacteria has now been found to calm the inflammatory storm of bowel disorders in adults, and is highly recommended for use by infants and young children, especially in the first years of life as their immune system matures.

Probiotics do not take up permanent residence in the digestive tract and requires repeated supplementation. Bifidobacterium infantis strain 345624 should be continually replaced, especially when antibiotics are used, when babies are born by Cesarean delivery, when there is other infection during pregnancy (herpes, hepatitis, HIV), when traveling (especially overseas), when children receive immunizations, when diarrhea arises, when children are weaned from breast milk, and by all individuals who are immune compromised (described above).

Bifidobacterium infantis is only available from one source, Natren, as LifeStart probiotic.

LifeStart® powder can be added to infant formula or other beverages. To find out more about LifeStart®, visit www.natren.com or call a probiotic counselor at 1-866- 4-Natren (1-866-462-8736).

CHAPTER 14

Herbs

p 432 - 492

Herbs

INTRODUCTION

Cancer researchers are beginning to expand their thinking. Plant-derived molecules may finally gain a place in modern cancer therapy. There is resistance, especially from sectors of the cancer industry dominated by vested interests. Researchers are now saying that plant-derived, anti-cancer agents have *"compelling preventive action,"* and *"it is the ability of these agents to exhibit multi-mechanisms of action whereas conventional single-action drugs have disappointed in the past."* [Current Medical Chemistry Anti-Cancer Agents 5: 201-13, 2005]

This chapter will first present information on the secret of plant extracts as anti-cancer weapons. Second, we will discuss herbal ingredients that affect an enzymatic liver detoxification system known as the cytochrome p450 system. Many herb-derived molecules inhibit the production of cytochrome p450 enzymes and therefore may either enhance or inhibit the activity of other anti-cancer molecules in drugs or herbal remedies. Third, the leading anti-cancer herbs will be presented along with recent scientific studies concerning their effectiveness. Among these are allicin from garlic, curcumin from turmeric, indole-3 carbinol from broccoli, green tea, soy phytoestrogens, flaxseed lignans, red grape/wine resveratrol, ellagic acid from pomegranate, oleuropein from olive trees and quercetin from red apples and onions.

It is literally impossible to mention every potential herbal anti-cancer remedy. There are some 250,000 species of flowering plants that could serve to provide anti-cancer molecules. There are an abundance of laboratory dish studies of herbal ingredients that have been shown to inhibit the growth of cancer. Which ones should be investigated? Can we assume from lab dish studies that humans should begin to treat cancer with a particular herb?

A study of the herb *Cymbopogon citratus*, or lemon balm, will serve as an example. It is known that mortality from cancer of the digestive tract is low in Thailand compared to Japan. Lemon grass is commonly used in the diet and as a medicine in Thailand. Studies reveal lemon grass inhibits various chemicals that can cause genetic mutations that can lead to cancer. [Carcinogenesis 18: 949-55, 1997]

Lemon grass extract has been shown to reduce the number, but not the size, of chemically-induced liver tumors in mice. [Cancer Letters 183: 9-15, 2000] But this experiment was conducted with a specially prepared extract, not raw lemon grass. Citral, a molecule in lemon grass, may be the primary anti-cancer ingredient. Concentrations of citral, comparable to that found in a cup of lemon grass tea prepared from one gallon of lemon grass, has been shown to promote tumor cell death in laboratory dishes. [Planta Medica 71: 484-48, 2005]

What this tells us is that lemon grass may be a good preventative against gastric cancer. In a tea, a hot water extract, it may be effective. But it is unknown if there is enough active ingredient in tea to treat growing tumors. Possibly, in the future, citral extract will be proven as a treatment for existing tumors. For now, lemon balm tea should be considered a healthy drink that reduces the risk for gastric cancer.

Whole herbs may be found to have cancer-inhibiting properties, but extracts of molecules within herbs are more likely to provide the concentrated doses required to treat already existing tumors. While some herbs many provide multiple anti-cancer molecules, because most tumors are composed of more than two billion cells, it is unlikely that whole herbs will be able to exhibit sufficient anti-cancer activity even when consumed in large amounts. On the other hand, the inclusion of fruits, vegetables and spices in the diet in aggregate may serve to prevent or reduce the risk for cancer. Simply said, it is easier to prevent than it is to treat cancer. Human populations that consume more plant foods have lower rates of cancer. This should not be construed to mean all herbal remedies prevent cancer. For example, the Chinese herb, Aristolochia fangchi, has been shown to promote the development of tumors in humans. [Toxicology 181-182:577-80, 2002]

> Here is how one researcher explained cannabis and cancer:
> *"Cannabis has been shown to inhibit the growth of tumour cells in lab dishes and animal studies. Cannabis is usually well tolerated, and does not produce the generalized toxic effects of conventional chemotherapies. So, could cannabis be used to develop new anticancer therapies?"*
> *Source: Nature Review Cancer 3: 745-55, 2003*

There are also many distractions in the pursuit of herbal molecules that fight cancer. Cannabis, or marijuana, serves as an example. There is no secret that, in addition to cannabis' ability to prevent nausea and vomiting induced by chemotherapy drugs, to block pain caused by cancer, and to stimulate appetite in wasting cancer patients, that it also has anti-tumor properties.

But all is not rosy when it comes to cannabis. There is no evidence cannabis has anti-cancer properties in humans. It is said that some studies indicate cannabis may impair the immune response to cancer. [Schmerz. 2004 Jun18(3):203-10, 2004] But there is little evidence of this response in humans, and certainly not as an injected drug, and smoking marijuana may irritate cells lining the throat. [Schmerz 18: 203-10, 2004]

Researchers conclude that *"medical, legal, and regulatory obstacles hinder the smoking of cannabis for medical purposes."* [Lancet Oncology 6: 35-42, 2005] Cancer patients have no time to become distracted with the arguments for or against cannabis. There are other herbal remedies with far greater promise of a cure. Though, for the cancer patient in pain, a cannabis-based drug would eliminate the temptation to smoke marijuana.

The Secret of Extracts

Which is better for optimal health, consumption of fresh fruits, vegetables and herbs, or the extracts of these herbs, often provided as liquid or powdered dietary supplements? Let's investigate.

Recently Cornell University food researchers claimed *"an apple a day can help keep breast cancer away."* Well, to be more precise, more like six apples a day. Rats fed extracts from apples were protected from developing breast cancer. The equivalent of one, three or six apples reduced the incidence of breast tumors by 17, 39 and 44 % and the number of tumors by 25, 25 and 61%. The study used *"whole apple extracts."*

Cornell researchers concluded: *"Our findings suggest that consumers may gain more significant health benefits by eating more fruits and vegetables and whole grain foods than in consuming expensive dietary supplements, which do not contain the same array of balanced, complex components. This balanced natural combination of phytochemicals present in fruits and vegetables cannot simply be mimicked by dietary supplements."* [Journal of Agriculture & Food Chemistry, March 2005]

So, should you forget the pills and engorge yourself in more and more food? That would make apple growers, who sponsored the above study, very happy. The problem is that the study used extracts of whole apples, not apples themselves. Beneficial nutrients are extracted from apples usually via alcohol extraction methods. The fermentation by alcohol solubilizes, withdraws and concentrates the fruit, vegetable or herbal ingredients. That, in reality, is quite different than eating whole apples.

Which is more healthful: soybeans or soybean paste soup?

An interesting study recently was conducted in Japan, a country known for its soy consumption and low rate of breast cancer. When Japanese researchers finished analyzing the results of a survey of 209,354 persons regarding their soy consumption, it was found that soy foods did not confer a reduction in breast cancer risk, but frequent consumption of miso soup did. With each bowl of miso soup consumed on a daily basis there was a greater reduction in breast cancer risk. But miso is soy. What's the difference? Miso is a fermented soy bean paste, sometimes mixed with rice barley or wheat. Miso is fermented with yeast mold (koji) and aged from one month to three years, for enhancement of taste. The fermentation process of making miso concentrates the molecules found in soy beans. [Journal National Cancer Institute 95: 906-13, 2003] Americans hear of the benefits of soy, so they drink soy milk, and eat soy cereal and soy burgers. But the Japanese don't eat these foods, they eat fermented sources of soy. There is an obvious difference. Fermented soy extracts and concentrates beneficial molecules from the soybean.

Tea: hot water extraction

Another common practice throughout the world is the consumption of hot tea. Tea drinkers appear to have a lower risk for simple infections and chronic diseases, including cancer, coronary heart disease, stroke, and osteoporosis. Tea is a hot water extract of tea leaves. [Antioxidant Redox Signaling 6: 571-86, 2004] The beneficial effects of tea drinking were recently demonstrated in a study of Chinese women with ovarian cancer. Almost 80 % of women who drank tea survived three years following their diagnosis compared to just 49 % of non-tea drinkers. By brewing tea, these Chinese women were making their own medicinal hot-water extracts. [Asia Pacific Journal Clinical Nutrition 13: S116, 2004]

Alcohol or water extracts?

Herbal extracts available commercially are either water or alcohol extracts. Alcohol is the preferred method of extraction because it is more efficient. For example, researchers in Taiwan compared freshly made water and alcohol extracts of Giant Knotweed (botanical name, *Polygonum multiflorum*). Mice who had these extracts added to their diet exhibited less cellular debris in their brain and better response to mental tests, with the beneficial effects observed more often in the mice who received the alcohol extracts. [Journal Nutrition Science Vitaminology 48: 491-97, 2002]

Olive washings

Olives are known to be healthy and olive oil is extolled as a key part of the Mediterranean Diet. But the primary molecules in olive oil that are credited with providing its healthy properties are from its polyphenols, not its oil content. [Nutrition Reviews 56:142-7, 1998] During olive oil production, large volumes of water are generated and subsequently discarded. Water washings of olives remove or extract some of these antioxidant polyphenols. Although polyphenols are present in the extracted olive oil, the water of the olives contains even higher concentrations of these polyphenols. [J Agriculture Food Chemistry 47:3397-401, 1999] The polyphenol/antioxidant content of the best olive oil is deemed too low to make a significant contribution to overall antioxidant protection. [European J Clinical Nutrition 58:955-65, 2004] Only olive oils with very a high polyphenol content are likely to produce health benefits. [European Journal Nutrition 43:140-7, 2004]

While high quality, extra virgin olive oils may contain between 100 and 300 mcg of polyphenols per liter of oil, the concentration of these same polyphenols is 300 to 500 times higher in olive water.

The olive water can then be dehydrated into a polyphenol-rich powder. One company, CreAgri, has developed a pill (Olivenol™) that provides as much antioxidants as 4 to 6 ounces of extra virgin olive oil without the fat and calorie content. A special extra concentrated olive extract yields a potent antioxidant called hydroxytyrosol, known as Hidrox™ commercially. Some time ago, olive oleuropin, a precursor to hydroxytyrosol was introduced in the US as a dietary supplement. But it is poorly absorbed compared to hydroxytyrosol.

Wine: an extract from grapes

Consuming grapes, grape juice and raisins promote health. But only wine produces exceptional health qualities. Wine is simply an alcohol extract of grape skins. The fermentation process in winemaking draws beneficial antioxidant nutrients like resveratrol and quercetin from the skin of the grape, and then the bottling process goes a step further in preserving the extracts in a dark, airtight bottle [J Agriculture Food Chemistry 52:5747-5751, 2004]

Recognize how powerful the red wine effect is. The red-wine drinking French consume 3.8 times more butter and 2.8 times more lard, and exhibit higher serum cholesterol levels and higher blood pressure than do Americans, yet have a 2.5-fold lower death rate due to coronary heart disease. Known as *"the French paradox,"* this puzzling effect obviously points to something in red wine that virtually erases the deleterious effects of an otherwise unhealthy diet. The only thing that keeps health authorities from recommending wine drinking for all is its undesirable calorie and alcohol content.

A comparison of alcoholic spirits versus wine reveals the importance of grape extract. Adhesion of white blood cells (monocytes) to cells that line the inner artery (endothelium) facilitates the formation of undesirable blood clots. In a human study published in 2004, the adhesion of monocytes to artery walls was partly inhibited when gin was consumed as an alcoholic beverage, but was almost completely abolished when red wine was consumed. [Am J Clinical Nutrition 80:225-30, 2004] Something remarkable occurs through the consumption of red wine, but not other alcoholic beverages.

Red wine pills

So, what about concentrating red wine molecules into a pill? Then the alcohol could be avoided.

In a recent study, Danish researchers provided humans with red wine, red grape extract tablets or drinking water. The tablets were not graded for resveratrol content, thought to be the primary molecule in red wine responsible for the French paradox. Red wine produced a significant increase (11-16%) in HDL *"good"* cholesterol, a reduction (8-15%) in fibrinogen (blood clotting factor), and had no effect upon blood pressure or total cholesterol. Surprisingly, the red grape extract tablets produced no significant difference in HDL *"good"* cholesterol and actually raised fibrinogen by about 10 % compared to water consumption. [European Journal Clinical Nutrition, January 2005]

Another study tells us why the red wine tablets didn't work. Researchers in Italy provided rats with a standard diet or a high-cholesterol diet and then added red wine or alcohol-free red wine to their daily regimens. An artificial artery was placed into the abdominal aorta of the animals and the time for a blood clot to block the synthetic artery was clocked. (A slower clotting time is preferable.) In animals with the normal diet, 50% experienced a blood clot that blocked the false artery in 120 hours. In the animals given a high-cholesterol diet, the false artery was blocked in half of the animals in 72 hours. When wine was given to the animals with the high-cholesterol diet, the clotting time reverted back as if the animals were on a normal cholesterol diet. Animals given the alcohol-free red wine experienced a similar reversion of clotting time (about 120 hours). The alcohol-free red wine delayed or prevented the blockage of the artificial artery in a similar manner to alcoholic red wine, without affecting cholesterol or triglyceride numbers. Researchers concluded that the effect of red wine is *"attributable to polyphenolic compounds (i.e. resveratrol, quercetin- author's emphasis) modulating blood clotting function."* [Journal Thrombosis and Haemostasis 3: 346, 2005] What can be concluded from these two experiments is that red wine molecules are preserved in a wine bottle but not in tablet form.

Preserving red wine molecules in pills

Wine is placed in dark-colored bottles to retard spoilage by light, and these bottles are airtight and devoid of oxygen to inhibit oxidation. Bottles should be kept in a cool environment. One patented technology fills gelatin capsules with liquid herbal extracts under a nitrogen-air environment and then seals the capsule to create an airtight pill.

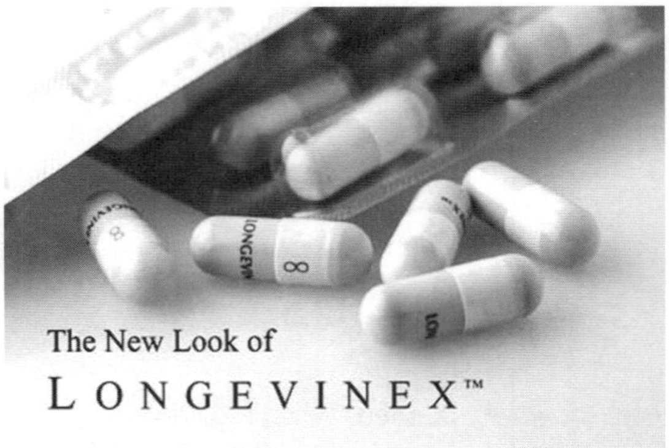

When red wine molecules (resveratrol, quercetin) are preserved inside a capsule they exhibit beneficial gene-switching qualities not commonly produced by conventional red wine pills. One such red wine pill, Longevinex™, has already been introduced using the airtight technology. (www.longevinex.com)

Summary: So far, we've learned that extracts of plants, in soup, tea, wine and dietary supplements produce far more concentrated forms of beneficial molecules than do fresh raw plant foods that are widely promoted for health. This may help explain why some fermented foods exhibit health benefits. Dietary supplements are often devalued or belittled while fresh foods are widely promoted. In some instances, herbal extracts are unfairly characterized as potentially toxic. Devotees of dietary supplements often believe pharmaceutical companies may be behind these anti-supplement sentiments. But in fact, as revealed in this report, it is often food companies that exert their influence over researchers and public health authorities to continually disparage dietary supplements. Plant extract dietary supplements offer health benefits that simply cannot be achieved with foods. While pills do not replace food, food is not always superior to botanical extracts.

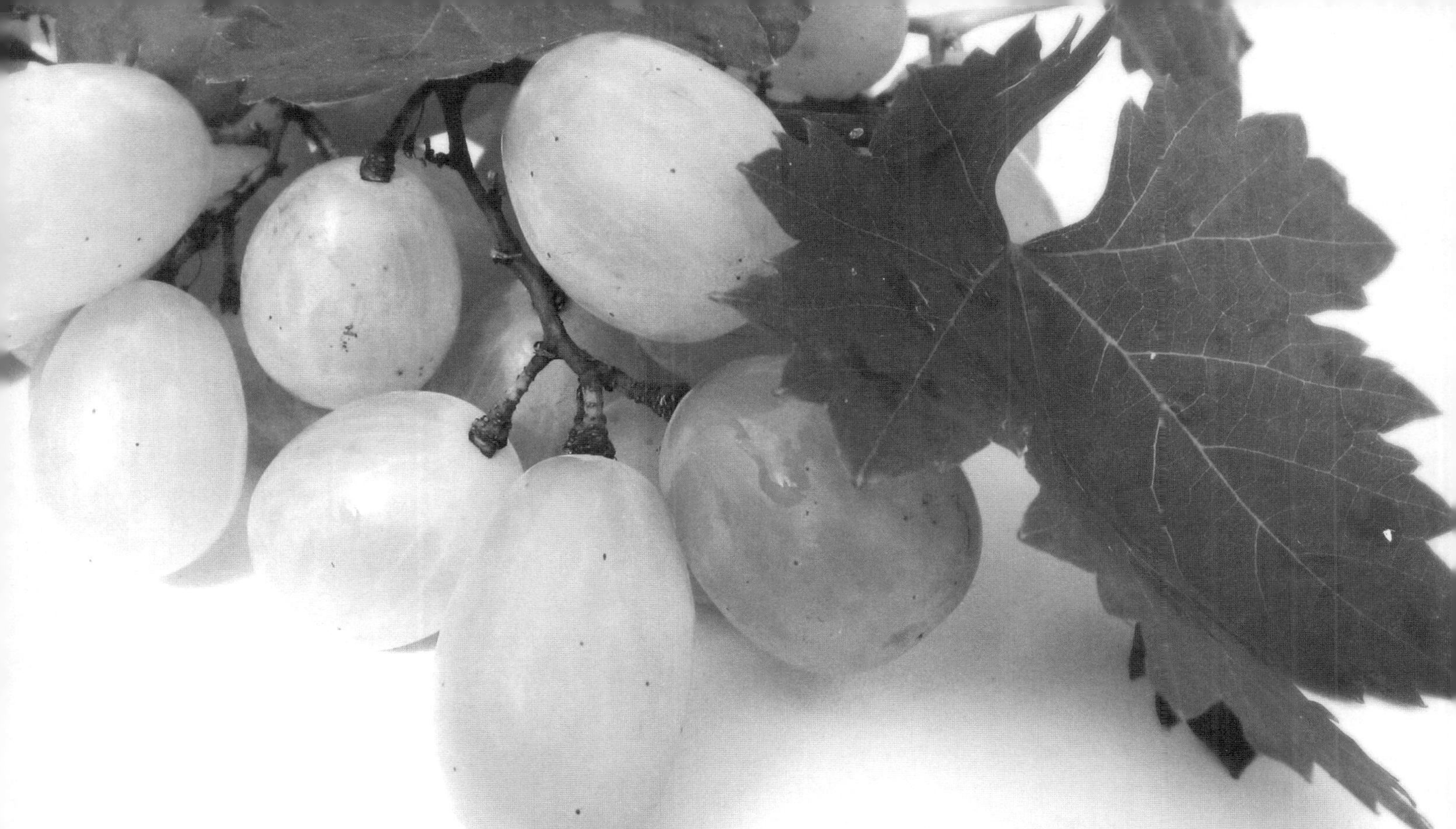

Cruciferous vegetables and cancer

In his treatise on medicine, Cato the Elder (234-149 BC), wrote: *"If a cancerous ulcer appears upon the breasts, apply a crushed cabbage leaf and it will make it well."* Crushing a cabbage leaf converts it into a potent anti-cancer molecule called indole-3 carbinol.

Diets high in cruciferous vegetables – broccoli, cauliflower, cabbage, bok choy, and Brussels sprouts – are known to prevent cancer. Indole-3 carbinol was identified as the primary anti-cancer agent in these plant foods. However, there is no indole-3 carbinol in cruciferous vegetables. It is formed only when crushed such as in chewing or macerating foods. Once in the stomach, hydrochloric acid then converts indole-3-carbinol to diindolymethane, believed to be the most potent anti-cancer end product of metabolism after consumption of cruciferous vegetables.

How does indole-3 carbinol work? In 1997, researchers at Rockefeller University discovered that diindolymethane alters estrogen so it converts into a weak form, thus stopping human tumor growth and inducing cancer cells to die off naturally. The vege-molecules also increase the activity of detoxification enzymes in the liver as well as increase antioxidant enzymes. Furthermore, they have recently been found to inhibit growth factors that accelerate cancer growth. [J Agric Food Chemistry 53:5 64-9, 2005]

The question arises, can humans get the full benefits of cruciferous vegetables from a pill? The answer is a qualified *"no."* Not only does dietary intake of cruciferous vegetables decrease the risk for cancer, high intake levels even reduce mortality rates from all causes. [Int J Vitamin Nutrition Research 73:135-43, 2003; Am J Epidemiology 160:1223-33, 2004] Furthermore, cruciferous vegetables provide other nutrients, namely sulfur and selenium, which have strong anti-cancer properties. [Integrative Cancer Therapy 3:5-12, 2004]

The cruciferous vegetable assault on cancer should actually be termed the Brussels sprouts cure since this vegetable provides three times more molecules glucosinolates) that convert to indole-3 carbinol than any other vegetable in its class.

However, there is evidence that concentrated forms of indole-3 carbinol can inhibit cancer more effectively than hefty intakes of fruits and vegetables. [Integrative Cancer Therapy 3:5-12, 2004]. Nonetheless, this doesn't diminish the impact of a diet rich in cruciferous vegetables.

Investigators examined studies and determined that it takes 200 to 400 mg of indole-3 carbinol to be optimally efficacious for prevention. This is far beyond what most plant food diets provide. It would require 130 raw Brussels sprouts or one quarter of a head of raw cabbage to obtain sufficient amounts of indole-3 carbinol to prevent cancer. [Gynecologic Oncology 78: 123-29, 2000; Nutrition & Cancer 16: 59-66, 1991] This means concentrated indole-3 carbinol supplements would be beneficial. Here is where an argument arises. If taking a pill that attempts to duplicate cruciferous vegetable intake, does a person take indole-3 carbinol, or its breakdown product, diindolymethane?

How do you determine whether to take indole-3 carbinol or diindolymethane supplements? For women who are overweight, and therefore have extra fat cells to produce estrogen, and do not have a diet rich in cruciferous vegetables, a dietary supplement would certainly be in order. Men, too, experience a rise in estrogen levels with advancing age and would benefit from taking supplements to protect from prostate cancer.

Instability, particularly following exposure to light, has been brought up as a criticism of indole-3 carbinol dietary supplements. But this does not appear to have hampered its effectiveness in human studies. Indole-3 carbinol as a dietary supplement has been shown to be effective. Upcoming studies with diindolymethane will likely yield similar results.

It's puzzling why, with the revelation that Brussels sprouts provide three times the cancer- fighting molecules as any other cruciferous vegetable, consumption of this single vegetable is not emphasized.

Knowing that indole-3 carbinol and diindolymethane are vulnerable to degradation from exposure to light, it is strange that suppliers of these supplements don't encapsulate the products in opaque capsules.

To preserve glycosinolates in foods like Brussels' sprouts, cabbage and cauliflower, these foods must be steamed or microwave cooked, as boiling results in 90% loss of the active ingredient. [Food Chemistry Toxicology 45: 216-24, 2007]

BroccoSprouts® Broccoli Sprouts are the only product that guarantees a consistent level of sulforaphane GS, a natural compound found in broccoli and other cruciferous plants that supports the body's own antioxidant function. Developed by scientists at Johns Hopkins University School of Medicine, the Broccoli Sprouts and Sprout Blends are now available in supermarkets throughout the country.

	Indole-3 carbinol	Diindolymethane
Shown to prevent cancer in human studies	Yes	Studies underway
Dosage	200-400 mg/day; ~ 30 times dietary intake	30-40 mg; ~ 3 times dietary intake
Requires stomach acid for action	Yes (antacids may negate action)	No
Absorption	Good	Poor, but enhanced with vitamin E derivative
Compatibility with other drugs	Compatible with tamoxifen. May reduce drug resistance	Not reported
Side effects	Nausea, vomiting, dizziness at 800-1,200 mg dose	None
Reduces breast pain	Yes	Yes

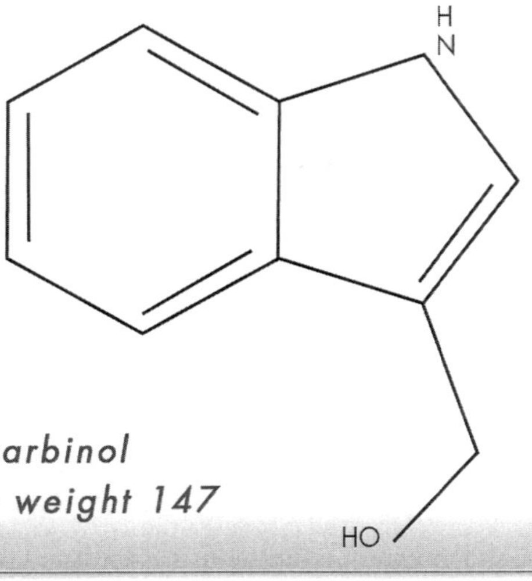

Indole-3 carbinol
Molecular weight 147

Artemisia

Artemisinin, a compound derived from the Chinese herb *qinghaosu*, known as wormwood, is the most overlooked anti-cancer, herbal drug. Varieties of wormwood have been used for centuries, both as a moth repellant and pesticide, but also as a medicinal tea. Sadly, world health authorities have dragged their feet in using artemisinin to treat malaria, which has cost millions of lives, and are now snubbing artemisinin as a promising anti-cancer drug.

Artemisia is the starting material for the semi-synthetic artemisinin that is used to treat malaria. Artemisinin was isolated from wormwood in 1972 and researchers at the Walter Reed Army Institute crystallized the active component in 1984, as announced in the May 31st issue of Science magazine a year later. [Science 238:1049, 1985] In modern times, Chinese army researchers first began using artemisinin to treat malaria in the jungles of Vietnam in the early 1990s. Its first mention as an anti-cancer agent appears in the National Library of Medicine in 1992 and 1993. [Zhongguo Yao Li Xue Bao 13:541-3, 1992; Journal Natural Products 56:849-56, 1993] Artimisinin has been used in Asia for 30-40 years as an anti-cancer treatment.

Yet, in 2001, researchers in Germany acted surprised when they discovered that artesnunate, a semi-synthetic form of artemisinin derived from Artemisia annua, is active against cancer. It was shown to be most active against leukemia and colon cancer cells. [International Journal Oncology 18: 767-73, 2001] More than a decade after artemisinin was first reported as an anti-cancer agent, researchers at the University of Washington claim *"only recently have additional uses for artemisinin as an anticancer drug been discovered."* [Anticancer Research 24: 2153-60, 2004]

Inexpensive, considered nontoxic, and relatively available, there are no obvious reasons why artemisinin has been slow to be considered as an anti-cancer agent. Concern over artemisinin's solubility and absorption were overcome by the development of dehydroartemisinin, a more water-soluble version. [Cancer Chemotherapy Pharmacology, August 2005] Researchers claim that *"artemisinin and its chemical derivatives possess potent activity against tumor cells in very low concentrations."* [Drug Resistance Update 8: 85-97, 2005]

Artemisinin is known to inhibit new blood vessel formation (angiogenesis) that feeds tumor cells. [Cancer Chemotherapy Pharmacology 53: 423-32, 2004] It induces otherwise immortal cancer cells to die off (apoptosis). [Anticancer Research 24: 2277-80, 2004] Artemisinin is described as a *"remarkable drug with low toxicity to humans"* that may be a *"promising and novel candidate for cancer chemotherapy."* [Pharmacological Research 48: 231-36, 2003] It does not develop drug resistance as do many current anti-cancer drugs. [Biol Pharm Bulletin 25: 1555-61, 2002] Yet there has been no fast-track urgency to test this drug in human trials.

What is intriguing is how artemisinin kills cancer cells. Artemisinin generates free radicals and kills cancer cells by oxidation, similar to the way a rusty nail can kill germs in water. Cancer cells utilize a large amount of iron for their growth. Artemisinin has an affinity for iron and enters tumor cells where it literally causes tumor cells to explode. [Expert Opinion Therapeutic Targets 9: 995-1007, 2005] In fact, one animal experiment showed that the provision of iron with artemisinin effectively killed cancer cells whereas the provision of artemisinin or iron alone did not significantly inhibit tumor cell growth. [Cancer Letters 98: 83-87, 1995] Cancer researchers at the University of Washington report that artemisin, by itself, "*is about 100 times more selective in killing cancer cells as opposed to healthy cells.*" One artemisinin compound tested was 34,000 times more potent in killing cancer cells than normal cells. [University of Washington Bulletin, Feb. 20, 2005]

Doctors in Erlangen, Germany, report on the first use of artemisinin for human cancer cases. A patient with metastatic melanoma at the back of the eyes, for whom chemotherapy was ineffective, was given artemisinin on a compassionate basis. Regression of cancer in the lungs and spleen were reported. The patient was still alive 47 months following treatment whereas median survival is usually only 2 to 5 months. [Oncology Reports 14: 1599-603, 2005]

It is artemisinin's use as an anti-malarial drug that may really upset the apple cart when it comes to anti-cancer drugs. World health authorities claim artemisinin's cost, $2.40 per course of therapy, is costlier than other inexpensive drugs now used to treat malaria, as ineffective as they may be. A $42 million grant from the Bill and Melinda Gates Foundation to the Institute for One World Health, the first non-profit drug company in the U.S., will make it possible to synthesize artemisinin molecules by fermentation processes so their cost can be reduced to well under a dollar. [UC Berkeley Web, Dec. 13, 2004] What if the world discovers artemisinin is the tremendous anti-cancer agent it appears to be? It would make most, if not all, of the current pharmaceutical anti-cancer drugs antiquated. This is another natural anti-cancer molecule that cancer patients have direct access to via dietary supplementation.

Tea and cancer

- They have been shown to inhibit cancer in population studies.
- They have been shown to inhibit cancer in laboratory dish studies.
- They have been shown to inhibit cancer in animal studies.
- They have been shown to inhibit cancer in human studies.
- They are the molecules in green tea.

A compelling study, conducted in Japan among 8,500 adults over a nine-year period, found that those with the highest green tea intake (more than ten cups per day) had a significantly lower relative risk of cancer than those consuming fewer than three cups per day, even when adjustments were made for cigarette smoking and alcohol intake. For heavy tea drinkers, the average age of onset of cancer was remarkably delayed, by three years for men and almost nine years for women. [Preventive Medicine 26: 769-75, 1997]

Another remarkable study in Japan revealed that the mean age at death for male smokers who consumed 10 or more cups of green tea was 75.2 years, compared to non-smokers who drank less than 3 cups of green tea per day. [Ageing Research Reviews 2: 1-10, 2003]

A study of 309 patients with confirmed epithelial ovarian cancer, were recruited in a study during 1999-2000, and were followed for a minimum of three years. Among green tea drinkers, 79.6% survived the three-year study period compared to just 49.0% of non-tea drinkers. Researchers concluded that regular consumption of green tea post-diagnosis can enhance epithelial ovarian cancer survival. [Asia Pacific J Clinical Nutrition 13:S116, 2004]

A survey of 1,124 newly diagnosed stomach cancer patients found that smoking and alcohol use increased the risk for this type of cancer, especially males, compared to adults

Green tea has been specifically shown to:

- Protect DNA from damage that can lead to cancer. [Nutrition Cancer 34: 83-87, 2000]
- Promote the death of cancer cells (apoptosis) [Journal National Cancer Institute 89: 1881-86, 1997]
- Favorably control hormone levels involved in the progression of breast cancer. [Nutrition Cancer 30: 21-24, 1998]
- Inhibit the formation of new blood vessels that feed tumors (angiogenesis). [Journal Nutritional Biochemistry 16:1-8, 2005]
- Selectively inhibit the growth of tumor cells but not healthy cells. [Cancer Letters 129: 173-79, 1998]
- Block signals between cancer cells and normal cells that cause tumors to spread. [Mutation Research 555:3-19, 2004]
- Inhibit the spread of cancer to other organs (metastasis).[J Cell Biochemistry 83:631-42, 2001]
- Inhibit anticancer drug resistance. [J Pharm Pharmacology 56:1307-14, 2004]

who abstain from either substance. This is explained by the fact that males have higher iron loads than females (iron is a growth factor for cancer). The startling finding was that green tea consumption reduced the risk for stomach cancer, even among males who consumed alcohol and smoked tobacco. [Cancer 77: 2449-57, 1996]

Some researchers claim that *"green tea is now accepted as a cancer preventive on the basis of numerous in vitro, in vivo and epidemiological studies. We found an apparent delay of cancer onset/death associated with increased consumption of green tea, specifically in those under 79 years of age in a prospective study of a Japanese population with 13-year follow-up data."* [Preventive Medicine 26:769–775, 1997] That statement was made in 1997. Since then, contrary data has arisen.

All that glitters is not green tea

The Food & Drug Administration has given a thumbs-down on the idea that green tea is a cancer fighter. [FDA Bulletin, July 6, 2005] Food and dietary supplement companies are forbidden from saying green tea is beneficial for any health condition. Here's why.

An FDA reviewer says the current scientific evidence from human studies doesn't support the claim that green tea prevents cancer. The research on stomach cancer – done in Japan – was not considered because the nature of the disease and salt intake differs in the Japan and the U.S. The FDA says there is "*no credible evidence*" supporting green tea as a fighter of other cancers, including lung, gastric, colon, rectal, pancreatic, esophageal, skin, ovarian, or liver cancers.

With all of the positive news reports surrounding green tea, here are some of the negative reports.

- In a study conducted in Japan among adults age 40-79 years, the consumption of green tea, 10 cups or more a day, did not reduce the risk for stomach cancer. [British Journal Cancer 90: 135-38, 2004] In a review of studies involving green tea and stomach cancer published in 1998, six studies suggested green tea reduces the risk while three studies indicate it might increase the risk for stomach cancer. [Nutrition & Cancer 31:151-9, 1998]

- A study that spanned a period of 7-9 years among 66,000 adults in Japan did not reveal a reduced risk for colon cancer. [Journal Epidemiology 15: 118-24, 2005]

- Researchers at the University of Mississippi have found that a major green tea component (epicatechin-3-gallate) strongly activates a gene that causes oxygen conditions characteristic of tumor cells. These results suggest that intended cancer prevention with high-dose green tea extracts may be compromised by the ability of tea molecules to promote tumor cell survival. [Journal Natural Products 67: 2063-69, 2004] It's a disturbing finding. However it's just a lab dish study.

- A review of studies involving breast cancer was also not glowing. Green tea may prevent recurrence of early-stage breast cancer, but the data from other prevention studies is not conclusive. Researchers say that "*conclusions as to the potential therapeutic application of green tea are currently impossible to make due to the small number of studies conducted, the lack of any clinical trial evidence, and the lack of a consistent dose-response relationship.*" [Integrative Cancer Therapy 4:144-55, 2005]

- In another study involving 35,004 Japanese women, green tea intake, five or more cups per day, was not associated with a significant reduced risk for breast cancer. [British Journal Cancer 90: 1361-63, 2004]

- Researchers in Japan gave high oral-dose (~2000 mg) green tea extract to 17 patients with advanced lung cancer for 16 weeks. The patients also underwent chemo and radiation therapy. Lung cancer progressed in all of the patients and some experienced side effects from the caffeine in the green tea (nausea, diarrhea, anxiety, lack of sleep). It was concluded that high-dose green tea extract "*may not be warranted*" for therapy in advanced cases of cancer. [Cancer Chemotherapy Pharmacology 55: 33-38, 2005]

It is easy to see how difficult it is to draw conclusions on the use of green tea for cancer prevention or treatment. But there are some reasons for the failed studies. One, it is not likely that any single agent, certainly not cups of tea, will be able to treat tumors that are billions of cells in size. Green tea, when combined with other cancer fighting molecules, may be efficacious. Two, dosage in some of these studies was not sufficient to produce a therapeutic effect. Three, there are ways to enhance the effect of green tea that were not employed, as explained below. Adequate dosage, enhanced absorption, avoidance of caffeinated sources, use of concentrated capsules rather than weak tea, and use after fasting, can vastly improve the effect.

Examples of the use of green tea combined with other cancer fighting molecules have recently been published. In an animal study, green tea combined with the anti-cancer drug Adriamycin improved effectiveness and decreased side effects. [Clinical Cancer Research 4: 153-56, 1998] The idea of combination therapy is further confirmed by research conducted by Matthias Rath, MD, a former Linus Pauling Institute scientist. Rath has developed a multi-targeted approach to cancer using natural substances that enhance the strength and stability of the material (collagen, also called extracellular matrix) that surrounds cancer cells. Green tea is utilized with collagen boosters, the amino acids lysine and praline, along with vitamin C. In lab dishes, this combination exhibits effective anti-cancer activity. In a mouse study, this combination inhibited tumor growth and spread by 53 %. [Oncology Reports 14:807-15, 2005]

Drawbacks of green tea

There are some nagging drawbacks to green tea.

Most of the side effects of green tea are the result of its caffeine content. Most green tea supplements contain small amounts of caffeine, about 5 to 6 mg in two 250 mg pills. One cup of brewed tea, however, has about 40 mg of caffeine. But this is half as much as coffee. If you drink excessive amounts of brewed tea, you may experience caffeine-related irritability, sleeplessness, irregular heartbeat, dizziness, vomiting, diarrhea, headache, or loss of appetite.

Green tea is an iron binder. [Chinese J Physiology 41: 189-94, 1998] Green tea molecules inhibit the absorption of iron from plant foods. Green tea does not inhibit iron absorption from iron pills or meat. [Am J Clinical Nutrition 73:607-12, 2001]

Fluoride content of green tea is of concern. It is difficult to state the fluoride content of green tea bags or extracts because of variable fluoride content. Generally, the younger the tea leaves, the less fluoride and the more antioxidant polyphenols it contains. [J Agriculture Food Chemistry 52: 4472-76, 2004]

There are false claims that green tea, by virtue of its vitamin K content (vitamin K is a blood clotting vitamin), may interfere with blood thinners. But the amount of vitamin K in green tea is negligible.

Studies show that green tea inhibits the utilization of vitamin B1 (thiamin). [Plant Foods Human Nutrition 41: 337-53, 1991] Most cancer patients using green tea may need to take supplements. However, very high-dose vitamin B1 (thiamin, 12.5 and 250 times the recommended dietary allowance), has been shown to stimulate tumor growth. [European J Biochemistry 268:4177-82, 2001] The RDA for males is 1.4 mg per day and females 1.0 mg per day.

Green tea has ingredients, such as caffeine and theanine, which may induce weight loss. This may be desirable for healthy middle-aged adults, but is probably not advised for senior adults, especially those battling cancer. Cancer is a wasting disease. [Obesity Research 13: 1195-204, 2005]

In a study of 19 patients with prostate cancer who took 250 milligram capsules of green tea extract per day, 12 reported side effects, mostly associated with the caffeine. [Urological Oncology 23: 108-13, 2005]

One of the ways green tea may hinder tumor cell growth is that it depletes tissues of folic acid. The anti-cancer drug methotrexate is an anti-folic acid drug. Folic acid is needed for DNA repair. Without folic acid, cancer cells fall apart. But this is not a selective cancer therapy. Healthy cells are affected in the same manner. Depletion of folic acid would increase the risk for birth defects among offspring of females. [Cancer Research 65: 2059-64, 2005]

Green tea has beneficial health properties. But this has to be taken into perspective. Jeffrey Blumberg, a researcher at Tufts University says green tea might modestly reduce some people's chances of developing lung cancer. But if a person continues to smoke cigarettes, there is little benefit. Blumberg estimates smoking increases the risk for lung cancer by 15 times while green tea might reduce that risk to 14.8 times. [Washington Post, March 21, 2000]

How to make green tea capsules work for you

Green tea capsules can contain anywhere from 50% to 90% polyphenols, depending on the brand. Find the brands that are 90% polyphenols. Only use decaffeinated products. Ten cups (150 ml per cup) of green tea contain 2.0–2.5 grams (2,000-2,500 mg) of green tea extract. Capsules contain 400–750 mg total tea polyphenols and are used as the standard daily dose for clinical trials in the U.S. and Japan. For cancer prevention, about 250 mg of polyphenols twice a day (500 mg) is recommended. For cancer treatment, between 2,000-2,500 mg per day is needed.

There are ways to significantly enhance the effect of green tea. Green tea molecules are better absorbed from capsules than from tea. [American Journal Clinical Nutrition 80: 1558-64, 2004] Consumption of milk or sugar at the same time as green tea may negate its effects. If green tea capsules are consumed first thing after awakening in the morning on an empty stomach, that is, after an overnight fast, there is a 350% increase in the blood plasma concentrations compared to being consumed with a meal. [Clinical Cancer Research 11: 4627-33, 2005]

Other teas

Two other teas of note in regard to cancer are rooibos and Essiac. Essiac tea, named after Canadian nurse Renée Caisse (Essiac is Caisse spelled backwards), is a combination of burdock root, Indian rhubarb, sorrel and slippery elm, though over the years others have made other versions of this tea. Caisse claimed a patient passed the formula on to her in 1922 after the patient's breast cancer had been cured. The original tea recipe was attributed to an unknown native American healer in Canada. There is little evidence that Essiac tea is beneficial, but its ingredients do have some documented anti-cancer properties. [Journal Alternative Complementary Medicine 10: 687-91, 2004; Journal Ethnopharmacology Oct 12, 2005] While Essiac has been shown to have strong antioxidant activity [Journal Ethnopharmacology Oct 12, 2005], and in a lab dish may inhibit prostate cells from replicating [J Alternative Complementary Medicine 10: 687-91, 2004], human studies using Essiac have not been performed. There are many anecdotal reports that Essiac is beneficial for cancer patients. [Phytotherapy Research 14: 1-14, 2000]

Another promising and popularized tea is red rooibos tea, which also has anti-cancer properties. [Cancer Letters 77: 33-38, 1994; Bioscience Biotechnology Biochemistry 65: 2137-45, 2001] In one study, tea extracts were applied to the skin. Green tea inhibited tumor formation 100% and processed rooibos by 75%. [Cancer Letters 224: 193-202, 2005]

Curcumin for cancer

Your kitchen spice rack probably holds a jar of turmeric, an East Indian spice that contains curcumin, a well-studied molecule in regard to cancer. It has been under scientific investigation since the 1970s.

There are many laboratory dish studies that show cancer cell growth is inhibited when curcumin is added. But these studies fall short of being equivalent to a human cure for cancer. Certainly, numerous studies point to curcumin as being efficacious, safe and non-toxic. It is an excellent anti-inflammatory agent. It specifically works on cancer cells without harming healthy cells. It blocks several cell-signaling pathways that promote cancer cell growth. But its future will likely be confined to prevention or treatment of colon and rectal cancer because of its poor absorption and bioavailability. [European Journal Cancer, August 1, 2005] It may also have potential in the treatment or prevention of prostate cancer since it was shown to be effective after oral consumption in animals. [Prostate 47: 293-303, 2001]

Of course, it is tempting for cancer patients to go to the health food store to purchase crude turmeric powder that is labeled for its curcumin content, while the same turmeric powder can be purchased for a lower price at the grocery store as a spice. Dietary supplements that provide standardized extracts of curcumin are required for any reliable health benefits. Somewhere between 1,500 and 3,600 mg of curcumin per day (only about 2% of turmeric is curcumin) is considered a typical oral dosage. For treatment of tissue in the liver and gastric tract, 3,600 mg has been determined to be an effective oral dose. [Cancer Epidemiology Biomarkers Prevention 14: 120-25, 2005] Consumption of other antioxidants, such as vitamin C, N-acetyl cysteine and glutathione, potentiate curcumin. [Pharmazie 60: 57-61, 2005]

While it is said that adequate doses of curcumin beyond the digestive tract are not likely to be achieved in humans, researchers have dismissed curcumin too quickly. It is stated that curcumin is complexed with other molecules (sulfur, glucuronic acid) once it reaches the liver, which renders it biologically unavailable. [British Journal Cancer 90: 1011-15, 2004] However, the liver metabolism preserves curcumin from degradation and extends its lifetime in the body.

Monoclonal Antibodies for Cancer Treatment	Trade Name	Used to Treat:	Approved in:
Rituximab	Rituxan	Non-Hodgkin lymphoma	1997
Trastuzumab	Herceptin	Breast cancer	1998
Gemtuzumab ozogamicin*	Mylotarg	Acute myelogenous leukemia (AML)	2000
Alemtuzumab	Campath	Chronic lymphocytic leukemia (CLL)	2001
Ibritumomab tiuxetan*	Zevalin	Non-Hodgkin lymphoma	2002
Tositumomab*	Bexxar	Non-Hodgkin lymphoma	2003
Cetuximab	Erbitux	Colorectal cancer	2004
Bevacizumab	Avastin	Colorectal cancer	2004

Furthermore, when piperine, a pungent extract derived from black pepper, is combined with curcumin, it decreases the intestinal production of glucuronic acid, thus making more curcumin available. A 20 milligram dose of piperine (Bioperine®, Sabinsa) can increase curcumin's bioavailability twenty-fold. [Planta Medica 64: 353-56, 1998]

Curcumin can be an irritant to the digestive tract and can increase stomach acid, which may be intolerable for some individuals.

Medicinal mushrooms

There is little question that boosting the human immune system is an effective way of preventing and treating the recurrence of cancer. The immune system doesn't stop cancer cells from arising, but it can intercept them once they are released into the blood circulation. The question is how to do this.

Doctors prescribe drugs, but there are other just as promising, if not more effective, immune boosters, available directly to cancer patients in the form of medicinal mushrooms and purified mushroom-like molecules called beta glucan.

Although the Mayo Clinic regards the use of medicinal mushrooms as more traditional than scientific, they operate in a manner similar to prescription drugs known as monoclonal antibodies (see chart above). Despite their unimpressive track regard, they have been a remarkably profitable class of drugs and doctors have not abandoned their use. Their effect wears off over time. [International Journal Hematology 76: 394-400, 2002]

Normally, when substances such as viruses, bacteria and tumor cells invade the body the immune system responds by producing natural killer cells and thymus cells (T-cells). Antibodies to specific antigens are also produced, to destroy cancer cells. With monoclonal antibodies, the antibodies are made in large quantities outside the body (in a laboratory) rather than by a person's immune system.

Scientists can make monoclonal antibodies that react with specific antigens on certain types of cancer cells.

Profits or cures?

Cancer patients need to understand the disconnect between the supposed mission to cure cancer and the objective of the companies that make monoclonal antibodies, which appears to be profits above delivery of an effective treatment. The total therapeutic monoclonal antibodies market was estimated at $296 million in 2002, and was projected to surge to $2.8 billion by 2010. Because pharmaceutical companies were being financially rewarded for these drugs, there was little impetus to abandon them.

Here is an excerpt from a report published in Scientific American magazine:

Unfortunately, people who received infusions of the early therapeutic monoclonal antibodies tended to develop their own antibodies against the foreign ones, which caused them to become even sicker for reasons that are not entirely clear. And the liver showed a predilection for these early monoclonals, sopping them up before they could target their quarries. Clinical trials failed. Stocks plunged. Millions of dollars were lost. And a generation of scientists and biotechnology businesspeople developed the skepticism shared only by the once burned, twice shy. [Scientific American September 19, 2001]

Notice, no disappointment was expressed for the cancer patients who were given ineffective monoclonal antibody drugs since the 1980s. It's all about money and stock prices, not cures. The pharmaceutical industry responds by saying there are newer types of monoclonal antibodies under development or in clinical testing. But the simple fact remains, cancer patients are guinea pigs and the FDA approves ineffective therapies for cancer.

In contrast to the failures of monoclonal antibody drugs, a recent report says *"it is well established that mushroom-extracted compounds are commonly used as immune boosters" ... and that "over 30 mushroom species have shown anticancer action in animals."* [Applied Microbiology Biotechnology 67: 453-68, 2005] The critics will claim medicinal mushrooms are unproven. So oncologists continue to prefer disproven monoclonal antibodies over unproven mushroom extracts.

In fact, a number of mushroom molecules have proceeded through phase I, II, and III clinical trials. (Phase I tests a new drug or treatment in a small group; Phase II expands the study to a larger group of people; Phase III expands the study to an even larger group of people; and Phase IV takes place after the drug or treatment has been licensed and marketed.) Mushroom extracts have been employed on thousands of cancer patients, often with considerable success. Lentinen, an extract from Shitake mushroom, has been approved for clinical use in Japan for many years and is manufactured by several companies. Lentinen has proved successful in prolonging the overall survival of cancer patients, especially gastric and colorectal cancer patients. [International Journal Medicinal Mushrooms 3: 86, 2001]

Other mushroom extracts that have been shown to have clinical effectiveness against human cancers are D-fraction extracted from the Maitake mushroom, and extracts from the split gill, turkey tail and Reishi mushrooms. In 1998, Maitake Products received FDA approval for an Investigational New Drug Phase II pilot study of maitake mushroom extract in the treatment of advanced breast and prostate cancer.

Dietary mushrooms and cancer

There is also some evidence that the consumption of mushrooms in the diet may ward off cancer. A 15-year study of 174,505 mushroom farmers in Japan concluded that mushroom intake reduced the cancer death rate from 160 per 100,000 non-mushroom farmers to 97 per 100,000 among the growers of these fungi. [International Journal Medicinal Mushrooms 3: 291-98, 2001] Another small study in Korea also found a reduced risk for gastric cancer among adults who consume mushrooms. [International J Cancer 97:531-5, 2002]

Another study documents the ability of mushroom extracts to raise immunity. The normal range of natural killer cells in humans is about 5 to 20 % of the white blood cell population, or about 75-1,800 cells per cubic millimeter. Treatment with extracts from coriolus mushroom extract raised natural killer cell count from 129 to 175, an increase of 35 %. [Archives Environmental Health 58:533-7, 2003]

Mushroom extracts sometimes disappoint

But not all studies using mushroom extracts have been shown to be effective. A controlled study among 68 patients with advanced stage non-small cell lung cancer did not produce any complete or partial responses to Coriolus versicolor mushroom extract. The patients received three 340 milligram capsules daily. Other studies using Reishi or Shiitake mushroom extract also did not produce any partial or complete remissions. [Experimental Biology Medicine 229: 393-406, 2004]

There are a number of reasons why studies using mushroom extracts have failed in cancer trials.

One, mushroom extracts may degrade if exposed to heat and light. Mushroom extract that is not properly preserved and stored may spoil and lose its activity. [Journal Agriculture Food Chemistry 47: 1530-32, 1999]

Two, many studies that cancer patients read about mushrooms and their effectiveness involve injected mushroom extracts, not orally consumed mushroom extract. [Oncology Reports 13:497-502, 2005]. Or, if oral doses are used, they are so large as to be impractical for many cancer patients. For example, in one study, maitake mushroom given orally to mice inhibited tumors by up to 38 %, but the mice were given the human equivalent of 3,500-10,500 mg per day. [Zhong Yao Cai 26: 31-32, 2003]

Another study describes cancer patients who took 35-70 mg of the maitake extract called D-fraction, and 4,000-6,000 mg of maitake mushroom powder per day. This is equivalent to taking 25 commercially available maitake mushrooms pills at a cost of about $3 per day. Tumor regression and symptom improvement was recorded in 11 of 15 breast cancer patients, 12 of 18 lung cancer patients and 7 of 15 liver cancer patients, and pain reduction was noted in 83% of patients taking maitake extract and raw powder. [Journal Orthomolecular Medicine 12: 43-49, 1997] As impressive as this appears, no data was provided regarding survival. Radiation and chemotherapy also shrink tumors, but they rarely prolong survival in any meaningful way.

A promising type of mushroom extract, derived from *Agaricus balzei Murill Kyowa*, is a much smaller molecule than what is found in other mushrooms. But again, the literature describes an Agaricus extract 20,000 Daltons in molecular weight that had to be injected to produce results in one study. [Anticancer Research 19:113-8, 1999]

The higher the molecular weight (size) of the mushroom extract molecules, the greater the anti-tumor effect, but the lower the absorption when taken orally.

AHCC

Active Hexose Correlated Compound (AHCC) is a cultivated product that enzymatically modifies several species of mushrooms, which are grown in rice bran extract. AHCC is known as a booster of natural killer cells. In animal studies, AHCC appears to produce good results in preventing metastases. [Anticancer Drugs 9: 343-50, 1998] Among 269 patients who had undergone liver surgery for cancer, 113 were given AHCC and experienced a longer survival period and less recurrence. [Journal Hepatology 37: 78-86, 2002]

Beta glucan extracts

Most medicinal mushrooms are labeled for their beta-D-glucan content, which is believed to be the active substance that boosts immunity. Beta-D-glucans are indigestible sugar-like molecules (called polysaccharides) and in addition to mushrooms are also found in grains, yeast, bacteria and algae. In yeast cells, beta-D-glucans are primarily located in the cell walls. Beta-D-glucan derived from baker's yeast (Saccharomyces cerevisiae) is marketed as a nutritional sup-

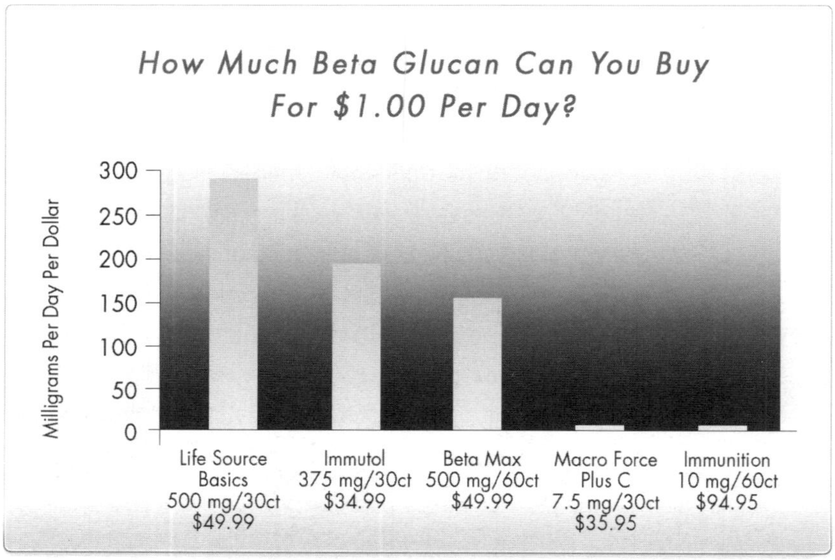

plement and its molecular weight and purity can be maximized for optimal effect. Beta glucan with molecular weights below 20,000 daltons, have been detected in the serum of animals, as well as of humans, following oral consumption. (Note, there is no remaining yeast in these supplements.) Beta-D-glucan supplements may be superior to medicinal mushrooms in their immune-boosting properties.

For example, Biothera produces a food-grade ingredient that contains beta glucan extracted from Baker's yeast (*Saccharomyces cerevisiae*). Biothera's WGP 3-6 is the purest beta glucan, and it is manufactured to deliver 1-2 micron-size beta glucan particles for optimal effect and absorption. The suggested human oral dosage is 2 mg per 2.2 pounds of body weight, or about 90 mg for a 100-pound person, 145 mg for a 160-pound person, and 180 mg for a 200-pound person. Biothera WGP 3-6 beta glucan is marketed under Life Source Basics and Imucell WGP brand names, and is included in other immune-boosting supplements as well. There are many beta glucan products offered. Few offer the dosage, molecular weight, or proven science as does Biothera WGP 3-6.

It appears mushroom extracts and beta glucans will be relegated to playing second fiddle in the war against cancer. They are being studied for use with monoclonal antibodies. Mice with tumors survive longer when administered monoclonal antibodies with beta glucan. [Cancer Immunology Immunotherapy 51: 557-64, 2002; Leukemia Research 29: 679-83, 2005] However, beta glucan may overcome a flaw in monoclonal antibody drugs such as Herceptin, Erbitux, Campath and Rituxin, and finally facilitate their successful use in cancer treatment. [Journal Immunology 174: 7050-56, 2005]

Aloe and cancer

Aloe is known as a soothing topical remedy for sunburn. It may serve as a laxative for cancer patients undergoing treatment. It is also frequently ingested orally as a tonic for health. There is evidence that aloe concentrates (70% or more) may exhibit germ-killing properties. [International Journal Dermatology 30: 679-83, 1991] Aloe extract has been shown in humans to have some ability to inhibit the growth of Helicobacter pylori, a bacterium that causes gastric ulcers and stomach cancer. [Planta Medica 64: 176-78, 1998] An experimental study published in 2000 suggests aloe has anti-tumor activity. [Cancer Research 60: 2800-04, 2000] Another study suggests aloe may protect liver cells. [Pharmacological Toxicology 90: 278-84, 2002] Yet another study showed that rodents intentionally exposed to a cancer-causing chemical that usually induces liver cancer, suppressed tumor formation. [Nutrition 14: 846-52, 1998] Human studies are lacking, but a study of rodents given aloe vera showed that life-long aloe consumption was not harmful and reduced mortality. [Phytotherapy Research 16: 712-18, 2002] Every-day use as a dietary supplement may work as a cancer preventive agent. [Phytotherapy Research 16: 491-93, 2002] There is an intriguing human study where 50 patients suffering from advanced solid tumors (lung, breast, brain, gastric tract) were given 20 mg of melatonin and aloe prior to bedtime, which improved one-year survival rates in 4 of 26 who received a melatonin supplement to 9 of 24 given melatonin and aloe. Cancer patients should not be persuaded that aloe is asole cure for cancer, but it may have beneficial properties, especially in dealing with the side effects of treatment and stabilizing their disease, especially for patients who have no other remaining therapeutic options. [Nature Immunology 16: 27-33, 1998]

Chaparral and cancer

Would you use a traditional herbal remedy for cancer that the U.S. Food & Drug Administration has banned? Many people do every day in Mexico. It is chaparral which is used as a medicinal tea.

Reports of cancer cures surround chaparral, also known as the creosote bush, but so do reports of its toxicity. Numerous cases of liver toxicity over the years have been well documented. What is a cancer patient to think?

The information surrounding this herb is an example of the misinformation surrounding many herbal remedies. The pro-toxic drug, anti-herbal stance of the FDA is unconscionable. To digress for a moment, the FDA continues to ignore the 70,000 confirmed cases of liver toxicity that occur annually from acetaminophen pain relievers. The American Poison Control Centers count about 70-100 deaths per year from acetaminophen poisoning. More than 8 billion acetaminophen pills are sold annually. But the FDA chooses to issue a warning about chaparral, not acetaminophen (Tylenol).

Acetaminophen overdose results in more calls to poison control centers in the United States than does overdose with any other pharmacologic substance. [Am J Health System Pharm, Volume 56, June 1999] The American Liver Foundation reports that 35% of cases of severe liver failure, which may require organ transplantation, are caused by acetaminophen poisoning [USA Today, August 13, 2001]

Chaparral is widely used as a medicinal tea, and has also been widely used as a dietary supplement. An extract of chaparral has been used as a food preservative. Its widespread use speaks for some level of safety. Liver toxicity associated with chaparral is explainable. Many herbal remedies, and even prescription drugs, contain molecules that inhibit detoxification liver enzymes (called cytochrome p450 enzymes). These enzymes dull the effects of medicines, herbs and food ingredients so they don't overwhelm the body. But if these enzymes are inhibited, as they are by chaparral, then any medicine, food or herbal product taken simultaneously may cause a heightened reaction to the second agent. Chaparral inhibits detoxification enzymes in the liver and can potentiate any other food, drug or herb. [Drug Metabolism Disposition 19: 620-24, 1991] Like grapefruit components, chaparral inhibits drug oxidation (breakdown), allowing more of a drug to be bioavailable. [Drug Safety 28:677-94, 2005] The same problem is documented when taking grapefruit juice with a blood pressure pill. The blood pressure drug may work too well, resulting in an inordinate drop in blood pressure and dizziness experienced by the patient. The FDA hasn't banned grapefruit juice; it just instructs users of drugs to avoid simultaneous consumption of grapefruit with certain drugs. Chaparral may be unfairly characterized as a liver toxin when it is no more harmful than grapefruit. This may explain the inconsistent reports of liver toxicity. A 78-page report issued by the Institute of Medicine and National Research Council on chaparral in 2004 explains many of the promises and problems associated with chaparral., but it is probably too lengthy a document for cancer patients to wade through.[Dietary Supplements: A Framework for Evaluating Safety, Institute of Medicine, National Research Council, 2004]

Surprisingly, after years of condemnation by the Food & Drug Administration, a report issued at the International Conference on Head and Neck Cancer in 2004 by researchers at the Medical University of South Carolina indicates an extract from chaparral seems to be *"completely safe as well as beneficial."* The extract, M4N (which stands for tetramethyl-O-nordihydroguaiaretic acid, a derivative of a powerful antioxidant called nordihydroguaiaretic acid, or NDGA), is now being studied by the National Cancer Institute. Such a turnaround was unexpected for an herb that the FDA has condemned and the American Cancer Society said has shown no proof that it is an effective treatment for cancer or any other disease.

Certainly chaparral wouldn't be a good herb to take if a person has a diseased liver. Nor would it be advisable to take chaparral with alcohol or acetaminophen. Hopefully, the extract of chaparral will proceed through successful clinical trials and contribute as a meaningful cancer remedy in the near future.

Pure NDGA from chaparral is a topical drug (Masoprocol) that is used on the skin and some studies indicate it may be effective as an oral anti-diabetic agent as well. [Journal Ethnopharmacology 98: 231-39, 2005

Ginkgo biloba

Ginkgo biloba is a drug in Europe and a dietary supplement in the U.S. It is widely used for cardiovascular problems, improvement of circulation in small blood vessels in the brain, eyes, and ears, and may improve memory among compromised individuals. While there are over 1,000 published reports involving ginkgo biloba, only a handful involve cancer. A somewhat recent report said ginkgo biloba extracts are in an "*infancy stage*" regarding their role as cancer treatment or prevention. Lab dish studies shows ginkgo inhibits cancer cell growth. [Fundamental Clinical Pharmacology 17: 405-17, 2003] Ginkgo may inhibit tumor growth by gene switching. [Cellular Molecular Biology 48: 655-62, 2002] Ginkgo biloba may also be helpful in preventing the toxic cardiac side effects of certain chemotherapy drugs (Adriamycin). [Research Communications Molecular Pathology Pharmacology 106: 181-92, 1999]

Plant estrogens (phytoestrogens) molecularly appear like real estrogen, though they have a much weaker biological effect.

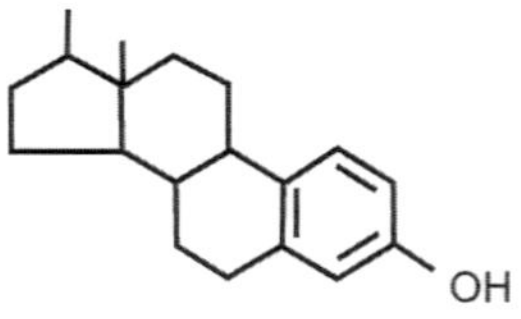

Estrogen

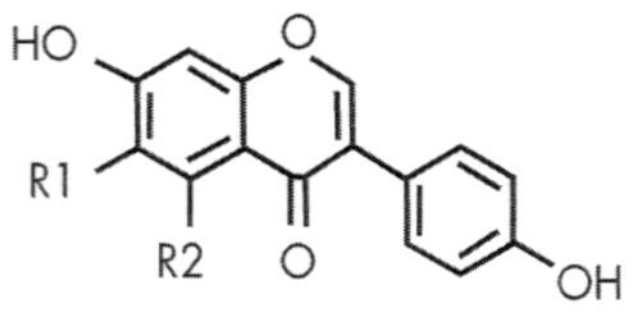

Isoflavone

The phytoestrogens

Estrogen is recognized as a promoter of breast cancer. Both elevated concentrations of estrogen and hormone replacement therapy with estrogen for menopause are associated with an increased risk of breast cancer. Plant estrogens (called phytoestrogens) are appealing because they inhibit the development and growth of hormone-related (breast, uterine, prostate) cancer. Phytoestrogens work by blunting the effect of a woman's naturally produced estrogen, and blocking its entry into a cell (blocking the estrogen receptor). Phytoestrogens are 1/1000th the strength of a woman's natural estrogen.

Women seeking alternatives to hormone replacement may find phytoestrogen supplements appealing, especially when suffering symptoms of the change of life. The potential of these herbal remedies to prevent bone loss, heart disease, menopausal symptoms and breast cancer has been a focus of attention since hormone replacement therapy has gone out of vogue.

Much more is said about the role of anti-estrogens, or plant phytoestrogens, in the section in this book on breast cancer. These herbal remedies will be addressed as a group in this chapter.

There are many herbs that have mild estrogen-like activity, including rosemary, licorice, red clover, flaxseed, soy, coffee, kudzu, black cohosh, onions and grapes. The active estrogen-like molecules in these plants are lignans (flax, rye), quercetin (onions), resveratrol (grapes, wine), formononetin (clover), glabridin (licorice), and isoflavones (soy), to name a few. Which of these plant hormone-like molecules are best for humans?

The three major classes of phytoestrogens are isoflavones, which are concentrated in soybeans and soy products but are also found in other legumes; lignans, which are distributed in seeds, whole grains, berries, fruit, vegetables, and nuts; and coumestans, which are found in broccoli and sprouts. These three classes of phytoestrogens, individually or in combination, are most likely the primary types of plant estrogens that deliver health benefits since other components are not provided in plant food diets in high amounts.

Researchers point to numerous population studies which suggest that diets rich in phytoestrogens, particularly soy and unrefined grain products, may be associated with low risk of some cancers, especially sex-hormone related breast and prostate tumors. [Anticancer Research 25:2357-66, 2005]

Actually, North Americans consume plant estrogens every day, just not very much. Breast cancer rates in the United States are 4–7 times greater than in Asia. This has historically been attributed to soy consumption in Asian countries. Asians consume 20-80 mg of plant estrogens per day compared to North Americans who consume less than 1% of that. [American Journal of Clinical Nutrition 79:183-184, 2004]

The daily dietary intake of phytoestrogens among white women in the U.S. has been estimated to be less than 1 mg, with 80% from lignans (flax, rye), 20% from isoflavones (soy), and less than 0.1% from coumestans (broccoli). [Journal Nutrition 131: 1826–32, 2001]

A recent report says:

"Women, especially those at high risk, want to know whether phytoestrogens decrease or increase breast cancer risk. If phytoestrogens are indeed protective, are soy and isoflavone nutraceuticals that are designed to supply phytoestrogens at 50 mg/day, an intake comparable with that of an Asian diet, required to guarantee sufficiently high dosages?"
American Journal of Clinical Nutrition 79:183-184, 2004

That's not an easy question to answer.

Although most animal studies have shown cancer-preventive effects, a few recent studies suggest that soy phytoestrogens may stimulate breast cancer cell growth under certain circumstances.

Imagine you hired someone knowledgeable to review all of the current and past reports regarding plant estrogens and cancer. You asked them to report back to you on what these reports suggest. Most likely the person you hired would throw up her hands and become perplexed.

Cancer researchers can't make up their minds whether phytoestrogens are good or bad. So how are cancer patients supposed to know what to do?

Here are some examples of the indecision regarding phytoestrogens and cancer:

A report issued by researchers at the University of Rochester Medical Center says: *"Despite great promise, it is difficult to make many specific recommendations about their (isoflavones') use at the current time. No recommendation regarding soy isoflavones can be made based on the current data. Also, soy isoflavones should not be taken by postmenopausal women for the specific purpose of decreasing their risk of breast or endometrial cancer."* This is very puzzling, given the fact that the American Heart Association says the inclusion of soy protein foods as part of an otherwise healthy diet is well justified. Good for the heart but unclear for breast health. [Endocrinology 1:293-311, 2002]

Another report says: *"Of current concern is the effect of phytoestrogen compounds on the growth of pre-existing breast tumors. Data are contradictory, with lab dish studies reporting both the estrogenic stimulation of estrogen receptor-positive breast cancer cells and well as antagonism of tamoxifen activity at physiological phytoestrogen concentrations. Conversely, phytoestrogen ingestion by rodents is associated with the development of less aggressive breast tumors with reduced metastatic potential. Despite the present ambiguity, current data do suggest a potential benefit from use of phyto-estrogens in breast cancer chemoprevention and therapy."* [Breast Cancer Research 6:119-27, 2004]

In 2004, the *Journal of Nutrition and Cancer* published the first report of a positive link between plant estrogen intake and pre-cancerous changes in cervical tissue of women. [Nutrition & Cancer 49:109-24, 2004]

The case of a man diagnosed with breast cancer whose history is notable because he extensively used supplemental phytoestrogens, and had no family history of breast cancer or genetic predisposition, is of significance. [European Journal Cancer Prevention 13:481-4, 2004]

Here are more examples of ambiguous or confusing reports concerning phytoestrogens.

→ *"The increasing popularity and availability of phytoestrogen dietary supplements necessitates additional research in order to counsel patients regarding their safety and efficacy."* [European Journal Cancer Prevention 13:481-4, 2004]

→ *"Consensus in the biomedical community has been hampered by conflicting data from various in vitro and in vivo models of estrogenic activity."* [Integrative Cancer Therapy 2:120-38, 2003]

→ *"The relevant research is complicated, inconsistent, and inconclusive. At present, scientific research does not support increasing phytoestrogen intake among US women to Asian levels, nor does it suggest that the typical US phytoestrogen intake is problematic for healthy women."* [American Journal of Clinical Nutrition 79:183-184, 2004]

→ *"Although these compounds have a great potential for improving health, there is still not enough evidence to recommend the routine use of phytoestrogens."* [Rev Med Chile 131:1321-8, 2003]

→ A study of 15,555 Dutch women aged 49-70 years found a high intake of soy isoflavones or mammalian flaxseed and other lignans is not significantly related to breast cancer risk. [American J Clinical Nutrition 79:282-8, 2004]

→ The strongest data show that phytoestrogens reduce the number and intensity of hot flashes, although the reduction is a modest 10-20%. [Journal Nutrition 133:1983S-6S, 2003]

→ A review of published dietary intake studies involving prostate cancer did not show any protective action from phytoestrogens. [Preventive Medicine 41:1-6, 2005]

Here's another problem. Population and rodent studies suggest that breast cancer chemoprevention by dietary phytoestrogen compounds is dependent on ingestion before puberty, when the mammary gland is relatively immature. However, phytoestrogen supplements are commercially marketed for use by postmenopausal women as natural and safe alternatives to hormone replacement therapy. [Breast Cancer Research 6:119-27, 2004]

This just doesn't sound like a glowing report about phytoestrogens, and it certainly is confusing.

Phyto-nutrients	Flaxseed meal 2 tablespoons	Soy protein concentrate dose?
Weak estrogen-like molecules	50+ mg lignans	
Omega-3 oil	3,000 mg	57% omega 3 fatty acids vs 16% omega-6
Phenolic Acids	100 mg	
Flavonoids	5 mg	
Phytic Acid	320 mg	Whole raw soy beans, 3.5 oz. 1,000-1,470 mg
Iron	-	14.50 mg
Folic acid	-	340 mcg

Similarity Of Molecules
Enterodiol - Enterolactone - Estradiol

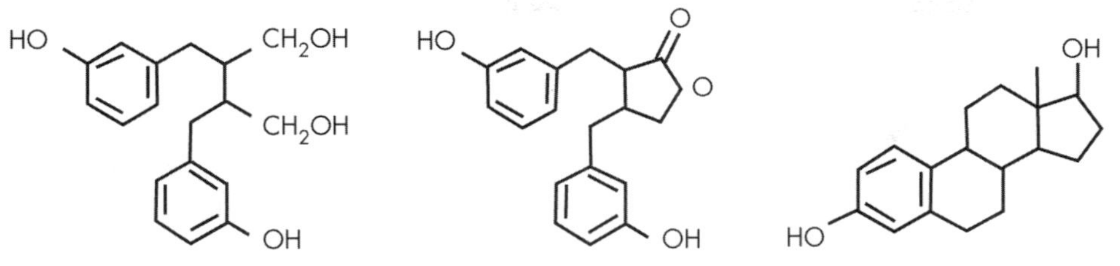

Enterodiol Enterolactone Estradiol

The primary problem in understanding phytoestrogens is that they have a dual nature In animal models and in lab dish studies, phytoestrogens bind weakly to estrogen receptors on living cells and can either produce or inhibit estrogen effects. [Journal Nutrition 131:3095S–108S, 2001]

While this author often promotes the idea of extracts from herbal products as providing superior biological effects, in this case, plant estrogens really should be considered in the context of the whole herbs they emanate from. When the anti-cancer effects of phytoestrogens are examined, it can clearly be seen that other important anti-cancer molecules are complexed naturally with in the plant. Some phytoestrogens, such as red clover, are said to combat symptoms of menopause and are not strongly promoted for anti-cancer effects. The two most often cited sources of phytoestrogens involving cancer are soy and flaxseed. Both of these botanical sources have similar anti-cancer molecules. Soybeans and flaxseed contain omega-3 oil, an iron-binder called IP6 phytate, and mild, estrogen-like molecules. That's three major cancer fighters from just one botanical source. Flaxseed is superior in this regard, since it provides the most concentrated source of omega-3 oil and IP6 compared to other seed grains.

A study involving flaxseed, flaxseed oil and flaxseed extract (lignans) confirms that all the components of flax together maximize the effect of phytoestrogens. All of the components of flaxseed, individually and combined, have been found to inhibit tumor growth. [International J Cancer 116:793-8, 2005] However, one study indicates higher lignan (enterolactone) urinary excretion (a marker of consumption of lignans) was associated with a slight increase in breast cancer risk. [Cancer Epidemiology Biomarkers & Prevention 10: 223-228, 2001] Only one of the three published U.S. studies that estimated dietary lignan intake found a protective effect. [Journal Nutrition 132:3036–41, 2002]

Sources of Lignans	Typical quantity µg/g
Linseed meal	675-808
Linseed flour	527
Linseed oil	17
Oat bran	7
Oatmeal	2
Wheat	5
Lentil	8
Asparagus	3
Carrot	4

Sources of Isoflavones	Typical quantity µg/g
Textured soybean	1136
Soy flakes	501-566
Tofu	417-494
Soy flour	1338
Tempeh	430
Soya sauce	23

Animal studies

Animal studies using flaxseed have produced remarkable outcomes.

One approach to cancer prevention is to determine which foods prevent genetic damage, which is an indication of a predisposition to cancer. Researchers are York University in Toronto, Canada, set out to do just that. They measured chromosome fragments that are not incorporated into the nucleus at cell division, called micronuclei, and other markers of genetic instability, in rodents. Of the 26 food supplements tested (cabbage, spinach, asparagus, Brussels sprouts, carrots, lentils, broccoli, soybeans, rye, flaxseed and others), flaxseed and rye were found to be the strongest genetic stabilizers. [Mutation Research 551:213-22, 2004] The diet can prevent spontaneous gene mutations, and flaxseed and rye in particular, can accomplish this. The researchers attributed this protective effect to the lignans or phenols in these seeds, but they overlooked IP6 phytate which is the most stable antioxidant in nature.

In animals, exposure to flaxseed or its lignan extract due to breast feeding suppresses breast tumor development later in life in female offspring. [Experimental Biology Medicine 228: 951-58, 2003]

Supplementation of 10% flaxseed, the richest source of mammalian lignans, to mice with established human breast tumors not only reduced tumor growth, but also inhibited metastasis. [Cancer Letters 185:31-7, 2002]

Flax oil by itself exerts anti-cancer properties. In rats fed corn oil or flaxseed oil and then injected with tumor cells underneath their skin, colon tumors developed in 100% of the mice on corn oil and only 54% of the mice on flaxseed oil. Tumors were larger and more numerous in the corn oil-fed animals. There were about three tumors per corn oil-fed animal, compared to about one tumor in the flaxseed oil-fed animals. [Nutrition Cancer 51:52-8, 2005]

Flaxseed works well with tamoxifen, an anti-cancer drug. In rodents who had their ovaries removed, and had tumors implanted with low-dose estrogen, subsequent treatment with flaxseed reduced tumor size by 74%. Tamoxifen initially shrunk the tumor but later induced a larger malignancy. However, tamoxifen plus flaxseed shrunk tumors by 53%. With high estrogen levels, flaxseed reduced tumor size by 22%, tamoxifen by 41% and flaxseed plus tamoxifen by 50%. Flaxseed appears to enhance tamoxifen treatment. [Clinical Cancer Research 10:7703-11, 2004]

Flax also inhibits the spread of cancer. In one experiment, mice were fed a standard lab diet with or without flaxseed. The flaxseed-fed mice were fed a diet of 2.5, 5 or 10% flaxseed for two weeks before and after the intravenous injection of melanoma cancer cells. The number of tumors that spread to the lungs fell by 32, 54 and 63% with increasing amounts of flaxseed in the diet. This study shows that flaxseed inhibits metastasis. [Cancer Letters 124:181-6, 1998]

In animal studies, flax lignans appear to inhibit the earlier growth of tumors, whereas flaxseed oil appears to be more effective at the stage when tumors begin to metastasize. [Carcinogenesis 17:1373-6, 1996]

In another animal study, flaxseed and its components (oil and lignans) inhibited the spread of breast tumors but not their recurrence after surgical removal. [Cancer Letters, May 20, 2005]

Human studies

Does flaxseed have the potential to reduce tumor growth, not just in animals, but in women with breast cancer? When 25 grams of flaxseed was added to the diet of women who were newly diagnosed with breast cancer, they exhibited favorable changes in tumor markers. [Clinical Cancer Research 11:3828-35]

A survey of a few hundred women in Germany found women who consume flaxseed are less likely to exhibit dense mammograms, a marker for breast cancer. [European Journal Medical Research 10: 389-94, 2005]

In 28 postmenopausal women who consumed 0, 5 or 10 grams of ground flaxseed per day, blood serum estrogen concentrations dropped. [Nutrition & Cancer 39:58-65, 2001]

Flax among men

How about males and prostate cancer?

Flaxseed works to prevent prostate cancer as well as breast cancer.

A daily diet containing four slices of a bread rich in soy grits favorably influences the PSA level and the free/total PSA ratio in patients with prostate cancer. This study provides some evidence to support epidemiologic studies claiming that male populations who consume high phytoestrogen diets have a reduced risk of development and progression of prostate cancer. [Urology 64:510-5, 2004]

Among 39 men with prostate cancer who were given 100 mg of soy isoflavone (Novasoy) taken by mouth twice daily for a minimum of three or maximum of six months, their mean PSA score stabilized in 83% of patients in the hormone-sensitive group and in 35% of the non-hormone sensitive group. [Nutrition & Cancer 47:111-7, 2003]

Fifteen men who were scheduled to undergo repeat prostate biopsy were instructed to follow a low-fat, flaxseed-supplemented (30 grams/day) diet for six months. PSA was reduced (from about 8.5 points to about 5.75 points). Tumor growth slowed significantly. [Urology 63:900-4, 2004]

Among men awaiting prostate surgery, a low-fat diet with 30 grams of flaxseed meal per day for 21-77 days experienced a drop in testosterone; PSA scores remained about the same, but Gleason scores dropped. [Urology 58:47-52, 2001]

Flaxseed, flax oil or flax lignans?

Which is the most beneficial way to acquire the therapeutic and preventive benefits of flaxseed? The question arises, is it flaxseed, or its lignan or oil fractions, that most inhibit cancer? Rodents were given these three dietary ingredients or corn oil 13 weeks following administration of a cancer-causing chemical. After seven weeks, breast tumor volume was more than 50% smaller in flaxseed, flax oil, and lignan-fed animals than in animals fed corn oil. New tumor number and volume were lowest in the flaxseed and lignan-fed animals. [Carcinogenesis 17:1373-6, 1996]

Studies reveal that flaxseed feeding of rodent offspring during breast feeding favorably alters the cells in breast tissue. In a study of rodents after weaning from breast milk, and then exposed to a cancer-causing chemical, the flax-fed animals exhibited 31% fewer tumors, and the flax-extract (SDG) 42% fewer tumors. The size of the tumors was 51% and 63% less, and tumor number was 47% and 45% less. There was not much difference in the numbers between flaxseed and its extract. [Experimental Biology Medicine 228:951-8, 2003]

In another study, flaxseed, flaxseed oil, and flaxseed extract called lignans (lignan secoisolaric resinol diglycoside) all exhibited the ability to inhibit tumor growth in animal studies. However, one study showed a weaker effect for lignan alone than when given in combination with flaxseed oil or whole flaxseed. [International Journal Cancer 116: 793-98, 2005]

Researchers at the University of Toronto again attempted to determine exactly what it is in flaxseed that prevents tumors, this time colon tumors. In a study of rodents fed flaxseed, or defatted flaxseed, or flaxseed extract, there were four small adenomas and two polyps observed in rodents on a regular diet, but not in the flax-treated groups. There were no significant differences between the flaxseed and the corresponding defatted flaxseed groups. The researchers concluded that flaxseed has a colon cancer protective effect, that is due in part, to the lignans within flaxseed. The mechanism attributed to this anti-cancer effect with flaxseed is the elevation of an enzyme called glucuronidase. [Carcinogenesis 17:1343-8, 1996] The activity of the enzyme beta-glucoronidase increases in many pathological conditions such as inflammation, infection and cancer. Without glucuronidase, flax and other phytoestrogens cannot efficiently enter the blood circulation. [Forum Nutrition 57: 100-11, 2005]

However, the flaxseed lignan extract (secoisolariciresinol diglycoside) has been shown by itself to inhibit the number of tumors that develop in rodents after they are given a cancer-causing chemical. [Nutrition & Cancer 26:159-65, 1996]

Feeding rats 5% flaxseed flour after exposure to a cancer-causing chemical, reduces tumor size by 67%. However, the effect of flaxseed is not consistent throughout all stages of cancer. [Nutrition Cancer 17:153-9, 1992] Lignans are reduced in flax flour compared to crushed flaxseed meal.

But again, in a contrary finding, since lignans have been suggested to have some cancer-protective effects, flaxseed, the most abundant source of lignan precursors, was tested for its effect on early markers of risk for mammary carcinogenesis. Supplementation of a high-fat diet with flaxseed flour or defatted flaxseed meal (5% or 10%) was provided to animals. Flaxseed flour appeared to be superior to defatted-flaxseed meal in inhibiting cancer in the breast of rodents. [Cancer Letters 60:135-42, 1991]

Whole grains consistently test positively as cancer prevention agents. Whole grains contain IP6 phytate, more so than other plant foods. The intake of the whole grain, with bran that provides IP6, is emphasized for optimum human health. [Critical Review Food Science Nutrition 34:473-97, 1994] Animal studies unfailingly confirm that IP6 has widespread and profound anti-cancer properties. [Complementary Therapy Medicine 10:229-34, 2002] Whole grain consumption by itself may not be a protective factor for breast cancer. [Cancer Causes Control 12:917-25, 2001] Health benefits are attributed to the whole array of nutrients found in whole grains (lignan, vitamin E, phenols, selenium, and IP6 phytate) is, especially the reduced risk of breast cancer with whole grain intake. [Critical Review Food Science Nutrition 34:473-97, 1994] The anti-cancer properties of whole grains are often mistakenly attributed to fiber rather than IP6 phytate. [Cancer 56:717-8, 1985]

For examination, look at the array of nutrients in crushed flaxseed in the chart displayed on this page. [Data: Barlean's Forti-Flax]

Two tablespoons of flaxseed meal is suggested for all females and males to normalize hormone levels throughout adulthood. Flaxseeds can also be crushed in a coffee grinder (uncrushed seeds are of little value). Flaxseed meal should be stored in a dark container in the refrigerator. Other phytoestrogens, such as red clover and black cohosh, are more appropriate for the symptoms of menopause than for cancer prevention or treatment.

Supplement Facts

Flaxseed meal

Suggested use: 2-4 tablespoons daily
Serving Size 2Tbsp (15 g)
Servings Per Container 30
Amount Per Serving
Calories 70 Calories from Fat 45

Amount Per Serving

Total Fat 5 g
Saturated Fat 0 g
Polyunsaturated Fat 3.5 g
Monounsaturated Fat 1 g
Cholesterol 0 mg
Sodium 0 mg
Total Carbohydrate 6 g
Dietary Fiber 3 g
Insoluble Fiber 2 g
Soluble Fiber 1 g
Trace Vitamins
Vitamin C 75 mcg
Folic Acid 16 ug
Niacin 480 mcg
Pantothenic Acid 85 mcg
Vitamin B-1 (Thiamin) 79 mcg
Vitamin B-2 (Riboflavin) 34 mcg
Vitamin B-6 (Pyridoxine Hcl) 90 mcg
Tocopherols (Vit. E)
Alpha-Tocopherol 8 mcg
Delta-Tocopherol 6 mcg
Gamma-Tocopherol 4 mcg
Trace Minerals
Calcium 30 mg
Alanine 125 mg
Amino Acids (Protein) 3000 mg
Arginine 270 mg

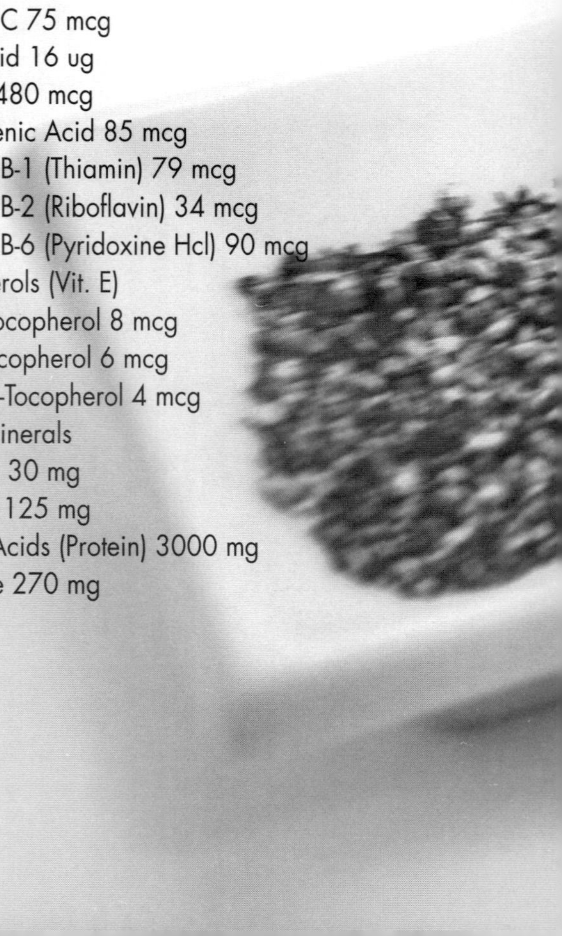

Aspartic Acid 270 mg
Copper 150 mcg
Cystine 30 mg
Glutamic Acid 580 mg
Glycine 170 mg
Histidine 60 mg
Isoleucine 115 mg
Leucine 170 mg
Lysine 115 mg
Methionine 40 mg
Phenylalanine 130 mg
Proline 100 mg
Serine 130 mg
Threonine 1000 mg
Tryptophan 50 mg
Tyrosine 60 mg
Valine 130 mg
Essential Fatty Acids
Omega-3 (alpha-linolenic acid) 3,000 mg
Omega-6 (linoleic acid) 1,000 mg
Monounsaturated Fatty Acids
Omega-9 1,000 mg
Phyto-nutrients
Lignans > 50 mg
Flavonoids 5 mg
Phenolic Acids 100 mg
Phytic acid (IP6) 320 mg
Barlean's Forti-Flax

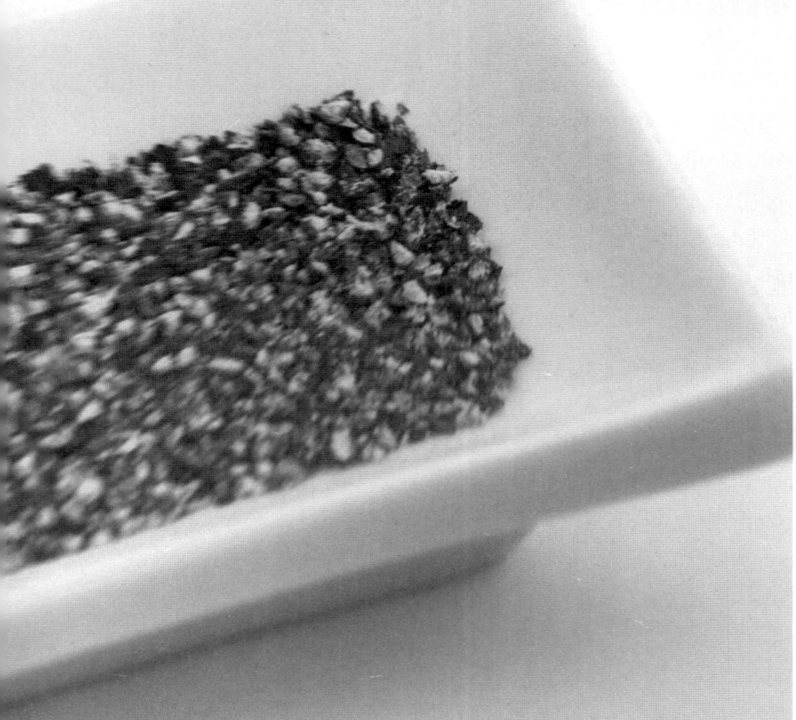

Pomegranate

It certainly has a lot of seeds in it. Pomegranates are those red, hard-shelled fruits that squirt juice everywhere when you peel them open. But recent studies indicate this fruit and its extracts, at the very least will be cancer preventive agents, and maybe even mainline cancer therapy some day. *"Mother Nature has an unusual plant that punches all of the right mechanistic buttons to kill a tumor cell,"* says a recent report published in the Journal of the National Cancer Institute.

While there were only 38 papers published on pomegranates from 1975 to 1999, they are all trumped by an endorsement from a higher authority – the Bible. Numerous scientific studies are now underway, and they describe some potent antioxidants like ellagic acid, and some unusual ingredients, such as punicic acid, an oil that rarely occurs in nature. [Journal National Cancer Institute 95: 346-48, 2003] This oil has achieved an 87% reduction in tumor size in an animal study involving breast cancer. [European Journal Cancer Prevention 13: 345-48, 2004] One journal says pomegranate ingredients could be classified as new anti-cancer drugs. [Investigative New Drugs 23: 121-22, 2005] The juice appears to have superior qualities over pomegranate fruit extract. [Journal Nutritional Biochemistry 16: 360-67, 2005] Numerous reports extol pomegranate for prostate, colon and skin cancer. Its one drawback is that ellagic acid, a primary antioxidant in pomegranate, is poorly absorbed. However, it still has potency against colon cancer. [Clinical Chim Acta 348: 63-68, 2004]

Ellagic acid, found in pomegranate and red raspberries, inhibits an enzyme, topoisomerase, that breaks DNA strands that can produce cancer. Ellagic acid mimics the cancer drug etoposide (Etopophos, vepesid). [Nutrition & Cancer 23: 121-30, 1995] If pomegranate juice were a drug, its dry, tart sweetness would be missed. Pomegranate is a good cancer preventive agent today, and a promising drug for tomorrow.

Graviola (Paw Paw)

Oh the promises of another cancer cure, this one from a *"miraculous Amazon tree."* The manufacturer of this herb offered testimony from a 26-year-old mother of three children, diagnosed with cervical cance.r According to the promotion, treatment was ineffective and the patient lost appetite and began to lose weight. Down to 80 pounds, she began to take the rain forest elixir. What other options did she have at that point? She regained her energy, gained 10 pounds, her sleep improved and her pain subsided.

This online report, part of an advertisement for the herbal extract known as paw paw, or graviola, is likely to be grasped like a straw by any desperate cancer patient. But the online report never indicates whether the patient survived. Survival is the only gold standard by which to evaluate cancer therapies. For instance, surgery shrinks tumors, in fact it removes them, but may not prolong life.

Paw paw extracts became available in 2003 and soon thereafter were promoted as a cancer cure. This herbal extract is said to be more potent than the cancer drug cisplatin (which is very toxic), and is reported to shrink human tumors, according to Dr. Jerry McLaughlin, PhD, the Purdue University researcher who first published reports about paw paw extracts and cancer in 1997. The paw paw extract, bullatacin, was shown to reduce cell energy selectively in cancer cells, but not in healthy cells. Without energy, the tumor cells could not pump out anti-cancer drugs and develop drug resistance. It was quite a startling laboratory experiment. [Cancer Letters 115: 73-79, 1997]

In a subsequent study, a molecule that resembles bullatacin was found to be as much as 250 times more potent than adriamycin (another very toxic cancer drug). [Journal Medicinal Chemistry 40: 2102-06, 1997] Even more recent research confirms that another similar paw paw molecule, squamocin, *"is a potentially promising anticancer compound."* [Life Sciences, Sept. 7, 2005]

There is an unsettling report where paw paw fruit was associated with an unusual Parkinsons disease-like movement disorder among consumers of this tree fruit. [Movement Disorders 20: 1629-33, 2005]

It's a big jump, from test tube to humans. Desperate cancer patients don't have the time for another decade of research before molecules like these are ever tested in humans. So they may just hyper-space the research and make themselves guinea pigs. It's all part of the desperation caused by the failings of modern medicine to find a real cure for cancer. As easy as it is to criticize this yet unproven cancer cure, can anyone fault a dying cancer patient for trying?

Ginseng

After population studies conducted in Korea found that users of ginseng exhibit lower cancer rates, it has become apparent that ginseng may be a useful dietary measure to prevent cancer. [Journal Korean Medical Society 16: S19-27, 2001] Ginseng extract and powder appear to be more effective than fresh sliced ginseng, or ginseng tea. [International Journal Epidemiology 19: 871-76, 1990]

Cancer prevention almost appears to be an afterthought in the cancer industry. Most efforts are made to treat cancer rather than prevent it. Ginseng exhibits broad, non-organ specific, anti-cancer activity. [Lancet Oncology 2: 49-55, 2001] Molecules called ginsenosides have been identified as the primary anti-tumor agents in this herbal remedy. [Mutation Research 523: 63-74, 2003]

Beyond cancer prevention, ginseng has been shown to make cancer cells more vulnerable to radiation treatment. [Am Journal Chinese Medicine 29: 517-24, 2001] Ginseng, especially its Rh2 ginsenoside, makes it easier for cancer drugs like paclitaxel to kill cancer cells, especially drug-resistant cancers. [Canadian Journal Physiology Pharmacology 82: 431-37, 2004]

A review of published studies involving ginseng and cancer published from 1983-1998 led researchers to conclude that available evidence for ginseng in cancer prevention is not conclusive. [Cancer Causes Control 11: 565-76, 2000] There may be good reasons why.

The majority of the studies for ginseng as a cancer preventive agent have been conducted with Panax ginseng, (C.A. Meyer) Other types of ginseng (American, Siberian) may not work as well. [Public Health Nutrition 3: 473-85, 2000]

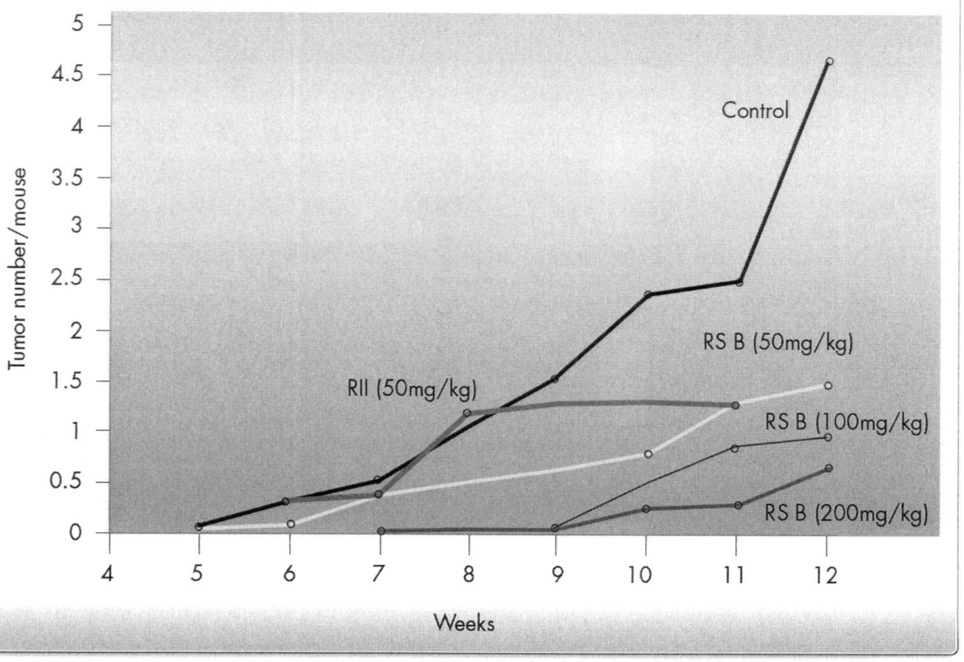

Effect of red ginseng extract B (RS B) on tumor number per mouse over time at varying oral doses (50 to 200 mg per kilogram/2.2 pounds of body weight).
Journal Ethnopharmacology 60: 71-78, 1998

Not all ginseng products deliver the ginsenoside active ingredients required to quell cancer. A study conducted in the United States of 25 commercial brands of ginseng found the ginsenoside content varied by as much as 15 to 36 times in capsules and liquids. [American Journal Clinical Nutrition 73: 1101-06, 2001] The possibility for cancer prevention may be nullified in this case by inferior products. Second, the dosage used in various studies, animal and human, is wide ranging, it is difficult to determine what an adequate daily dose is. One study that used Panax ginseng in mice at a human equivalent dosage range from 70 to 700 mg oral dose per day (calculated for a 160-pound human), which was successful in reducing tumor incidence. [Phytotherapy Research 19: 65-71, 2005] Another animal study employed the human equivalent of 3,500-28,000 mg per day. [Journal Ethnopharmacology 60: 71-78, 1998]

A study comparing animal and human response to Panax ginseng is telling. In mice, Panax ginseng that was aged six years exhibited far stronger ability to inhibit tumor formation than younger ginseng roots. Among two groups of 905 adults each, 562 (62%) developed cancer among the ginseng users compared to 674 (74%) among non-users. [Nutrition Reviews 54: S71-81, 1996]

In conclusion, red Korean Panax Ginseng (C.A. Meyer) is an herb that functions as a cancer preventive agent and as a companion to conventional cancer therapy. If using commercial ginseng extracts, search for products that accurately label the minimum amount of ginsenosides (active ingredient). Most brands range from 2 to 8 % ginsenosides.

Ginger

Cancer patients frequently experience nausea and constipation as side effects from chemotherapy. Anti-nausea drugs (anti-emetics) are frequently prescribed. However, high doses of anti-nausea drugs like metoclopramide may induce other side effects.

Ginger is widely known as an anti-nausea remedy, for motion sickness and nausea of pregnancy. Ginger has been found to be helpful in these instances. [Pharmazie 60: 83-96, 2005] In one study, ginger juice produced better reversal of symptoms than did ondansetron, a drug commonly used to overcome nausea during chemotherapy. [Journal Ethnopharmacology 62: 49-55, 1998]

Ginger root has been shown to inhibit the growth of tumors in the colon in animal studies. [Clin Chim Acta 358: 60-67, 2005] Ginger root extract (gingerols) inhibits the growth of

Helicobacter pylori in the digestive tract, which is a bacterium known to cause stomach cancer. [Anticancer Research 23: 3699-702, 2003]

Ginger is also a potent anti-inflammatory agent. [Journal Environmental Pathology Toxicology Oncology 18: 131-39, 1999] Recall that anti-inflammatory drugs like aspirin and ibuprofen are considered anti-cancer agents.

Olive leaf extract

Olive leaf extract will serve as an example of a safe and remarkable way of quelling cancer that is just now being fully understood.

In recent years cancer researchers have become aware of the fact that 90% of cancer mortality is due to the development of many distant tumors (metastasis) rather than the initial tumor. Cancer cells must be able to migrate in order to produce a colony elsewhere in the body. Various drugs attempt to either inhibit the degradation of *"goo"* (collagen) that surrounds cancer cells, or inhibit the adherence of tumor cells to tissues, in order to stop tumor cell movement and invasion. There has been disappointment with these efforts.

Tumor cells actually crawl, like a snail, utilizing their backbone, or what is called their cytoskeleton for movement. The backbone of cells is comprised of actin. [Cancer Sci. 96:379-86, 2005] *"Break the back"* of actin and tumor cells can't move or migrate. A number of actin breaker drugs are under investigation. Natural small molecules, called polyphenols, may be able to specifically target the cytoskeleton of cancer cells.

One such class of natural molecules, that have been rearranged to make patentable drugs, is taxanes (docetaxel/Taxotere, paclitaxel/Taxol). Taxanes are anti-cancer drugs that interfere with the 'scaffolding' that cancer cells need to help them multiply. [International Journal Oncology 27:247-56, 2005] Taxanes are primarily used as a secondary drug treatment since they produce significant side effects.

Taxol

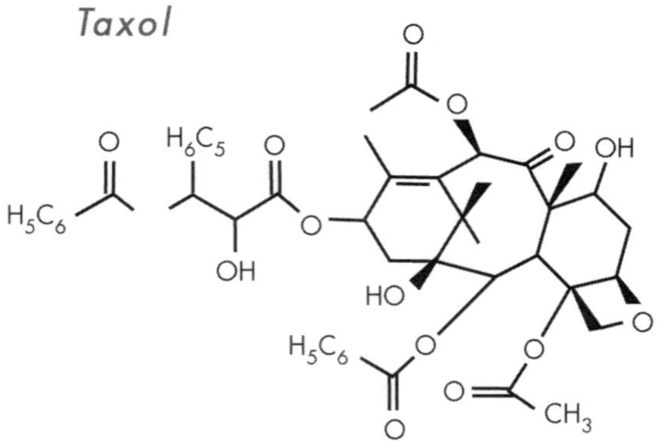

A natural molecule of similar structure to taxol is oleuropein, the bitter component in olives, which has gained the attention of cancer researchers because of its various health-promoting properties. [Life Sciences 62:541-6, 1998]

There is something unusual about olives – they can be placed in a dish and remain intact without the fungal spoilage experienced by most other foods, for over a year.

Structure Of Oleuropein

O - $C_6H_{11}O_5$ is O - ß - D - glucopyranose

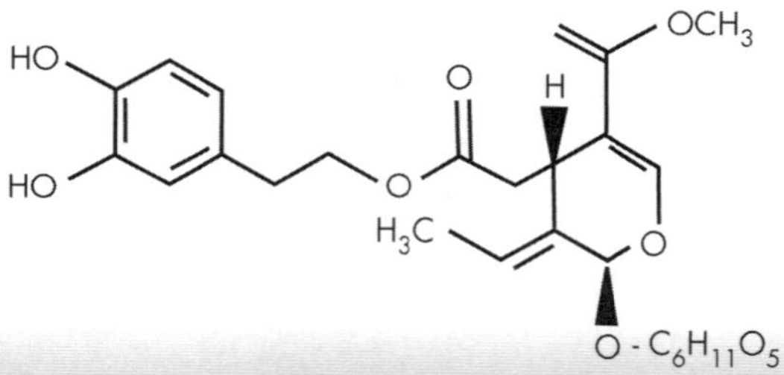

A remarkable study conducted by researchers Hamdi Hamdi and Raquel Castellon provides the first evidence of the powerful manner in which oleuropein works to *"cure"* cancer. This study is drawing worldwide attention, even though it was conducted in animals and hasn't entered human trials as yet. The reason is the way oleuropein eradicated cancer cells.

Here are the exact words the researchers used to describe their animal experiment:

"Here, we show it to be a potent anti-cancer compound, directly disrupting actin filaments in cells and in a cell-free assay. Oleuropein inhibited the growth and migration of advanced-grade tumor cells in a dose-responsive manner. In a novel tube-disruption assay, oleuropein irreversibly rounded cancer cells, preventing their replication, mobility, and invasiveness. These effects were reversible in normal cells. When administered orally to mice that developed spontaneous tumors, oleuropein completely regressed tumors in 9-12 days. These observations elevate oleuropein from a non-toxic antioxidant into a potent anti-tumor agent with direct effects against tumor cells. Our data may also explain the cancer-protective effects of the olive-rich Mediterranean diet."

Source: Biochemical Biophysical Research Communications 334:769-78, 2005

Taxol causes cancer cells, and normal healthy cells to turn into a round shape. They then die off, but not in a selective manner. Healthy cells are killed off with the malignant cells. Using oleuropein, both healthy and tumorous cells appeared rounded after treatment, but the healthy cells then reverted back to their normal shape without toxicity. Oleuropein is a remarkably selective tumor cell destroyer.

Here is a graphic presentation of what these researchers discovered.

Oleuropein from olives selectively disrupts the cytoskeleton of tumor cells, which leads to cell death without harming healthy cells. Oleuropein produces non-toxic tumor cell death.

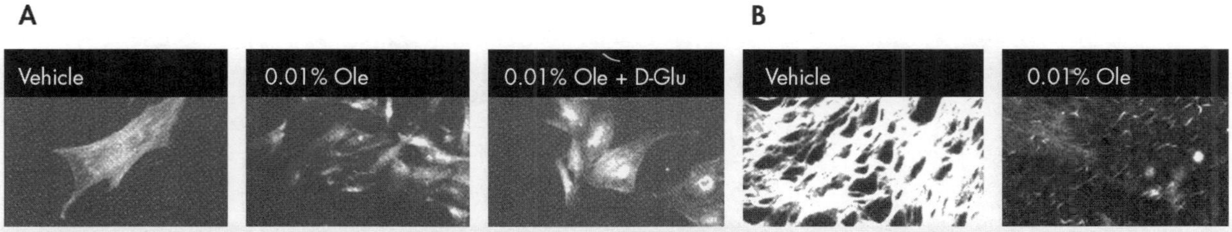

Tumor cells are always on the move. They migrate quickly. In the experiment below, left, tumor cells were placed within a circular ringand quickly migrated towards the edge of a lab dish. On the right, the lab dish was pre-treated with oleuropein, which completely blocked tumor cell migration.

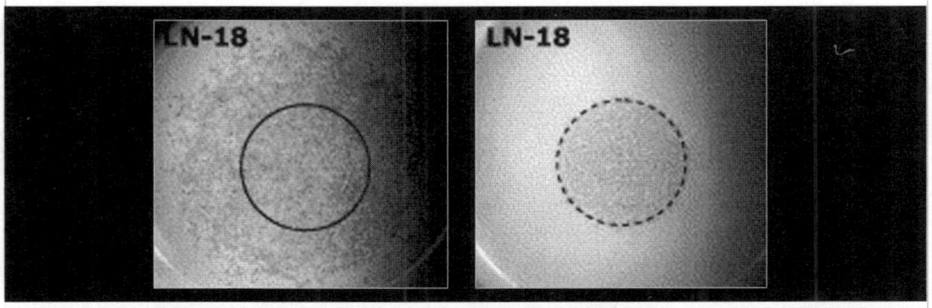

The animal shown on the left has visually observable tumors on its back. After oleuropein treatment, the tumor disappeared within 9-12 days, shown on the right.

Source: Biochemical and Biophysical Research Communications 334: 769-78, 2005

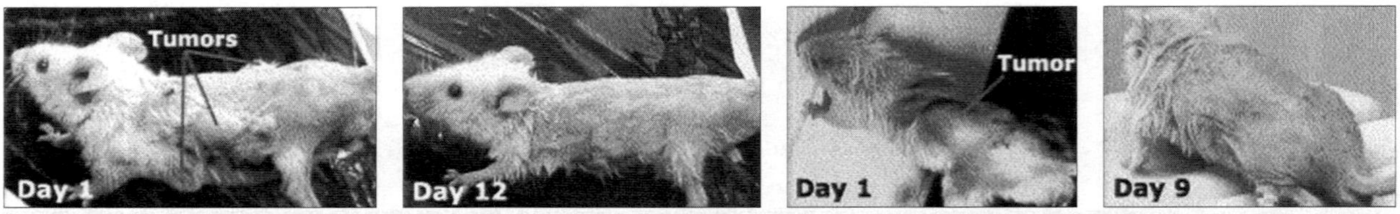

Experimental outcomes and survival for control and oleuropein-treated mice			
Mouse number	Oleuropein treatment (9–12 days)	Experimental outcome	Survival (months)
1	None	Increased tumor	0
2	None	Increased tumor	0
3	None	Increased tumor	0
4	None	Increased tumor	0
5	None	Increased tumor	0
6	Oral (ad libitum)	Complete regression	18+
7	Oral (ad libitum)	Complete regression	14
8	Oral (ad libitum)	Complete regression	18+
9	Oral (ad libitum)	Complete regression	18+
10	Oral (ad libitum)	Complete regression	12
11	Oral (ad libitum)	Complete regression	18
12	Oral (ad libitum)	Complete regression	12
13	Oral (ad libitum)	Complete regression	15+
14	Oral (ad libitum)	Complete regression	14+
15	Oral (ad libitum)	Complete regression	14+
16	Oral (ad libitum)	Partial regression	3
17	Oral (ad libitum)	Early resection	N/A
18	IP injection	Early resection	N/A

Diagram showing the filaments that comprise the cytoskeletonor "backbone" of living cells

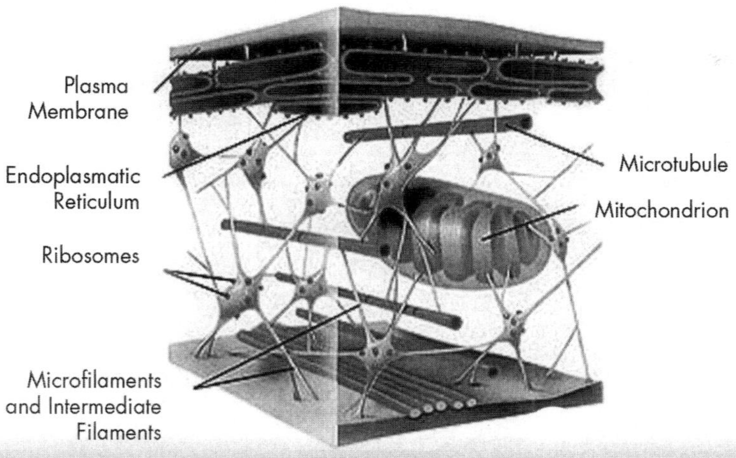

Note: these are laboratory experiments. It cannot be directly construed that oleuropein cures cancer. The oleuropein used in the laboratory tests was a pure grade. Oleuropein only represents a small amount of the olive. Olive leaf extracts, as dietary supplements, also provide small amounts of oleuropein and often to do not provide the amount of oleuropein listed on the label.

Killing cancer cells is not the *"gold standard"* to measure effectiveness of proposed cancer cures. Survival is the only valid measure of the effectiveness of a given cancer treatment. Harsh treatments such as radiation or chemotherapy kill many cancer cells, but their side effects often lead to the demise of the patient. In an experiment rodents who had experimental tumors were then given 1% oleuropein in their drinking water. Tumors regressed and disappeared. The unusual high survival rate is noted in the chart on the opposite page. Some animals continued to produce offspring after treatment.

Lycopene

This is another molecule, mostly derived from tomatoes, that is fast becoming the first molecule to conquer prostate cancer, and it's not a drug. Modern pharmacology doesn't have a molecule to compare to it. However, despite its remarkable performance so far in controlled studies, there are reasons why it hasn't reached its full potential to prevent or treat prostate cancer. In this report you will find how to make lycopene work for you, what dosage to consume, how to take lycopene for optimal absorption, and where you can obtain the most concentrated sources.

Lycopene provides the redness in tomatoes, watermelons and pink grapefruits, and is found in over 40 different plants. There is a plant source that can deliver 17 times more lycopene than tomatoes, but few prostate cancer patients know about it. It could save the lives of many prostate cancer sufferers. You'll find out more about that lycopene source below.

Lycopene is a targeted, fat-soluble antioxidant that protects fatty tissues, such as the breast, testes, liver and adrenal glands. In nature, it protects fruits from destruction by solar radiation. In humans, it has exhibited remarkable properties. Here is what lycopene has accomplished so far in the war against prostate cancer.

→ When 30 mg of lycopene were given to men with newly diagnosed prostate cancer, they had smaller tumors than men who weren't given lycopene and their tumors were more likely to remain localized rather than spread. [Experimental Biology Medicine 227: 881-85, 2002]

→ Two to four servings of tomato sauce, rich in lycopene, per week, results in a significant drop in prostate cancer risk. [Experimental Biology Medicine 227: 852-509, 2002]

→ The consumption of 30 mg of lycopene per day results in less DNA damage to prostate tissues. Prostate Specific Antigen (PSA), a marker of prostate inflammation, dropped by 17.5%. [Experimental Biology Medicine 227: 886-93, 2002]

→ The provision of tomato powder to rodents, equivalent to 910 mg of lycopene in a 160-pound human, reduced the risk of dying from chemically induced prostate cancer. [CA Cancer Journal Clinicians 54: 68-69, 2004] The aggressiveness of prostate tumors is associated with low consumption of lycopene. [Cancer Research 59: 1225-30, 1999]

→ While other colored plant pigments are powerful antioxidants, such as beta carotene and lutein, only lycopene exerts protection against prostate cancer. [Journal National Cancer Institute 87: 1767-76, 1995]

→ Lycopene works by interference with growth signals (insulin growth factor-1) in prostate cancer cells. [Nutrition Cancer 36: 101-11, 2000]

→ A group of men with diagnosed prostate cancer underwent surgical removal of their testicles plus lycopene supplementation, or surgery alone. Six months following surgery, PSA levels were almost three times lower (9.1 versus 26.4) in the group that consumed lycopene. In the six-month period, 22% of the men who underwent surgery died, compared to only 13% who underwent surgery plus lycopene supplementation. [British Journal Urology 92: 375-78, 2003]

→ Lycopene appears to take the aggressiveness out of prostate cancer. There is a greater reduction in mortality and risk for aggressive prostate cancer with increasing lycopene intake. [American Journal Epidemiology 155: 1023-32, 2002]

→ Lycopene also inhibits parathyroid hormone. Elevated levels of this hormone accelerate cancer cell growth. [J Medicinal Food 6:69-78, 2003]

→ The provision of just 4 mg of lycopene to men with pre-cancerous prostate cells, delays or prevents fully developed prostate cancer without side effects. [Urological Oncology 23: 383-85, 2005]

→ In China, a study found that the highest consumption of lycopene conferred an astounding 82% relative risk reduction for prostate cancer among those in the highest intake group. [International Journal Cancer 113: 1010-14, 2005]

Scientists have already confirmed the superiority of lycopene in the prostate gland. Among all antioxidants analyzed, only blood plasma lycopene concentration is significantly lower in prostate cancer cases than in healthy males. [Journal Nutrition 134: 3486-92S, 2004; Cancer Research 59: 1225-30, 1999]

Some of the prostate cancer rates around the world are:

Country	Incidence Rate of Prostate Cancer (per 100,000)	Blood Plasma lycopene concentration**
U.S. (African American)*	137	
U.S. (Caucasian) *	101	
Canada	65	
Sweden	55	0.52
Australia	53	
Norway	48	
U.S. (Japanese)	47	
France	44	
Finland	41	
Germany	36	0.59-0.63
Denmark	31	0.59-0.63
England	28	0.72 1.01 vegetarian
Spain	27	
Israel	24	
Yugoslavia	21	
U.S. (Chinese)	20	
Italy	12	1.02-1.30
China	10	
Japan	9	
India	8	

**Higher numbers may be explained in part by better detection methods*
*** Journal Nutrition 135: 2032S, 2005*

Lycopene disappoints

Lycopene Intake – Relative Risk Of Prostate Cancer					
Relative risk of prostate cancer	1	0.9	0.94	0.89	0.79
Daily lycopene intake	Less than 2.2 mg	2.2-3.6 mg	3.4-4.6 mg	4.6-6.5 mg	More than 6.5 mg

According to the above chart, the relative risk of prostate cancer is only moderately reduced with increasing lycopene consumption. A downward trend is established with greater daily lycopene intake. But how far down could these numbers go if a potent lycopene supplement were offered that was highly absorbable?

Surprisingly, a study involving data from 44 countries found no correlation between tomato consumption and prostate cancer. [International Journal of Cancer, 98: 262-267, 2002] The problem with this kind of study is that it often hides subgroups within countries that exhibit significantly lower prostate cancer risk. For example, tomato consumption in Italy ranges from 49 to 175 grams annually, a three-fold variation. Furthermore, Italians are likely to use processed tomatoes, such as tomato sauce or paste, which provides more concentrated sources of lycopene and use olive oil with their meals, which enhances absorption of lycopene.

When researchers combined the results of 21 studies they found lycopene plays a preventive role against prostate cancer, but the effect was statistically modest. [Cancer Epidemiology Biomarkers Prevention 13: 340-45, 2004] There is good reason for this.

First, most of these are dietary intake studies. Data on dietary consumption of lycopene is inconsistent. Some sources estimate daily consumption to be as much as 16.15 mg per day; others say 8 mg, 5.2 mg or 3.7 mg. These are trivial amounts and would hardly be expected to weigh in against prostate tumors that have been developing for decades. Yet, about 20 to30% of males have pre-cancerous cells in the prostate gland by age 30.

Blood levels of lycopene

Blood plasma levels of lycopene vary by a factor of four (0.22 to 1.06 nanomole/ milliliter). Intake of tomatoes may not deliver significant amounts of the right form of lycopene to the prostate gland because of the type of tomato product (processed or raw), co-administration with oil or fat for absorption, and number of cholesterol particles available for transport.

Other studies state the lycopene concentration in blood serum has been recorded as high as 2.58 nanomole from foods. But supplementation could potentially raise this figure even further. [Archives Biochemistry Biophysics 336: 1-9, 1996] Furthermore, lycopene from tomato paste raises blood levels 2.5 times greater than eating fresh tomatoes. [Proc Society Exp Biology Medicine 218: 121-23, 1998]

Dietary lycopene intake

The majority of lycopene intake (~82%) by American men is from a single source, tomatoes.

According to the U.S. Department of Agriculture, the average American consumes about 18 pounds of fresh tomatoes and 69 pounds of processed tomato products annually. Watermelon, pink grapefruit and other fruits also provide

Product	Lycopene Milligrams per 100 grams	Serving Size b	Lycopene (mg /serving)
Tomato Juice	9.3	240 mL (1 cup)	22.9
Tomato Ketchup	17	15 mL (1 tbsp)	2.9
Spaghetti Sauce	16	125 g (1/2 cup)	20
Tomato Paste	29.3	30 g (2 tbsp)	8.8
Tomato Soup (Condensed)	10.9	245 g (1 cup prepared)	13.1
Tomato Sauce	15.9	60 g (1/4 cup)	9.6
Watermelon	4.9	280 g (~1/16 of a watermelon)	13.6
Pink Grapefruit	1.5	154 g (1/2 medium)	2.3
Raw Tomato	3	148 g (1 medium)	4.5

Sources: USDA-NCC Carotenoid Database for U.S. Foods – 1998 and other sources

small amounts of lycopene. Just 2-4 servings of tomatoes per week, or just 6-8 mg of lycopene per day, has a preventive effect. [Journal Nutrition 134: 3486-92S, 2004]

Lycopene prostate concentration

There is about a 10-fold variance in lycopene concentration in the prostate gland. There is significant inter-individual variation, meaning these are ways to enhance utilization and delivery of lycopene to the prostate gland. [Cancer Epidemiology Biomarkers Prevention 5: 823-33, 1996] Learning how to preserve, enhance absorption and transport lycopene to the prostate gland might save your life.

Stability of lycopene

Lycopene only has a 10 -14-day half life (time it takes for half of it to degrade). If it is consumed, it will remain in the body for about two weeks.

Lycopene powder degrades when exposed to light, oxygen and heat, by as much as 40 % in two days when placed in a lab dish. [Journal National Cancer Institute 95: 1578-86, 2003]

U.S. Department of Agriculture experts declare that "*extraction, storage, handling and analysis of lycopene have to be carried out under controlled environmental factors not only to minimize oxidative degradation, but also to avoid the introduction of other isomers. Exposure of extracted lycopene to light should be avoided, and only yellow or red lights used. Other antioxidants should be used for stabilization. Nitrogen should be used to flush air space in containers.*" But is any of this meticulously attended to in the production of lycopene supplements? These protective measures are not evident in current products. Significant loss of lycopene in tomato pulp samples occurs in the presence of oxygen, with or without light. Lycopene is more stable in native fruit tissues than in purified form. However, the heating of tomato into a paste increases its concentration and bioavailability when consumed with oil. [Food Technology 53: 38-45, 1999]

There are various forms, or what are called isomers, of lycopene. The two major forms are called *cis* and *trans.*

Tomato products primarily consist of all-*trans* lycopene (35-96%). Cis lycopene accounts for 79-88% of the total lycopene in malignant tissues. [Journal Nutrition 134: 3486-92S, 2004] This is probably because all-*trans* lycopene has been altered into the cis form.

Dosage of lycopene

Forms of lycopene

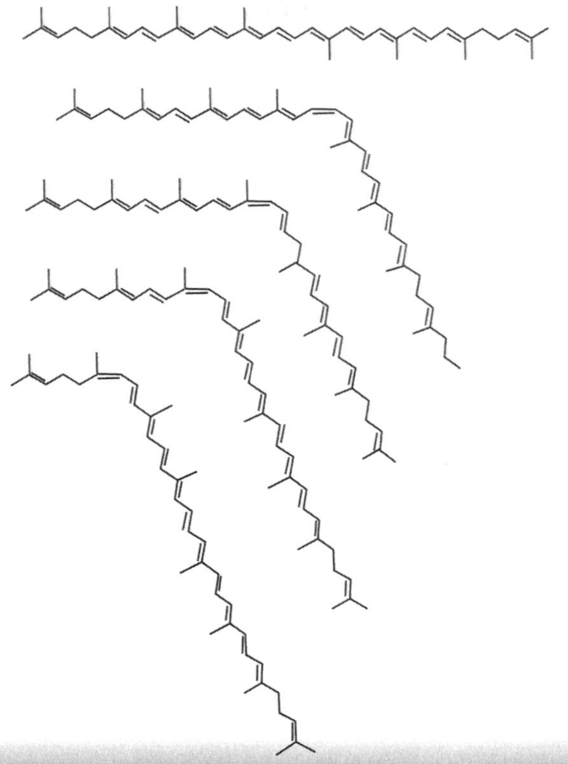

Studies appear to confirm that *trans* lycopene is the desired form of lycopene in the body. When no lycopene is consumed, all-trans lycopene levels decrease while cis lycopene increases. When tomato products are resumed, this is reversed. [Journal Nutrition 134: 3486-92S, 2004] There is some evidence that trans lycopene converts to cis lycopene in the body. [Journal of the American College of Nutrition 19: 563-569, 2000] However, trans lycopene is poorly absorbed, which has led researchers into thinking the cis form in dietary supplements is more desirable.

Trans lycopene should be considered the preferred form since it is predominant in food and the most heat stable. The provision of oils with trans lycopene can enhance absorption.

A recent study showed that 10 mg of lycopene given to males with metastatic prostate cancer produced a significant drop in PSA count. [Urological Oncology 22: 415-20, 2004]

However, according to Dr. Venket Rao of the University of Toronto, daily consumption of tomato products providing at least 40 mg of lycopene through processed tomato products substantially reduces low-density lipoprotein oxidation. [Lipids 33:981-4, 1998] LDL cholesterol is what transports lycopene. The two nutrients work hand-in-hand. Obviously, lycopene is a strong antioxidant that offers health benefits beyond cancer prevention.

One study showed that men who consumed 18.78 mg of lycopene daily reduced their relative risk for prostate cancer by 16 % compared to men who consumed just 3.42 mg. [Journal National Cancer Institute 94: 391-94, 2002] The American diet provides ~8 mg of lycopene daily, so supplements would appear to be beneficial, though tomato paste and tomato juice are excellent sources as well.

Thirty-milligrams of lycopene daily obtained from a variety of food sources has been shown to increase blood levels by three times. [Canadian Journal Dietary Practice Research 65: 161-65, 2004]

With all of these reports to analyse, readers are likely to ask, *"so how much lycopene do the studies say to consume?"* The answer is, as much as you can get, in highly absorbable forms.

Sources of lycopene

According to the US Department of Agriculture, tomato paste provides 29 mg of lycopene per 100 grams (~3.5 oz), compared to 16 mg in tomato sauce, 17 mg in ketchup and just 3 mg in a raw tomato. [Journal Nutrition 135: 2042S-45, 2005]

Food	Serving	Lycopene (milligrams)
Tomato juice	1 cup	20 mg
Pasta sauce	½ cup	19 mg
Tomato puree	½ cup	18 mg
Tomato sauce	½ cup	17 mg
Tomato soup	1 cup	12 mg
Tomato paste	1 ounce	8 mg
Watermelon	4 ounce	6 mg
Fresh tomato	4 ounce	4 mg
Pink grapefruit	4 ounce	2 mg

Lycopene from tomato paste is 2.5 times more bioavailable than fresh tomatoes. [American Journal Clinical Nutrition 66: 116-22, 1997]

Absorption of lycopene

About 10% to30% of lycopene is absorbed from foods. This is a wide variation and suggests there must be influencing factors.

Absorption of lycopene is enhanced when consumed with oil or fat. Lycopene supplements that are encapsulated in soft-gel capsules and are accompanied by oil will exhibit better absorption.

Alcohol lowers concentrations of lycopene in prostate tissue. [Cancer Epidemiology Biomarkers Prevention 5: 823-33, 1996]

The lycopene content of tomato products remains unchanged during the production of juice or paste and remains stable for up to 12 months of storage at ambient temperature. However, subjecting tomato juice to cooking temperatures in the presence of corn oil results in the formation of the cis isomeric form, which is more bioavailable, but not necessarily the most desirable form. [Journal Medicinal Food 4: 9-15, 2001]

In a controlled study, healthy adults were given lycopene-rich tomato juice, tomato oleoresin or a lycopene beadlet supplement containing 70-75 mg lycopene, for four weeks for each source. The concentration of lycopene in the oral tissues (cheek) doubled over this time period with beadlet and oleoresin forms of lycopene, but not with tomato juice treatment. [American Journal Clinical Nutrition 70: 490-94, 1999]

Companion nutrients

It is difficult to expect a single nutrient like lycopene to eradicate prostate cancer. In one lab dish study, lycopene was not found to be a potent inhibitor of prostate cancer cells, but when vitamin E was simultaneously added to lycopene, a strong inhibition of cancer cell multiplication, nearly 90%, was observed. [Biochemistry Biophysical Research Communications 250: 582-55, 1998]

Not only does olive oil enhance absorption of lycopene, with its antioxidant polyphenols, it also works synergistically to raise antioxidant power when combined with lycopene. [Free Radical Biology Medicine 29: 1051-55, 2000]

Hormonal factors

To underscore the importance of combining other therapies with lycopene to enhance its effectiveness, researchers at the University of Illinois in Urbana report that castration of male rodents *"profoundly increases lycopene levels in the liver."* Castration also decreases food consumption. Food restriction further reduces testosterone levels and increases liver lycopene levels. Castrated rodents accumulated nearly twice as much lycopene in their liver as untreated animals. Lycopene must reach the liver in order to be transported to distant tissues like the prostate. [Journal Nutrition 131: 1746-52, 2001] The co-provision of lycopene with dietary supplements that inhibit testosterone levels, such as lignans from flaxmeal, may be desirable.

Lycopene supplements

In one study, the provision of tomato powder and pure synthetic lycopene tomato beadlets produced the same blood concentrations even though the beadlets (small beads rather than fine powder) contained 10 times more lycopene. The tomato powder was made from tomato paste that included seeds and skins and included a small amount of fat, which probably aided absorption. [Journal National Cancer Institute 95: 1578-85, 2003] In an animal study, the tomato powder produced a 26% drop in the lethal form of prostate cancer versus only a mild decline with the tomato supplement beadlets. [Journal National Cancer Institute 95: 1563-65, 2003] This report speaks loudly to say that lycopene supplements leave something to be desired. It spawned news headlines that said: *"Tomato supplements may not affect cancer."* - Reuters Nov. 4, 2003

When dietary supplement manufacturers submitted an application to the Food & Drug Administration regarding a claim that lycopene inhibits prostate and other malignancies, the application was turned down. The supplement companies cried foul.

The FDA responded to the appeal by saying that it is mulling over the idea of accepting a health claim for lycopene as follows: *"Prostate Cancer - Very limited and preliminary scientific research suggests that eating one-half to one cup of tomatoes and/or tomato sauce a week may reduce the risk of prostate cancer. FDA concludes that there is little scientific evidence supporting this claim."* [FDA Docket No. 2004Q-0201]

The supplement manufacturers can't figure out why their health claims have been denied when it's obvious their lycopene products aren't stable and don't provide the same consistent benefits as tomato paste or tomato paste-powder.

So what should a cancer patient do? There are some other ways to optimize lycopene for health.

One is to incorporate tomato paste and other processed tomato products into the diet, and use with oils like virgin olive oil, along with vitamin E and flaxseed meal, to enhance absorption and antioxidant activity while calming hormone levels.

Another option is to find more concentrated sources of lycopene. Agricultural researchers were caught unawares when they found a fruit that contains 17 times more lycopene than tomatoes. The fruit is autumn olive (botanical name: *Elaeagnus Umbellata)* that produces a small red berry that grows like a shrub. It is native to China but also grows on the east coast of the United States. Autumn olives contain 30 to 50 mg of lycopene per 100 grams, or about 20% of its total weight is lycopene, and it is high in phenols, other potent antioxidants. For comparison, 100 grams of tomatoes provide about 4.2 mg of lycopene. [US Agriculture Research Service, 2001]

Garlic

The public popularly believes garlic is good for health and helps prevent cancer. This is true. But the use of garlic pills comes into question for cancer prevention or treatment because most don't release much allicin, its major anti-cancer ingredient. However, there are other anti-cancer molecules in garlic and there are ways that cancer patients can enhance garlic's properties.

As early as 1949 it was demonstrated that garlic has anti-cancer properties. [Preventive Medicine 19: 346-61, 1990] Yet garlic is not employed in prevention or treatment regimens. There may be good reasons why.

Garlic has tremendous potential to prevent and treat cancer. But it often falls short of accomplishing this because of processing, heating, acidity and other factors.

Dietary studies

Garlic in foods is good for cancer prevention. Population studies as well as laboratory studies have shown that garlic consumption reduces certain cancer incidences in the stomach, colon, breast, and cervix, etc. [Critical Review Food Science Nutrition 44:479-88, 2004]

A number of studies indicate the consumption of garlic reduces the risk of stomach cancer. [Asian Pac J Cancer Prevention 6:387-95, 2005] Both raw and cooked garlic appear to protect against colon/rectal cancer. [American Journal Clinical Nutrition 72: 1047-52, 2000]

In areas of China where high amounts of garlic are consumed, there is a much lower rate of gastric cancer (3.45 per 100,000 in high-garlic consumption areas versus 40.0 per 100,000 in low-garlic consumption areas). [Medical Tribune, August, 12, 1981]

It has been said that humans would have to eat their own weight in garlic before gaining any health benefits. However, researchers at the Ruakura Agricultural Research Centre in New Zealand dispel this notion, and show that just a half a clove a day of raw garlic exhibits anti-cancer properties. If cooked, 4-5 cloves of garlic would be needed. The active ingredient was identified as diallyl sulfide, which increased the levels of protective detoxifying enzymes (quinone reductase and glutathione transferase) by up to 60 % in animals. [Nutrition & Cancer 34: 42-48, 1999]

Garlic's action

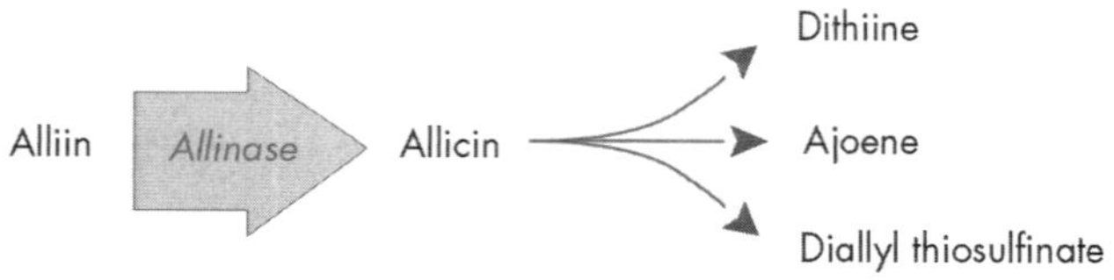

When a garlic clove is crushed, compartments within the clove that contain alliin are mixed with the enzyme alliinase to form allicin, the main, but not sole, active ingredient in garlic.

Allicin is a stealth molecule, able to penetrate through all cell membranes, which is why garlic odor is apparent on the skin hours after consumption. Researchers at Ben-Gurion University in Israel have demonstrated that allicin inhibits the ability of cancer cells to multiply by its ability to selectively deplete glutathione from inside tumor cells. [Nutrition & Cancer 38: 245-54, 2000] Glutathione is a sulfur-based antioxidant produced within cells.

The anti-tumor effect of allicin is also related to its immune-stimulatory properties. [International Immunology 16:275-81, 2004] Allicin, being a small molecule, can enter cellular machinery and influence a gene known as p21, which stimulates the immune system by increasing white blood cell production. [International Immunology 16: 275-81, 2004]

Allicin Diallyl thiosulfinate

Allicin Diallyl thiosulfinate

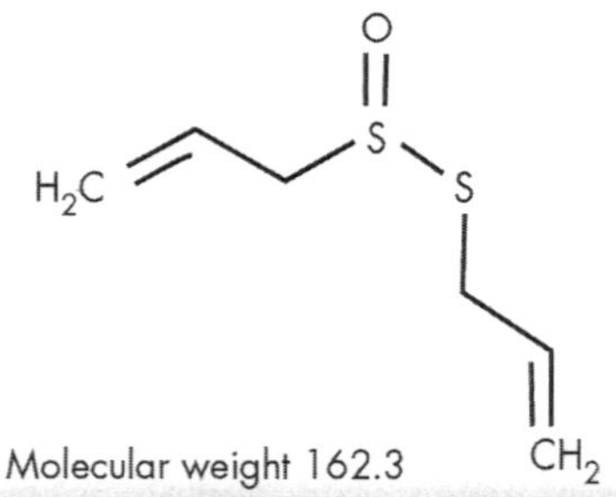

Molecular weight 162.3

Weaponizing allicin

In recognition of the known anti-cancer action of allicin, researchers at the Weizmann Institute of Science in Israel recently developed a targeted way to utilize allicin in cancer therapy. But they had to overcome the rapid degradation of allicin by stomach acid. To do this, first, they chemically attached alliinase with an antibody. Alliinase is the enzyme required with alliin to produce allicin. The alliinase plus antibody was injected into tumor cells in a lab dish.

The antibody was specific for a tumor antigen on the surface of the tumor. This would aim the alliinase directly at tumor cells and not healthy cells. Then alliin was introduced into the lab dish, mimicking what happens in a garlic clove when it is crushed and the alliin/ alliinase mix produces allicin. [Molecular Cancer Therapeutics 2: 1295-1301, 2003] Hopefully this can become a new cancer treatment in the near future.

Other garlic molecules

Garlic (*Allium sativum*) is metabolized into a dizzying list of other molecules (N-aceryl-S-allyl cysteine, allyl mercaptan, diallyl disulfide, diallyl sulfide, diallyl sulfoxide, diallyl sulfone, and allyl methyl sulfide). [Critical Review Food Science Nutrition 44:479-88, 2004] While allicin is considered to be the chief active molecule in garlic, other sulfur molecules, especially diallyl disulfide, also exhibit anti-cancer properties. [Neoplasma 48: 307-12, 2001]

Diallyl disulfide (DADS), one of the major components of garlic, is well known to have anti-cancer properties. [Food Chemistry Toxicology 42:1543-52, 2004] In rodents, DADS inhibits chemically induced carcinogenesis in the colon. DADS anti-promoting effect may result partly from its ability to inhibit tumor cell multiplication. DADS may also influence the expression of a subset of genes. [Carcinogenesis 25:1227-36, 2004]

DADS also inhibits estrogen-positive breast tumor growth. Diallyl disulfide also works synergistically with omega-3 oils to inhibit breast cancer cell growth. [Carcinogenesis 22: 891-97, 2001]

Researchers in India found diallyl disulfide inhibits the growth of prostate cancer cells in a dose-dependent manner. Diallyl disulfide worked by inducing apoptosis, the slow die- off of prostate cancer cells. [Biological Pharm Bulletin 28:740-3, 2005]

Aged garlic

Aged garlic has a major antioxidant compound (S-allylcysteine) that inhibits the growth of chemically induced tumors in animals. [Current Cancer Drug Targets 3: 67-81, 2003] Aged garlic extract (AGE) has been shown to inhibit both the growth and migration of tumor cells in a laboratory dish. [International J Molecular Medicine 9:641-3, 2002]

In order to confirm the effects of AGE on colon/rectal adenomas (benign epithelial tumors having a glandular origin and structure), researchers provided 2.4 and 0.16 milliliters of AGE per day to patients diagnosed with adenomas. The number and size of these pre-cancerous tumors were determined before and 12 months after intake by direct observation with a colonoscopy. Nearly 48% of the high-AGE group, and 67% of the low AGE group developed at least one new adenoma within the first year. The results of this study suggest the possibility of preventive and therapeutic effects of AGE on colorectal adenomas, though it is necessary to investigate these in larger-scale and longer-term trials. [Hiroshima J Medical Science 53:39-45, 2004]

Garlic and H. pylori

A bacterium called *Helicobacter pylori* is the major cause of gastric ulcers and stomach cancer. Allicin and other allicin breakdown molecules (allyl-methyl plus methyl-allyl thiosulfinate from acetonic garlic) inhibit the growth of H. pylori. Exposure of allicin to heat will negate its ability to kill *H. pylori.* [Biotechnol Progress 20:397-401, 2004]

Consumers may read that garlic oil may kill *H. pylori.* While undiluted garlic oil does exhibit the ability to kill off *H. pylori* in a laboratory dish [Applied Environmental Microbiology 66: 2269-73, 2000], actual human use of garlic oil does not inhibit *H. pylori.* [Helicobacter 6: 249-53, 2001]

Drug resistance

Tumor cells develop resistance to anti-cancer drugs. They do this by overproducing a protein (P-glycoprotein) that energizes tumor cells so they can efficiently pump out anti-cancer drugs as they enter. Diallyl sulfide, a breakdown product of allicin, decreases P-glycoprotein activity back to normal in a laboratory study. This garlic component could be coupled with anti-cancer drugs to inhibit drug resistance. [Carcinogenesis 25: 941-49, 2004]

Garlic, blood clotting and cancer

Micro blood clots facilitate the spread of cancer by creating a stoppage of cancer cells within small blood capillaries, which then causes tumor cells to accumulate and invade surrounding tissues, what is known as a metastasis. It is critical to prevent metastasis because it is the chief mortality factor in 90% of cancer cases.

Garlic is known as a good blood clot inhibitor. Thromboxane is a factor that facilitates the clotting of blood. When a fresh clove of garlic was given to middle-aged males there was an 80% reduction in thromboxane. [Prostaglandins Leukot Essent Fatty Acids 53:211-2, 1995]

It is difficult to ascertain the blood-clot inhibiting properties of most garlic pills. [Thrombosis Research 65: 141-56, 1992] Garlic is a more potent blood clot inhibitor in its raw form. [Prostaglandins Leukotrienes Essential Fatty Acids 60: 43-47, 1999] Raw garlic exhibits a blood thinning effect for up to 12 hours after ingestion. [Atherosclerosis 38: 417-21, 1981]

Telomeres, garlic and cancer

Telomeres, the "end caps" of chromosomes
Image credit: Robert Moyzis,
University of California, Irvine, CA;
U.S. Department of Energy Human Genome Program,
http://www.ornl.gov/hgmis.

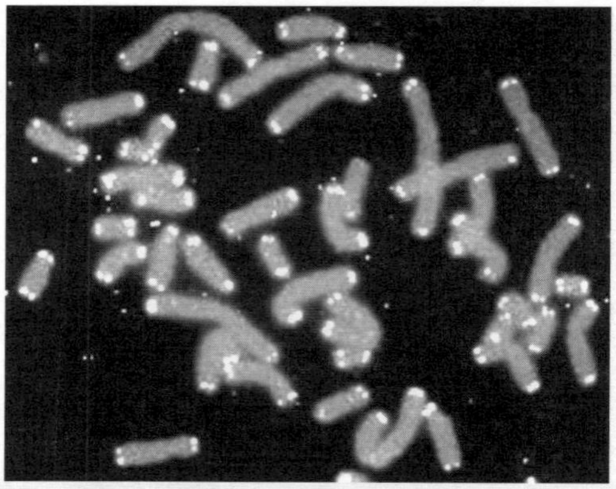

Chromosomes have end caps called telomeres. Telomerase is an enzyme that repairs broken telomeres and extends the life of cells. Since cancer cells are immortal, the inhibition of telomerase could induce cell death and combat a widely variety of cancers. Allicin effectively inhibits telomerase, blocks the division of tumor cells and can be used to treat cancer. In lab studies, allicin reduces tumor incidence and survival is prolonged. Allicin induces apoptosis, the slow die off of tumor cells. Of additional interest, the anti-cancer/ anti-HIV drug AZT also inhibits telomerase. Allicin is superior to AZT and is far less expensive. [World Journal Gastroenterology 9: 1930-34, 2003]

Garlic and medications

Garlic inhibits detoxifying enzymes in the liver (cytochrome p450) and therefore may be beneficial or harmful when simultaneously taken with medications. The medications may work too well and cause side effects, or be more effective, depending upon the drug. [Journal Pharmaceutical Sciences 4: 176-84, 2001]

Garlic tolerability

Home production of fresh crushed garlic may provide very potent allicin dosage, more potent than most garlic pills. However, pure allicin is a strong oxidant and can damage the lining in the stomach, which is why the consumption of a fresh clove of garlic is often following by a painful stomach ache. Liquid lecithin, a neutral pH emulsifying agent, may help to buffer the pungency of fresh crushed garlic. Cuisinart® Custom Prep 11TM Food Processor is able to process a clove of garlic.

Which garlic product?

Various garlic preparations exhibit anti-cancer properties, including fresh crushed garlic cloves, fresh garlic extract, aged garlic, garlic oil, and other sulfur compounds derived from garlic.

The question is, which is the best way to consume garlic: fresh, cooked or aged? [Critical Review Food Science Nutrition 44:479-88, 2004]

Garlic processing

A study was designed to compare several garlic powders with various levels of alliin, a precursor of active sulfur compounds, for their ability to prevent cancer. Rodents were fed diets with three garlic powders with various alliin contents. The garlic powders were obtained from bulbs grown on soils with different levels of sulfur fertilization. A cancer-causing chemical (aflatoxin) was injected into the animals. A strong reduction of pre-cancerous growths was observed in rodents fed garlic powder that contained the highest level of alliin. This study highlights the possibility of controlling the cultivation conditions to improve the cancer-fighting properties of garlic. [Carcinogenesis 25:1953-59, 2004]

Garlic pills

Most garlic pills have a very different composition than what is claimed by their manufacturer. Some claim to provide allicin, or "*certified allicin*," or "*allicin potential*." But the fact is, garlic pills don't have any real allicin in them.They have the potential to produce allicin once they enter the digestive tract, if stomach acid doesn't destroy the alliinase enzyme that is needed to make allicin.

Allicin production in garlic pills is determined by dissolving powdered garlic in water at room temperature and measuring the allicin content after 30 minutes. But the stomach is acidic, not like water which has a neutral pH. So this measurement is flawed. Allicin is stable at the higher pH (above pH 4.0) found in the intestine, but decomposes readily at a stomach pH of 1.2-2.0 to 5% of initial levels after 30 minutes. (Journal of Nutrition. 131:968S-971S, 2001.)

At pH 3 or below, the acidic environment usually found in the stomach, alliin cannot be converted to allicin because the alliinase enzyme is destroyed by stomach acid. Most garlic pills are tested in water for allicin yield, not under the acidic conditions found in the stomach. Heating garlic before it is consumed also destroys alliinase. [Journal Nutrition 131: 1054-57S, 2001] Garlic pills are usually coated to pass through the acid stomach before they begin to mix alliin and alliinase in the intestines to produce allicin.

Enteric-coated garlic pills are usually not well formulated. Many pass all the way through the digestive tract before opening up. Most brands yield less than 15% of their labeled potential. Garlicin is one brand of garlic pill that did pass tests. [Journal Agriculture Food Chemistry 49: 2592-99, 2001]

Even if garlic pills contain stable allicin, they lose their potency over time on the store shelf. Most garlic pills lose more than 50% of their effectiveness over a period of 18 months. [Journal Pharmaceutical and Biomedical Analysis 37: 963-70, 2005]

To product allicin, the main cancer-fighting molecule in a garlic clove, the clove must be crushed to mix alliin with alliinase to produce allicin. A crushed glove of garlic will yield about 5,000 mcg of allicin, and if processed in a food blender, about 12,000 mcg of allicin will be produced.

Once allicin is formed by crushing a fresh clove of garlic, it is unstable and half of it will disappear within 2-16 hours; as garlic juice it may last up to 2.4 days. Refrigeration increases the life of allicin by a factor of 20.

A remarkable new type of garlic powder, called Garli-eze® (Nutra Products®) is derived from high-allicin yield garlic powder mixed with a patented array of alkaline minerals to buffer the contents of a garlic pill as it enters the acidic stomach. The alkaline minerals prevent stomach acid from destroying alliinase long enough for allicin to be produced. This is a world's first. Garli-eze garlic powder has been shown in independent lab testing to produce as much allicin as a fresh clove of garlic (around 5,000 mcg per garlic pill). This is the first time a garlic pill has reliably been shown to produce allicin without the need for enteric coating of the capsule.

Mistletoe (Iscador)

Cancer patients often wonder whether there are more effective treatments available outside their own country. Once such treatment, which originates from Germany, is mistletoe extract. A survey in Germany showed up to 50 % of women with cancer who used alternative cancer treatments used mistletoe extract. [Archives Gynecology Obstetrics 258: 81-88, 1996]

Mistletoe extract, also called Iscador, Helixor, Eurixor, and Isorel, works by elevating natural killer cell and interleukin activity. Natural killer cells and interleukin are a natural part of the human immune system. [Toxicology 207: 105-16, 2005]

In animal tests, rodents lived 71% longer and experienced shrinkage of experimental tumors when injected with mistletoe extract. [Anticancer Drugs 8: S15-16, 1997] In another animal study, the feeding of oral mistletoe extract resulted in the disappearance of experimentally induced non-Hodgkin's lymphoma tumors in 4 of 15 mice. [Cancer Detection Prevention 28: 52-56, 2004]

Use of mistletoe extract for cancer patients has never been shown to be harmful, but its effectiveness has been questioned.

In 1983, the American Cancer Society claimed it did not have evidence that treatment with mistletoe extracts are beneficial for patients with cancer and *"strongly urged individuals afflicted with cancer not to participate in treatments using mistletoe."* [CA Cancer Journal Clinicians 33: 186-88, 1983] This is an example of the duplicity exhibited by cancer authorities. The unproven is dismissed in favor of the disproven. Twenty years later intensive study of mistletoe is underway because conventional cancer treatments have failed miserably.

In 1989, British surgeons reported that a patient with small cell lung cancer, which is usually very aggressive, opted to receive mistletoe extract instead of chemotherapy and survived five years and seven months beyond the date of diagnosis, far longer than expected. [Thorax 44: 1047-48, 1989] So, despite its skeptics, mistletoe therapy persists.

A crude survey of patients with blood and lymphatic cancer showed that patients lived 11.4 years after mistletoe extract treatment and only 8.6 years without it, but it is not known whether the patients in both groups were in similar stages of cancer. [Forsch Komplementarmed Lkass Naturheilkd 7: 139-46, 2000]

In another study where cancer patients were matched in pairs for type and stage of cancer, the patients receiving mistletoe extracts survived about 4.23 years compared to 3.05 years among patients who didn't receive mistletoe extract. [Alternative Therapy Health Medicine 7: 57-66, 68-72, 2001] For comparison, some widely promoted anti-cancer drugs like Erbitux only extend life by an average of four months and cost $48,000.

A survey of German physicians found that the probability to achieve complete or partial remissions with mistletoe extract was estimated to be 6% and 15% respectively. [Disch Med Wochenschr 125: 1222-26, 2000]

A study of patients who had undergone bladder cancer surgery did not find that mistletoe extract significantly delayed recurrence of cancer. [Journal Urology 168: 72-75, 2002]

In 2002, a German medical journal reported that mistletoe therapy has not gained an established placed in the treatment of cancer and no overall improvement in survival had been reported. [Onkologie 25: 374-80, 2002]

However, a review of 23 published studies suggests further investigation of mistletoe extract be continued [European Journal Medical Research 8: 109-19, 2003], and a study using genetically engineered mistletoe has entered human clinical trials. [Drug Discovery Today 8: 52-53, 2003]

More recently, researchers in Germany instilled mistletoe extract into the bladder of patients who had undergone bladder cancer surgery and reported that it was equally as effective in preventing recurrence of bladder tumors as another widely used drug (bacillus Calmette-Guerin BCG). [Journal Urology 174: 76-79, 2005]

Then again, German researchers confirmed that mistletoe therapy is relatively safe, prolongs survival among malignant melanoma patients and even prevents the spread of tumors to other locations. [Arzneimittleforschung 55: 38-49, 2005]

Some 85 years after mistletoe was first proposed for the treatment of cancer by Rudolph Steiner, an Austrian Swiss Physician, mistletoe is slowly becoming a part of modern cancer treatment. While not generally considered a complete cure for cancer, it exhibits ability to shrink tumors and prevent metastasis.

Licorice

Licorice is an herbal medicine that has multiple applications against cancer. [Nutrition & Cancer 39: 1-11, 2001] It inhibits the growth of *H. pylori*, the bacterium that causes gastric ulcers and tumors. [Life Sciences 71: 1449-63, 2002] Licorice inhibits the growth of viruses, and therefore may be beneficial for individuals with herpes or papilloma viruses that can sometimes trigger tumors. Some researchers now think licorice kills viruses rather than just keeping them dormant. [Journal Clinical Investigation 115: 591-93, 2005] Licorice inhibits testosterone, so it may have applications for the treatment or prevention of prostate cancer. [European Urology 43: 580-86, 2003] Since licorice molecules inhibit the production of melanin, it may be beneficial in the treatment or prevention of melanoma. [Pigment Cell Research 11: 355-61, 1998]

Licorice has some drawbacks. High doses of licorice (50,000 mg) could raise blood pressure and deplete potassium. [Journal Human Hypertension 9 345-48, 1995] But most licorice supplements are relatively safe.

Milk thistle

This is a traditional herbal remedy for liver problems that is just now getting recognition for its cancer-fighting properties. A primary way it works against cancer is to bind to loose iron. [Gastroenterology 109: 1941-49, 1995] Surprisingly, silibinin, the active ingredient in silymarin, the extract of milk thistle, is now considered a cancer-preventive agent for skin, cervical, prostate and breast cancer. [Molecular Carcinogenesis 26: 321-33, 1999] It is now in Phase I study for human prostate cancer. [Current Cancer Drug Targets 4: 1-11, 2004]

Researchers now believe silymarin from milk thistle will play a useful role in cancer therapy. [Journal Alternative Medicine 9: 411-16, 2003] It can be used simultaneously with other anti-cancer drugs. [Clinical Cancer Research 8: 3512-19, 2002]

Tumor cells don't grow very well in a lab dish when exposed to silibinin. [Carcinogenesis 23: 499-510, 2002] But this doesn't mean silibinin is a singular cure for cancer.

Milk thistle extract's ability to reduce PSA levels in males is a strong point for this herb. [Journal Urology 171: 1934-38, 2004] Furthermore, it inhibits survivin, a factor that causes tumors to thrive. [Biochemical Biophysical Research Communications 312: 1178-84, 2003] It also has no apparent toxicity. [Mutation Research 555: 21-32, 2004]

Topical applications of silibinin inhibit skin cancer. [International Journal Oncology 26: 169-76, 2005]

Oral silibinin both inhibits tumor growth and counters the toxicity of anti-cancer drugs that are co-administered. [Clinical Cancer Research 10: 8641-47, 2004] Researchers conclude that milk thistle extracts have a *"strong potential to prevent skin cancer."* [European Journal Cancer 41: 1969-79, 2005]

Silymarin is also helpful in preventing toxic side effects from radiation treatment. [Pharmacological Research 45: 447-54, 2002]

Milk thistle is considered an adjunct (secondary) therapy for patients with liver cancer. [Journal Alternative Complementary Medicine 9: 411-16, 2003] It can be used simultaneously with other anti-cancer drugs. [Clinical Cancer Research 8: 3512-19, 2002] It has also been shown to be beneficial for prostate cancer. [Mutation Research 555: 21-32, 2004]

Standardized milk thistle should be used for reliable dosing. Extracts containing 70-80% silymarin are available. Silymarin is a mixture of three herbals: silibinin, quercetin and other plant molecules.

Resveratrol

> *"Ask not what resveratrol can do; ask rather, what resveratrol cannot do."*
> *Source: D. M. Goldberg and G.J. Soleas, Resveratrol: biochemistry, cell biology and the potential role in disease prevention, in Wine, A Scientific Exploration, Sandler and Pinder, Taylor & Francis, New York, 2003.*

A primary theme of this book is that cancer patients have, for the first time, access to more potent anti-cancer molecules than any oncologist can prescribe. It's an unforeseen development, one that even pharmaceutical companies and doctors have not yet fully recognized. A natural molecule called resveratrol serves as a primary example.

Will cancer patients welcome the availability of super anti-cancer molecules that they can purchase off the shelf? It's not a situation many cancer patients or their families are likely to feel comfortable with. If cancer patients elect to wait until their doctor prescribes resveratrol, well, they are going to have a long wait, and they simply haven't the time.

A major task of this book is to get cancer patients to see that modern cancer treatment has failed, that mortality rates are often higher from treatment than from cancer itself, and that they might be better served embarking upon their own treatment regimen. But again, many cancer patients want someone to hold their hand, and a doctor with an MD behind his name provides that level of comfort. Few patients and their families realize that most cancer treatment is designed to shrink tumors, not prolong survival, or is palliative, designed to reduce pain, not to cure the disease. A third of newly diagnosed cancer patients have tumors that have spread to other organs (metastasis), but there is no effective treatment for metastasis. Ninety percent of cancer patients die of metastasis, not the initial tumor. Cancer patients don't know this going in to the doctor's office.

The professor finds a cure for his leukemia

When Professor Hubert, age 87, a retired university professor of plant genetics, was diagnosed with a leukemic condition, he was told he had only weeks to live. Blood transfusions would buy him some time– build up his blood count so he could function. A drug called epoietin was also prescribed to build up his red cells. But he had already lost much of his side vision. He couldn't walk up stairs without feeling faint. He had to stop driving. His hematocrit, a measure of the percent of whole blood that is red blood cells, was down to 7. Normal range for men is 14 to 18.

Professor Hubert said he made a deal with his doctor. He prodded his doctor to tell him his prognosis. *"He showed me the table they use to predict my remaining lifespan,"* he said. That was something that isn't often shared with patients.

> *"None of the doctors have been able to do much. The doctors have been only able to estimate how long I will live, and can only make me comfortable," he said. "I still can't lift anything or walk upstairs. I stumbled at an outdoor event and my friend asked what was wrong. I explained I had cancer."*

Professor Hubert was angry over past events. He had had a kidney failure two years previously from taking too much of a heartburn remedy. *"The pharmaceutical companies didn't tell the doctors a certain number of people would develop kidney problems. So I was placed on EPO (epoetin)."* (This is a drug that boosts red blood cells.)

A friend began sending him emails about resveratrol. *"I asked seven or eight doctors. I have a nephew who is a doctor. None of them knew about it,"* he said.

He read of a European study where resveratrol was being used to prevent cancer. He read of a woman, Johanna Brandt, who wrote a book many years ago entitled *The Grape Cure*, and how grapes cured cancer. What did he have to lose at that point? He began, on his own, to take mega-doses of resveratrol pills. It was March of 2005. He chose a special pill that included resveratrol, quercetin and rice bran extract (Longevinex). When he reached 16 pills a day his hematocrit began to rise.

> *"After I began taking the extra-high doses, I began to improve. I just felt different. I was still weak, but I could go up the stairs without collapsing. I was driving to the hospital and I felt very alert, and seeing more than I had in a long time. My peripheral vision was improved."*

His hematocrit rose above 10, and then to 12, but doctors initially believed this was due to good transfusions. Fewer and fewer blood transfusions were needed. Then the doctors stopped ordering more blood and watched as Professor Hubert went into remission. It was beyond their comprehension. His case was so unusual, one of his doctors wanted to write up the remission and submit it to a medical journal. Leukemia doesn't do an about-face on its own. It was now Christmas and Professor Hubert was feeling well enough to visit art galleries, and enjoy life. Resveratrol was extending his life beyond that of any known technology. How much longer, no one knows. His story is ongoing. He has been in remission now for over over two years.

Professor Hubert is just one of the cancer patients beginning to benefit from discoveries that can only be explained with superlatives.

Small molecules rule

Why did resveratrol work in such a dramatic fashion to reverse Professor Hubert's leukemia? Just a few years ago the entire human genome was mapped. Surprisingly, humans have only 30,000 genes, far less than expected. Small molecules can switch these genes on or off, called gene expression or silencing. Resveratrol is one of these small molecules.

A landmark report in *Nature Magazine* recently stated that most diseases involve many genes. Only one percent of diseases are single-gene disorders. Single-gene targeted anti-cancer drugs like Iressa (gefitinib) and Tarceva (erlotinib) have been disappointing. The report in *Nature Magazine* suggests drugs be used that target many genes.

Resveratrol is one such molecule. It is very small, and is able to be readily absorbed, pass through the cell wall and enter the nucleus of cells where it can manipulate gene expression or silencing. It can cause bundles of genes, called chromatin, to curl up to the point where they are like a computer file that is locked and cannot be read. Resveratrol can put cancer genes to sleep. Hundreds of genes that are required for tumor cells to divide and replicate can be shut off. One cancer researcher described the ability of resveratrol to influence gene-controlled tumor growth as a *"biologically specific tsunami."* [Cancer Biology Therapy 3:889-90, 2004]

Natural compounds from plants like resveratrol address whole mechanisms and sets of pathways that interfere with tumors rather than single enzyme inhibition accomplished through the use of synthetic drugs.

> *"Natural compounds (like resveratrol) .... offer a less specific but perhaps more effective strategy for cancer therapy by inducing combinations of effects that may counteract the metabolic alterations related to cancer promotion,"* says Paolo Signorelli and Riccardo Ghidoni, researchers at San Paolo University Hospital, School of Medicine, in Milan, Italy. [Journal Nutritional Biochemistry 16: 449-66, 2005]

Researchers at the University of Illinois state that *"resveratrol holds great promise for future development as a chemopreventive agent that may be useful for several disorders."* [Annals NY Academy Sciences; 957: 210-29, May 2002]

Given that most cancer patients succumb to the toxic effects of treatment rather than their disease itself, resveratrol's non-toxic and selective ability to kill cancer cells makes it the most desirable of treatments. Resveratrol blocks the three stages of cancer genesis: initiation, promotion and progression. No anti-cancer drug comes even close to doing this. Resveratrol is as close as biologists have come to a cure for cancer. [Journal Nutritional Biochemistry 16: 449-66, 2005]

Resveratrol tackles lymphoma

For Mack, a 57-year-old stock broker, resveratrol was more than reaching for a straw. He had a recurrence of lymphoma that was visible on his neck. He heard the news reports and even spoke with a Harvard professor about resveratrol. Would it be a cure for his lymphoma? It was worth a try. But shortly after he began to take resveratrol pills, a news story claimed red wine pills were not biologically available. A month later another researcher claimed resveratrol could actually cause cancer. He was alarmed. He called this author, practically spitting the resveratrol pills out of his mouth. With assurances, he continued taking the resveratrol, timidly, just one pill a day. [Personal communication]

Months went by. The visible growth on Mack's neck was 3.2 centimeters in size, more than an inch. His doctor had nothing to offer him other than the chemotherapy that didn't work before. He began to learn about nutrition, taking green tea, grape seed, more vitamin D and vitamin C. Then he overcame his fear and began taking more resveratrol pills, three a day. Within three weeks the growth on his neck had shrunk to half its size.

Who spread the falsehoods?

But if resveratrol is so miraculous, why did researchers claim it was ineffective or even could cause cancer?

In the first instance, the researcher involved in spreading this rumor was being backed by a billion-dollar pharmaceutical company that had a secret project underway to develop a resveratrol-like drug for cancer. If Americans began taking resveratrol dietary supplements on their own, they could likely discover it cures cancer, and this would interfere with their efforts to introduce a resveratrol-like drug.

The other researcher, who was quoted in news reports as saying resveratrol could cause cancer, later had a plausible denial. He claimed he said resveratrol could cure cancer, but alcohol in wine could cause cancer. He claimed he was misquoted, but never made any effort to correct the mistaken news reports. Consumers were frightened away from resveratrol pills just after news stories had told of its great promise. The public is going to have to catch on to these efforts of dissuasion.

Many pathways blocked by resveratrol

There isn't a known biological mechanism that prevents or interferes with cancer that resveratrol doesn't promote. Like some other molecules found in olives and berries, resveratrol hinders all three major steps involved in cancer – the initiation (gene mutation), growth and spread (metastasis) of tumor cells, something no existing cancer drug does. It is a small molecule that can enter into the genetic machinery of living cells and favorably switch certain genes on or off. [Journal Nutritional Biochemistry 16: 449–66, 2005]

One cancer researcher calls the gene switching properties of resveratrol enormous. That statement is attributed to Dr. John Pezutto of the University of Illinois who was commissioned to travel the world to identify the most promising anti-cancer molecules in nature. His investigation assayed over 30,000 molecules found in plants. He found a particular molecule in a crude extract of the roots of a tree collected in Peru. Working under a grant from the National Cancer Institute which involves screening for cancer-inhibiting compounds from plants, Pezutto focused his attention on resveratrol. According to Pezzuto, "*Of all the plants we've tested for cancer chemopreventive activity and all the compounds we've seen, this one has the greatest promise.*" [Science 275: 218, 1997]

A recent research study involving resveratrol showed that it switched hundreds of genes at one time. [Cancer Biology Therapy 3: 882–89, 2004] Commenting on that study, Dr. Pezutto likened resveratrol to a "*whiff that induces a biologically specific tsunami.*" [Cancer Biology Therapy 3: 889–90, 2004] Those are strong words from a usually reserved investigator.

This method of action is different than that of the new anti-cancer drugs, like Iressa, Erbitux, and Herceptin, which target a small number of genes that are responsible for cancer cell replication.

Researchers Paolo Signorelli and Riccardo Ghidoni of the University of Milan question whether drugs singularly targeted at certain genes will ever work. So far, they have only added a few months of survival to cancer patients' lives, at great expense and with side effects.

> "*Natural compounds... offer a less specific but perhaps more effective strategy for cancer therapy by inducing combinations of effects that may counteract the metabolic alterations related to cancer promotion,*" says Signorelli and Ghidoni.
> *Source: Journal Nutritional Biochemistry 16: 449-66, 2005*

Resveratrol: the nine ways it fights cancer

Research report after research report extols the many cancer-inhibiting properties of resveratrol. While pharmaceutical companies endeavor to test drugs that block cancer growth in specific ways, resveratrol remarkably appears to inhibit the formation of tumor cells at every stage of cancer.

1 Resveratrol is involved in inhibiting the first step in cancer formation, the DNA mutations and abnormalities within the energy-producing centers of living cells (the mitochondria) that initiate the signals for cell growth to go awry.

2 Resveratrol interrupts chemical signals between cells that promote cancer cell growth.

3 Resveratrol inhibits gene-controlled proteins that cause tumor cells to become starved for oxygen, which then triggers the undesirable production of new blood vessels (angiogenesis) that feed tumors.

4 Resveratrol knocks cancer cells out of their immortal state and induces them to die off, a process called apoptosis, that is, the maturation and death of cells. [Experimental Molecular Medicine 32: 88-92, 2000] Resveratrol promotes tumor cell "*suicide*" by its ability to inhibit the production of a protein called survivin. [Cancer Research 64:337-46. 2004]

5 Resveratrol calms down inflammation which is involved in all tumor environments.

6 Resveratrol inhibits Hypoxia Inducible Factor-1, a protein that is activated by a lack of oxygen in cancer tissues. Hypoxia Inducible Factor-1 protein is needed for tumors to expand.

7 Resveratrol helps to prevent blood clots which serve as spawning grounds for tumors to spread and metastasize to other organs in the body.

8 Resveratrol activates the Sirtuin 1 DNA repair gene. [Oncogene Sept. 19, 2005]

9 Resveratrol inhibits for production of an enzyme (matrix metalloproteinase) that degrades collagen, thus limiting the spread of cancer by locking tumor cells within their collagen surroundings. [Oncogene 23: 1845-53, 2004]

Virtually every pathway for tumor growth and propagation is blocked by resveratrol. [Drugs Today 2002; 38: 571-80, 2002]

Researchers appear to have developed a consensus that low concentrations of resveratrol can *"not only counteract tumor initiation.... but can inhibit tumor cell survival."* Resveratrol targets the very machinery inside cells that promote tumor cell survival. It appears to be able to concentrate its action on tumor cells rather than healthy cells. Resveratrol has also has the ability to induce cancer cells, but not normal cells, to die off. [Bone Marrow Transplantation 2000; 25: 639-45, 2000]

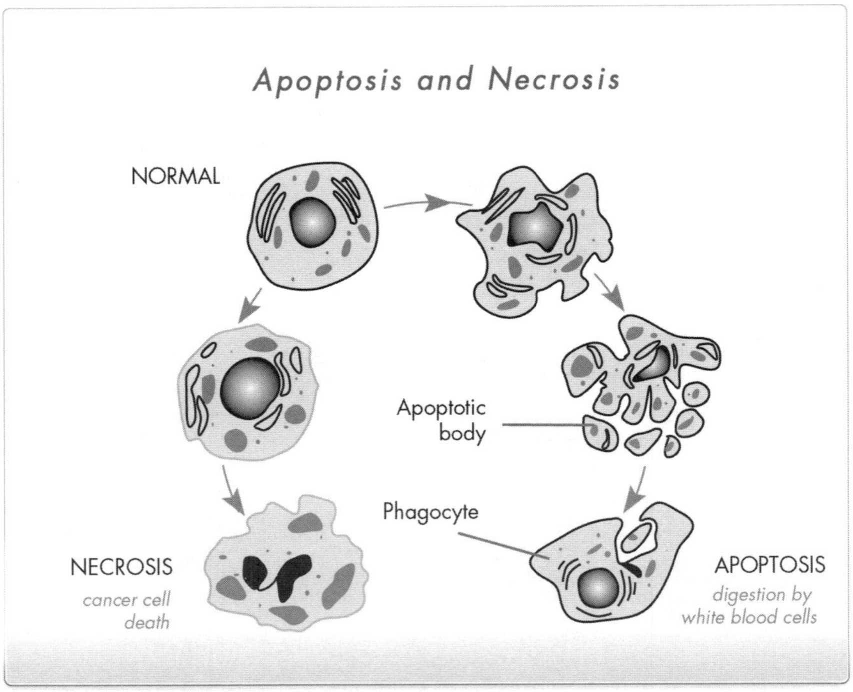

How resveratrol gently kills cancer cells

Resveratrol induces cancer cells to die off in a preferred manner so their cellular debris will be digested by white blood cells called phagocytes.

Cancer cells are immortal. They refuse to grow up (mature) and die off in a gradual manner as do normal cells. The normal process of cell death is called apoptosis (ay-pa-tow-siss). Toxic methods of killing cancer cells, such as radiation and chemotherapy, harshly destroy cancer cells by causing them to break open, release their contents and damage neighboring cells and provoke inflammation. This is why cancer treatment is fraught with side effects. The way that cancer cells are killed determines the severity of treatment-induced side effects and the survival of the cancer patient.

The discovery that resveratrol exerts the profound ability to induce apoptic cell death was described in the Federation of American Societies for Experimental Biology Journal in 2003 (volume 117, p 2340). Resveratrol facilitates apoptosis by converting lipids (fats) in the outer membrane of tumor cells into molecules called ceramides. A more recent report shows that resveratrol, and some altered resveratrol-like molecules, causes aggressive breast cancer cells to die off in a preferred manner. [Journal Medicinal Chemistry 48: 6783-86, 2005]

Warburg Effect Reversed

Researchers at the University of Southern California report that a molecule found in red wine inhibits a protein that controls the rapid growth of tumors [Molecular Cancer Therapeutics 4: 1465-74, October 2005]

Since the work of Nobel Prize winner Otto Warburg in the 1930s, it has been known that tumor cells are hypoxic, that is, they no longer utilize oxygen to produce energy, and rather produce energy through fermentation. In search of a supply of oxygen, tumor cells then relentlessly proceed to migrate and send signals for new blood vessels to grow towards the tumor (a process called angiogenesis). In so doing, the tumor obtains nutrients and grows at an accelerated pace.

Tumor cells produce a gene-controlled protein called hypoxia inducible factor-1 (HIF-1) that facilitates this whole process. The loss of HIF-1 activity dramatically decreases tumor growth, new blood vessel formation and energy metabolism.

A major reason for treatment failure is that the most aggressive tumors over-produce HIF-1. If just 10% of malignant cells over-activate HIF-1 the tumor is more likely to resist radiation treatment. [Molecular Cancer Therapeutics 3: 647-54, 2004]

Cancer investigators believe HIF-1 inhibiting drugs may overcome the problems posed by fast-growing solid tumors. Researchers claim that *"the most exciting possibility would be the discovery of small-molecule inhibitors of HIF-1."* [Nature Medicine 9: 677-84, 2003] Small molecules would be able to penetrate inside the nucleus of tumor cells, to inhibit the activity of HIF-1. [Current Cancer Drug Targets 3: 391-405, 2003]

Researchers now believe hypoxia-inducible factor-1 is a promising drug target, and that resveratrol, a red wine molecule, appears to be the small molecule they were searching for since it *"dramatically inhibits the stimulatory effects of hypoxia on invasive tumor cells."* [Molecular Cancer Therapeutics 4: 1465-74, October 2005] Once tumor cells no longer exhibit high HIF-1 activity, blood vessels that supply nutrients to these malignant cells begin to recede, the tumor cells begin to utilize oxygen once again, and these otherwise immortal cells begin to age and die off.

Resveratrol and the p53 gene

Early on, in the months following revelations by Harvard Medical School researchers late in 2003, that the red wine molecule resveratrol could possibly extend the human life span by as much as 50 years, a scientific cloud lingered over resveratrol. In the laboratory, resveratrol switched on DNA repair enzymes controlled by the Sirtuin 1 gene, but also turned off the p53 tumor suppressor gene. Scientists wondered if it would be premature to tell people to reach for bottles of red wine or red wine pills in a quest for longevity only to find that this increased their risk of developing cancer. The p53 gene is inactivated in over half of all human cancers.

Now researchers at the Salk Institute for Biological Studies in La Jolla, California, report that the *"Cancer related gene p53 is not regulated as indicated by previous tissue culture research."* Moving research out of lab dishes and into live animals, Salk Institute investigators conclude that what has been previously learned about the regulation of p53 activity from lab dish (in vitro) studies may not be relevant to living, breathing organisms. *"It came as a complete surprise. This study caused a big shift in how we think about p53,"* said Kurt Krummel, lead researcher. [Proceedings of the National Academy of Sciences 102: 10188-93, 2005]

Resveratrol and the bax gene

Another tumor-regulating property that resveratrol has is the ability to turn on the bax gene which causes the otherwise immortal tumor cells to die off. It does this by making the membranes surrounding the energy-producing organelles (mitochondria) within cells more permeable. This leads to the death of the tumor cell. Resveratrol, in concentrations available in some foods, can produce these anti-cancer effects. In a study of mice, resveratrol prevented the formation of colon and small intestinal tumors. Resveratrol is being discussed as a sole or companion *"drug"* to treat cancer. [BMC Cancer 2: 27, 2002]

Resveratrol and tumor necrosis factor

The body mounts its own defense when challenged with cancer. One important inborn anti-cancer fighter is a protein called tumor necrosis factor (TNF). It is primarily produced by white blood cells called macrophages and T cells. Although TNF can effectively kill off cancer cells, it can also over-respond to the tumor and trigger excessive inflammation. This same process occurs in the autoimmune disease rheumatoid arthritis. Attempts to use TNF as a treatment for cancer have been problematic for obvious reasons. TNF is also a factor in blood vessel disease. TNF can promote plaque or blood clots to stick to the inside of blood vessel walls. Resveratrol, at concentrations achieved by moderate wine consumption, has been shown to inhibit the TNF-related inflammation and resultant blood vessel abnormalities. [Therapie 56: 613-16, 2001]

Blocking the spread of cancer

Cancer itself is horrendous, but its spread (metastasis) to other organs is what causes mortality. Modern cancer therapy has no treatment to stop tumors from spreading.

U.S. scientists say they have discovered how tumors control the development of secondary cancers in the body.

Chemical signals make the target sites for secondary tumors sticky and direct bone marrow cells to them to secure a foothold for roaming tumor cells. Initially, growth factors released by the primary tumor trigger the production of an adhesive protein called fibronectin on the surface of cells at the target site.

Resveratrol has been found to inhibit endothelial cell attachment to basement membrane components fibronectin and laminin, and can theoretically block the spread of cancer.

Resveratrol also blocks the formation of new blood vessels (angiogenesis) that feed tumor growth. [Journal Asian Natural Product Research 7:205-13, 2005; Journal Nutritional Biochemistry 13: 380-90, 2002]

Resveratrol as estrogen blocker

With the loss of estrogen production in the ovaries that occurs at menopause, females often experience shrinkage of vaginal tissues with accompanying symptoms of itching, dryness, bleeding and painful intercourse. Estrogen replacement therapy has been the standard therapy in the past but now is called into question because of increased risks for breast and ovarian cancer. Drugs like raloxifene (Evista) and tibolone (Livial) are sometimes prescribed with varying degrees of relief for menopausal changes in vaginal tissue.

Researchers at the Inonu University Medical Faculty in Turkey compared resveratrol against two drugs (raloxifene, tibolone) and estrogen replacement therapy in rodents whose ovaries had been removed. Resveratrol was found to offset the aging effects of the vaginal tissues in a superior manner to the two drugs and hormone therapy. Researchers explained that *"resveratrol has the potential to be developed into drugs superior to raloxifene and tibolone in regards to prevention of vaginal changes."* [Gynecology Obstetrical Investigation 60: 186-91, 2005]

Resveratrol is considered an orally available molecule that binds to estrogen entry sites on cells with an affinity 1/7000th the strength of estrogen. So it has a very mild estrogen-like effect, which speaks for its safety.

Researchers used the human equivalent of 800 mg of resveratrol in the animal experiment cited above. [Gynecology Obstetrical Investigation 60: 186-91, 2005]

Resveratrol and types of cancer

Despite resveratrol's many mechanisms of action against all types of cancers, patients and their families always want to know, could it work for their specific type of cancer? Here is a list of the cancers that resveratrol may be effective against. And, resveratrol's ability to fight cancer is not limited to just those mentioned below.

Types of cancer resveratrol has been shown to be active against	
Types of Cancer	Reference
Colon	Int J Molecular Medicine 2002; 10: 193-99
Leukemia (cancer of the blood)	Bone Marrow Transplantation 2000; 25: 639-45
Lung	Journal Nutrition 2001; 131: 1844-49
Liver	Biochem Biophys Res Commun 1999; 254: 739-41
Oral cancer	Anticancer Drugs 1999; 10: 187-93
Uterine	Cancer Research 2001; 61: 6137-44
Esophageal	World Journal Gastroenterology 2003; 9: 408-11
Thyroid	J Clinical Endocrinology Metab 2002; 87: 1223-32
Breast	Clinical Cancer Research 2000; 6: 2921-30
Cervical	Cancer Letters 2002; 175: 165-73
Pancreatic	Pancreas 2002; 25: 71-76
Prostate	Journal Nutrition. 2003;133:2440S-2443S
Neuroblastoma	Neurochemistry International 2003;42:419-29
Skin (melanoma)	International Journal Cancer 2000; 87: 595-600

1. Resveratrol and prostate cancer

Stanford University School of Medicine researchers report profound anti-prostate cancer properties for resveratrol [Cancer Epidemiology Biomarkers & Prevention 14: 596-604, 2005] The Stanford researchers employed gene expression, cell cycle and prostate specific protein analysis. As evidenced by the chart below, resveratrol, in concentrations achievable in humans, inhibited prostate cancer cell growth by 16% at 24 hours and 83% at 60 hours, after instillation of purified resveratrol into cell dishes.

Stanford researchers said *"Dramatic gene expression changes accompany this cell cycle arrest and are distributed throughout all phases of the cell cycle."*

A marker of inflammation that is used to determine if tumors are present in the prostate gland is called the prostate specific antigen test, or PSA. High PSA scores often indicate there is a need for further testing, usually a biopsy of the prostate tissue, to determine if a tumor is present.

PSA (prostate specific antigen), a well-characterized male sex hormone-regulated gene, was also repressed by greater than two-fold 12 hours after treatment with resveratrol. (See chart)

The Stanford researchers go on to say that *"animal and human studies have shown that resveratrol is rapidly absorbed in the gut, attaining highest concentration in the blood in one hour,"* and that desirable changes in gene expression were obtained with concentrations of resveratrol attainable in rodents. *"However, the levels of resveratrol used in this study that result in gene expression modulation in vitro may or may not be attainable in man. At the very least, the relatively low concentration of resveratrol in grapes or wine will likely make it necessary for it to be given as a dietary supplement."* [Cancer Epidemiology Biomarkers & Prevention 14: 596-604, 2005]

Among many nutraceuticals now being considered, resveratrol has gained the attention of urological doctors for its unusual properties. [Urology Oncology 7: 223-27, 2002]

In fact, researchers at the Department of Cancer Biology, University of Texas, M.D. Anderson Cancer Center in Houston, state that *"resveratrol may be especially suitable as a lead agent for prostate cancer prevention given its ability to (a) inhibit each stage of cancer; (b) scavenge populations of hormone-sensitive cancer cells; (c) reduce populations of prostate cancer cells by short-circuiting the chemicals responsible for tumor cell growth."* [Journal Nutrition 133: 2440-43S, 2003]

It is becoming more and more apparent that natural molecules can effectively influence the genetic-controlled production of proteins and enzymes. The American Health Foundation in Valhalla, New York, screened a library of

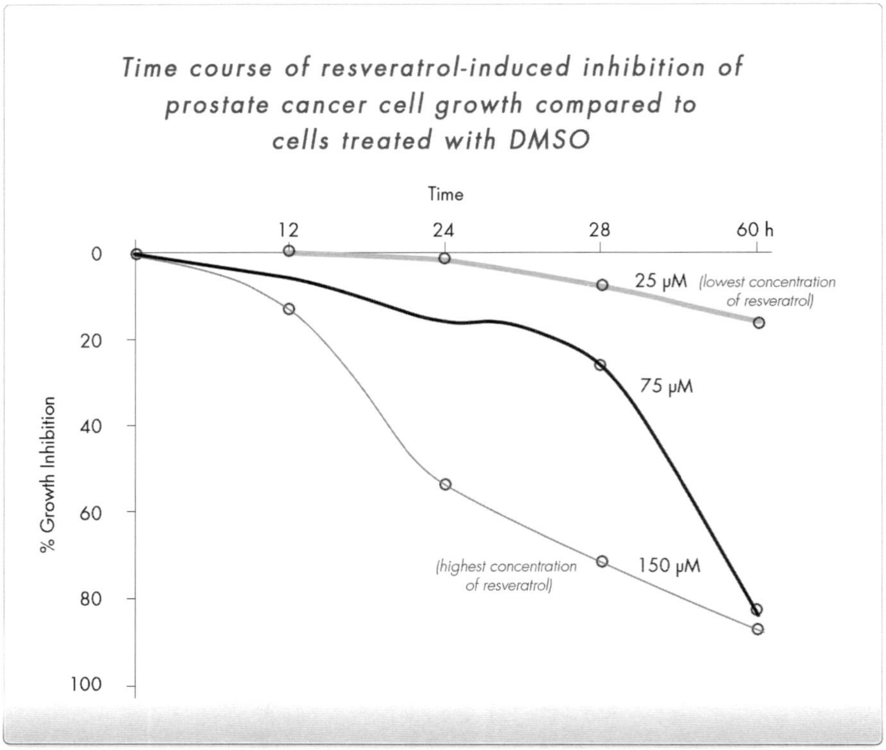
Time course of resveratrol-induced inhibition of prostate cancer cell growth compared to cells treated with DMSO
Time
12
24
28
60 h
0
20
40
60
80
100
% Growth Inhibition
25 μM (lowest concentration of resveratrol)
75 μM
150 μM
(highest concentration of resveratrol)

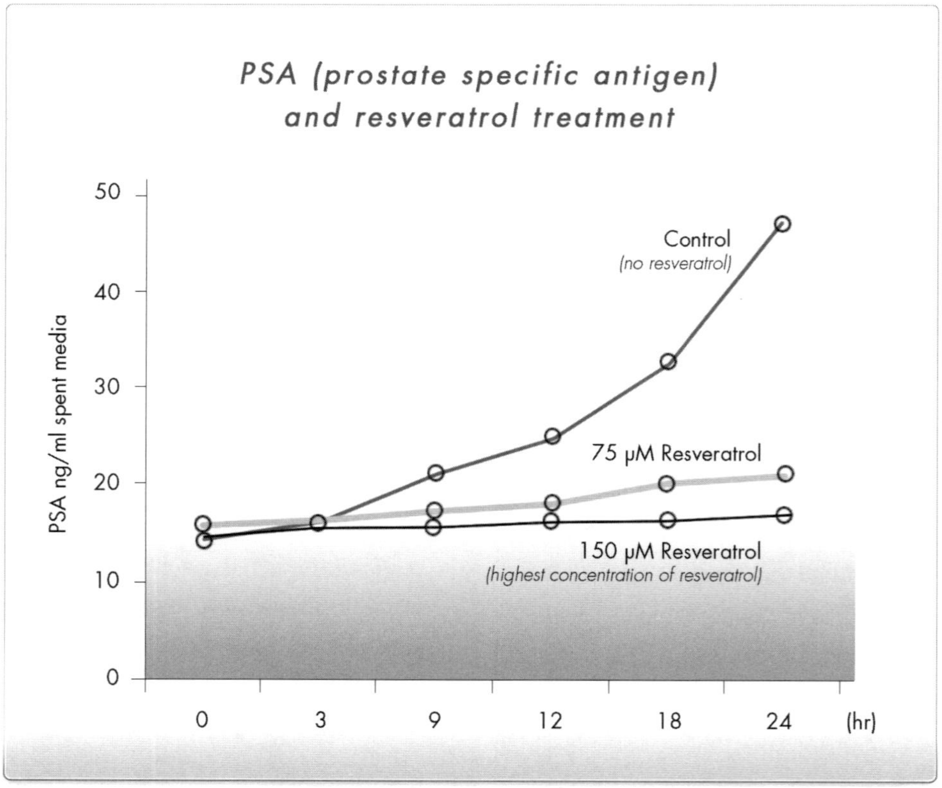
PSA (prostate specific antigen) and resveratrol treatment
50
40
30
20
10
0
PSA ng/ml spent media
Control
(no resveratrol)
75 μM Resveratrol
150 μM Resveratrol
(highest concentration of resveratrol)
0
3
9
12
18
24
(hr)

genes in prostate cancer cells to determine how many were influenced by resveratrol or ellagic acid (a natural molecule found abundantly in red raspberries and pomegranate). Both natural molecules doubled the ability of more than 500 genes to produce biologically active proteins, a process called gene expression. [Life Sciences 70: 1821-39, 2002]

Resveratrol causes prostate cancer cells in the laboratory to die off more rapidly by its influence on the p53 tumor suppressor gene. [Journal Urology 168: 748-55, 2002]

It is now known that resveratrol exhibits the *"unique ability"* to control processes involved in prostate tumor cell growth. [Cancer Research 62: 2488-92, 2002]

In fact, components of red wine, such as resveratrol and quercetin, were found to be potent inhibitors of prostate cancer cell growth at low concentrations achievable by diet (red wine) or supplements. [Nutrition Cancer 37: 223-33, 2000]

In laboratory studies using prostate cancer cells, resveratrol exhibits the ability to reduce PSA secretion and inhibit cell growth independent of any influence over male hormones. [Experimental Cell Research 249: 109-15, 1999] Resveratrol has been found to be toxic to prostate cancer cells regardless of whether or not they grow in response to male hormones. [Prostate 2002; 52: 319-29, 2002]

Researchers have discovered that resveratrol reduces the level of PSA secreted by prostate cells by 80 %. [Anticancer Research 20: 225-28, 2000]

Researchers in Italy claim that resveratrol may be used as an alternative to a common drug used to treat prostate cancer. [Oncological Research 14: 415-26, 2004]

2. Resveratrol and brain cancer

Neuroblastoma is a particularly difficult form of cancer to treat as it typically strikes babies and young children. It often emanates near the adrenal glands on top of the kidneys and by the time it is diagnosed is has often spread to various other organs. The search for a cure is urgent and the number of effective treatments small. The combination of resveratrol with quercetin, both red wine antioxidants, has been shown to inhibit the growth of this type of tumor cell, with both of these wine constituents producing greater effect than either alone. [Pharmazie 57: 556-58, 2002]

While only a laboratory test using neuroblastoma cells, this preliminary experiment sheds light on the potential therapeutic effects of resveratrol for this very disturbing type of cancer.

3. Liver cancer

"Resveratrol might be a new potent chemopreventive drug candidate for liver cancer." [Life Sciences 22: 23-34, 2002] Resveratrol appears to have an affinity for liver cells more so than cells in the colon, and thus would be more biologically active in the liver. [International Journal Molecular Medicine10: 755-60, 2002]

4. Uterine cancer

Resveratrol inhibits the growth of uterine (endometrial) cancer cells. [International Journal Oncology 23: 1167-72, 2003]

5. Pancreatic cancer

Another type of cancer that is in desperate need of a cure is pancreatic cancer. Early diagnosis is not common and survival is usually limited to less than six months. A laboratory study using human pancreatic tumor cells indicates that resveratrol has potent abilities to kill off pancreatic tumor cells and say researchers, *"is likely to be valuable for the management and prevention of human pancreatic cancer."* [Pancreas 25: 71-76, 2002]

6. Lung cancer

"Resveratrol has strong potential for development as an agent for prevention against human lung cancer." [International Journal Molecular Medicine10: 755-60, 2002]

A remarkable report, published by the Cancer Drug Discovery Group in Great Britain, indicates resveratrol is altered by an enzyme found in human tumors and this form of resveratrol is the actual agent that prevents cancer. This would means resveratrol could serve as a common antioxidant until tumors develop, and thereafter it works as an anti-tumor agent. [British Journal Cancer 86: 774-78, 2002]

Cells in breast and prostate tissues have receptor sites or what might be called parking spaces for estrogen to bind and enter the cells. Resveratrol is considered a phytoestrogen, that is, an estrogen-like molecule that also binds to and activates the estrogen receptors. In doing so resveratrol can both mimic estrogen and inhibit the action of estrogen by limiting the number of receptor sites estrogen has access to in a cell. Because phytoestrogens exhibit very mild hormonal action– about 1/1000th that of natural estrogen-- they have the ability to improve health and reduce the risk of hormonal-related cancer. To more fully understand how plant estrogens can be beneficial, the need for estrogen in the body needs to be recognized. Without estrogen, the bones begin to wither as calcium is lost and mental depression may set in. It's important for women and men to maintain small amounts of estrogen or estrogen-like molecules in their system throughout life.

The exact effect of phytoestrogens on breast cancer cells and tumors depends upon their concentration. At low concentrations they have been shown to possibly stimulate growth whereas at higher concentrations they inhibit tumor growth. This laboratory finding is backed by population studies which show that women who consume more plant estrogens in their diet, up to a point, appear to derive protection against breast cancer.

Resveratrol from red wine differs from soybean phytoestrogens. The soybean-based plant hormones may increase some chemical pathways, known as Akt and FAK, that promote breast cancer cell survival and invasion, whereas red wine resveratrol inhibits the activity of both of these chemicals. [Journal Nutrition 132: 3482-89S, 2002]

Paclitaxel (Taxol) is a quite toxic chemotherapy drug, derived from the yew tree, which is intravenously administered to treat various forms of cancer. One of the reasons for the lack of effectiveness of this drug is that once introduced, it may be metabolically converted into inactive forms, rendering it less useful for cancer treatment. Researchers have found that quercetin and resveratrol are among two red wine molecules that inhibit the metabolic conversion of paclitaxel. Therefore, resveratrol may prove to be an effective companion to paclitaxel therapy. [N S Archives Pharmacology 368: 200-09, 2003]

7. Stomach cancer

A diet rich in resveratrol has been suggested to prevent stomach cancer. [American Journal Physiology Gastrointestinal Physiology 282: G809-16, 2002].

Wine appears to inhibit the growth of *Helicobacter pylori* and the primarily active ingredient is resveratrol. [Microbios 104: 79-85, 2001]

8. Colon cancer

Resveratrol is active against colon cancer. [International Journal Molecular Medicine 10: 193-99, 2002] A comparative test found resveratrol far more powerful at inhibiting colon tumor cell growth than a commonly used drug, and at a much lower dose. [Journal Nutrition132: 2082-86, 2002]

In an animal test conducted in France, mice genetically predisposed to develop intestinal tumors were given small amounts of resveratrol in their drinking water. The resveratrol reduced small tumors by 70 %. [Nutrition Cancer 39: 102-07, 2001]

9. Breast cancer

Resveratrol is a unique molecule for study in regard to breast tissue because its structure resembles estrogen, making it a phytoestrogen (plant-based). Additionally, it is a potent antioxidant (breast tissue preserver) and blocker of abnormal cell growth.

In rats given a cancer-causing chemical, resveratrol "*produced a striking reduction*" in the incidence and number of breast tumors. It does this by inhibiting an enzyme called NF-kappaB. [Cancer Research 62: 4945-54, 2002]

Vitamin D is known to inhibit breast cancer cell growth. Resveratrol (from wine) and genistein (from soy) are comparable molecules known as phytoestrogens. In a laboratory cell study, both have been shown to increase the receptor sites for vitamin D to enter cells, but genistein increases breast cancer cell growth while resveratrol does not. [Journal Steroid Biochemistry Molecular Biology 84: 149-57, 2003] Resveratrol has been found to be a very strong inhibitor (87.5% inhibition) of chemically induced breast tumors in laboratory mice. [Nutrition Cancer 40: 173-79, 2001]

It has been repeatedly demonstrated that breast cancer cells grow rapidly in a corn oil environment (linoleic acid). Resveratrol antagonizes this effect, blocking the growth of both estrogen positive and negative types of breast tumor cell growth. Therefore, researchers are describing resveratrol as a *"promising anti-cancer agent for both hormone-dependent (estrogen positive) and hormone-independent (estrogen negative) breast cancers,"* and it may counter the undesirable effects of the western diet which is rich in these cancer-promoting oils. [Journal Cancer Research Clinical Oncology 127: 258-64, 2001]

Resveratrol and other antioxidants like quercetin found in red wine work at very low concentrations to inhibit breast cancer. [Journal Cell Biochemistry 78: 429-41, 2000] Animal studies confirm that resveratrol significantly inhibits breast tumor cell growth. [Cancer Letters 23: 113-22, 2006]

10. Leukemia

There are a flurry of research reports regarding resveratrol and leukemia. Seven of the nine reports listed by the National Library of Medicine on resveratrol and leukemia have been published in the last two years.

Resveratrol inhibits the propagation of leukemia cells grown in a laboratory dish. [International Journal Hematology 75: 528-33, 2002] Because of its low toxicity, investigators believe resveratrol deserves further research as an anti-leukemia agent. [Leukemia Lymphoma 2002; 43: 983-87, 2002]

11. Radiation therapy

Gamma rays or x-rays are directed at tumors in what is known as radiation therapy. Intense therapeutic radiation then can generate inflammation at the site of the treated tumor, which further exacerbates the tumor environment. Sometimes non-steroidal anti-inflammatory drugs such as ibuprofen or indomethacin are used to reduce inflammation associated with tumor therapy. It has already been demonstrated that anti-inflammatory agents appear to reduce the risk of cancer. It is possible they can also be used to reduce the toxic side effects of radiation therapy. When tumor cells are pre-treated with resveratrol, they are more sensitive to the destructive radiation treatment. Therefore, not only does resveratrol patrol the body and inhibit inflammatory reactions that trigger or enhance tumor growth, during radiation treatment it has the potential to inhibit tissue damage caused by gamma radiation and enhance the effect of treatment as well. [Cancer Letters 175: 165-73, 2002]

This dual nature of resveratrol is what intrigues researchers. While, in many instances, oncologists advise patients to stop consumption of all vitamin and herbal products during cancer therapy, it appears resveratrol would be an exception.

12. Resveratrol compared to anti-cancer drug

Two antioxidant anti-cancer agents were recently tested. Deferoxamine (drug name: Desferal) isolated from the bacterium *Streptomyces pilosus*, commonly used in cancer treatment, and resveratrol. Research-grade trans resveratrol was used and stored frozen for the study. Blood samples were obtained from healthy adults and mixed with deferoxamine or resveratrol. Researchers at the University of Lodz (Poland) tested the ability of the two agents to inhibit damage to proteins in blood platelets caused by the reactive oxygen species known as peroxynitrite.

At concentrations that correspond to those achievable in humans, resveratrol *"had a very similar inhibitory effect"* to deferoxamine, said researchers. *"Resveratrol seems to have protective effects against impairment of plasma proteins caused by a strong biologic oxidant,"* they added. [Journal Nutritional Biochemistry, 17: 96-102, 2006]

Deferoxamine (Desferal)	Resveratrol
Molecular description	
Deferoxamine mesylate is N -[5-[3-[(5-aminopen tyl)hydroxycarbamoyl]propionamido] pentyl]-3-[[5-(N - hydroxyacetamido) pentyl]carbamoyl] propionohydroxamic acid monomethanesulfonate (salt).	/active form trans-3,4′,-5-trihydroxystilebene
Molecular configuration	
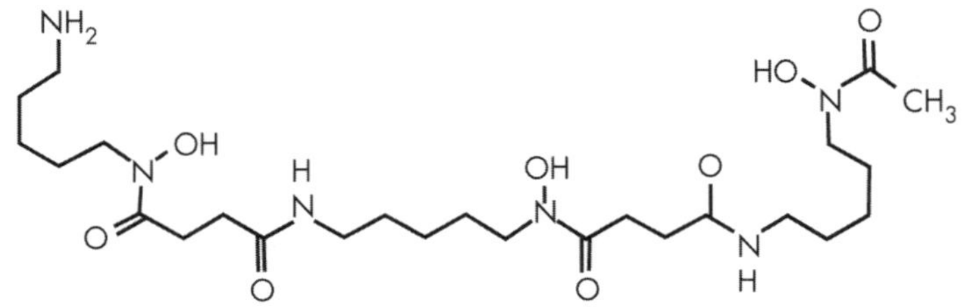	Resveratrol 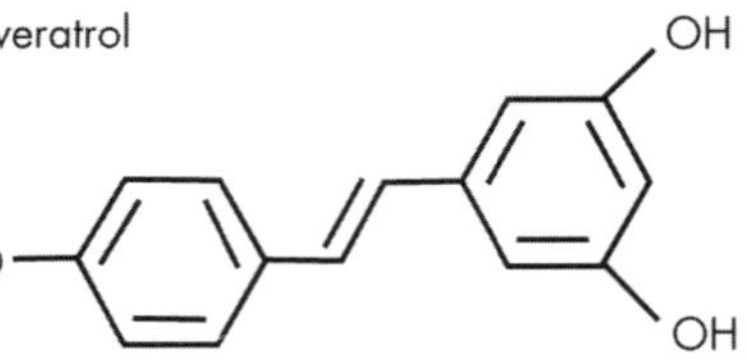
Molecular designation	
$H_2N(CH_2)_5\underset{OH}{N}\overset{O}{C}(CH_2)_2\overset{O}{C}NH\ (CH_2)_5\underset{OH}{N}\overset{O}{C}(CH_2)_2\overset{O}{C}NH(CH_2)_5\underset{OH}{N}\overset{O}{C}CH_3\ \ CH_3SO_3H$	C14H12O3
Molecular weight	
656.79	228.2
Administration	
Intravenous	Oral
Side effects	
Bluish fingernails, lips, or skin; blurred vision or other problems with vision; convulsions (seizures); difficulty in breathing (wheezing), or fast breathing; fast heartbeat; hearing problems; pain or swelling at place of injection; redness or flushing of skin; skin rash, hives, or itching; diarrhea; difficult urination; fever; leg cramps; stomach and muscle cramps; stomach discomfort; unusual bleeding or bruising	May interfere with some medications, otherwise side effects are rare

For comparison, deferoxamine is a drug that must be administered intravenously and is fraught with side effects. Resveratrol is an economically available dietary supplement with few reported side effects other than drug incompatibilities.

How much resveratrol is being used in cancer studies?

Therapeutic doses of resveratrol may be required for active forms of cancer. In a study conducted in Japan, the equivalent human dose of 2.5 mg per kilo of body weight (175 mg of resveratrol/160 lb human) reduced the size, weight, and spread of lung tumors in mice whereas a 42 milligram equivalent human dose (based on a 160 lb human) was not effective. [Journal Nutrition 131: 1844-49 2001]

However in another study, very low dose resveratrol, 200 mcg per kilo of body weight (equivalent to 14 mg for a 160 lb human), inhibited colon cancer in rodents. [Carcinogenesis 21: 1619-22, 2000]

A daily dose of 40 mg per kilogram of body weight (2,800 mg for a 160lb human) remarkably increased survival rates in mice with brain tumors (neuroblastomas) from zero to 70%. [Surgery 136: 57-66, 2004]

Safety

Because resveratrol disables detoxification enzymes produced in the liver, it may interfere with certain medications and should not be used at the same time as blood pressure, cholesterol or other drugs.

Up to 300 mg of resveratrol per kilogram of body weight (21,000 mg human equivalent) showed no detrimental effect upon animals. [Toxicological Science 82: 614-19, 2004]

Resveratrol has passed the safety arm of three human clinical studies including two ongoing cancer studies.

Resveratrol dietary supplements

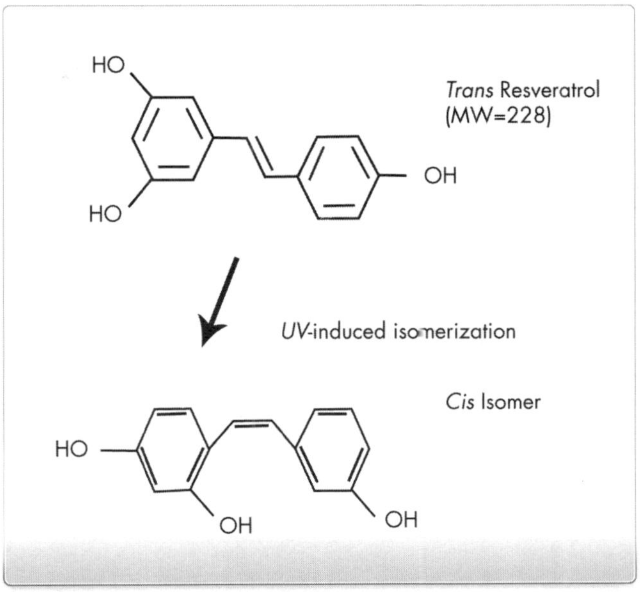

All of the cancer research studies have been performed with trans resveratrol. However resveratrol, as a drug or dietary supplement, synthetically produced or extracted from botanical sources, is subject to isomerization that is, a change in molecular structure from the *trans* to the *cis* form. *Trans* resveratrol is considered the major active form. Exposure to ultraviolet light, heat or oxygen may accelerate isomerization to cis resveratrol which is less biologically active. [Journal Agriculture Food Chemistry 44: 1253-57, 1996; Electrophoresis 22: 2574-79, 2001; J Agriculture Food Chemistry 51:1653-7, 2003] To make raw extracted resveratrol into a reliable and effective dietary supplement, it would need to be adequately preserved following extraction and then placed in an opaque, airtight capsule without significant exposure to light or oxygen during processing. One brand of resveratrol pills, Longevinex®, is never exposed to oxygen, heat or light during production and is sealed in an airtight capsule (Licaps®, Capsugel®)* [*The author has a financial interest in this product. www.longevinex.com]

Once captured and stabilized, either in wine or a dietary supplement, resveratrol is ready for human use. Dietary supplements and wines are restricted to making claims that they solely promote health and do not prevent or treat any disease. Dietary supplements must confine their product claims to structures and functions in the human body. So if readers want conclusive evidence that resveratrol prevents or treats cancer, they will have to wait for human studies with synthetically produced resveratrol molecules manufactured by pharmaceutical companies. That is likely to take years.

Is resveratrol biologically available?

Some researchers misleadingly claim resveratrol, when orally absorbed, is subsequently metabolized by the liver (complexed with glucuronic acid or sulfated with sulfur), and is therefore not biologically available. Therefore, it cannot work as a dietary supplement.

Resveratrol has a short half life of around 15 minutes. In less than an hour it would degrade in the body. But contrary to what some researchers have claimed, the process of glucuronidation in the liver actually preserves resveratrol, keeping it intact for up to nine hours. Sites of inflammation, infection or malignancy in the body produce an enzyme called glucuronidase, which releases resveratrol from its carrier molecule, and delivers it at the right time in precisely the right place. [J Pharmacology Experimental Therapy 302:369-73, 2002; Drug Metabolism Disposition 32: 1377-82, 2004]

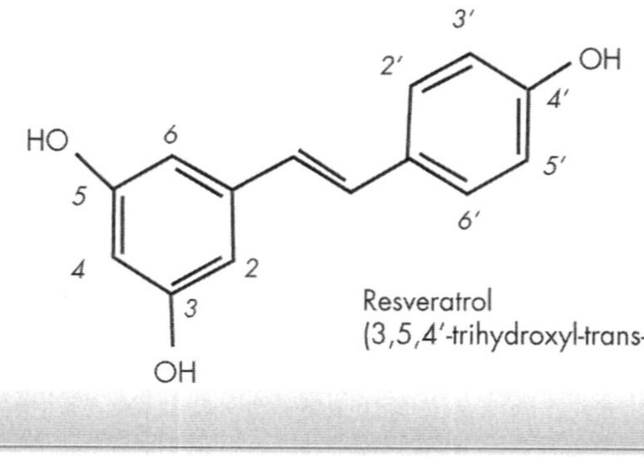

Resveratrol
(3,5,4′-trihydroxyl-trans-stilbene)

Pharmacologists actually utilize this process as a delivery system for prescription drugs. The researchers were being disingenuous. They knew this all along, but the misinformation effectively served to steer the public away from resveratrol pills.

Furthermore, it was shown in a laboratory experiment that sulfated resveratrol fully actives the Sirtuin 1 gene, believed to be responsible for many of the anti-cancer properties of resveratrol. [DA Sinclair, K Howitz, in Handbook of the Biology of Aging, 6th edition, Academic Press, 2006, p. 89] The argument over resveratrol's bioavailability is now moot.

Resveratrol for cancer prevention

What about taking resveratrol pills for cancer prevention? Dr. Nihal Ahmad and colleagues, at the University of Wisconsin Medical Science Center, write that conventional and therapeutic surgical approaches have *"not been able to control the incidence of most types of cancer."* Therefore, *"there is an urgent need to develop approaches for the management of cancer. Non-toxic agents are one such approach."*

An ideal cancer prevention agent should: (a) have little or no toxic effects in normal healthy cells; (b) be effective for all types of tumors; (c) be easily consumed orally; (d) have a known mechanism of action; (e) be low in cost; (f) and be accepted by the public. Resveratrol meets all of these requirements. [International Journal Oncology 23: 17-28, 2003]

For prevention, dosages in the range of 30-50 mg are suggested, while for cancer treatment, doses above 300 mg are consistent with current studies.

What do the researchers say?

One of the questions that arises when talking to cancer patients and their families is how they intend to evaluate what is told to them about cancer. Will they blindly accept everything they are told about cancer from their doctors? If they seek alternatives to conventional treatment, what kind of evidence for alternative treatment would be convincing? What if you were like Hubert and Mack. Their doctors knew nothing about resveratrol.

As encouraging as the existing data is on resveratrol, most studies either involve experiments conducted in laboratory dishes with living cells (called in vitro studies), or animal experiments. However, readers need to examine the enthusiasm that scientists have for this molecule and the breadth of its applications.

So some quotations from medical journals regarding resveratrol are provided below, for your examination. Here's what the experts have to say.

"It is urgent that more efforts be made to investigate newer therapies employing antioxidants for the chemoprevention of cardiovascular disease and cancer."
- Researchers at Taiwan University, Taipei. Lin JK, Tsai SH, Chemoprevention of cancer and cardiovascular disease by resveratrol, Proceedings National Science Council Republic China B 1999; 23: 99-106.

"Resveratrol merits investigation as a potential cancer chemopreventive agent in humans."
- Jang M, Cai L, Udeani GO, Cancer chemopreventive activity of resveratrol, a natural product derived from grapes, Science 1997; 275: 218-20.

"Resveratrol holds great promise for future development as a chemopreventive agent that may be useful for several disorders."
- Bhat KP, Pezzutto JM, Cancer chemopreventive activity of resveratrol, Annals NY Academy Science 2002; 957: 210-29.

"Resveratrol may be considered for use as a strong cancer chemopreventive agent in humans."
- Chun YJ, Kim MY, Guengerich FP, Resveratrol is a selective human cytochrome P450 1A1 inhibitor, Biochemical Biophysical Research Communications 1999; 262: 20-24.

Researchers call resveratrol *"an important new cell cycle blocker as well as a cancer chemopreventive agent."*
- Park JW, Choi YJ, Jang MA, Chemopreventive agent resveratrol, a natural product derived from grapes, reversibly inhibits progression through S and G2 phases of the cell cycle in U937 cells, Cancer Letters 2001; 163: 43-49.

"Resveratrol exerts a strong inhibition of human colon and rectal tumor cells."
- Delmas D. Passily-Degrace P, Jannin P, Resveratrol, a chemopreventive agent, disrupts the cell cycle control of human SW480 colorectal tumor cells, Int J Mol Med 2002; 10: 193-99.

"Clearly, the studies with resveratrol provide support for the use of resveratrol in human cancer chemoprevention and in combination with chemotherapeutic drugs."
- Cal C, Garban H, Jazirehi A, Resveratrol and cancer: chemoprevention, apoptosis and chemo-immunosensitizing activities, Curr Med Chem Anti-cancer Agents 2003: 3: 77-93.

"The remarkable message is that exquisitely low daily doses of resveratrol (between 14 and 140 mg in a 160 pound human) will suffice to exert potent cancer chemopreventive efficacy and pharmacodynamic activity. These animal studies render resveratrol one of the most potent diet-derived chemopreventive dietary polyphenols ever described."
– Andreas J, Gescher and William P Steward, Department of Oncology, Leicester, United Kingdom, in Cancer Epidemiology, Biomarkers and Prevention, 2003; 12: 953-57.

"Perhaps the greatest therapeutic advantage of these small natural molecules is that they can be administered orally without causing severe side effects."

- Cao Y, Cao R, Brakenhielm E, Antiangiogenic mechanisms of diet-derived polyphenols, J Nut Biochem 2002; 13: 380-90.

These are strong words from scientists who are usually reserved in their comments. Here are the many reasons why scientists worldwide are eager to study resveratrol.

Summary

In summary, as promising as resveratrol is in the war against cancer, there are only two human trials underway, one in Europe using a high-dose (500 mg) pill for cancer prevention among healthy adults and another in California for colon cancer.

If resveratrol lives up to its promise, it will put the entire cancer care industry out of business, usher in an era of true cancer prevention, and save billions of dollars in health care costs.

CHAPTER 15

Nutrition Regimen

p 494 - 508

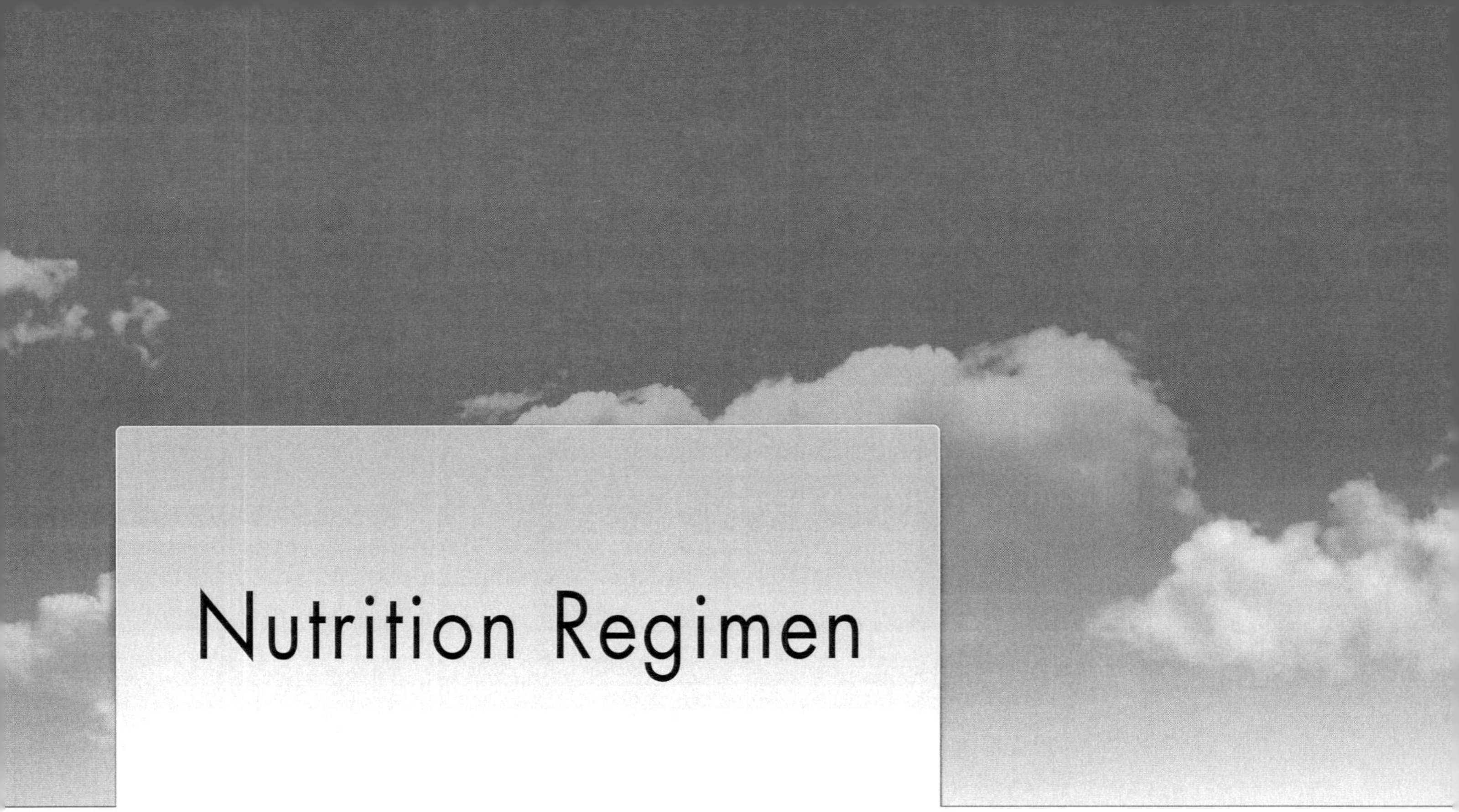

Nutrition Regimen

Universal dietary and supplement regimens to successfully fight cancer

Cancer authorities now speak of universal mechanisms that can be manipulated to block the growth, spread and recurrence of cancer. This can be accomplished through the informed use of foods and dietary supplements years in advance of the discovery of a tumor, during conventional treatment, as stand-alone cancer treatment, or when cancer is in remission to prevent recurrence.

This chapter provides you with a universal regimen of foods and dietary supplements which may be able to effectively prevent, treat, cure and thwart the recurrence of cancer far better than toxic chemotherapy drugs or medicinal immune boosters such as interferon or monoclonal antibody drugs like Herceptin, Avastin, Erbitux that temporarily infuse targeted antibodies into a tumor. Anti-cancer mechanisms within your own body can be activated to put a stop to cancer in a continual manner that exceeds that of anti-cancer drugs.

The unproven versus the disproven

If you ask your doctor about dietary and food supplement regimens, his or her most likely response will be that these methods to fight cancer are unproven. The American Cancer Society recommends that "*nutritional cancer cures*" be avoided. [CA Cancer Journal Clinicians 43: 309-19, 1993] The American Cancer Society says: "*If a supplement is taken, the best choice is a balanced multivitamin/mineral supplement containing no more than 100% of the Daily Value of most nutrients, because high doses of some nutrients can have harmful effects.*" [American Cancer Society 2006] So therefore, are we to illogically consent to surgery, chemo and radiation therapy, which have been disproven?

The medicine cupboard is bare when it comes to cancer cures. To cite a recent report: *"For many human cancers, chemotherapy can often significantly reduce systemic cancer burdens (size and number of tumors), but unfortunately, for most advanced metastatic solid organ cancers, such as cancers of the breast, colon, and prostate, drug treatments generally fail to effect cancer cures."* [International Journal Oncology 12:161-70, 1998] Such admissions aren't likely to come from the lips of your oncologist, who will be reticent to tell you the disappointing truth: conventional cancer therapy is useless against most cancers.

Ineffective cancer treatment prolongs life for only a short time and temporarily shrinks tumors until drug resistance sets in. The preference for toxic chemo and radiation therapy diminishes the paramount role of nutrition in conquering cancer. The prevailing idea is that nutrients conflict with toxic cancer treatment, but the exact opposite is true. There can be no such thing as integrative medicine, when useless cancer treatment is combined with nutritional approaches to cancer. Nutritional approaches to cancer, which activate the body's own defenses against cancer, cannot be effectively mixed with toxic cancer treatment. After six decades, conventional cancer care does not hold the scientific high ground. It only has a legacy of failure. Decades of different mixes and doses of chemo, radiation and surgery have not significantly improved survival rates.

Physicians not likely to be swayed

All of the documented evidence provided in this text is not likely to sway any physician to believe nutritional therapy is of any value to cancer patients. Some doctors have had the gall to tell their patients to take Flintstones children's vitamins if they want to take vitamin pills. The position of the American Cancer Society, to take dietary supplements that don't exceed 100% of the Daily Value, because of the potential for side effects, is mistaken advice because side effects don't begin until five times greater dosage than the Safe Upper Limit is consumed. Furthermore, the Daily Value and Recommended Daily Allowance are intended for totally healthy adults, not for patients at risk for or battling cancer. Physicians often lump nutrition therapy in with snake oil remedies of the past. The thousands of references cited in this book in favor of dietary and food supplement therapy for cancer makes this approach stand apart from the pseudo-science that prevails throughout alternative medicine.

The futility of removing or killing cancer cells

Cancer patients want cancer cells out of their bodies, by whatever means. Most cancer patients have the overly simplistic belief that if the entire tumor is removed or every cancer cell is killed, you no longer have cancer. But efforts to eradicate tumor cells do not address what caused cancer in the first place. You can kill off every cancer cell, but the cancer will usually come roaring back at some time in the future.

Cancer is prevalent

You may be surprised to learn that many millions of American adults over age 50 have cancer cells in their body. These cells may survive for a time and then die off. As long as they are cemented in place by surrounding connective tissue (collagen), they cannot obtain sufficient nutrients to grow and migrate to other locations.

For example, based upon autopsy studies, there are an estimated 16 million American women with undiagnosed breast cancer in the population (2003 estimate). About 180,000 of these women are diagnosed with breast cancer annually (about 1% of the pool of women with breast cancer). While the annual death toll from breast cancer is 40,000, this represents less than 3/10ths of one percent of all women with cancer cells in their breast tissue. Similarly, males have cancerous cells in the prostate gland beginning at age 30 and yet the lives of most men diagnosed with prostate cancer will never be threatened by cancer.

Obviously, something keeps these cancer cells in check in the vast majority of adults. The collagen network and the human immune system play dominant roles in this regard. The innate immune system is of primary importance too. This opens the door for nutritional therapy that can help maintain collagen barriers and boost immunity.

Does every cancer patient need treatment?

It is widely believed that cancer begins years in advance of symptoms or detection. By the time cancer can be detected by any means, it is usually too large and has often spread too far to mount an effective defense against it. It is foolish to believe every person entering the cancer era of their lives, from age 50 on, should continually be subjected to screening radiation (X-rays, mammograms, CT scans) and invasive needle biopsies, in a futile attempt to detect cancer at its earliest stage. Paradoxically, all these screening methods only serve to increase the risk for cancer.

Among women with detected breast cancer, 88% have not spread and 12% are invasive tumors. It would take 400 years for the 16 million U.S. women with undiagnosed breast cancer to die of the disease at the current mortality rate of 40,000 per year. There is no justification for treating every breast cancer detected and no sense in detection until the few breast cancers that threaten women can be distinguished from the rest.

In an overlooked report published in the Journal of the American Medical Association, researchers at the Norwegian Institute of Public Health, Oslo, Norway, find that three times more breast cancers are detected on the first mammogram than in subsequent screenings. If none of the miniscule tumors that cannot be detected by mammography undergo remission, but rather accumulate over time, then one would expect the incidence of breast cancer to increase and be about three times what is observed. The only explanation for the findings of the Norwegian Institute is that undetectable tumors disappear spontaneously, without treatment. [Journal American Medical Association 292: 2579-80, 2004]

Drs. John K. Whiteford, MD, and John Ryan Whiteford, MD, of Verona, Pennsylvania, emphasize that most women with breast cancer survive without treatment. [Annals Internal Medicine 138:768-9, 2003] The same is true for many other types of cancer.

If far more cancers exist than are detected and treated, this speaks for the need to boost natural defenses against cancer.

Undetectable metastases

The mortal form of cancer is when it spreads to other tissues and organs from its original site of origin. This is called metastasis. Cancer researchers have shown there are micrometastases that are too small to be seen or detected on x-ray film or by other conventional methods. Micrometatases are about ½ of 1 millimeter in size. Even with the best cancer treatment, some cancer cells escape and threaten to arise elsewhere at a later time.

For example, researchers conducted a study of breast cancer patients. Prior to surgery, 51% of patients displayed evidence of scattered cancer cells in the bone marrow. Following surgery, tissue samples were taken from bone marrow and blood samples where cancer is likely to spread. Four years after post-operative chemotherapy, up to 87% of patients had tumor cells (micrometastases) that had spread beyond the breast. [International Journal of Cancer, 114: 94-100, 2005]

Micrometastases are found in 15% of early-stage cancer patients. [Obstetrics & Gynecology 103:1204-1210, 2004]It makes a big difference in survival rates if micrometastases can be blocked. A study of colon/rectal cancer patients provides an example. Surgical treatment of colon/rectal cancer calls for follow-up chemotherapy for patients with Stage III disease, which means they have cancer cells that have already spread to surrounding lymph nodes.

About 20 % of Stage II patients, who have no detectable cancer cells that have spread to the lymph nodes, and do not receive chemotherapy, succumb to this disease. An analysis of 192 lymph nodes from 26 consecutive patients with Stage II colorectal cancer, found micrometastases in one or more lymph nodes from 14 of 26 patients. The 5-year survival rate was 50 % in this group, whereas in the 12 patients without micrometastases, the survival rate was 91 %. [New England Journal Medicine 339:223-228, 1998]

An effective treatment is needed to cleanse the body of micrometastases in order to improve the cure rate achieved with surgical removal of cancer. Efforts are currently underway to find such a therapy. [Charles H Weaver MD, CancerConsultants.com 2004] However, none are claimed to be available yet.

This is difficult to believe, since the medical literature clearly explains why micrometastases occur and how to stop them.

Immunity and micrometastases

A weak immune system facilitates micrometastases. It is imperative that the immune system be addressed since surgery, chemo and radiation therapy impair the immune system, making micrometastases more of a threat. [Cancer 43: 945-51, 1979; Cancer 68: 482-88, 1991; Journal Immunology Letters 80:55-66, 2002; Journal Veterinary Internal Medicine 20:342-7, 2006]

Stop metastases!

Regardless of the stage of your cancer, even hidden yet-to-be-diagnosed cancer, the primary objective is to stop metastases, which is the chief threat to life. You cannot rely on your oncologist to prescribe a drug or therapy that prevents metastasis, and in fact, all conventional methods of cancer treatment increase the risk for metastasis.

There are numerous ways to inhibit metastatic cancer that are at hand, without prescription. Following are 12 ways of halting the spread of cancer and the natural products that are most likely to accomplish this:

1 Elevation of the immune system by boosting natural killer cell activity (resveratrol, vitamin D, vitamin E, beta glucan, beta carotene, IP6 rice bran

2 Maintenance of the collagen that surrounds malignant cells so they cannot spread (vitamin C, the amino acids proline and lysine, chondroitin, hyaluronic acid, resveratrol)

3 Inhibition of blood clots so roaming tumor cells cannot stagnate and begin a new colony (allicin/garlic, vitamin E, omega-3 oil, resveratrol and nattokinase enzymes).

4 Prevention of the adhesion of roaming cancer cells to the wall of blood vessels, and colonization (nattokinase, resveratrol and other nutrients).

5 Cessation of activity of cancer-causing genes (resveratrol and HDAC inhibitors)

6 Selective destruction of cancer cells (allicin from garlic, vitamin C, IP6 rice bran)

7 Escalation of cellular energy by burning oxygen in cancer cells (coenzyme Q10, magnesium, lipoic acid, acetyl L carnitine, resveratrol).

8 Utilization of agents that target cancer cells only (allicin from garlic, IP6 phytate, vitamin C, resveratrol).

9 Destruction of cancer-causing germs (allicin from garlic, quercetin, resveratrol).

10 Prevention of angiogenesis (resveratrol, green tea, curcumin, vitamins C and D, quercetin, proline, lysine, omega-3 oils).

11 Limitation of iron and copper in the body (IP6 rice bran, magnesium, resveratrol, tea extracts, zinc).

12 Normalization of hormonal activity (fermented sources of soy: miso, tofu, flaxseed meal or lignan extracts, resveratrol).

Natural killer cells

A particular type of white blood cell, called natural killer cells, inhibits micrometastases. Natural killer cells are a type of white blood cell that contains enzymes that can kill tumor cells or germ cells.

Mice with very high natural killer cell activity are very resistant to metastasis. [Cancer Metastasis Review 1: 45-64, 1982] An experiment was conducted with mice with melanoma of the eye, to determine its spread to the liver as micrometastases. Groups of mice were made deficient or fully depleted of natural killer cells using toxic chemicals.

In this mouse experiment, interferon was used to boost natural killer cell activity which decreased micrometastases in the liver. [Investigative Ophthalmology Visual Science 45: 2056-64, 2004] Interferon is a biologic therapy that stimulates the immune system but is fraught with side effects. Interferon induces a severe vitamin C deficiency [American Journal Clinical Nutrition 54: 1292-97S, 1991] which in healthy individuals results in a decline in natural killer cells. Supplemental vitamin C can restore natural killer cell activity but is not usually utilized. [Immunopharmacology Immunotoxicology 19: 291-312, 1997]

Monoclonal antibodies can also be employed. Monoclonal antibodies are made in a laboratory and infused into tumors, but they are not able to adequately penetrate bulky tumors. [Proceedings National Academy Science 92: 8999-9003, 1995]

There are few studies that have been conducted to show that boosting natural killer cell activity reduces micrometastases. However, researchers in Japan inoculated mice with kidney cancer cells and then gave them vitamin D. Vitamin D inhibited tumor micrometastases and growth and prolonged the life span of tumor-bearing mice. [Journal Urology 160: 247-51, 1998]

Meanwhile, a number of nutritional factors have been shown to boost natural killer cell activity:

- Resveratrol
  Life Sciences 70:81-96, 2001
- Vitamin D
  Mechanisms Ageing Development 102:279-92, 1998
- Rice bran extract (IP6)
  Carcinogenesis 10:1595-8, 1989
- Vitamin C
  Immunopharmacology Immunotoxicology 19: 291-312, 1997
- Vitamin E (tocotrienols 10 times more than tocopherols)
  International Journal Food Science Nutrition 51: S13-20, 2000
- Beta carotene *International Journal Food Science Nutrition 51: S13-20, 2000*
- Beta glucan
  Journal Medicinal Food 8:154-8, 2005
- Healthy bacteria (Bifidobacteria)
  European Journal Clinical Nutrition 54:849-55, 2000
- Zinc
  American Journal Clinical Nutrition 71: 590-98, 2000
- Selenium
  Z Emahrungswiss 37: 50-56, 1998
- N-acetyl cysteine (sulfur)
  Experimental Gerontology 34:675-85, 1999
- Nucleotides (parts of RNA and DNA, available as a dietary supplement)
  Journal Parenteral Enteral Nutrition 14: 18-22, 1990

Folic acid and natural killer cells

Folic acid, known as vitamin B9, is widely used in dietary supplements and is required for DNA repair. Folic acid is often used by fertile females to prevent birth defects. It is also known as a cancer fighter by virtue of its ability to raise natural killer cell activity among individuals who are deficient in folic acid. [Journal Nutrition 132: 1361-67, 2002]

However, there is justified concern over provision of too much folic acid. At about 200 mcg per day, folic acid will begin to overwhelm the enzymatic metabolism of folic acid to methylfolate. At 400 mcg intake there is saturation and much of the folic acid enters the blood circulation unmetabolized. In a study of postmenopausal women, 54% of whom who took multivitamins, 78% had unmetabolized folic acid in their blood serum and experienced about a 23% reduction in natural killer cell activity. [Journal Nutrition 136: 189-94, 2006] Health authorities are concerned that this may cause symptomless, undetected micrometastatic cancer to begin to spread and become deadly.

A study of postmenopausal women taking high-dose folic acid found a very slight increased risk for breast cancer (about 2/10ths of 1 percent difference between women whose intake of folic acid was less than 335 mcg compared to over 853 mcg). While not alarming, it does show a trend that is of concern. [American Journal Clinical Nutrition 83: 895-904, 2006]

However another study employing much larger doses found that 5,000 mcg of folic acid given 3 times a day for six months to 43 subjects at risk for laryngeal (throat) cancer produced promising results. At the end of the study, 12 patients (28%) no longer had pre-cancerous lesions, and 19 patients had the size of their lesions reduced by half or more. The remaining 12 patients experienced no change in the size of their lesions. [Institute of Otolaryngology, Universita Cattolica del Sacro Cuore, Rome, Italy, 2006]

While high intake levels of folic acid are desirable, the drawback of diminished natural killer cell activity needs to be addressed. The answer is to use a type of folic acid supplement called Metafolin (Merck) that is pre-metabolized. It is widely available as a dietary supplement.

Up to 40% of adults are genetically flawed so that they are unable to convert folic acid to its active form. [Journal Nutrition 129: 919-22, 1999] These individuals may be at increased risk for micrometastases. However, high-dose folic acid supplementation may exacerbate the problem, not improve it. The new understanding that high-dose supplemental folic acid may caused unmetabolized folic acid to enter the blood circulation and impair natural killer cell-derived immunity, may explain why some health-minded individuals who take dietary supplements are observed to have difficulty controlling cancer while others are able to maintain dormant tumors that never cause symptoms during their lifetime.

Strengthening collagen

There is yet another mechanism to control cancer that is not employed by conventional cancer therapy. The stimulation of collagen formation, with vitamin C and the amino acids proline and lysine, can *"wall off"* tumors. The provision of antioxidants can prevent the breakdown of collagen/hyaluronic acid, and thus control cancer. [Alternative Medicine Review 3: 174-86, 1998]

A mixture of vitamin C, two amino acids (lysine, proline) and antioxidants (green tea) have repeatedly been shown by Dr. Matthias Rath to inhibit the breakdown of collagen and prevent the spread of cancer. [Experimental Lung Research 32:69-79, 2006; Medical Oncology23:105-11, 2006; In Vivo 20:25-32, 2006; Oncology Reports 14:807-15, 2005; International Journal Gastrointestinal Cancer 35:97-102, 2005; In Vivo 19:179-83, 2005]

Blood clots and sticky cancer cells

Oncologists are fully aware of the link between blood clots and cancer. Cancer patients tend to form clots, but cancer doctors believe this is a result of, not a cause of, metastasis. Once cancer cells have escaped from their mother tumor and enter the blood circulation they need to stop for a period of at least 20 minutes so they can begin to accumulate and invade through the blood vessel wall to establish another colony. To do this cancer cells must either adhere to the wall of blood vessels or find their way into the tiniest of blood vessels (capillaries) where blood clots have formed.

Clot-busting agents

It has long been known that the tendency to form blood clots facilitates the spread of cancer. The use of blood thinners (anti-clotting agents) has been shown to inhibit metastasis. [Minerva Medicine 97: 175-89, 2006] There are numerous anti-blood clotting agents.

Anti-blood clotting agents

- Omega-3 oils
  Arteriosclerosis Thrombosis Vascular Biology 24:1734-40, 2004
- Garlic
  Prostaglandins Leukotrienes Essential Fatty Acids 53:211-2, 1995
- Magnesium
  Thrombosis Haemostasis 86:1292-5, 2001
- Vitamin E
  Thrombosis Research 79:109-23, 1995
- Nattokinase
  Biochem Biophys Res Communications 197:1340-7, 1993

Block cancer cell adhesion

Certain enzymes can be consumed that will literally break up blood clots. One natural food supplement, the soy enzyme nattokinase, is such an agent. Because of nattokinase's long-acting, clot-busting activity, it is the most desirable of enzymes. [Acta Haematologica 84:139-43, 1990]

Resveratrol and quercetin inhibit cancer cells from adhering and creating new colonies. [Oncogene 24: 3274-84, 2005; J Asian Natural Product Research 7:205-13, 2005; Neoplasia 7:37-47, 2005]

Putting cancer cells to sleep

Cancer reearchers are raving about molecules that can literally put cancer cells to sleep. By inhibition of an enzyme, histone deacetylase, certain molecules can make cancer-causing genes cease activity. When the histone deacetylase enzyme is inhibited, gene strands remain tightly coiled and their genetic instructions cannot be read. Cancer researchers say histone deacetylase inhibitors (HDACs) *"have become one of the hottest targets in drug development today."* [Clinical Lung Cancer 7: 309-12, 2006] Unlike conventional chemotherapy drugs, HDAC inhibitors work on solid tumors. [BMC Genomics 7:90, 2006] HDACs are many cancer drugs in one, suppressing cancer cell migration, invasion, metastasis, blood supply, and angiogenesis. [Cancer Treatment Review 32:157-65, 2006]

There is a race to introduce HDAC drugs to treat cancer. HDACs are found in nature and can be synthetically produced as patentable drugs. [Current Medicinal Chemistry 13:935-58, 2006] Cancer patients needn't wait for HDAC inhibitors to become approved drugs.

How tumors become metastatic (spread)

1. Local invasion- breaks through collagen barriers
2. Tumor cells enter blood or lymphatic vessels (called intravasation)
3. Begins to roam through circulatory system
4. Adheres to wall of blood vessel or stops in small capillaries that have blood clots
5. Invasion into surrounding tissues (called extravasation)
6. Reproduction and growth of tumor, accomplished by acquisition of nutrients from newly formed blood supply (angiogenesis)

Resveratrol, available as a dietary supplement, is a strong enzyme inhibitor and virtually silences the genes that are involved in cancer growth. [Journal Biological Chemistry 280:17187-95, 2005] Because resveratrol is virtually non-toxic, anyone wishing to prevent or treat cancer can begin using it immediately. There are efforts to mislead the public into thinking resveratrol is not bioavailable as a dietary supplement, but in fact it is the same molecule being used successfully in oral-dose animal and human experiments.

Other HDAC inhibitors found in nature are butyrate, the garlic sulfur compound diallyl disulfide, and sulforaphane found in cruciferous vegetables. [Molecular Carcinogenesis 45:443-6, 2006]

It is challenging to write about resveratrol because it virtually blocks cancer by every known mechanism. Here is what researchers in France have to say about resveratrol and cancer:

Resveratrol acts on the process of carcinogenesis by affecting the three phases: tumor initiation, promotion and progression and suppresses the final steps of carcinogenesis, i.e. angiogenesis and metastasis. It is also able to activate apoptosis (causes cancer cells to die off gradually) and to arrest the cell cycle (stop cancer cell growth). Interestingly, resveratrol does not present any toxicity in animal models. Moreover, concentrations of resveratrol in blood seem to be sufficient for anti-invasive activity. The recirculation or resveratrol may contribute to delayed elimination from the body and bring about a prolonged effect. Interestingly, low doses of resveratrol can sensitize to low doses of toxic anti-cancer drugs and so provide an innovative strategy to enhance the effectiveness of anticancer therapy in various human cancers. By these properties, resveratrol appears to be a good candidate in prevention as well as therapy and is believed to be a novel weapon for new therapeutic strategies. [Current Drug Targets 7:423-42, 2006]

Selectively kill cancer cells (spare the healthy cells)

There are at least four agents in nature that selectively kill cancer cells. Modern chemotherapy drugs are toxic to cancerous and healthy cells, and thus cause many side effects that even threaten the life of the patient. While cancer researchers say they are desperately searching for agents that target cancer cells only, four already exist in nature:

- **Allicin** from garlic works by depleting antioxidants from cancer cells. [Nutrition & Cancer 38: 245-54, 2000] Allicin works by literally causing cancer cells to commit suicide. [Nutrition & Cancer 38:98-105, 2000]
- **Vitamin C** given intravenously (but not orally) transiently creates hydrogen peroxide which kills cancer cells without harm to normal cells. [Proceedings National Academy Science 102:13604-9, 2005]

- **Rice bran extract (IP6)** kills cancer cells by depriving them of iron and copper, their primary growth factors. [Anticancer Research 25:2891-903, 2005]

- **Resveratrol** selectively silences thousands of gene-controlled growth mechanisms in cancer cells. [Cancer Epidemiology Biomarkers Prevention 14:596-604, 2005; Cancer Biology Therapy 3:882-8, 2004]

Experiment after experiment shows that when omega-3 oils (flaxseed, fish) predominate over omega-6 oils (corn oil) in the diet, cancer cell growth is inhibited. [World Review Nutrition Dietetics 94:158-65, 2005] Remarkable tumor remissions have been documented with high-dose omega-3 oil intake (12,000 mg/day). [Nutrition & Cancer 52:121-9, 2005] Omega-3 oils have been shown to increase survival when combined with chemotherapy drugs. [Cancer 88:1916-28, 2000]

Kill cancer-causing germs

Address the germ theory of cancer by consumption of natural agents that kill bacteria, viruses and fungi.

- **Garlic/allicin** by virtue of its ability to kill all known viruses, bacteria, fungi. [Planta Medica 58:417-23, 1992; Mycoses 48:95-100, 2005] Papilloma virus causes cervical cancer. Lymphomas are known to be of viral origin. [Current Opinion Hematology 13:254-259, 2006] Allicin kills *Helicobacter pylori*, the bacterium involved in gastric cancer. [Biotechnology Progress 20:397-401, 2004]

- **Resveratrol** inhibits growth of bacteria (*H. pylori* involved in gastric cancer), viruses and fungi. [American Journal Gastroenterology 98:1440-1, 2003; Pharmacological Research 45:499-505, 2002; Archives Pharmacological Research 28:557-60, 2005]

- **Quercetin**, found naturally in red onions, is available as a dietary supplement, and when combined with vitamin C is known to be active against most viruses. [Journal General Virology 69:1749-51, 1988]

Increase cellular energy naturally

Cancer cells do not rely upon utilization of oxygen for cellular energy, but rather produce energy by fermentation of sugars within tumor cells. Various strategies are being developed to increase cellular energy by burning oxygen in cancer cells. [Science 312: 1158-59, 2006] Natural agents that increase cellular energy are:

- **Coenzyme Q10**
- **Magnesium**
- **Lipoic acid**
- **Acetyl L carnitine**
- **Resveratrol** (inhibits tumor hypoxia factor- lack of oxygen in cells that causes cancer cells to ferment sugars for energy, which creates lactic acid outside the cell)

Stop angiogenesis naturally

As a small tumor begins to grow it obtains nutrients like other cells. But once a tumor has reached a certain size, about 1-2 millimeters, it must develop access to nutrients (oxygen, growth factors) via direct blood supply. At this stage, cancer cells will secrete substances (angiopoietin-1, fibroblast growth factor, vascular endothelial growth factor) employed in normal wound healing, to promote the formation of new blood vessels. This is called angiogenesis. In normal wound healing these blood vessels recede after 2-3 weeks. These new blood vessels do not normally recede after a tumor is formed. The body produces its own angiogenesis inhibitors (angiostatin, endostatin) that are obviously overwhelmed as tumors grow.

There is a question of whether a small non-metastatic tumor should be operated upon. Surgery creates a wound that must be healed, so growth factors are secreted which can then cause the tumor from newly formed blood supply and begin to spread. If undergoing surgery, utilize natural anti-angiogenesis agents.

- **Resveratrol, green tea and curcumin** from turmeric inhibit angiogenesis. [Journal Physiology Pharmacology 56: 51-69, 2005]

- **Vitamin D** inhibits angiogenesis and metastasis. [Carcinogenesis 26: 1044-54, 2005]

- **Quercetin** inhibits angiogenesis [British Journal Nutrition 95:1016-23, 2006]

- **Vitamin C, proline, lysine, antioxidant combination**

- **Omega-3 oils (flaxseed)** [Med Hypotheses 66:1121-4, 2004]

Limit iron and copper

Tumor cells rely upon iron and copper for growth. Chelation (removal) of metallic metals is important in cancer control. This can be accomplished by use of chelating molecules and other minerals. Cancer researchers report that *"chelators can now be designed to target molecules to induce specific effects, for instance, angiogenesis or metastasis suppression."* [Current Medicinal Chemistry 12:2711-29, 2005] Virtually all man-made chelators are toxic. Chelators that already exist in nature are non-toxic.

- **IP6 rice bran extract** removes metallic metals (tumor growth factor) [Biochemical Journal 294:929-34, 1993]

- **Magnesium, zinc** (to compete with iron absorption and utilization) and reduce cancer risk. [Epidemiology 17: 308-314, 2006]

Calm down the hormones

Calming (but not completely blocking) hormone production in sex gland cancers (prostate and breast tumors) inhibits tumor growth. Strong hormone blockers (Tamoxifen, aromatase inhibitors) or hormones themselves (estrogen, Lupron) are fraught with side effects. Without adequate hormones, bones will wither, mood will decline, and other side effects will occur. Normalize hormone levels with:

- **Fermented sources of soy**: miso, tofu

- **Flaxseed meal (lignans) or lignan extracts** (Prevail pill) [Annual Review Plant Biology 55:225-61, 2004]

- **Resveratrol**

Aid DNA repair and repair of tissues damages by cancer

- **Folic acid**

- **Vitamin B12**

- **Resveratrol**

- **Vitamin C**

- **Chondroitin sulfate**

Reduce tumor cell resistance against anti-cancer agents

Tumors resist drugs. The body will create defenses (P-glycoprotein, cytochrome p450 enzymes) against toxic drugs over time. Quercetin and resveratrol inhibit drug resistance and may be compatible with prescribed chemotherapy. These natural agents will enhance the effect of toxic drugs and therefore caution is advised. [Federation of European Biochemical Societies Journal 272: 4725-40, 2005]

Prevent side effects caused by chemo or radiation therapy

Various tissues in the body are at increased risk for damage while undergoing chemotherapy or radiation. Protection with antioxidants and other nutrients is advised.

- **Vitamin E**
- **Vitamin C, proline, lysine**
- **Resveratrol**
- **Folic acid**
- **Magnesium**
- **Vitamin C**
- **Acidophilus/Bifidus good bacteria** (10-50 billion count)

Many of the above factors or cancer processes are not even addressed by conventional cancer care. Furthermore, nutritional factors can accomplish more in this regard than can drugs or other conventional cancer treatment.

Stage 4 Advanced cancer care

Melatonin given to tumor-bearing animals increases their survival time. [Molecular Cell Biochemistry 278: 15-20, 2005] A review of all human studies involving supplemental melatonin and cancer reveals a consistent improvement in survival. The dosage used in most studies was greater than used for jet lag, about 20 mg per day (range 10-40 mg), taken prior to bedtime. [Journal Pineal Research 39: 360-66, 2005]

Anti-cancer diet

Diets that prevent cancer should be low in iron (less meat), rich in omega-3 oils, high in antioxidants like vitamin C and vitamin E, low in saturated fats; devoid of hydrogenated fats; high in dark-green leafy vegetables that provide folic acid, high in cruciferous vegetables; include fermented sources of soy (miso, tofu) and flaxseed meal; and be abundant in water-rich foods such as peaches, melon, grapes, apricots, etc., and sulfur-rich foods such as garlic, onions, asparagus and eggs.

It has been shown that various foods, spices and herbs can interfere with cellular pathways involved in the formation of cancer cells and tumors. Researchers at the MD Anderson Cancer Hospital in Houston, Texas identify these natural molecules. These natural agents include curcumin (turmeric), resveratrol (red grapes, peanuts and berries), genistein (soybean), diallyl sulfide (garlic, leek, onion, chive), S-allyl cysteine (garlic, leek, onion, chive), allicin (garlic), lycopene (tomato), capsaicin (red chilli), diosgenin (fenugreek), 6-gingerol (ginger), ellagic acid (pomegranate), ursolic acid (apple, pears, prunes), silymarin (milk thistle), anethol (anise, camphor, and fennel), catechins (green tea), eugenol (cloves), indole-3-carbinol (cruciferous vegetables), limonene (citrus fruits), beta carotene (carrots), and dietary fiber. These foods are targeted to fight cancer. [Biochemical Pharmacology 71:1397-421, 2006]

Recognize that an iron overloaded, folic acid, vitamin D and omega-3 oil deficient human body is a ripe field for cancer.

Food list (short list)

- Brussels' sprouts
- Garlic
- Onions
- Grapes
- Flaxseed meal
- Fermented soy (tofu, miso)
- Broccoli
- Spinach
- Kale
- Bran
- Melon
- Tomatoes
- Berries
- Pomegranate
- Citrus peel
- Olives
- Virgin olive oil or rice bran oil
- Avoid or limit red meat, hydrogenated fats

Personal Dietary Supplement Regimen

Nutrient, spice, herb	Preferred Forms	Typical Dosage Range	
		Prevention	**Therapeutic**
VITAMINS			
Vitamin A	Beta carotene	5,000 IU	10,000 IU
Vitamin C	Comfort-C if intolerant to acidity	2,000 mg	15,000 mg
Vitamin D	Vitamin D3 natural source	2,000 IU	4,000 IU +
Vitamin E	D-alpha tocopherol succinate, Now Foods E-Powder	200 - 400 IU	400 - 3,200 IU
Folic acid	Use Metafolin (Merck) only	400 mcg	400-800 mcg
MINERALS			
Selenium	SelenoExcel® - Natural Factors	200 mcg	200 - 3,200 mcg
Zinc	Zinc citrate- Natural Factors	15 - 25 mg	15 - 25 mg
Magnesium	Citrate or hydroxide best absorbed (oxide only 4% absorbed)	200 - 400 mg	200 - 400 mg
Boron		6 - 12 mg	12 - 20 mg
AMINO ACIDS			
Proline	Vita Cor Plus or Epican Forte- Dr. Rath formulas	500 mg	1,000 mg +
Lysine	Many brands	500 mg	1,000 mg +
OMEGA OILS			
Flaxseed meal	Vacuum container preferred; refrigerate (Barlean's)	1 tablespoon	1-2 tablespoons
Flaxseed oil	Barlean's for freshness	tablespoon 3,000 mg	12,000 mg

Personal Regimen

	AM	Midday	PM	Bedtime
VITAMINS				
Vitamin A				
Vitamin C				
Vitamin D				
Vitamin E				
Folic acid				
MINERALS	AM	Midday	PM	Bedtime
Selenium				
Zinc				
Magnesium				
Boron				
AMINO ACIDS	AM	Midday	PM	Bedtime
Proline				
Lysine				
OMEGA OILS	AM	Midday	PM	Bedtime
Flaxseed meal				
Flaxseed oil				

Personal Dietary Supplement Regimen

Nutrient, spice, herb	Preferred Forms	Typical Dosage Range: Prevention	Typical Dosage Range: Therapeutic
HERBALS			
Allicin/garlic	Garli-eze® proven allicin	400 mg	400 mg +
Quercetin	Many brands	100 mg	500 mg
Resveratrol	Trans resveratrol in sealed Licaps capsule (Longevinex®)	40 mg	300 mg +
CHELATORS			
IP6 Rice bran	Tsuno Foods IP6 (Jarrow, Source Naturals, Purity Products brand names)	400 - 800 mg	2,000-4,000 mg
PROBIOTICS			
	Natren	10 billion	50 billion
MISCELLANEOUS			
Indole 3-carbinol	Now Foods with flaxseed lignans	200 mg	200 mg
Beta glucan	Biothera- Imucell WGP or Life Source Basics	As directed	As directed
Chondroitin	Many brands	500 -1,500 mg	
Hyaluronic acid	Purity Products	100 - 200 mg	
Melatonin	Take at bedtime (esp if metastatic)	3-10 mg	20 mg +
Coenzyme Q10	In softgel caps	100 mg	100 - 500 mg
Lignans	Brevail	100 mg	100 mg
Nucleotides	Nucleotide Immune Formula- Lifespan Nutrition		

Personal Regimen

	AM	Midday	PM	Bedtime
HERBALS				
Allicin/garlic				
Quercetin				
Resveratrol				
CHELATORS				
IP6 Rice bran				
PROBIOTICS				
Natren				
MISCELLANEOUS				
Indole 3-carbinol				
Beta glucan				
Chondroitin				
Hyaluronic acid				
Melatonin				
Coenzyme Q10				
Lignans				
Nucleotides				

Success story:

To all of you who have shown concern for my health. As you all may well know, I was diagnosed with ovarian cancer on 9/11/06 & had some blood tests done and had surgery on 9/18/06. Total hysterectomy was done as well as removal of glands and a small part of my liver, and the fat layer as well as my appendix. The medical report was written in medical terminology but you get the picture.

Since the 1st of October I have been taking the following alternatives to help me.

Flaxseed oil 12,000 mg
Vitamin D 4000 iu
Quercetin + vitamin C 2000 mg 3-5 times day
Resveratrol 200 mg
IP6 rice bran extract
Vitamin K
Nattokinase enzymes
Flaxseed meal & plain yogurt
Melatonin
Cellular zeolite (mineral supplement)
NO REFINED SUGARS
NO ARTIFICIAL SWEETNENERS
NO TAP WATER
NO IRON RICH FOODS (RED MEAT)
NO IRON SUPPLEMENTS

AND HAVE BEEN GETTING AS MUCH SUNLIGHT AS POSSIBLE & EATING LOTS OF ORGANIC VEGETABLES & THANKING GOD FOR HIS DAILY BLESSINGS. I am feeling uplifted and can move much easier, no pain pills, and am able to sleep at night for longer periods. Most important of all, my husband Al and I have just thrown ourselves at the mercy of God and asked for his divine help.

I do not want to have the chemo therapy, after reading all the information on side effects as well as hearing about what it can do to other body parts and after all that the chances the medical practitioners give me are 35 to 40 percent chance!
I prefer to live my life happy without the anxiety of chemo. Some people do all the above & still do chemo. I realize we are not out of the woods yet, but on a new journey (with Jesus Christ as our best friend)

The first CA 125 (cancer test by blood sample) result was 372, which is elevated (35 is normal).

On 11/3/06 another blood test was taken by our local oncologist and the end result of the CA125 was THIRTEEN! PRAISE THE LORD FOR HIS MERCY.

I thank God for all your prayers and intercession to our LORD for me. God bless you all.

C S D

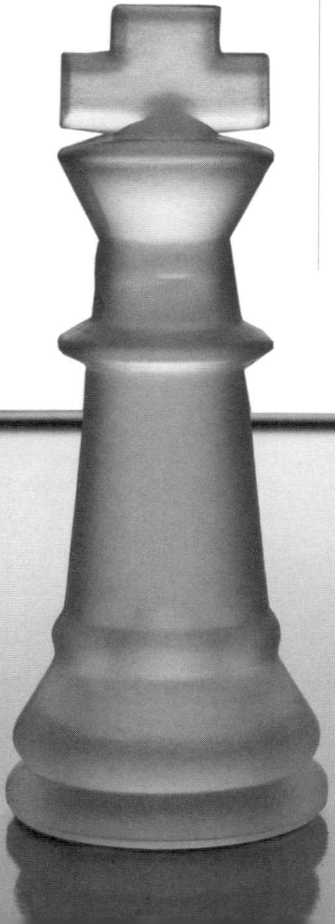

CHAPTER 16

The Cancer Care Industry

p 510 - 538

The Cancer Care Industry

INTRODUCTION

An army of doctors, pathologists, surgeons, radiologists, nurses, researchers, and pharmaceutical company personnel go to work every day in the war against cancer. They depend upon a steady stream of patients to keep the industry churning dollars rather than cures. This year some 1.4 million Americans will have a frightening diagnosis of cancer and enter a cancer care system that is dysfunctional if not outright fraudulent.

John C. Bailar III, a noted expert on cancer, says he is *"fed up with the constant procession of hopeful news stories" suggesting a cancer cure is just around the corner. Scientific American Magazine said in 1994 that "oncologists still cut, poison and burn."*

This chapter is frankly too upsetting for most cancer patients, and may only lead to confusion, conflicts or outrage by family members at a time when they must comfort the ailing cancer patient. Cancer patients and their families have little time to engage in philosophical, economic or ethical battles. Some patients decide they cannot handle any information that discredits their doctors. Where else are they to turn?

A major objective of this book is to urge cancer patients to back away from treatment that only harms, or in many instances, kills, and offers little if any benefits. Alternatives abound that go overlooked by modern medicine.

But, frankly, while cancer patients read of the failings of cancer therapy, few patients believe their trusted doctor has anything to do with this. The trust cancer patients have with their doctors is similar to the bond a crime victim makes when a criminal is pointing a gun at him and asking for money. Who would dare anger the doctor when he/she is needed to save your life? Certainly most patients are loyal to their doctors to a fault. They are reluctant to stand up to their doctor and asking questions would appear to be too con-

Cure For Cancer Worth $50 Trillion
A one percent reduction in mortality from cancer has a value to Americans of nearly $500 billion. A cure for cancer would be worth about $50 trillion.
Source: Kevin M. Murphy and Robert H. Topel. "The Value of Health and Longevity" Journal of Political Economy, May 2006

frontational. It's your life that is on the line. See if you can muster up a few good questions for your oncologist when you visit his/her office.

It's important for an author of a book on cancer not to prematurely form opinions for readers, or have an axe to grind. Authoritative sources are saying the cancer care industry is dysfunctional. After reading this book you may be better equipped to question which treatments are worthwhile and which are better to avoid.

Clifton Leaf of Fortune Magazine says: *"Experts offer testimony that, when taken together, describes a dysfunctional 'cancer culture'— a groupthink that pushes tens of thousands of physicians and scientists toward the goal of finding the tiniest improvements in treatment rather than genuine breakthroughs; that fosters isolated (and redundant) problem solving instead of cooperation; and rewards academic achievement and publication over all else."*

"At each step along the way from basic science to patient bedside, investigators rely on models that are consistently lousy at predicting success — to the point where hundreds of cancer drugs are thrust into the pipeline, and many are approved by the FDA, even though their proven 'activity' has little to do with curing cancer." [Fortune March 22, 2004]

Fortune Magazine published a long-running expose of the cancer industry in 2004. Clifton Leaf, a cancer patient himself, was designated to be the chief investigator. Here were some of the findings reported by Leaf.

Most recently, with media reports celebrating such revolutionary cancer medicines as Gleevec, Herceptin, Iressa, Erbitux, and the just-approved Avastin, the cure has seemed closer than ever. But it's not. Hope and optimism, so essential to this fight, have masked some very real systemic problems that have made this complex, elusive, relentless foe even harder to defeat. The result is that while there have been substantial achievements since the crusade began with the National Cancer Act in 1971, we are far from winning the war. So far away, in fact, that it looks like losing.

Living longer?

The National Cancer Institute just issued a news release claiming modest drops in cancer rates, just prior to the publication of this book. So, wait a minute, maybe the failures of the past can be forgotten if true advancements are being made now. Don't bet on it. As Clifton Leaf of Fortune Magazine said:

> *Researchers also say more people are surviving longer with cancer than ever. Yet here, too, the complete picture is more disappointing. Survival gains for the more common forms of cancer are measured in additional months of life, not years. The few dramatic increases in cure rates and patient longevity have come in a handful of less common malignancies—including Hodgkin's, some leukemias, carcinomas of the thyroid and testes, and most childhood cancers. But even using this analysis (in which the proportion of elderly is dialed back to what it was during the Nixon administration), the percentage of Americans dying from cancer is about the same as in 1970 ... and in 1950.*

Falsifying data

The cancer industry has even been caught rigging cancer rates to falsely show progress in the war on cancer. This is repeatedly done without correction or even apology. Congress is remiss for its lack of oversight, since most cancer research studies use public funds.

In 2002, *Wall Street Journal* reporter Sharon Begley reported that the National Cancer Institute (NCI) showed the incidence of several devastating cancers had leveled off or declined. The NCI's report was published in the *Journal of the National Cancer Institute.* The NCI initially declared breast cancer rates had been almost flat since 1987. But a re-analysis shows that breast-cancer rates actually have been rising 0.6% per year since 1987 to 2002. The NCI claimed melanoma rates were about the same, when they actually were soaring at a 4.1% increase per year since 1981. Prostate cancer was said to have fallen since 1995, but actually rose by 2.2% per year. Why the mistakes? The cancer registries have 19 months to submit data to the National Cancer Institute, but in fact many additions dribble in late, so that up to 12% of the cases may be reported late and not included in published statistics. [The Wall Street Journal, Oct. 18, 2002]

New anti-cancer compounds

Roughly 300 new anti-cancer drugs are in the development pipeline, about half of them are in the research and development stage.

The hope is that the new generation of targeted anti-cancer drugs might even replace toxic chemotherapy, says a report in *Business Week magazine. "It turns out, however, that most of the targeted cancer therapies coming down the research pipeline likely won't be the silver bullets investors and researchers had hoped for."* Notice patients are left out of Business Week's equation. All that counts is how much money investors have at risk, not patients' lives. [Business Week, March 5, 2003]

> *"Anytime someone standing near me talks about a 'new paradigm' in cancer treatment, I check my back pocket to see if my wallet is still there."*
> *Source: Dr. Ray Warrell, oncologist, Business Week, March 5, 2003*

Herceptin (trastuzumab) combats breast cancer

The attention given to Herceptin (trastuzumab) is just one example of the hype behind many of the so-called cancer breakthroughs. After the American Society of Clinical Oncology (ASCO) delivered its first-ever report on clinical cancer at the annual meeting in 2005, Dr. Sandra J. Horning, president of ASCO, described many of the advancements being made. [Annual meeting, ASCO, Abstract 555t, 2005] Here is what Dr. Horning had to say about Herceptin:

Up to 30% of breast cancer patients have malignancies that overproduce the HER-2 protein, and these cancers have been notoriously resistant to therapy. However, a recent study found Herceptin slashed cancer recurrence in this high-risk group by half. *"Many in the breast cancer community feel this is one of the most important breast cancer advances in decades,"* Horning said.

Long-term results indicate that the addition of Herceptin (trastuzumab) to Taxotere (docetaxel) improves long-term survival in patients with HER-2-positive metastatic breast cancer, from 22.7 months on Taxotere to 31.2 months with Herceptin. However, heart failure occurred with 2% of the patients treated with Herceptin.

Herceptin had previously been heralded as a breakthrough and even a *"cure"* for breast cancer. One study showed Herceptin increased survival from 20.3 to 25.1 months over the use of chemotherapy alone. [New England Journal Medicine 344: 783-92, 2001]

Here is the sleight of hand not mentioned in the news reports. If one is tabulating the increase in survival from breast cancer over a four-year period, Herceptin increased survival by 18.2%, but because Herceptin causes heart failure, overall, the survival rate was 94.3% among women taking Herceptin and 91.7% for women receiving chemotherapy alone. The headlines were all about a meaningless 2.5% difference in survival. [New England Journal Medicine Volume 353:1673-1684, 2005]

Joining in creating the excitement surrounding Herceptin was Gabriel N. Hortobagyi, MD, who declared the results of two studies published in the New England Journal of Medicine, on the use of Herceptin in the treatment of breast cancer *"stunning."* [New England Journal Medicine Volume 353:1734-1736, 2005]

All the hoopla over Herceptin promoted the following editorial in the British journal, The Lancet:

> *Promising results were initially presented at this year's American Society of Clinical Oncology annual meeting. In October, these studies were finally reported in the New England Journal of Medicine. In an accompanying editorial, Dr. Gabriel Hortobagyi described the results as "simply stunning" and "revolutionary". He even went so far as to say that Herceptin was "maybe even a cure" for breast cancer. Naturally this comment was picked up and repeated across the world, fuelling demand for rapid access to Herceptin. The excitement is premature. It is profoundly misleading to suggest, even rhetorically, that the published data may be indicative of a cure for breast cancer. [Lancet 366: 1673, 2005]*

Targeted therapies

Dr. Horning said many of the new cancer drugs fall into the category of *"targeted"* therapies, in which treatments are tailored to fight specific cancer types and used in patients with specific genetic profiles.

"This is what we call the 'individualization' of cancer therapy," Horning said. *"We're moving toward tailoring treatment for patients, based on a knowledge of their individual tumor and also their genetic predisposition to [drug] toxicity."*

But this isn't needed. There are already natural molecules that target a vast array of genes involved in cancer and no *"genetic tailoring"* is required.

A review of new anti-cancer drugs reaching the European market in the period 1995-2000 showed these new drugs offered few or no advantages over existing preparations, yet cost several times as much. New drug approvals, widely announced to the public to buoy stock prices and encourage public demand, may not be justified by the results of studies. For ethical reasons, new drugs should be compared with existing ones. An existing drug may be found to prolong survival times by six months and a new drug by nine months, which will likely be broadcast as a dramatic breakthrough increasing survival by 33-50%, depending how you compare the numbers (three months is half of six months, or a 50% increase; three months is a third of nine months, or a 33% increase). This sounds more appealing than *"90 days more of life"* for an extra $40,000, which is what some of these drugs cost.

Italian pharmacologists Silvio Garattine and Vittorio Bertele say: *"there is little to justify some of the promises made to the public."* [British Medical Journal 325: 269-71, 2002] Garattine and Bertele criticize the use of older data collected between 1970 and 1974. [British Medical Journal 325: 1302, 2002] Their criticism has been met with disagreement by some oncologists who maintain these Italian researchers did not consider the *"unprecedented advances that have been made in the treatment of common tumors, in both survival and quality of life at the end of the century."*

However, the older data must be used since recent data is misleading, producing the appearance of prolonged survival times because tumors are now being detected at earlier stages.

Many new cancer drugs obtain approval for their ability to slightly delay the time it takes for tumors to metastasize (spread), rather than to improve survival or quality of life. Some drugs, like monoclonal antibodies, are being utilized and patients want them because they hear they are new. However, they are unproven. In fact, monoclonal antibodies have surprisingly produced unfavorable safety profiles. *"It is widely expected that patients will gain no benefit from new anticancer drugs,"* says Garattine and Bertele. [British Medical Journal 325: 269-71, 2002]

Drug companies rewarded for failures

Are drug companies being rewarded for failure? It appears so. They are making more and more money for drugs that offer little or no benefit. The increasing prices of cancer drugs appear to be engineered to elevate stock prices, not reward true breakthroughs.

For example, the cancer drug Erbitux was heralded as a breakthrough and caused stock in ImClone System to rise dramatically, only to fall flat when the FDA rejected research studies on its effectiveness. (This is the drug that household television queen Martha Stewart sold off on an inside tip from Samuel D. Waksal, ImClone's chief executive.) Pharmaceutical companies have learned they can hype an upcoming cancer drug, and investors can reap benefits by buying and selling shares on speculation of the drug's approval. When the day of reckoning occurs, and the FDA rules, whoever is holding shares stands to lose or gain a bundle. Both investors and cancer patients are easily misled. Erbitux is not a stand-alone drug. It must be used with other cancer therapies and only adds a few months of life. Many executives involved in the $2 billion purchase of marketing rights for Erbitux by Bristol-Myers have resigned. [New York Times, Feb. 11, 2004]

What, no treatment for metastasis?

Again, Clifton Leaf of Fortune Magazine speaks out about the failings of cancer treatment.

> *In the end, it is not localized tumors that kill people with cancer; it is the process of metastasis—an incredible 90% of the time. That's because when most malignant solid tumors are diagnosed, they are typically quite large already—the size of a grape, perhaps, with more than a billion cells in the tumor mass.*
>
> *So you'd think that cancer researchers would have been bearing down on this insidious phenomenon for years, intently studying the intricate mechanisms of invasion. Hardly. According to a Fortune examination of NCI grants going back to 1972, less than 0.5% of study proposals focused primarily on metastasis—trying to understand, for instance, its role in a specific cancer (e.g., breast, prostate) or just the process itself. Of nearly 8,900 NCI grant proposals awarded last year, 92% didn't even mention the word metastasis.*
>
> *So pharma companies, quite naturally, don't concentrate on solving the problem of metastasis (the thing that kills people); they focus on devising drugs that shrink tumors (the things that don't).*
>
> *The second problem is even bigger: Clinical trials are focused on the wrong goal—on doing "proper" science rather than saving lives.*

Economic influence like this is probably what prompts political pressure on the FDA to eventually approve drugs so that investors can get their money back. The point of all this is, cancer treatment today is all about money, not patients.

False and misleading news reports

Samuel S. Epstein, MD, and Quentin D. Young, MD, write that while cancer is fast becoming the leading cause of death in the United States, the National Cancer Institute and the American Cancer Society have issued a *"steady stream of misleading press releases hailing major progress in the cancer war."* These include "*miracle*" breakthroughs in cancer treatment and that cancer mortality would be halved by the year 2000. In 1998, the NCI stated that the nation had "*turned the corner*" in the war on cancer. The American Cancer Society hired Schandwick International, a public relations firm, to help draft the National Cancer Control Act. Schandwick International also represents the R. J Reynolds Tobacco Co.

Breast cancer in Japan is four times lower than it is in the U.S. When Japanese women move to the U.S., they or their daughters eventually acquire the disease at North American rates.
Source: Scientific American, January 1994

More falsehoods and deceptions

Dr. Gabriella M. D'Andrea, Assistant Clinical Member, Department of Medicine, Memorial Sloan-Kettering Cancer Center, in New York City, wrote a scurrilous opinion in one of the leading cancer journals. Her words were picked up by the news media, though never challenged. Dr. D'Andrea wrote:

> *"Many patients being treated for cancer use dietary supplements, particularly antioxidants, in the hope of reducing the toxicity of chemotherapy and radiotherapy. However, mechanistic considerations suggest that antioxidants might reduce the effects of conventional cytotoxic therapies. Preclinical data are currently inconclusive and a limited number of clinical studies have not found any benefit. Clinicians should advise their patients against the use of antioxidant dietary supplements during chemotherapy or radiotherapy. Such caution should be seen as the standard approach for any unproven agent that may be harmful.*
>
> *Antioxidants might protect cancer cells, thereby reducing the oncologic effectiveness of cytotoxic therapy. This is the reason why most oncologists discourage patients from using antioxidants during treatment. Pending the publication of suitable trials, clinicians must be guided by existing data in the context of a fundamental principle of medicine, 'Primum non nocere.' There are reasons to believe that taking antioxidants concurrently with chemotherapy or radiotherapy might be harmful; therefore, patients should be advised against it."*
> [CA Cancer Journal for Clinicians 55:319-321, 2005]

Neil Levin, a certified nutritionist and watchdog of the cancer industry, wrote a rebuttal to Dr. D' Andrea's paper. Of course, the news media didn't print it, but the medical journal that published Dr. D' Andrea's paper said it would publish the rebuttal online. Here is Neil Levin's edited rebuttal.

Sent: Wednesday, November 09, 2005 5:25 PM

Dear colleagues and friends,
The American Cancer Society's cancer journal (*"CA"*) has agreed to e-publish my rebuttal to their well-publicized article that warned not to mix antioxidants with cancer therapies. That original article got exaggerated headlines telling us not to use supplements or vitamins along with cancer therapies.

Reviewing the original article, there are 29 references. Two refer to the number of cancer patients who use dietary supplements (50%), three references show how *"antioxidants can protect cells from radiation and chemotherapy"*, and the next five refer to evidence that antioxidants show promising evidence to *"reduce treatment-related toxicities"*. The next five references show that antioxidants *"can en-*

hance the effectiveness of chemotherapy and radiotherapy." In fact, only one reference specifically addresses using antioxidants during therapy and the effect on that therapy, which admittedly did not eliminate *"many confounding factors."* This was supposed to be the whole point of the article!

Was Dr. D' Andrea's report properly peer reviewed before it was published? Was Dr. D'Andrea admonished for her falsehoods? She works at the nation's designated cancer center. Where is the accountability?

The costs are calculated

The Journal of the National Cancer Institute asks *"When will the U.S. flinch at cancer drug prices?"* High hopes are pinned on targeted therapies, drugs that inhibit specific enzymes or pathways, such as Avastin, Erbitux, Tarceva and Iressa, which all became available with *"great fanfare."* Then came the sticker shock. These drugs are priced at thousands of dollars per month of treatment and are only effective when added to other treatments. *"Clinicians are wondering whether these new drugs are worth the cost,"* said the journal article. *"America is starving for effective therapies,"* says Bruce E. Hillner, MD, of Virginia Commonwealth University in Richmond. The drug companies counter by saying these drugs add precious time.

A Kaiser Family Foundation poll in 2005 found the public is not pleased with overall rise in drug prices. [Journal National Cancer Institute 97: 624-25, 2005] The public wants more regulation of drug prices, but the politicians are completely bought off in Washington by the pharmaceutical companies.

But when the failures of the cancer care industry are brought to the public's attention, the cry for more research funds is heard. The quoted figure is that only $30 billion has been spent in the war against cancer since 1971. However, the real figures are somewhat different.

Sales of anticancer drugs in the United States

Class of drugs	1994	2000
Cytotoxic drugs	$1.298 billion	$1.863 billion
Antimetabolites	$252 million	$338 million
Antitubulin drugs	$472 million	$783 million
Alkylating drugs	$210 million	$281 million
Antibiotics	$364 million	$461 million

Fortune Magazine reports that the budgetary outlay for cancer research was $4.74 billion in 2004, just a 3.3% increase over the previous year's budget.

However, the National Institutes of Health, the overseeing agency for the National Cancer Institute, provided an additional $909 million for cancer research through the National Institute of Environmental Health Sciences and other little-noticed grant mechanisms. Add another $457 million for the Department of Veterans Affairs. The Centers for Disease Control will spend an additional $314 million in outreach and education. Even the Pentagon gets involved with $249 million given in 2004 for research grants. Drug companies devote about $7.4 billion for cancer R & D. So Fortune Magazine estimated that taxes, donations, and private R & D, all totaled, in the war on cancer, piles up to $200 billion in inflation-adjusted dollars since 1971! That's a lot of money for no cures.

More tragic, virtually every cancer researcher concedes cancer is very difficult to treat and that cancer prevention programs would likely produce real declines in cancer mortality. Yet very little of the money spent on the war on cancer is devoted truly to prevention.

The money has produced knowledge, a great deal of it -- 1.56 million published papers at the National Library of Medicine – but few cures.

"The search for knowledge has become an end unto itself rather than the means to an end," says Clifton Leaf.

Much of the research money goes toward mouse studies. Homer Pearce, who once ran cancer research and clinical investigation at Eli Lilly and is now research fellow at the drug company, says mouse models are *"woefully inadequate"* for determining whether a drug will work in humans. *"If you look at the millions and millions and millions of mice that have been cured, and you compare that to the relative success, or lack thereof, that we've achieved in the treatment of metastatic disease clinically,"* he says, *"you realize that there just has to be something wrong with those models."*

Most cancer studies involve implanted tumors that have not spread to other locations. However, localized tumors do not kill people with cancer; it is the process of metastasis—an incredible 90% of the time. Aggressive cells spread to the bones, liver, lungs, brain, or other vital areas, wreaking havoc.

Fortune Magazine conducted a survey and found just 0.5% of NCI grants going back to 1972 deal with metastasis.

Cancer by the Numbers

- 180 Upper limit of median lifespan in days for those diagnosed with advanced pancreatic cancer
- 12.8 Days those individuals gain with the drug Tarceva
- $2,000 Cost in dollars of Tarceva per month
- 300 Anticipated annual sales in millions of dollars of the drug
- 6 Percentage rate of increase of stroke in those taking Tarceva

Source: Los Angeles Times

Doctors join in

A scheme between urologists and a pharmaceutical company to sell the anti-hormone drug Lupron, considered the primary treatment for advanced prostate cancer, came into public view recently. Physicians could purchase Lupron at low prices, and in turn were reimbursed at exorbitantly high prices by Medicare. Free samples (which were billed to Medicare at $1,200), resort trips, consulting services, debt forgiveness and educational grants were also used to entice urologists to prescribe Lupron.

Many urologists and oncologists earned an extra $100,000 annually in income with this program, and some of the busier urologists earned over $1 million.

One uncooperative urologist was found guilty of violating the Federal False Claims Act and sentenced to six months of home arrest, excluded from Medicare for five years, required to provide 600 hours of free medical care to indigent patients and patients covered by Medicare or Medicaid, and paid fines and restitution to the government. [Journal Clinical Oncology 23: 8894-905, 2005]

This mass-scale fraud has caused Medicare to downshift its reimbursement for Lupron and other cancer drugs. Many oncologists will earn 30 to 50% less a year as a consequence of the $1.1 billion Medicare fraud settlement.

The Pap smear

In 2004, investigators estimated 22 million U.S. women 18 years and older had undergone hysterectomy, representing 21% of the female population. However, the number of Pap smears to screen for cervical cancer did not change from the period 1992-2002 even with the increasing number of women who now had no cervix to conduct a Pap Smear.

Researchers estimated 10 million women who had undergone hysterectomy were being screened unnecessarily. Doctors were billing for Pap smears among women who were at no risk for cervical cancer. [Journal American Medical Assn 291: 2990-93, 2004]

This reveals the focus of doctors on billing rather than curing.

New cancer vaccine

While Pap smears have nearly eliminated cervical cancer in the developed world, the disease still kills thousands of women each year in poorer countries. However, two new vaccines appear to protect women against infection with the human papilloma virus, which is thought to trigger most cervical cancers.

But these vaccines will not likely influence mortality rates in the U.S. because most women get Pap smears and via early detection avoid death by surgical removal of the cervix. Furthermore, the vaccines are not foolproof and may give young women license to participate in more sexual activity that can breed transfer of cancer-causing viruses.

More misdirection

By late 2005 another misdirection was announced in the war on cancer. U.S. government researchers launched a pilot project to find all genetic changes that cause cancer in the hopes of opening *"a whole new world of targeted cancer therapy."* [Reuters, December 13, 2005]

> The news report says *"They hope to lay the groundwork for replicating the successes of a few targeted cancer therapies such as Herceptin, useful against one type of breast cancer, and Gleevec, a pill that revolutionized treatment of chronic myeloid leukemia."* But these pills have been abject failures.
>
> *"We are dealing with the tip of the iceberg,"* said Dr. Ron DePinho of Harvard Medical School and the Dana Farber Cancer Institute in Boston. *"There are a staggering number of genetic alterations that occur."* Yes, and they are addressed by small molecules, like resveratrol from red wine, allicin from garlic, and oleuropin from olives, that switch hundreds of genes at a time. No mention of these.
>
> *"I think this is a turning point in biomedical research and I think it is a turning point for medicine,"* said Anna Barker, deputy head of the NCI. In fact, it is tragic that no one confronts these health authorities on the misleading statements they continue to make.

Read the opening paragraph of this scathing report by Gardiner Harris in the New York Times:

> *"Despite promising discoveries and multibillion-dollar investments, cancer research is quietly undergoing a crisis. Few drugs are being marketed, and most of those that have been introduced are enormously expensive and provide few of the benefits that patients expect."* [New York Times, December 20, 2005]

Take for example, Nexavar, a drug described as a *"major advance"* in treating kidney cancer. X-rays showed that Nexavar doubled the time it took, from 84 to 167 days, for tumors to grow substantially in number or size. But if the study were to continue, it may turn out there is no increased survival in the long term with this drug.

Officials of the drug agency found the findings so compelling that they urged Bayer to stop the trial early and give Nexavar to subjects who had been taking placebos.

> Much work remains to be done, Harris said, adding: *"The crux of the crisis in oncology is that for years we have developed tremendous scientific advances in looking at how cancer develops, and that's not being translated into practical solutions that are benefiting patients at the pace you would expect. Look at what the government and all the drug companies are spending, and yet drugs are not reaching the market."*
>
> *"Drug companies have been promising for years that gene-hunting techniques would yield targeted nontoxic therapies that melt cancer, but few cancer medicines fit that profile,"* says New York Times reporter Gardiner Harris. *"True cancer cures are still exceptionally rare,"* he adds.
>
> *"There are all these myths having to do with cancer drugs,"* Dr. Steven Hirschfeld, an F.D.A. medical officer with expertise in cancer, said. *"That they're very targeted, when in fact all these drugs have multiple targets. That they're nontoxic, when in fact the latest ones have their own set of side effects. And that they're cures, when they are not."*

There is growing evidence that tumor size may not matter much. Small tumors can sometimes be as deadly as large tumors.

More false hopes

"I want to lead the National Cancer Institute on a mission to prevent the process (cancer) from occurring in the first place or detect the occurrence of cancer early enough to eliminate it with less morbidity."
Source: Andy von Eschenbach, director of the NCI

Another outrage, this time issued from the lips of Andrew von Eschenbach, director of the National Cancer Institute. He claims that *"Within 10 years, nobody will die of cancer; it may not be cured at that time. Drugs will be available to eliminate the pain, suffering, and death that cancer now dishes out."* As Dr. Eschenbach speaks, more die of cancer, fifteen hundred Americans every day. Cancer death rates have changed very little since 1950.

So, if in 55 years America has made almost no headway in the war against cancer, how can Eschenbach claim we will eliminate cancer deaths in ten years? The answer lies in what some refer to as the ***"Nanotech Revolution."***

The new technology Dr. Eschenbach speaks of is nanotechnology. Let's examine what it is. According to statements by the NCI, *"nanotech is a technology with major potential to drive new generations of cancer diagnostics and therapeutic products."*

Technology employs structures or devices that are so small they are only the size of atoms or molecules. Following are some of the new technology that Eschenbach and others say will revolutionize cancer care.

→ Quantum Dots
dramatically improves clinical diagnostic tests for early cancer detection. These tiny particles glow and act as markers on cells and genes, enabling doctors to visualize cancer when present or impending. Approval expected in five years.

→ Carbon Nanotubes
spots cancer lying in remission and determines if, and when it may flare up, and identifies new tumors as well. Development expected by 2008.

→ Lab-on-a-Chip
promises early detection of cancer, heart disease, Alzheimer's and other ills. Patients will one day walk into their doctor's office with this handheld device, give a few drops of blood, and in minutes, receive a complete health diagnosis.

Therapeutic systems destroy cancer cells non-invasively, without harming healthy cells; these include the following:

➤ Gold Nanoshells
enters into cancer cells, and when exposed to infrared light, explodes, killing cancer cells without harming healthy cells. Rice University researchers hope for human trials by 2006, available everywhere by 2008.

➤ Nanoparticles
combines hormones and cell-killing peptides that image, target, and destroy primary and metastatic breast cancer cells. Approval expected in five years.

➤ Nanocomplex
detects and destroys metastatic cancer cells. Its diagnostic and therapeutic functions utilize a microscopic, lipid-based liposome and an antibody, along with gene therapy; expected to enter clinical studies soon.

➤ Nanotube Bomb
enters cancer cells and when exposed to lasers, explodes along with the cancer cell. Scientists suggest this future scenario: *"after work, people take their 'Lab-on-a-Chip' to a clinic for a quick screen; if cancer is present they receive an injection of nanobombs, sit under the laser for a few minutes, and then go home".* Widespread use expected by 2010.

Will the fraudsters ever be punished?

One way to avoid being held accountable for fraud in the cancer industry is to keep moving. The former director of the National Cancer Institute from 1995 to 2001, Dr. Richard D. Klausner, who ended up in the employment of the Bill and Melinda Gates Foundation, has been under a long-running Congressional conflict-of-interest investigation. Dr. Klausner eventually resigned from Bill Gates' Foundation.

Dr. Klausner oversaw a $40 million contract the cancer institute awarded to Harvard Medical School while Klausner was a candidate for president of the university. After leaving the institute he took a board position with a company founded by Stuart Schreiber, a Harvard colleague who got the government contract to build the Molecular Target Laboratory.

To make matters worse, Dr. Klausner was also being investigated for dealings with the University of Pittsburgh, which presented him with the $40,000 Dickson Prize Award in 1997 for work he did before he became cancer institute director. At about the same time Dr. Klausner received the award, he approved a $300,000 government payment to help the University of Pittsburgh settle a $2.7 million lawsuit against the university.

Dysfunctional system

Clifton Leaf of Fortune Magazine speaks out again:

> *"Experts offer testimony that, when taken together, describes a dysfunctional "cancer culture"—a groupthink that pushes tens of thousands of physicians and scientists toward the goal of finding the tiniest improvements in treatment rather than genuine breakthroughs; that fosters isolated (and redundant) problem solving instead of cooperation; and rewards academic achievement and publication over all else."*

The cancer care industry is self serving, disingenuous, and insensitive, but its failings cannot be easily side stepped by cancer patients. Patients are caught in this system that controls how public insurance funds are utilized and has control over all the advanced tools, cat scans, ultrasound, mammograms, x-rays, that detect and monitor the occurrence and spread of cancer.

The only factor that keeps driving the failed and fraudulent cancer care industry is that patients and their families keep coming back for more treatment. If the public could only understand that modern cancer treatment is a killer in itself, patients would search elsewhere for cures. Instead, cancer patients are given the idea that any alternatives to the disproven therapies now in use represent nothing more than quackery.

Cancer patients and their families usually don't study up on the topic of cancer till it strikes. Then the volumes of information are just too large to know where to begin to investigate.

Be forewarned. When you or a loved one gets cancer, you will be entering the treacherous territory of the cancer industry. Cancer patients must learn how to navigate through this system, relying primarily on it for diagnosis rather than treatment, if they expect to survive. It's not likely many patients will accomplish this. Most patients and their families are not given to resisting their doctors. For most, the fraud and misrepresentations exist elsewhere, not with their trusted doctor. Cancer is upsetting enough, the realization that modern cancer care is bogus is too much for many patients to handle. It's easier to sign the treatment consent form than question the system. Many patients are so ill, and their families so distant, that there is no one to carefully analyze what cancer doctors prescribe.

Just count the bodies on the battlefield. In 2004, cancer will claim some 563,700 of your family, friends, co-workers, and countrymen. More Americans will die of cancer in the next 14 months than have perished in every war the nation has ever fought ... combined, says Clifton Leaf of Fortune Magazine, who wrote a documentary report on cancer.

Reliability of Cancer Detection Methods Recently dogs were trained to detect the scent of cancer patients. Their diagnostic accuracy is compared with other methods of cancer detection.	
Dogs, scent for lung cancer	99% accuracy
Dogs, scent for breast cancer	88% accuracy
Mammograms, detection of breast cancer	85% accuracy
PSA test for prostate cancer	Under re-evaluation; generally worthless
Occult blood/stool test	Under re-evaluation; generally worthless
Self-breast examination	Under re-evaluation; authorities suggest abandonment

Source: Integrative Cancer Therapy 5:30-9, 2006

Politics and cancer

Elected officials also share some of the blame for misdirected or ineffective cancer prevention and treatment programs. The United States spends about $2.4 billion a year on cancer research, compared to $16 billion a year for NASA's space exploration budget. A 2001 initiative only called for policymakers to streamline and accelerate approval of more and more ineffective drugs. Meanwhile, effective cancer prevention programs are almost nonexistent. Organizations intended to fight cancer also deserve some criticism. For the most part, donations to cancer treatment groups only fill the bank accounts of probably what are the wealthiest of disease clubs. It has been said there are so many people employed in the cancer industry that a bona fide cure would produce an unacceptable amount of unemployment. When more people live off of cancer than die of it, it becomes an ineffective system that traps many naïve cancer patients. Researchers seek endless studies that progress at a snail's pace, so as to ensure a lifetime of employment.

Cancer myths

Cancer myths abound. Yet, authorities on cancer appear to spread as many myths as the uninformed. The American Cancer Society has taken on the role of being the chief debunker of myths surrounding cancer care, but their list of common myths appears to be badly in need of updating.

Here is the American Cancer Society list of cancer myths, with critical analysis.

Does surgery spread or accelerate the growth of cancer?

According to a recent press release distributed by the American Cancer Society, 41% of Americans participating in a survey said they believed surgery can cause cancer to spread. The American Cancer Society says it is fiction. A physician spokesperson for the American Cancer Society says this myth *"really keeps patients from potentially receiving what could be a definitive, if not curative, surgery."* But surgery is not a cure for cancer, and there is published evidence surgery does indeed facilitate the spread of tumors.

Since 1958, it has been known that surgery accelerates existing cancer. A case where a limb was removed because of cancer, which subsequently triggered the spread of cancer to the lung, is cited. [Archives Surgery 77: 621-26, 1958]

In 1997, it was cited that women undergoing breast cancer surgery appear to develop a peak for relapse within three years after surgery and then again, a lesser peak some years later, which counters the idea that concealed small tumors (called micro metastases) continue to develop at a constant rate. Surgery seems to have an effect in inducing relapse. The use of chemotherapy prior to breast cancer surgery appears to counter some of the tumor-promoting effects of surgery. [European Journal Cancer 27: 2184-93, 2001]

It is said that surgery *"kick starts"* hidden small tumors. Surgeons know this and often prescribe pre-operative chemotherapy, or anti-estrogen drugs, to limit the effect surgery has upon accelerated growth of remaining small tumors following surgery. [Lancet 347: 260, 1996]

Another report says *"surgery may trigger tumor growth,"* and goes on to describe a patient who had been treated for a small cell lung cancer in 2001 and then experienced minor trauma to his head in a car accident 16 months later and developed a tumor at that location. [BMC Cancer 5: 94, 2005]

Tumors inhibit the growth of blood vessels that provide it with nutrients for growth by production of chemicals called angiostatins. Surgery triggers wound healing and repair chemicals that are the same as used to spur growth of a tumor. In eight cases where surgeons removed tumor cells from males with testicular cancer, surgery itself accelerated growth of remaining tumor cells. [Cancer 45: 1498-506, 1980]

In a controlled experiment, angiostatin, a chemical that inhibits the formation of new blood vessels that feed tumors, disappeared five days after animal tumors had been surgically removed. Tumor surgery *"accelerated the growth of other tumors"* says the report. [European Journal Cancer 37: 2283-88, 2001]

Even a simple biopsy is invasive enough to activate the wound-healing process and accelerate tumor progression. [Lancet 357: 1048, 2001] Abdominal surgery compared to less invasive procedures using a surgical scope induces a greater spread of tumors. [Archives Surgery 130: 649-53, 1995]

Before the era of modern surgery (anesthesia), it was known that, *"unless forced by the circumstances,"* surgery should be avoided for early stage tumors. There is question over the eagerness to operate on young women with early-stage breast cancer when there are indications tumors are spreading (positive lymph nodes). [European Journal Cancer 41: 508-15, 2005]

Researchers at Harvard Medical School clearly state that *"surgical wounding associated with the removal of experimental primary cancers can trigger angiogenesis (new blood vessels) in previously dormant micro-metastatic tumor deposits, which can result in the acceleration of relapse and death."* [Lancet 357: 1048, 2001]

In a report entitled *"Excisional surgery for cancer sure: therapy at a cost,"* researchers indicate there is *"strong"* evidence that tumor removal influences the growth of remaining tumors. [Lancet 4: 760-68, 2003]

A report in Medical Hypotheses states that *"surgery can increase the number of circulating tumor cells and induce an immunosuppressive effect that might facilitate metastatic spread. The process of wound healing can stimulate growth factors that have been shown to accelerate tumor cell growth. This situation is a double-edged sword."* [Medical Hypotheses 67: 1054-59, 2006]

Researchers in Ireland report that surgical removal of a primary tumor is often followed by a faster and more aggressive tumor at the same site. [Annals Thoracic Surgery 80: 1046-50, 2005]

Finally, Georgetown University doctors report that surgery carries an increased risk for cancer weeks or even years after an operation. [Anesthesiology Clinics North America, June 2006]

Is there a cancer cure cover-up?

Says the American Cancer Society: *"Another myth ... More than 25% of people think the medical industry is covering up a cure for cancer to increase profits."* That's nothing more than an *"urban legend"* says the ACS. *"Fiction,"* says oncologist Nikita Shah, M.D., from the M. D. Anderson Cancer Center in Orlando, who adds, *"if there were a cure, we'd know about it."*

Yet this book carefully documents the fact that the cancer industry not only has shunned more effective and less expensive treatments for cancer, but has actively participated in conducting fraudulent or flawed research to mislead the public.

Read the chapter in this book on vitamin C and how the Mayo Clinic conducted three flawed studies to dismiss the groundbreaking work of Drs. Ewan Cameron and Linus Pauling in the use of intravenous vitamin C to treat cancer patients.

Read how folic acid is being underutilized, not only as a nutrient that can prevent cancer, but how it is being overlooked by oncologists to prevent the relapse of cancer after treatment. Moreover, the FDA won't even mandate the inclusion of folic acid into birth control pills that deplete the body of folic acid and induce abnormal Pap smears.

Read how the cancer industry has overlooked vitamin D, purportedly because it causes over-calcification and that it is toxic in high doses, when it is perfectly safe in doses 1,000 times greater than the Recommended Daily Allowance. Instead, the American Cancer Society advocates the use of sunscreen lotions that have increased rates of malignant melanoma.

Read how the cancer industry today is attempting to steer the public away from resveratrol pills, a red wine molecule that is the most profound anti-cancer molecule ever discovered. In fact, three times the American Cancer Society has dismissed Johanna Brandt's book The Grape Cure, without any studies to invalidate the claim that grapes possess miraculous properties to prevent and treat cancer.

Read how Tsuno Foods and Rice Company in Japan has labored to tell the world of a cure for cancer from rice bran (IP6) based upon chelation (removal) of iron, but the National Cancer Institute has refused to launch any human trials.

The entire cancer care industry is involved in finding natural molecules that prevent or treat cancer, rearranging them solely to gain patents that ensure their ability to reap huge profits. These re-arranged molecules, called analogs, then produce side effects because the body does not accept them.

It's really quite enraging to read that the American Cancer Society says *"Fewer than half of all people with cancer in the U.S. actually die of the disease—and many who are not 'cured' of cancer still go on living for years with relatively few changes in their lives."* [American Cancer Society 12/19/2005] Death among cancer patients is often attributed to heart attack or other organ failures which are a result of harsh cancer treatments. So cancer itself doesn't appear as a statistical cause of death. It is disingenuous to say fewer than half of the patients with cancer will die of the disease. Yes, but how many die from the treatment?

The ACS goes on to say: *"Your doctor and the FDA, which must approve new drugs before they can be marketed, are your allies. As such, they make your safety a high priority."* However, recent revelations show the FDA approved relatively unsafe drugs (Vioxx COX-2 inhibitor) and at least five other drugs and continues to do little to remove these drugs from the marketplace.

Public Citizen, the Ralph Nader group, indicates 181 FDA-approved drugs should be recalled because they are not as safe as other drugs or are ineffective. An FDA drug reviewer, Dr. David Graham, had to publish his report on the hidden dangers of Vioxx outside of the country in the British Medical Journal.

Acetaminophen (Tylenol) causes thousands of reports of liver toxicity annually which results in liver transplants and death, all which could be avoided with the inclusion of a sulfur compound (N-acetyl cysteine) in pain pills, which the FDA refuses to consider. [British Medical Journal, Vol. 323, Sept. 15, 2001] Just the use of non-steroidal pain relievers like aspirin and ibuprofen cause an estimated 16,000 deaths annually. Side effects from properly used prescription drugs, administered by nurses in hospitals, result in over 100,000 deaths annually. The FDA approval process does not guarantee safety.

Does sugar cause cancer to grow?

According to the American Cancer Society, sugar doesn't make cancer grow faster. It is true that all cells depend upon sugar for energy, and that cancer cells produce their own form of sugar via fermentation.

According to the ACS:

This misconception may be based in part on a misunderstanding of positron emission tomography (PET) scans. Doctors use PET scans to help determine the location of a tumor and see if it has spread.

During a PET scan, your doctor injects a small amount of radioactive tracer — typically a form of glucose — into your body. All tissues in your body absorb some of this tracer. But tissues that are using more energy — exhibiting increased metabolic activity — absorb greater amounts.

Tumors are often more metabolically active than healthy tissues. As a result, they may absorb greater amounts of the tracer. For this reason, some people have concluded that cancer cells grow faster on sugar. But this isn't true.

However, upon further investigation, we find that high blood sugar levels are often manifested in cancer patients. High sugar diets are associated with the risk of getting cancer. But what about surviving cancer? Can cancer patients eat refined sugars without regard that this may cause tumors to grow faster? Dr. John T. Ely of the University of Washington decided to test whether sugar abets tumor growth. Dr. Ely found that patients in remission from tumors have lower blood sugar levels. [Integrative Cancer Therapy 4: 25-31, 2005]

Dr. Ely and colleagues went on to conduct an animal test. Mice were placed on three different diets designed to produce different blood sugar levels and then injected with highly aggressive breast tumor cells. Seventy days later 16 of 24 mice on a high sugar diet had succumbed to cancer, 8 of 24 mice on a normal sugar diet died and only 1 of 20 mice on a low-sugar diet died. [Biochemistry Biophysical Research Communications 132: 1174-79, 1985]

Dr. Ely has taken breast cancer patients, placed them on a low sugar diet, added supplemental vitamin C and treated their tumors with radiation, and demonstrated a prolonged survival.[Integrative Cancer Therapy 4: 25-31, 2005]

Hair dye and cancer

The American Cancer Society says hair dyes don't cause cancer. But this so-called myth persists. After examining 79 different studies, a report published in the Journal of the American Medical Association says *"We did not find strong evidence of a marked increase in the risk of cancer among personal hair dye users."* [Journal American Medical Assn 293: 2516-25, 2005]

However, a study conducted by the University of North Carolina School of Public Health found that the use of any hair dye in the month before and/or during pregnancy is associated with a modest increased risk of neuroblastoma in offspring. [Cancer Causes Controls 16: 743-48, 2005]

When data was pooled from different population studies, it was found that *"personal use of hair dye products increases bladder cancer risk by 22% to 50%."* [Public Health Reports 120: 31-38, 2005]

A recent study shows that the use of hair dyes is associated with adult acute leukemia and that more frequent use and long-term use increased the risks for this type of cancer. Non-permanent hair dyes were not associated with leukemia, but long duration of permanent hair dye *"may have an impact on the risk of leukemia."* [American Journal Epidemiology 160: 19-25, 2004]

Another study could not completely dismiss data linking hair dye use with a modest increased risk for bladder cancer. [International Journal Cancer 109: 581-86, 2004]

It's possible the hair care industry knows why hair dye is linked with cancer since a recent study shows that the increased risk for Hodgkin's lymphoma was only found among women who started using hair coloring products prior to 1980. [American Journal Epidemiology 159: 148-54, 2004] It's possible some carcinogens have been removed from currently made products.

The data is not clear enough to say no to the idea that hair dye may increase cancer risk, even if only by a modest degree. The American Cancer Society shouldn't give a green light to hair dyes until more is known. For now, hair dyes are in a yellow zone, proceed with caution. The risk is not a major one, like aging or smoking, but it may be a factor that promotes cancer.

Do anti-perspirants cause cancer?

According to the National Cancer Institute (NCI), there's no conclusive evidence linking the use of underarm antiperspirants or deodorants with breast cancer. A well publicized study by the American Cancer Society found no relationship between breast cancer and antiperspirant use. [Journal National Cancer Institute 94:1578-80, 2002]

Primarily at issue are parabens, estrogen-like molecules that could be implicated in breast tumor promotion, which are often used in antiperspirants.

Researchers compared parabens to the effect of estrogen. Parabens exhibit very mild estrogen-like effects, much like soy phytoestrogens and flaxseed lignans. Researchers conclude that *"it is biologically implausible that parabens could increase the risk of any male or female reproductive tract cancer. Parabens pose less of a risk than mild estrogen-like molecules in the diet."* [Critical Reviews Toxicology 35: 435-58, 2005]

The public is often confused here because doctors often speak out of two sides of their mouth in regard to estrogen and cancer. For years doctors prescribed estrogen replacement for menopausal women, before research found that it slightly increased the risk for cancer. Conventional medicine now prescribes anti-estrogens, like tamoxifen, or the newer aromatase inhibitors, to block breast cancer growth. But they often lump the weaker plant estrogens (called phytoestrogens) in with the stronger estrogen molecules. Phytoestrogens, by being 1/1000th the activity of estrogen, weaken the effect of naturally produced estrogen in the body. But physicians are often quick to warn patients away from these plant estrogens, while continuing to prescribe the stronger estrogens for symptoms of menopause. Modern medicine certainly has crossed wires here.

Another concern in anti-perspirants is aluminum content. Researchers in England report that aluminum in the form of aluminium chloride or aluminium chlorhydrate can interfere with the function of estrogen receptors on the surface of human breast cancer cells. *"This adds aluminum to the increasing list of metals capable of interfering with estrogen action and termed metallo-estrogens."* In other words, aluminum might actually work like the plant estrogens to dull the hormonal effects upon the growth of breast cancer cells. [Journal Inorganic Biochemistry 99: 1912-19, 2005]

However, a study of young women found that the frequency and early use of antiperspirants/deodorants with underarm shaving were associated with an earlier age of breast cancer diagnosis. The exact agents involved have not been identified. [European Journal Cancer Prevention 12: 479-85, 2003]

Aluminum is a metallic metal and is thus generally of concern. Studies show the brains of Alzheimer's patients have higher levels of aluminum and lower amounts of magnesium. [Journal Alzheimer's Disease 7, 273-84, 2005] Long-term exposure to low levels of aluminum in animals raises levels of an enzyme (acetycholinesterase) that facilitates memory loss in Alzheimer's disease. [Journal Inorganic Biochemistry 99:1865-70, 2005] Public health authorities may give aluminum a clean bill of health in regard to cancer, but need to warn the public there are other health concerns involving aluminum.

Is cancer contagious?

Well, cancer authorities say no, however they do indicate humans can transfer viruses that cause cancer, such as the papilloma virus during sexual contact, which can result in cervical cancer. Of interest are reports which show that a small percentage of patients receiving organ transplants develop tumors that originated from the implanted organ. [Transplantation 80: S164-6, 2005]

Do regular checkups detect all cancers in their early stage?

The American Cancer Society says: *"Regular checkups and today's medical technology can detect all cancer early. Routine screening has clearly led to an impressive decrease in deaths from several cancers, including cervical, breast and colon cancers. Although regular medical care can indeed increase your ability to detect cancer early, it can't guarantee it."*

This statement is misleading. Certainly, cancer is being detected at an earlier stage, which skews statistics and makes it appear cancer patients are living longer when in fact they are just having their cancer detected at an earlier stage. When cancers are first detected, about 30% have already spread to other organs. A tumor has to be a few billion cells in size to be detected with today's technology. Earlier cancer detection assumes there is safe and effective treatment available. In fact, for many types of cancer, there is no significant life-prolonging treatment. Cancer detection programs have become nothing more than ways for cancer hospitals and doctors to drum up more business.

For example, when Australian pop star Kylie Minogue was diagnosed with breast cancer at the age of 37, the cancer industry used her as an example for women to undergo frequent mammograms. Many women in her age group underwent mammogram screening after Ms. Minogue's announcement she had cancer. Doctors hailed Minogue for her public disclosure, saying it would result in the saving of many lives. However, women in Ms. Minogue's age group are not at high risk for breast cancer and the screenings are likely to result in little if any lives saved. But the self-serving cancer industry thinks it is a good idea to submit bills to insurance companies for more mammograms.

Does sunscreen use prevent skin cancer?

When Americans were surveyed, 43% said that sunscreen use can prevent skin cancer. The American Cancer Society says the public has a poor understanding of how to use sunscreens.

> The ACS says: *"The use of sunscreen on a daily basis is a good practice for reducing skin cancer risk. The problem with it is that it can sometimes give a false sense of security. Sunscreen needs to be reapplied, and even then it still only confers a certain amount of protection."*

Yet, when researchers scrutinized the issue of whether sunscreen use prevents skin cancer, they found that there is no association between sunscreen use and the development of malignant melanoma, the most feared form of skin cancer. [British Journal Dermatology 153: 378-81, 2005] When researchers analyzed data from many studies they concluded that *"the melanoma protective potential of sunscreens cannot be proven using the existing evidence."* [Photodermatology Photoimmunology Photomedicine 18: 153-56, 2002]

Have millions of Americans been applying sunscreens for no good reason? Well, not quite, sunscreen lotions do prevent sun burn.

The big shocker is that 95% of solar radiation is UV-A energy, while most sunscreens protect from the harsher UV-B rays. UV-A may also induce skin cancer. [Journal Investigative Dermatology 121:869-75, 2003] Oops! The latest study shows that UV-B rays only partially contribute to the development of melanoma. UV-A is also involved. [Journal of the National Cancer Institute, Vol. 97: 1822-1831, December 21, 2005]

SPF (sun protection factor) refers to the ability of a product to block out UV-B rays. So there was a flaw in the design of the sunscreen products themselves. [Postgraduate Medicine 116: July 2004]

There is a cozy relationship between the Skin Cancer Foundation, an organization funded by the sunscreen manufacturers, and the American Cancer Society as well as the American Academy of Dermatology. Melanoma was rare up until the 1950s when sunscreen use began as *"tanning lotions."* Now there are over 40,000 cases of melanoma and 7,000 deaths from melanoma reported annually. Rising trends in the incidence of and mortality from melanoma began in the 1970s and 1980s, when sunscreens with high sun protection factors were more widely used. [Annals Epidemiology 3: 103-10, 1993]

Sunscreen use is related to a decline in solar vitamin D production. [American Journal Clinical Nutrition 80: 1678-88S, 2004]

A report in Preventive Medicine reveals the following [Preventive Medicine 22: 132-40, 1993]:

1. Sunlight activation is the most effective source of vitamin D. The diet only contributes a small amount of vitamin D.

2. Regular sunlight/vitamin D *"intake"* inhibits growth of breast and colon cancer cells and is associated with substantial decreases in death rates from these cancers.

3. Metabolites of vitamin D beneficially alter leukemia and lymphoma cells to return to normal . Vitamin D prolongs the survival of leukemic mice, and produces complete and partial clinical responses in lymphoma patients.

4. Sunlight has a paradoxical relationship with melanoma, in that severe sunburning initiates melanoma, whereas long-term regular sun exposure inhibits melanoma

5. Sun phobia may be counterproductive. Frequent regular sun exposure acts to cause cancers that have a 0.3% death rate with 2,000 U.S. fatalities per year and acts to prevent cancers that have death rates from 20-65% with 138,000 U.S. fatalities per year.

6. Reports in the medical literature suggest that the 17% increase in breast cancer incidence during the 1991-1992 year may be the result of the past decade of pervasive anti-sun advisories from respected authorities, coinciding with effective sunscreen availability.

7. Trends in the epidemiological literature suggest that approximately 30,000 U.S. cancer deaths yearly would be averted by the widespread public adoption of regular, moderate sunning.

The American Cancer Society has taken a position that is unfounded by scientific studies, and only serves to provide a constant stream of new melanoma patients to dermatologists.

A recent study estimates that 50,000-63,000 individuals in the United States and 19,000-25,000 in Britain die prematurely from cancer annually due to insufficient vitamin D. [Photochemistry Photobiology 81: 1276-86, 2005]

Who is spreading myths about cancer?

It appears the American Cancer Society is the primary agency that spreads myths about cancer. Their information is badly in need of updating. There are obvious tragic consequences from heeding much of the information provided to the public by the American Cancer Society.

Cancer doctors

This year some 1.4 million Americans will hear words from their doctor of a frightening diagnosis of cancer.

The extended lifespan of Americans, the fact that cancer is largely an age-related disease, and the baby-boomers entering the *"cancer era"* of their lives, will increase the need for cancer doctors, called oncologists, in the United States. There are about 5,000 trained oncologists, or roughly 1.8 per 100,000 Americans, and the need is likely to double in coming years. [Journal National Cancer Institute 90: 567-69, 1998]

Oncologists will be challenged to deliver cancer care they haven't been trained to perform. Cancer care is largely a failure, prolonging life at great cost and suffering for only a few months in most instances. How oncologists will radically reform their own profession is preceded by the question of whether the profession even has a desire to do so. It is being rewarded handsomely for failure.

Sensitivity along with technology

On the front page of the New York Times a woman recently told her story of lying in her hospital bed the day after her breast cancer surgery and suddenly being confronted by her oncologist and a horde of other doctors. Her oncologist promptly proceeded to remove her hospital gown and begin chatting about her case as if she were a lawn mower that needed fixing. This is just one example of how impersonal cancer care has become. [New York Times, August 16, 2005]

Doctor, how long do I have to live?

"They deal with death every day, but doctors cannot bring themselves to tell terminally ill cancer patients the worst," says a Reuters News headline. According to a survey of cancer specialists, only 37% of doctors prefer to tell it to patients straight and 23% do not tell their patients at all about their fate. Most cancer doctors exaggerate how long a patient has to live. One study of 300 terminally ill patients found they lived a median of 26 days, but the forecasts by their doctors was 79 days and they were actually told they could expect to live 90 days. Another study found physicians overestimate survival in 52% of cases. [Reuters May 20, 2000]

One of the serious problems with delivering overly optimistic cancer survival times is that patients tend to opt for more aggressive treatment if they think they are going to live for six months. If they think their demise is more imminent, they are more likely to opt for hospice or palliative care. Terminal patients who opt for more aggressive care do not live longer and are more likely to require readmission to the hospital. Patients and doctors differ in their criteria used to go ahead with treatment. Patients are more likely to choose aggressive chemotherapy even if told it will only bring about a 10% reduction in pain and discomfort whereas doctors judge chemotherapy to be of value if it reduces symptoms by 50%.

A report in the Journal of the American Medical Association asks: *"Why do physicians provide treatment that does not improve survival and has unfortunate consequences?"* [Journal American Medical Assn 279: 1746-1748, 1998]

The answer to this question is that *"physicians find it too uncomfortable to tell patients that they cannot effectively fight their patients' cancer because it means that clinicians have failed. It is much simpler to give another round of chemotherapy."* The report goes onto to ask: *"Does this mean doctors must sit by the bedside, hold patients by the hand, and tell them that there is no way to control their cancer? The answer is yes, when it is the truth."* But at the same time, patients need to be assured they won't be abandoned and efforts to help them live as long as possible will be made.

DOCTOR, WOULD YOU TAKE YOUR OWN MEDICINE? Attitudes Toward Mild Chemotherapy Source: Chest 109: 80S, 1996			
	With 1% cure rate	With 3 month survival increase	With symptom relief
Cancer nurses	39%	25%	26%
General practitioners	44%	27%	21%
Radiation oncologists	27%	13%	2%
Medical oncologists	52%	45%	12%
Patients	67%	53%	59%

Source: Chest 109: 80S, 1996

Another problem is that patients who are diagnosed with cancer, but not told their prognosis, are more likely to be optimistic. Furthermore, the cancer patient doesn't know which questions to ask the doctor. When the doctor inquires whether they have any questions, this is a superfluous inquiry.

To add to the problem, families often insist that *"everything be done"* for the patient. Although patients do value their autonomy to make decisions on their own they need choices posed to them. Otherwise, without awareness of their options at hand, they are likely to ask their doctor: *"What should I do? What would you do?"* [Journal American Medical Assn 279: 1746-48, 1998]

Opinion Research Corporation reported that most Americans are skeptical about cancer diagnoses and believe that one third of all cancers in the United States are misdiagnosed. Sixty-two percent of Americans polled said they were not satisfied with the care provided to a relative who had cancer; 93% wanted to be told if they had cancer, rather than having the information withheld. [Health Management Technology 1997]

It was not long ago that doctors would not even discuss the diagnosis of cancer with an older patient. [Drugs & Aging 6: 351-57, 1995]

The results of the survey regarding who is most likely to consent to mild chemotherapy (lower dose, fewer sessions) was surprising. The health professional least likely to take chemo drugs was found to be radiation oncologists. Could it be because they view first-hand the devastation that this treatment causes?

After treatment is completed, then what?

It is estimated that there are more than 10 million Americans living with cancer. [Journal National Cancer Institute 96: 1412, 2004] An embarrassing, if not distressing, report reveals that doctors aren't providing adequate follow-up care after treatment. The problem, says a report from the National Cancer Policy Board of the Institute of Medicine, is that after treatment, patients are sent back to their primary care physicians, often without a plan for follow-up care. The big problem is that doctors aren't reimbursed for follow-up care, so it gets neglected. [CA Cancer Journal Clinicians 56: 65-67, 2006]

This is puzzling since a list of good health habits, dietary measures and dietary supplement regimens would suffice. A pre-printed sheet of paper with after-care instructions would go a long way. Once all the billing codes have been utilized for insurance claims, physicians virtually abandon patients in regard to secondary prevention. The message doctors are sending by this behavior is clear, if your cancer returns, then I will care for you again, otherwise you need to return to your family doctor. Patients who have completed treatment are literally left standing in the street with no plan to prevent cancer from recurring beyond troublesome drugs like Tamoxifen, or life-threatening drugs like COX-2 inhibitors.

Cancer patients

Patients – that's what cancer care is all about. Most cancer patients have no idea what they are facing when their cancer is diagnosed. Truly, regardless of the failings of modern cancer care and all the fraud involved in the industry, patients themselves carry a load of blame. The majority of the cancer burden upon society is produced by smokers and alcohol drinkers. How could any treatment or preventive measure overcome these health habits unless they are abandoned?

Even when confronted with the blunt facts, that modern cancer treatment is ineffective, most patients and their families are likely to still opt for treatment, hoping that somehow God has a miracle for them.

Risk factors, in the patient's mind

A survey released by the American Cancer Society indicates nearly half (47%) of Americans believe there is little or nothing they can do to reduce their risk of cancer.

Cancer patients and their family members tend to rank risk factors outside of their control ahead of ones that can be self managed.

Among 50 lung cancer patients surveyed, 8 were smokers (3 continued to smoke after cancer diagnosis; 3 others attempted to quit but later relapsed), 26 were ex-smokers and 16 never smokers. All but one patient had made prior attempts to quit using tobacco.

In a survey of cancer patients, here is how they ranked, in order, the importance of risk factors for cancer:

1. Stress
2. Bad luck
3. Heredity
4. Pollution
5. Smoking
6. Dietary fat
7. Passive smoking
8. Dietary fiber
9. Alcohol

Twenty-nine of the 50 patients changed their diet since their cancer diagnosis, 14 of whom decreased fat consumption and 5 who reduced or eliminated alcohol from their diet.

Only 12 of the 50 patients received a recommendation from their doctor that they quit smoking or change their diet. This was striking given the fact that 68% of these patients had a dietary-related cancer (colon).

Family members only modestly changed their dietary or smoking habits after their relative had been diagnosed with cancer, even though they often eat at the same table. [Preventive Medicine 25: 162-69, 1996]

Cancer reaction linked to gender

The diagnosis of cancer may be the same, but responses from male and female patients differ, according to a published survey. While men seek practical advice and the latest medical treatments, women look for emotional support, a study of internet postings suggests.

He defies his learned colleagues

A tutor in English at St. Catherine's College at Oxford, England, Michael Gearin Tosh became more widely known for his malignancy. At the age of 54 he was diagnosed with multiple myeloma, a virulent cancer of the bone marrow. After his doctor brusquely informed him there was no cure for his disease, but paradoxically scheduled him for chemotherapy the next week. Gearin-Tosh thought, for a disease you can't cure why should he undergo four months of dreaded chemotherapy? He paused.

He called a former professor at Memorial Sloan-Kettering Cancer Center who explained he was "a goner."

He turned his back on chemotherapy and elected for megadose vitamins, a raw food diet and other alternative cancer therapies. A world renowned meyloma expert courteously, but firmly told Gearin-Tosh that "nutrition has no place in the treatment of cancer." Eight years later his cancer saga was revealed in the New York Times. Though weak, anemic, and with brittle bones, he was alive. [New York Times, May 12, 2002] Some people can live for up to 7 years or more with multiple myeloma, but median survival is about 3 years. Gearin-Tosh lived for 12, without the harsh chemotherapy.

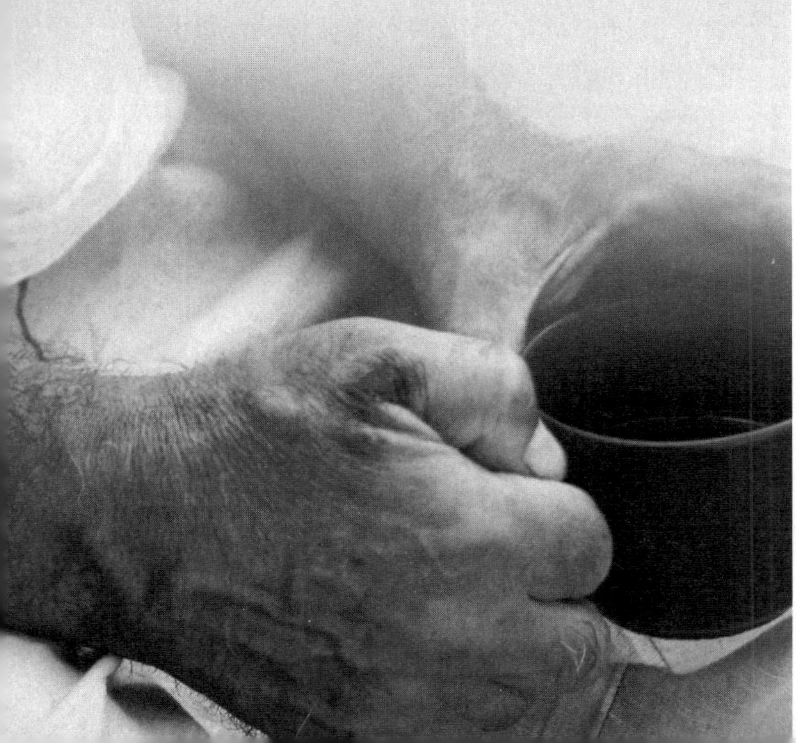

The survey found that men's primary concerns were treatments, tests, symptoms, procedures and side-effects of drugs. Women were more likely to seek social and emotional support, share personal experiences and talk about the impact of cancer on relationships and family. [Social Science & Medicine 62: 2577-90, 2006]

Left in the dark

There is so much information about cancer, yet so little attention given to what cancer patients experience. A recent survey indicates cancer patients are lost in a maze of information.

According to the survey:

- Almost two-thirds of cancer patients do not fully understand what their diagnosis means.
- Even when their doctor said *"the tumor is progressing,"* only half understood that was not good news.
- About 4 in 10 cancer patients said they didn't know what questions to ask about treatment options. [Cancer BACUP, November 15, 2005]

Do cancer patients want to be involved in treatment decisions?

A survey conducted some time ago showed that patients want to be informed, but not necessarily involved in making decisions regarding their care. Most surveys show older patients don't demand as much information from their doctors. [Archives Internal Medicine 156: 1414-20, 1996]

Cancer screening

Oddly enough, while studies show that people in higher income brackets are more likely to undergo mammography or sigmoidoscopy [used to detect colon/rectal cancer] [Preventive Medicine 23: 816-23, 1994], this has ended up as an exercise in finding more disease to treat rather than improving survival rates.

Mammography screening

According to a recent survey published in the Archives of Internal Medicine, women in their 40s want their family doctor to guide them through mammography screening, and want to know, in advance, how and when they would be notified of abnormal results and what steps to take thereafter. More than two out of three women undergoing first-time mammography wanted to know what the chances are for getting breast cancer during their lifetime and in the next ten years. In other words, they were asking, why undergo this test if the risks are very low? [Archives Internal Medicine, 165: 1370-1374, 2005]

It's not likely that doctors will tell women that mammography doesn't save or extend life, but it does permit earlier detection of tumors and create the statistical appearance that women live longer.

Doctors say terminal cancers overtreated

Explaining the disturbing trend for terminal cancer patients to receive chemotherapy and other aggressive but futile treatment in the last days of their lives, Dr. Roy Herbst of the MD Anderson Cancer Center in Houston aptly says: *"Patients don't like to give up."* A survey shows nearly 12% of cancer patients who succumbed to their disease received chemotherapy in the last two weeks of life. *"Overly aggressive treatment gives false hope and puts people through grueling and costly ordeals when there is no chance of a cure,"* say cancer specialists. [Dr. Craig Earle of the Dana-Farber Cancer Institute and Harvard Medical School, American Society of Clinical Oncology, Atlanta, June 2006; Associated Press, June 2, 2006]

Denial of treatment

With no treatment options remaining, and insurance companies withholding approval for experimental cancer treatments, cancer patients sometimes seek publicity in an attempt to pry loose insurance funds for care. Families of cancer patients often don't understand why insurance won't cover everything that can be tried, even unproven treatments, in an attempt to save the life of their loved ones.

Frequently, cancer patients become pawns of pharmaceutical interests, who want to force insurance companies to pay for unproven treatment. Such was the case in Scotland where health writer Richard Gray wrote the following report:

RICHARD GRAY HEALTH CORRESPONDENT
The Scotsman Nov 13, 2005

SCOTTISH cancer patients are being denied access to at least seven potentially life-saving new drugs on cost grounds and as a result of health service bureaucracy.

Scotland on Sunday can reveal that, since March, three key cancer-beating drugs have been rejected for use in the NHS because they were not considered *"cost-effective"*.

The failure to make these new treatments available on the NHS has been condemned as *"outrageous"* and could result in the needless deaths of hundreds of patients in the coming months.

Last week, Elaine Barber from Stoke-on-Trent, won her court battle to be prescribed the breast cancer 'wonder drug' Herceptin, which carries a price tag of £21,000 per treatment.

But an investigation by this newspaper has revealed that within the past week, officials at the Scottish Medicines Consortium turned down the NHS use of another new wonder drug, Taxotere, for treating prostate cancer as they did not consider it cost-effective at £6,000 a treatment.

They said that while the drug could improve the survival of 365 Scottish patients by an average of 2.4 months, improve pain control and the quality of life, costs would stretch to more than £3m over five years.

Earlier this year the authority also rejected the breast cancer drug Gemzar and the colorectal hormone therapy Erbitux on similar grounds.

Unfortunately, none of the above drugs are a cure for cancer and would, at best, give cancer patients an additional two or three months of life.

Survey finds a common belief that cancer cure withheld

A telephone survey of 957 Americans who have never been diagnosed with cancer reveals that about 1 in 4 (27%) of respondents believe there is a known *"cure"* for cancer that is being withheld from the public by a self-serving conspiracy of drug companies, doctors and hospitals.

Only 7% of respondents believed *"cancer is something that cannot be effectively treated."* However, as revealed in this book, most modern cancer treatments do not significantly prolong human life.

The survey also revealed that 40% of respondents believe surgery can spread tumor cells and worsen the disease by spreading malignant cells. [Cancer 104:653-60, 2005]
Pop pills to prevent cancer

Oddly enough, a survey conducted by the American Institute for Cancer Research (AICR) indicates older Americans would rather pop vitamin pills to prevent cancer than eat a healthy diet. Researchers said they found this *"worrying."* How so? I would ask. What's wrong with taking vitamins, which are safe, and have been shown to reduce the risk of certain cancer?

"The fact that so many Americans, especially older Americans, are seeking cancer protection in pills and powders is alarming," said one spokesperson for the AICR. The survey found:

- 13% of Americans age 18-35 years take supplements to lower their risk for cancer
- 24% of Americans age 55 to 64 and 54% over age 65 took vitamins with the specific aim of lowering cancer risk. [Reuters, August 31, 2000]

What cancer patients face when they elect to utilize alternative therapies

An Australian study found 4 in 10 cancer patients did not discuss the alternative therapies they used with their doctors. [Medical Journal Australia 165: 545-48, 1996]

To show how out of touch conventional medicine is with cancer patients, a survey conducted at a California Cancer Center found that 85% of patients wanted alternative therapy offered at the center, even though only 16% said they used alternative therapies after their first diagnosis and only 6% actually saw an alternative physician. [Cancer 6: 176-81, 1998]

A survey of prostate cancer patients found 43% used some form of alternative therapy and 3 out of 4 didn't tell their doctors about this. [Cancer 86: 2642-48, 1999]

Results of a survey of 100 cancer patients using alternative therapies:	
Used alternative therapies	80%
Used vitamins	81%
→ Multivitamin	65%
→ Vitamin C	39%
→ Vitamin E	31%
Used herbal product	54%
Used relaxation techniques	30%
Used massage therapy	20%
Used home remedies	10%

Source: Oncology 15: 1267-72, 2001

A survey of cancer patients in Spain revealed the following:

- 81% wanted to know their diagnosis
- 69% chose the doctor to tell them

If the person affected was a family member:

- 47% would always tell the person
- 39% would tell only if asked
- 9% would never tell
- The greatest fear was pain (44%)

Source: Aten Primaria 33: 368-73, 2004

Patients forced to hide alternative therapies from their doctors

When doctors surveyed 487 cancer patients at a clinic and over the internet about their use of alternative cancer therapies, they found that they are out of touch with their patients and not offering answers to their questions.

Knowing that their doctors will cast a dismissive eye upon alternative therapies, many cancer patients hide their use of alternative treatments from their doctors. Among the patients surveyed, almost half (48%) of cancer patients treated with chemotherapy and radiation used at least one type of complementary and alternative medical therapy treatment, and a majority of them (75%) didn't tell their doctors.

The study shows alternative therapies are used almost twice as often among patients treated only by chemotherapy (65%), compared to those treated only by radiation (35%). Most (88%) patients claim they are satisfied with using alternative therapies as a cost-effective method of cancer treatment with vitamin, herbal and botanical supplements being the most popular therapies. Only a little more than a third (36 %) said their doctors are an important source of information on alternative therapies. [American Society for Therapeutic Radiology and Oncology's 47th Annual Meeting in Denver; Science Daily Oct. 17, 2005]

In many instances, alternative therapies are even recommended by integrative physicians.

A study in Argentina found that 14% of cancer patients used alternative therapies before conventional treatment, 61% used alternative treatment with conventional therapy, and 25% used alternative cancer treatments only after conventional treatment was completed. [Tumori 82: 215-17, 1996]

While many alternative cancer therapies are recommended by doctors themselves, the objection to alternative treatments is widespread. In Italy, doctors there said: *"We hope that medical associations of each country declare it unethical to market questionable cancer treatment and expel members who do so. Considerable damage can be done by publishing stories that give false hope."* [Tumori 82: 215-17, 1996]

Can cancer patients refuse treatment?

What about the option of no treatment? Well, modern medicine considers anything less than surgery, chemo or radiation therapy as *"refusal for treatment."* When a 13-year-old Canadian boy elected to use herbal supplements rather than face amputation for a tumor on his leg, a court ordered treatment over the objections of the young patient who said he preferred prayers and herbs. His family supported him. The parents were characterized as *"fundamentalist Christians."* [Associated Press July 2, 1999]

"This year an additional 1.4 million Americans will have that most frightening of conversations with their doctor."

Cancer survivors

There are an estimated 10 million cancer survivors alive in the United States. A survey of 752 of these survivors ranked the most common problems they face. Here is a partial list of problems facing cancer survivors.

- 68.1% Feeling fearful that my illness will return
- 67.1% Fatigue
- 59.8% Concern about relapse
- 47.9 % Sleep problems
- 41.2% Less physically able to have sexual intercourse
- 38.5 % Preoccupation with being ill
- 36.6% Feeling vulnerable
- 32.7% Feeling angry

Source: Cancer 104: 2565-76, 2005

Living longer than anticipated

An article in the Los Angeles Times indicates cancer patients are beginning to strike out on their own, shunning expensive cancer drugs that often induce severe side effects and prolong life for only a short time, to leave their lives *"in the hands of fate."* Newspaper columnist Art Buchwald, at age 80 years, opted out of medical treatment, lived a year longer than anticipated, and said his final months were spent *"having a great time."*

"In our culture, we have a unique, almost religious, faith in medical technology," says Diane Meier, director of the Center to Advance Palliative Care at Mt. Sinai School of Medicine in New York. More patients are opting for no care rather than being tethered to a machine in their last days, she says.

Unanticipated survival can be treacherous. Failure to die poses problems. What is prompting gripes and distress is that terminal cancer patients enter hospice care when their prognosis is six months or less. Patients get kicked out of hospice if they lave past a predetermined point. Buchwald cracked, in a March 7, 2006, column: *"I've gotten so well Medicare won't pay for me anymore."* [Los Angeles Times, Feb. 5, 2007]

A striking finding is that terminal hospice patients who forgo treatment are living longer by days to months than patients who elect to undergo treatment. [Journal Pain Symptom-Management, Sept. 2004]

Patients talk

E-mail from a breast cancer patient

I have a healthy lifestyle, take vitamins. I was diagnosed with breast cancer 8/19/05 - stage 2 Lumpectomy performed on 9/26/05 and sentinel node procedure. Scheduled first chemo treatment 11/2 - cancelled - blood clot...due to injury to foot - they believe.

Just came home from hospital yesterday - as they found the blood clot had not moved... thought there might be an infection due to a cortisone shot 10/31. All I know is that from the beginning I did not want chemo but decided do the first treatment... from there... I haven't been able to walk on my left foot due to the neuromas... the swelling in my leg has gone down...

I have an open MRI scheduled for today to find out what is wrong with the foot as it turns blue when I stand up though it looks as though it's getting better since the anti-biotic was introduced...

Meanwhile I was put on two blood thinners, taken off one... after the situation in the hospital - which began on Friday as my leg was swollen again, blood clot checked still there... I was sent to the hospital... taken off coumadin...

I left the hospital yesterday as I told them there was nothing more they could do for me that I couldn't do at home... I'm on coumadin 3 mg.

I don't want to go back to chemo I want a safer more natural way to deal with this cancer... I have started taking essiac tea, as I've done research and I believe the body accepts it as it is not toxic...

Journal entries from a cancer patient

"I turned to my boyfriend and said, "This doctor is crazy. I'm 36 and in love. How could I possibly have cancer?"

"On Saturday I went to the synagogue. I prayed to God: 'All I ask is a fighting chance.'"

"It was decision time. Surgery was a definite; a mastectomy would be scheduled. Radiation and more chemo were probable. A bone-marrow transplant was possible. Other than that, it was up to me."

"Great news, the scans were clear. One year after diagnosis, I was officially declared NED (no evidence of disease)."

"Hearing that you have multiple lesions in your brain is not an easy thing. I took the news with eerie calm. We spent a few minutes holding each other, crying...."

"I went to bed weeping. I was tired of fighting. It wasn't me, it was some other woman in a deteriorating body. I asked God to bring me a quick and painless end."

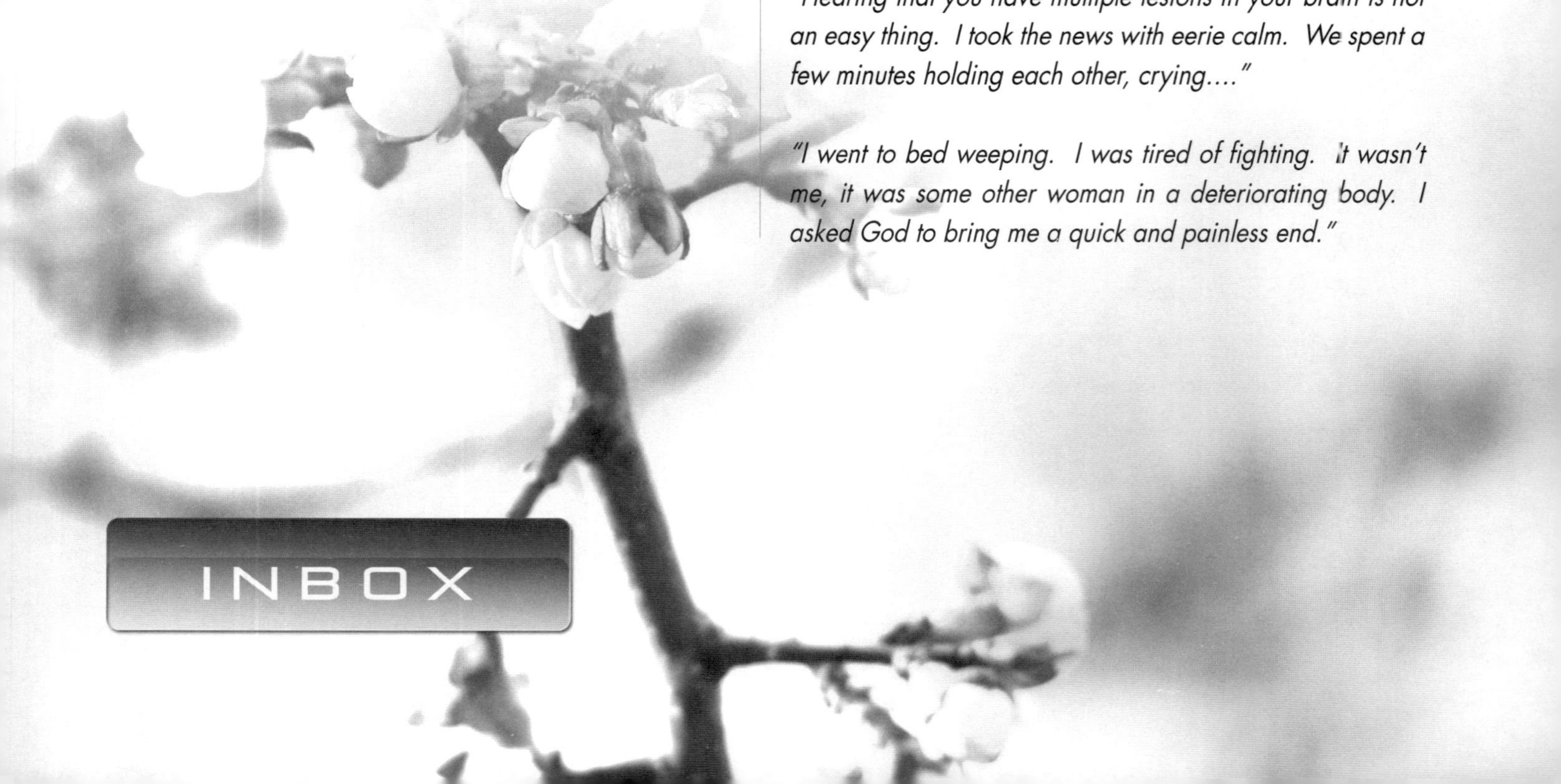

Do Unto Others...

Craig C. Earle, of the Dana-Farber Cancer Institute, Boston, Massachusetts, writes about cancer patients and how they choose chemotherapy treatment in the Journal of Clinical Oncology. This author has not read such a compassionate and frank discussion as Earle's anywhere else. This is what he said (abbreviated version):

> *'Doc, what would you do?' We do not usually offer our advice to patients facing treatment decisions for a terminal diagnosis in the form of 'If I were you, I'd do this...'*
>
> *We are concerned that we cannot be objective when imagining scenarios that involve our loved ones or ourselves. However, it is a reasonable question from the patient's perspective, as in knowing the stocks your broker is buying, or on which house your real estate agent would put an offer.*
>
> *A research study finds patients choose chemotherapy for much smaller improvements in outcome than would health care providers. A common interpretation of this finding is that we should not impose our opinions on patients because we have a different perspective than they do... But why are our patients choosing a course that we ourselves would not take? An alternative interpretation of the findings is that we are not communicating to them the information that leads us to choose differently. Is this because we are unable? Do we lack the tools to convey the pros and cons of treatment? Or do we find it too emotionally distressing? Is it because we choose not to be completely honest in an attempt to preserve hope? Or is it because patients are unable to accept what we are telling them?*
>
> *Patients generally are not experts in oncology, and yet they have to make decisions without knowing what the whole course of their illness will be. We, on the other hand, have shepherded many patients through this journey toward death.*
>
> *–Bereaved family members interviewed 6 months after the death of their loved one had a very different perspective: "think the earlier the doctor mentions [hospice], the better it is ... because the patient could plan for things ahead, rather than to spend so much time doing the treatment." Similarly, physicians reflecting on anticancer treatment agreed 'there is a time to stop.' Perhaps, then, if patients could look back from the grave, they would have chosen differently. With this knowledge, why is there this gap between these informed opinions and the decisions our patients make?*
>
> *Certainly we have all encountered patients who prefer not to know anything about their prognosis or refuse to believe it once it is conveyed. However, surveys suggest that the majority of patients do want an accurate estimate of prognosis, even if it is poor. Physicians, on the other hand, have reported a reluctance to provide survival estimates to patients, and that the majority of the time they would consciously over- or underestimate what they believed to be the facts. In most cases, this is done to preserve hope. There was a time in the not too distant past when patients often were not even told they had cancer because of a fear that they could not cope with the diagnosis. It turns out most can cope.*
>
> *Well-intentioned mistruths can actually be detrimental to patients. Data are presented in the article that patients with unrealistic expectations were more likely to choose aggressive antineoplastic treatment, but lived no longer and were more likely to die in intensive care on life support. An overly rosy prognosis deprives patients of the ability to make truly informed decisions about whether to take chemotherapy rather than a final, important, and meaningful trip. [Journal of Clinical Oncology, 24:3331-3332, 2006]*

Index

Symbols

A

B

C

D

E

F

G

H

I

J

K

L

M

N

O

P

Q

R

S